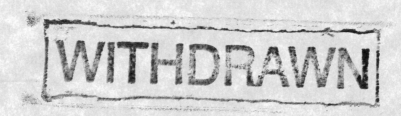

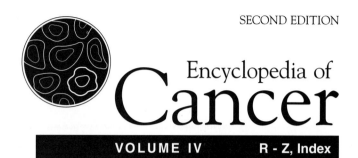

SECOND EDITION

Encyclopedia of
Cancer

VOLUME IV   R - Z, Index

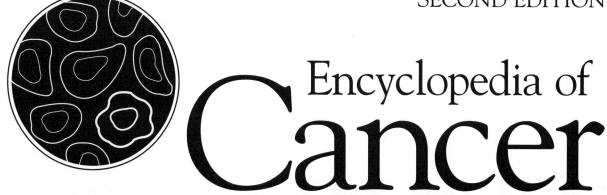

SECOND EDITION

Encyclopedia of Cancer

VOLUME IV **R - Z, Index**

Editor-in-Chief

Joseph R. Bertino

The Cancer Institute of New Jersey
Robert Wood Johnson Medical School
New Brunswick, New Jersey

ACADEMIC PRESS

An imprint of Elsevier Science

Amsterdam Boston London New York Oxford Paris San Diego San Francisco Singapore Sydney Tokyo

Requests for permission to make copies of any part of the work should be mailed to:
Permissions Department, Academic Press, 6277 Sea Harbor Drive,
Orlando, Florida 32887-6777

Academic Press
An imprint of Elsevier Science
525 B Street, Suite 1900, San Diego, California 92101-4495, USA
http://www.academicpress.com

Academic Press
84 Theobalds Road, London WC1X 8RR, UK
http://www.academicpress.com

Library of Congress Catalog Card Number: 2002102352

International Standard Book Number: 0-12-227555-1 (set)
International Standard Book Number: 0-12-227556-X (Volume 1)
International Standard Book Number: 0-12-227557-8 (Volume 2)
International Standard Book Number: 0-12-227558-6 (Volume 3)
International Standard Book Number: 0-12-227559-4 (Volume 4)

PRINTED IN THE UNITED STATES OF AMERICA
02 03 04 05 06 07 MM 9 8 7 6 5 4 3 2 1

Contents

VOLUME II

D

E

N

O

P

Contents by Subject Area

VIRAL CARCINOGENESIS

Contributors

Sanjiv S. Agarwala
University of Pittsburgh Cancer Institute
Melanoma: Epidemiology

Siamak Agha-Mohammadi
University of Pittsburgh
Cytokine Gene Therapy

Jaffer A. Ajani
University of Texas M. D. Anderson Cancer
Center
Gastric Cancer: Epidemiology and Therapy

Anthony P. Albino
The American Health Foundation
Multistage Carcinogenesis

Jeffry R. Alger
University of California, Los Angeles Medical
Center
Brain Cancer and Magnetic Resonance Spectroscopy

Robert Amato
Baylor College of Medicine
Testicular Cancer

Howard Amols
Memorial Sloan-Kettering Cancer Center
*Dosimetry and Treatment Planning for
Three-Dimensional Radiation Therapy*

Darrell E. Anderson
Scientific Consulting Group, Inc., Gaithersburg,
Maryland
*Cancer Risk Reduction (Diet/Smoking
Cessation/Lifestyle Changes)*

Cristina R. Antonescu
Memorial Sloan-Kettering Cancer Center
TLS-CHOP in Myxoid Liposarcoma

Wadih Arap
University of Texas M. D. Anderson Cancer Center
Vascular Targeting

Ralph B. Arlinghaus
University of Texas M. D. Anderson Cancer
Center
BCR/ABL

Georg Aue
University of Pennsylvania School of Medicine
Antisense Nucleic Acids: Clinical Applications

Nicholas R. Bachur
University of Maryland Cancer Center
Anthracyclines

Richard Barakat
Memorial Sloan-Kettering Cancer Center
Endometrial Cancer

Fred G. Barker II
Massachusetts General Hospital
Brain Tumors: Epidemiology and Molecular and Cellular Abnormalities

Frederic G. Barr
University of Pennsylvania School of Medicine
PAX3–FKHR and PAX7–FKHR Gene Fusions in Alveolar Rhabdomyosarcoma

Michael T. Barrett
Fred Hutchinson Cancer Research Center
Esophageal Cancer: Risk Factors and Somatic Genetics

P. Leif Bergsagel
Weill Medical College of Cornell University
Multiple Myeloma

Leslie Bernstein
University of Southern California Keck School of Medicine
Non-Hodgkin's Lymphoma and Multiple Myeloma: Incidence and Risk Factors

Sandra H. Bigner
Duke University Medical Center
Genetic Alterations in Brain Tumors

R. Michael Blaese
ValiGen, Inc., Newtown, Pennsylvania
Suicide Genes

Eda T. Bloom
U.S. Food and Drug Administration
Gene Therapy Vectors, Safety Considerations

Clara D. Bloomfield
Roswell Park Cancer Institute
Chromosome Aberrations

Peter Blume-Jensen
Serono Reproductive Biology Institute
Kinase-Regulated Signal Transduction Pathways
Signal Transduction Mechanisms Initiated by Receptor Tyrosine Kinases

Paolo Boffetta
International Agency for Research on Cancer, Lyon, France
Lung, Larynx, Oral Cavity, and Pharynx

Melissa Bondy
University of Texas M. D. Anderson Cancer Center
Brain and Central Nervous System Cancer

David Boothman
University of Wisconsin–Madison
Radiation Resistance

Ernest C. Borden
Taussig Cancer Center
Interferons: Cellular and Molecular Biology of Their Actions

George J. Bosl
Memorial Sloan-Kettering Cancer Center
Germ Cell Tumors

Marc E. Bracke
Ghent University Hospital
Molecular Mechanisms of Cancer Invasion

Patrick J. Brennan
University of Pennsylvania School of Medicine
Her2/neu

Ricardo R. Brentani
Ludwig Institute for Cancer Research, Sao Paulo
Cell–Matrix Interactions

Norman E. Breslow
University of Washington, Seattle
Wilms Tumor: Epidemiology

Ronald Breslow
Columbia University
Differentiation and the Role of Differentiation Inducers in Cancer Treatment

Jacqueline F. Bromberg
Memorial Sloan-Kettering Cancer Center
STAT Proteins in Growth Control

Steven J. Burakoff
Dana-Farber Cancer Institute
T Cells and Their Effector Functions

Barbara Burtness
Yale Univesity School of Medicine
Head and Neck Cancer

Anna Butturini
Children's Hospital of Los Angeles
BCR/ABL

Blake Cady
Brown University School of Medicine
Endocrine Tumors

José Campione-Piccardo
National Laboratory for Viral Oncology, Canada
Viral Agents

Judith Campisi
Lawrence Berkeley National Laboratory
Senescence, Cellular

Eli Canaani
Kimmel Cancer Center
ALL-1

France Carrier
University of Maryland
Ataxia Telangiectasia Syndrome

JoAnn C. Castelli
University of California, San Francisco
HIV (Human Immunodeficiency Virus)

Webster K. Cavenee
University of California, San Diego
PTEN

R. S. K. Chaganti
Memorial Sloan-Kettering Cancer Center
Germ Cell Tumors

Roger Chammas
Ludwig Institute for Cancer Research,
Sao Paulo
Cell–Matrix Interactions

Paul B. Chapman
Memorial Sloan-Kettering Cancer Center
Anti-idiotypic Antibody Vaccines

Irvin S. Y. Chen
University of California, Los Angeles School of
Medicine
Human T-Cell Leukemia/Lymphotropic Virus

Seng H. Cheng
Genzyme Corporation, Framingham,
Massachusetts
Cationic Lipid-Mediated Gene Therapy

David A. Cheresh
The Scripps Research Institute
Integrin-Targeted Angiostatics

Rajas Chodankar
University of Southern California Keck School
of Medicine
Ovarian Cancer: Molecular and Cellular Abnormalities

Ting-Chao Chou
Memorial Sloan-Kettering Cancer Center
Chemotherapy: Synergism and Antagonism

Edward Chu
Yale University School of Medicine
*Resistance to Inhibitor Compounds of
Thymidylate Synthase*

John A. Cidlowski
National Institute of Environmental Health Sciences
Corticosteroids

Lena Claesson-Welsh
Uppsala University
*Anti-Vascular Endothelial Growth
Factor-Based Angiostatics*

Bayard Clarkson
Memorial Sloan-Kettering Cancer Center
*Chronic Myelogenous Leukemia: Etiology, Incidence,
and Clinical Features*
*Chronic Myelogenous Leukemia: Prognosis and
Current Status of Treatment*

Jack S. Cohen
The Hebrew University
*Magnetic Resonance Spectroscopy and Magnetic
Resonance Imaging, Introduction*

Peter Cole
Cancer Institute of New Jersey
Folate Antagonists

Susan P. C. Cole
Queen's University, Canada
Multidrug Resistance II: MRP and Related Proteins

Jerry M. Collins
U.S. Food and Drug Administration
PET Imaging and Cancer

O. Michael Colvin
Duke University
Akylating Agents

Raymond L. Comenzo
Memorial Sloan-Kettering Cancer Center
Stem Cell Transplantation

Abigail A. Conley
The Mayo Clinic
*Pancreatic Cancer: Cellular and
Molecular Mechanisms*

Louis Constine
University of Rochester Medical Center
Late Effects of Radiation Therapy

Leslie C. Costello
University of Maryland, Baltimore
*Metabolic Diagnosis of Prostate Cancer by Magnetic
Resonance Spectroscopy*

Wendy Cozen
University of Southern California Keck School of
Medicine
*Non-Hodgkin's Lymphoma and Multiple Myeloma:
Incidence and Risk Factors*

Carlo M. Croce
Kimmel Cancer Center
ALL-1

Stanley T. Crooke
Isis Pharmaceuticals, Inc.
*Antisense: Progress toward Gene-Directed
Cancer Therapy*

Lloyd A. Culp
Case Western Reserve University School
of Medicine
*Extracellular Matrix and Matrix Receptors:
Alterations during Tumor Progression*

Thomas J. Cummings
Duke University Medical Center
Genetic Alterations in Brain Tumors

David T. Curiel
University of Alabama at Birmingham
Targeted Vectors for Cancer Gene Therapy

Tom Curran
St. Jude Children's Research Hospital
fos Oncogene

George Q. Daley
Whitehead Institute
Cytokines: Hematopoietic Growth Factors

Chi V. Dang
The Johns Hopkins University School of
Medicine
c-myc Protooncogene

James E. Darnell, Jr.
Rockefeller University
STAT Proteins in Growth Control

Michael David
University of California, San Diego
Jak/STAT Pathway

Roger G. Deeley
Queen's University, Canada
*Multidrug Resistance II: MRP and
Related Proteins*

Samuel R. Denmeade
Johns Hopkins University School of Medicine
Hormone Resistance in Prostate Cancer

Christopher T. Denny
University of California, Los Angeles School
of Medicine
EWS/ETS Fusion Genes

Channing J. Der
University of North Carolina at Chapel Hill
Ras Proteins

Mark W. Dewhirst
Duke University Medical Center
Hyperthermia

Frederick A. Dick
Massachusetts General Hospital Cancer Center
Retinoblastoma Tumor Suppressor Gene

John P. Dileo
University of Pittsburgh
Liposome-Mediated Gene Therapy

Eugene P. DiMagno
The Mayo Clinic
Pancreatic Cancer: Cellular and Molecular Mechanisms

Clark W. Distelhorst
Case Western Reserve University
Steroid Hormones and Hormone Receptors

Ethan Dmitrovsky
Dartmouth Medical School
Chemoprevention, Pharmacology of

M. Eileen Dolan
University of Chicago
Resistance to DNA-Damaging Agents

Alessia Donadio
Memorial Sloan-Kettering Cancer Center
Germ Cell Tumors

Zhongyun Dong
University of Texas M. D. Anderson Cancer
Center
Macrophages

Harold O. Douglass, Jr.
Roswell Park Cancer Institute
Pancreas and Periampullary Tumors

Louis Dubeau
University of Southern California Keck School
of Medicine
*Ovarian Cancer: Molecular and
Cellular Abnormalities*

Anita K. Dunbier
University of Otago
Gastric Cancer: Inherited Predisposition

Nicholas J. Dyson
Massachusetts General Hospital Cancer Center
Retinoblastoma Tumor Suppressor Gene

Timothy J. Eberlein
Washington University School of Medicine,
St. Louis
T Cells against Tumors

Randa El-Zein
University of Texas M. D. Anderson Cancer
Center
Brain and Central Nervous System Cancer

Elaine A. Elion
Harvard Medical School
MAP Kinase Modules in Signaling

Volker Ellenreider
The Mayo Clinic
Pancreatic Cancer: Cellular and Molecular Mechanisms

Paul F. Engstrom
Fox Chase Cancer Center
Hepatocellular Carcinoma (HCC)

Zelig Eshhar
Weizmann Institute of Science
Antibodies in the Gene Therapy of Cancer

Conrad B. Falkson
McMaster University
Malignant Mesothelioma

Geoffrey Falkson
University of Pretoria
Malignant Mesothelioma

Gerold Feuer
State University of New York Upstate
Medical University
Human T-Cell Leukemia/Lymphotropic Virus

Isaiah J. Fidler
University of Texas M. D. Anderson Cancer
Center
Macrophages

Mary E. Fidler
The Mayo Foundation
Renal Cell Cancer

Richard Fishel
Thomas Jefferson University
*Hereditary Colon Cancer and DNA
Mismatch Repair*

David FitzGerald
National Cancer Institute
*Antibody–Toxin and Growth Factor–Toxin
Fusion Proteins*

Hernan Flores-Rozas
Ludwig Institute for Cancer Research
Mismatch Repair: Biochemistry and Genetics

Albert J. Fornace Jr.
National Cancer Institute
Ataxia Telangiectasia Syndrome

Ruben C. Fragoso
Dana-Farber Cancer Institute
T Cells and Their Effector Functions

Thomas S. Frank
Myriad Genetic Laboratories, Salt Lake City
*Hereditary Risk of Breast and Ovarian
Cancer: BRCA1 and BRCA2*

R. B. Franklin
University of Maryland, Baltimore
*Metabolic Diagnosis of Prostate Cancer by Magnetic
Resonance Spectroscopy*

Eric O. Freed
National Institute of Allergy and Infectious
Diseases
Retroviruses

Michael L. Freeman
Vanderbilt University School of Medicine
Hyperthermia

Krystyna Frenkel
New York University School of Medicine
*Carcinogenesis: Role of Active Oxygen and Nitrogen
Species*

Frank B. Furnari
University of California, San Diego
PTEN

Robert Peter Gale
Center for Advanced Studies in Leukemia,
Los Angeles
BCR/ABL

Susan Gapstur
Arizona Cancer Center and Southern Arizona
VA Health Care System
*Nutritional Supplements and Diet as
Chemoprevention Agents*

Lawrence B. Gardner
The Johns Hopkins University School of
Medicine
c-myc Protooncogene

Harinder Garewal
Arizona Cancer Center and Southern Arizona
VA Health Care System
*Nutritional Supplements and Diet as
Chemoprevention Agents*

James E. Gervasoni, Jr.
Robert Wood Johnson Medical School
Endocrine Tumors

Pär Gerwins
Uppsala University
*Anti-Vascular Endothelial Growth
Factor-Based Angiostatics*

Alan M. Gewirtz
University of Pennsylvania School
of Medicine
Antisense Nucleic Acids: Clinical Applications

John F. Gibbs
Roswell Park Cancer Institute
Pancreas and Periampullary Tumors

Anna Giuliano
Arizona Cancer Center and Southern Arizona
VA Health Care System
*Nutritional Supplements and Diet as
Chemoprevention Agents*

R. A. Gjerset
Sidney Kimmel Cancer Center
p53 Gene Therapy

Peter S. Goedegebuure
Washington University School of Medicine,
St. Louis
T Cells against Tumors

Jason S. Gold
Memorial Sloan-Kettering Cancer Center
Cell-Mediated Immunity to Cancer

Ashwin Gollerkeri
Yale University School of Medicine
*Resistance to Inhibitor Compounds of
Thymidylate Synthase*

Jesús Gómez-Navarro
University of Alabama at Birmingham
Targeted Vectors for Cancer Gene Therapy

Ellen L. Goode
University of Washington
Genetic Predisposition to Prostate Cancer

Richard Gorlick
Memorial Sloan-Kettering Cancer Center
Bone Tumors

Kathleen Heppner Goss
University of Cincinnati College of Medicine
*APC (Adenomatous Polyposis Coli) Tumor
Suppressor*

Michael M. Gottesman
National Cancer Institute
Multidrug Resistance I: P-Glycoprotein

Joseph P. Grande
The Mayo Foundation
*Kidney, Epidemiology
Renal Cell Cancer*

Ellen Graver
Arizona Cancer Center and Southern Arizona
VA Health Care System
*Nutritional Supplements and Diet as
Chemoprevention Agents*

F. Anthony Greco
Sarah Cannon–Minnie Pearl Cancer Center
Neoplasms of Unknown Primary Site

Mark I. Greene
University of Pennsylvania
School of Medicine
Her2/neu

Peter Greenwald
National Cancer Institute
*Cancer Risk Reduction (Diet/Smoking
Cessation/Lifestyle Changes)*

John R. Griffiths
St. George's Hospital Medical School, London
*Magnetic Resonance Spectroscopy of Cancer: Clinical
Overview*

Joanna Groden
University of Cincinnati College of Medicine
*APC (Adenomatous Polyposis Coli)
Tumor Suppressor*

Jun-Lin Guan
Cornell University College of
Veterinary Medicine
Integrin Receptor Signaling Pathways

Udayan Guha
Albert Einstein Cancer Center
Transgenic Mice in Cancer Research

Parry J. Guilford
University of Otago
Gastric Cancer: Inherited Predisposition

Anjali Gupta
University of Pennsylvania Hospital
Molecular Aspects of Radiation Biology

John D. Hainsworth
Sarah Cannon–Minnie Pearl Cancer Center
Neoplasms of Unknown Primary Site

Joshua W. Hamilton
Dartmouth Medical School
Chemical Mutagenesis and Carcinogenesis

Joyce L. Hamlin
University of Virginia School of Medicine
Drug Resistance: DNA Sequence Amplification

Kenneth R. Hande
Vanderbilt University School of Medicine
Purine Antimetabolites

J. Marie Hardwick
Johns Hopkins School of Public Health
Caspases in Programmed Cell Death

Louis B. Harrison
Beth Israel Medical Center
Brachytherapy

Lynda K. Hawkins
Genetic Therapy Institute, Gaithersburg, Maryland
Replication-Selective Viruses for Cancer Treatment

Lifeng He
Albert Einstein College of Medicine
Taxol and Other Molecules That Interact with Microtubules

Stephen S. Hecht
University of Minnesota Cancer Center
Tobacco Carcinogenesis

Ingegerd Hellström
Pacific Northwest Research Institute
Tumor Antigens

Karl Erik Hellström
Pacific Northwest Research Institute
Tumor Antigens

Kurt J. Henle
University of Arkansas for Medical Sciences
Hyperthermia

Meenhard Herlyn
The Wistar Institute
Melanoma: Biology

Masao Hirose
Nagoya City University Medical School
Antioxidants: Carcinogenic and Chemopreventive Properties

Dah H. Ho
University of Texas M. D. Anderson Cancer Center
L-Asparaginase

Samuel B. Ho
University of Minnesota Medical School
Glycoproteins and Glycosylation Changes in Cancer

F. Stephen Hodi
Dana-Farber Cancer Institute
Interleukins

Kyle Holen
Memorial Sloan-Kettering Cancer Center
Colorectal Cancer: Epidemiology and Treatment

Julianne L. Holleran
Case Western Reserve University School of Medicine
Extracellular Matrix and Matrix Receptors: Alterations during Tumor Progression

Waun Ki Hong
University of Texas M. D. Anderson Cancer Center
Chemoprevention Trials

Susan Band Horwitz
Albert Einstein College of Medicine
Taxol and Other Molecules That Interact with Microtubules

Alan N. Houghton
Memorial Sloan-Kettering Cancer Center
Cell-Mediated Immunity to Cancer
DNA-Based Cancer Vaccines

Jane Houldsworth
Memorial Sloan-Kettering Cancer Center
Germ Cell Tumors

Franklyn A. Howe
St. George's Hospital Medical School, London
Magnetic Resonance Spectroscopy of Cancer: Clinical Overview

H.-J. Su Huang
University of California, San Diego
PTEN

Leaf Huang
University of Pittsburgh
Liposome-Mediated Gene Therapy

James Hulit
Albert Einstein Cancer Center
Transgenic Mice in Cancer Research

Tony Hunter
The Salk Institute
Kinase-Regulated Signal Transduction Pathways
Signal Transduction Mechanisms Initiated by Receptor Tyrosine Kinases

Mark D. Hurwitz
Harvard Medical School
Bladder Cancer: Assessment and Management

David H. Ilson
Memorial Sloan-Kettering Cancer Center
Esophageal Cancer: Treatment

Katsumi Imaida
Nagoya City University Medical School
Antioxidants: Carcinogenic and Chemopreventive Properties

Harry L. Ioachim
Lenox Hill Hospital
Immune Deficiency: Opportunistic Tumors

John T. Isaacs
Johns Hopkins University School of Medicine
Hormone Resistance in Prostate Cancer

Mark A. Israel
University of California, San Francisco
Brain Tumors: Epidemiology and Molecular and Cellular Abnormalities

Nobuyuki Ito
Nagoya City University Medical School
Antioxidants: Carcinogenic and Chemopreventive Properties

Helen A. James
University of East Anglia
Ribozymes and Their Applications

Gail P. Jarvik
University of Washington Medical Center
Genetic Predisposition to Prostate Cancer

Alan M. Jeffrey
Columbia University
Carcinogen–DNA Adducts

D. Joseph Jerry
University of Massachusetts, Amherst
TP53 Tumor Suppressor Gene: Structure and Function

Eric Johannsen
Harvard Medical School
Epstein–Barr Virus and Associated Malignancies

Ricky W. Johnstone
Peter MacCallum Cancer Institute, East Melbourne
P-Glycoprotein as a General Antiapoptotic Protein
Wilms Tumor Suppressor WT1

Douglas J. Jolly
Chiron Viagene, Inc., San Diego, California
Retroviral Vectors

Peter A. Jones
University of Southern California
DNA Methylation and Cancer

V. Craig Jordan
Northwestern University Medical School
Estrogens and Antiestrogens

Ellen D. Jorgensen
The American Health Foundation
Multistage Carcinogenesis

Jacqueline Jouanneau
Institut Curie
Tumor Cell Motility and Invasion

Raymond Judware
Case Western Reserve University School of Medicine
Extracellular Matrix and Matrix Receptors: Alterations during Tumor Progression

Joseph G. Jurcic
Memorial Sloan-Kettering Cancer Center
Monoclonal Antibodies: Leukemia and Lymphoma

Joanna Kaczynski
The Mayo Clinic
Pancreatic Cancer: Cellular and Molecular Mechanisms

William G. Kaelin, Jr.
Harvard Medical School
von Hippel–Lindau Disease

Dhananjaya V. Kalvakolanu
Greenebaum Cancer Center
Interferons: Cellular and Molecular Biology of Their Actions

Barton A. Kamen
Cancer Institute of New Jersey
Folate Antagonists

Mark P. Kamps
University of California, San Diego School of Medicine
Differentiation and Cancer: Basic Research

Gary D. Kao
University of Pennsylvania Hospital
Molecular Aspects of Radiation Biology

Johanne M. Kaplan
Genzyme Corporation, Framingham, Massachusetts
Cationic Lipid-Mediated Gene Therapy

Emmanuel Katsanis
University of Arizona
Neuroblastoma

Frederic J. Kaye
National Cancer Institute
Lung Cancer: Molecular and Cellular Abnormalities

Michael J. Keating
University of Texas M. D. Anderson Cancer Center
Chronic Lymphocytic Leukemia

David Kelsen
Cornell University Medical College
Esophageal Cancer: Treatment

Nancy Kemeny
Memorial Sloan-Kettering Cancer Center
Colorectal Cancer: Epidemiology and Treatment

Fadlo R. Khuri
University of Texas M. D. Anderson Cancer
Center
Chemoprevention Trials

Se Won Ki
University of California, San Diego
Cellular Responses to DNA Damage

Edward S. Kim
University of Texas M. D. Anderson Cancer
Center
Chemoprevention Trials

Young S. Kim
University of California, San Francisco
*Glycoproteins and Glycosylation Changes
in Cancer*

Sol Kimel
Sheba Medical Center, Israel
*Photodynamic Therapy: Basic Principles and
Applications to Skin Cancer*

Timothy Kinsella
University of Wisconsin–Madison
Radiation Resistance

John M. Kirkwood
University of Pittsburgh Cancer Institute
Melanoma: Epidemiology

David Kirn
Kirn Biopharmaceutical Consulting
*Replication-Selective Viruses for
Cancer Treatment*

Jan Kitajewski
Columbia University
Wnt Signaling

George Klein
Karolinska Institute
Tumor Suppressor Genes: Specific Classes

Priit Kogerman
Case Western Reserve University School
of Medicine
*Extracellular Matrix and Matrix Receptors:
Alterations during Tumor Progression*

Richard D. Kolodner
Ludwig Institute for Cancer Research
*Mismatch Repair: Biochemistry
and Genetics*

Genady Kostenich
Sheba Medical Center, Israel
*Photodynamic Therapy: Basic Principles and
Applications to Skin Cancer*

Robert J. Kreitman
National Cancer Institute
*Antibody–Toxin and Growth Factor–Toxin
Fusion Proteins*

J. Kurhanewicz
University of California, San Francisco
*Metabolic Diagnosis of Prostate Cancer by Magnetic
Resonance Spectroscopy*

Alexander E. Kuta
U.S. Food and Drug Administration
Gene Therapy Vectors, Safety Considerations

Mark Ladanyi
Memorial Sloan-Kettering Cancer Center
TLS-CHOP in Myxoid Liposarcoma

Michael M. C. Lai
University of Southern California Keck School
of Medicine
Hepatitis C Virus (HCV)

Wayne D. Lancaster
Wayne State University School of Medicine
Viral Agents

Jean-Baptiste Latouche
Memorial Sloan-Kettering Cancer Center
*Cancer Vaccines: Gene Therapy and Dendritic
Cell-Based Vaccines*

John S. Lazo
University of Pittsburgh
Bleomycin

Derek Le Roith
National Institutes of Health
Insulin-like Growth Factors

Jane S. Lebkowski
Applied Immune Sciences, Inc.,
Santa Clara, California
*Adeno-Associated Virus: A Vector for
High-Efficiency Gene Transduction*

Linda A. Lee
The Johns Hopkins University School
of Medicine
c-myc Protooncogene

Loïc Le Marchand
Cancer Research Center of Hawaii
Lung, Larynx, Oral Cavity, and Pharynx

Alexandra M. Levine
University of Southern California Keck School
of Medicine
*Neoplasms in Acquired
Immunodeficiency Syndrome*

Alexander Levitzki
The Hebrew University of Jerusalem
Protein Kinase Inhibitors

Jay A. Levy
University of California, San Francisco
HIV (Human Immunodeficiency Virus)

Runzhao Li
Medical University of South Carolina
ETS Family of Transcription Factors

Nicole T. Liberati
Duke University Medical Center
TGFβ Signaling Mechanisms

David C. Linehan
Washington University School of Medicine,
St. Louis
T Cells against Tumors

Stephen J. Lippard
Massachusetts Institute of Technology
Cisplatin and Related Drugs

Philip O. Livingston
Memorial Sloan-Kettering Cancer Center
Carbohydrate-Based Vaccines

Jay S. Loeffler
Harvard Medical School
Proton Beam Radiation Therapy

W. Thomas London
Fox Chase Cancer Center
Liver Cancer: Etiology and Prevention

Dan L. Longo
National Institute on Aging
Lymphoma, Non-Hodgkin's

Ti Li Loo
George Washington University Medical Center
L-Asparaginase

Michael T. Lotze
University of Pittsburgh
Cytokine Gene Therapy

Henry T. Lynch
Creighton University School of Medicine
*Colorectal Cancer: Molecular and
Cellular Abnormalities*

Wendy J. Mack
University of Southern California
Thyroid Cancer

Robert G. Maki
Memorial Sloan-Kettering Cancer Center
Sarcomas of Soft Tissue

David Malkin
University of Toronto School of Medicine
Li-Fraumeni Syndrome

Yael Mardor
Sheba Medical Center, Israel
*Magnetic Resonance Spectroscopy and Magnetic
Resonance Imaging, Introduction*

Marc M. Mareel
Ghent University Hospital
Molecular Mechanisms of Cancer Invasion

Paul A. Marks
Memorial Sloan-Kettering Cancer Center
*Differentiation and the Role of Differentiation
Inducers in Cancer Treatment*

Peter M. Mauch
Harvard Medical School
Lymphoma, Hodgkin's Disease

Harold M. Maurer
University of Nebraska Medical Center
Rhabdomyosarcoma, Early Onset

George Mavrothalassitis
University of Crete
ETS Family of Transcription Factors

William H. McBride
University of California, Los Angeles
Radiobiology, Principles of

Thomas S. McCormick
Case Western Reserve University
Steroid Hormones and Hormone Receptors

Charles J. McDonald
Brown University Medical School
Skin Cancer, Non-Melanoma

Sharon S. McDonald
Scientific Consulting Group, Inc.,
Gaithersburg, Maryland
*Cancer Risk Reduction (Diet/Smoking
Cessation/Lifestyle Changes)*

Clare H. McGowan
The Scripps Research Institute
Cell Cycle Checkpoints

Melissa S. McGrath
Memorial Sloan-Kettering Cancer Center
Resistance to Antibody Therapy

W. Gillies McKenna
University of Pennsylvania Hospital
Molecular Aspects of Radiation Biology

Paul M. J. McSheehy
St. George's Hospital Medical School, London
*Magnetic Resonance Spectroscopy of Cancer:
Clinical Overview*

Peter W. Melera
University of Maryland School of Medicine
Resistance to Inhibitors of Dihydrofolate Reductase

Richard A. Messmann
National Cancer Institute
Targeted Toxins

Paul A. Meyers
Memorial Sloan-Kettering Cancer Center
Bone Tumors

Carson J. Miller
Case Western Reserve University School
of Medicine
*Extracellular Matrix and Matrix Receptors:
Alterations during Tumor Progression*

Amin Mirhadi
University of California, Los Angeles
Radiobiology, Principles of

Elizabeth Moran
Temple University School of Medicine
DNA Tumor Viruses: Adenovirus

Thomas Moritz
University of Essen Medical School
*Transfer of Drug Resistance Genes to
Hematopoietic Precursors*

John C. Morris
National Cancer Institute
Suicide Genes

Krzysztof Mrózek
Roswell Park Cancer Institute
Chromosome Aberrations

Bijay Mukherji
University of Connecticut Health Center
Molecular Basis for Tumor Immunity

Annegret Müller
Thomas Jefferson University
*Hereditary Colon Cancer and DNA
Mismatch Repair*

Karl Münger
Harvard Medical School
Papillomaviruses

Tatsuya Nakamura
Kimmel Cancer Center
ALL-1

Hector R. Nava
Roswell Park Cancer Institute
Pancreas and Periampullary Tumors

Andrea K. Ng
Harvard Medical School
Lymphoma, Hodgkin's Disease

Jac A. Nickoloff
University of New Mexico School of Medicine
*Recombination: Mechanisms and Roles
in Tumorigenesis*

Garth L. Nicolson
Institute for Molecular Medicine
*Autocrine and Paracrine Growth Mechanisms in
Cancer Progression and Metastasis*

John L. Nitiss
St. Jude Children's Research Hospital
Resistance to Topoisomerase-Targeting Agents

Karin C. Nitiss
St. Jude Children's Research Hospital
Resistance to Topoisomerase-Targeting Agents

Philip D. Noguchi
U.S. Food and Drug Administration
Gene Therapy Vectors, Safety Considerations

Shoichiro Ohta
University of California, San Francisco
*Brain Tumors: Epidemiology and Molecular and
Cellular Abnormalities*

Arie Orenstein
Sheba Medical Center, Israel
*Photodynamic Therapy: Basic Principles and
Applications to Skin Cancer*

George A. Orr
Albert Einstein College of Medicine
*Taxol and Other Molecules That Interact
with Microtubules*

Keren Osman
Memorial Sloan-Kettering Cancer Center
Stem Cell Transplantation

Michelle A. Ozbun
University of New Mexico School of Medicine
*TP53 Tumor Suppressor Gene: Structure
and Function*

Robert F. Ozols
Fox Chase Cancer Center
Ovarian Cancer: Epidemiology

Kevin W. Page
Applied Immune Sciences, Inc.,
    Santa Clara, California
*Adeno-Associated Virus: A Vector for
    High-Efficiency Gene Transduction*

Tej Krishan Pandita
Columbia University
Telomeres and Telomerase

Renata Pasqualini
University of Texas M. D. Anderson Cancer
    Center
Vascular Targeting

Ira Pastan
National Cancer Institute
*Antibody–Toxin and Growth Factor–Toxin
    Fusion Proteins*

Frederica P. Perera
Mailman School of Public Health at Columbia
    University
Molecular Epidemiology and Cancer Risk

Richard G. Pestell
Albert Einstein Cancer Center
Transgenic Mice in Cancer Research

Anusch Peyman
Avetis Pharma Deutschland GmbH
Antisense: Medicinal Chemistry

Pieter Pil
Massachusetts Institute of Technology
Cisplatin and Related Drugs

Giuseppe Pizzorno
Yale University School of Medicine
Pyrimidine Antimetabolites

Miriam C. Poirier
National Cancer Institute
DNA Damage, DNA Repair, and Mutagenesis

Pamela M. Pollock
National Human Genome Research Institute
Melanoma: Molecular and Cellular Abnormalities

Randy Y. C. Poon
Hong Kong University of Science and Technology
Cell Cycle Control

Susan Preston-Martin
University of Southern California
Thyroid Cancer

Wendy Morse Pruitt
University of North Carolina at Chapel Hill
Ras Proteins

Amanda Psyrri
Yale University School of Medicine
Pyrimidine Antimetabolites

Harry Quon
Beth Israel Medical Center
Brachytherapy

Govindaswami Ragupathi
Memorial Sloan-Kettering Cancer Center
Carbohydrate-Based Vaccines

R. Beverly Raney
University of Texas M. D. Anderson Cancer
    Center
Rhabdomyosarcoma, Early Onset

Ritesh Rathore
Boston University School of Medicine
Vinca Alkaloids and Epipodophyllotoxins

Bandaru S. Reddy
American Health Foundation
Animal Models for Colon Cancer Chemoprevention

E. Premkumar Reddy
Fels Institute for Cancer Research and Molecular
    Biology
myb

John C. Reed
The Burnham Institute
*Bcl-2 Family Proteins and the Dysregulation of
    Programmed Cell Death*

Heinz R. Reiske
Cornell University College of Veterinary Medicine
Integrin Receptor Signaling Pathways

Victoria Richon
Memorial Sloan-Kettering Cancer Center
*Differentiation and the Role of Differentiation
    Inducers in Cancer Treatment*

Richard A. Rifkind
Memorial Sloan-Kettering Cancer Center
*Differentiation and the Role of Differentiation
    Inducers in Cancer Treatment*

Gert Rijksen
University Hospital, Utrecht, The Netherlands
Pyruvate Kinases

Paul F. Robbins
National Cancer Institute
Cancer Vaccines: Peptide- and Protein-Based Vaccines

Leslie Robinson-Bostom
Brown University Medical School
Skin Cancer, Non-Melanoma

Sara Rockwell
Yale University School of Medicine
Hypoxia and Drug Resistance

Charles E. Rogler
Albert Einstein College of Medicine
Hepatitis B Viruses

Ronald K. Ross
University of Southern California/Norris
Comprehensive Cancer Center
Bladder Cancer: Epidemiology

Astrid A. Ruefli
Peter MacCallum Cancer Institute,
East Melbourne
P-Glycoprotein as a General Antiapoptotic Protein

N. Saadatmandi
Sidney Kimmel Cancer Center
p53 Gene Therapy

Michel Sadelain
Memorial Sloan-Kettering Cancer Center
*Cancer Vaccines: Gene Therapy and Dendritic
Cell-Based Vaccines*

Ajay Sandhu
Eastern Virginia Medical School
Late Effects of Radiation Therapy

Kapaettu Satyamoorthy
Manipal Academy of Higher Education, India
Melanoma: Biology

Edward A. Sausville
National Cancer Institute
Targeted Toxins

David A. Scheinberg
Memorial Sloan-Kettering Cancer Center
*Monoclonal Antibodies: Leukemia and Lymphoma
Resistance to Antibody Therapy*

Charles A. Schiffer
Barbara Ann Karmanos Cancer Institute
Acute Lymphoblastic Leukemia in Adults

Cornelius Schmaltz
Memorial Sloan-Kettering Cancer Center
Graft versus Leukemia and Graft versus Tumor Activity

John D. Schuetz
St. Jude Children's Research Hospital
*Genetic Basis for Quantitative and Qualitative
Changes in Drug Targets*

Nicholas T. Schulz
University of Pittsburgh School of Medicine
c-mos Protooncogene

Shelley Schwarzbaum
Weizmann Institute of Science
Antibodies in the Gene Therapy of Cancer

Andrew D. Seidman
Memorial Sloan-Kettering Cancer Center
Breast Cancer

Victor Sementchenko
Medical University of South Carolina
ETS Family of Transcription Factors

Arun Seth
University of Toronto
ETS Family of Transcription Factors

George Sgouros
Memorial Sloan-Kettering Cancer Center
Radiolabeled Antibodies, Overview

Brenda Shank
University of California, San Francisco
Total Body Irradiation

Navneet Sharda
University of Wisconsin–Madison
Radiation Resistance

Yang Shi
Harvard Medical School
Wilms Tumor Suppressor WT1

Kang Sup Shim
Thomas Jefferson University
*Hereditary Colon Cancer and DNA
Mismatch Repair*

James D. Shull
University of Nebraska Medical Center
Hormonal Carcinogenesis

William M. Siders
Genzyme Corporation, Framingham, Massachusetts
Cationic Lipid-Mediated Gene Therapy

Alfred R. Smith
Harvard Medical School
Proton Beam Radiation Therapy

Judy L. Smith
Roswell Park Cancer Institute
Pancreas and Periampullary Tumors

Thomas Smyrk
Creighton University School of Medicine
*Colorectal Cancer: Molecular and
Cellular Abnormalities*

Mark J. Smyth
Peter MacCallum Cancer Institute,
East Melbourne
P-Glycoprotein as a General Antiapoptotic Protein

Robert J. Soiffer
Dana-Farber Cancer Institute
Interleukins

Michael B. Sporn
Dartmouth Medical School
Chemoprevention, Pharmacology of

Gerard E. J. Staal
University Hospital, Utrecht, The Netherlands
Pyruvate Kinases

Patricia S. Steeg
National Cancer Institute
nm23 Metastasis Suppressor Gene

Peter G. Steinherz
Memorial Sloan-Kettering Cancer Center
Acute Lymphoblastic Leukemia in Children

M. I. Straub
Connecticut Veterans Administration
Medical Center
Carcinogen–DNA Adducts

Dwayne G. Stupack
The Scripps Research Institute
Integrin-Targeted Angiostatics

Michael Wei-Chih Su
Dana-Farber Cancer Institute
T Cells and Their Effector Functions

Hubert Szelényi
Weill Medical College of Cornell University
Multiple Myeloma

Chris H. Takimoto
University of Texas Health Science Center
Camptothecins

R. V. Tantravahi
Fels Institute for Cancer Research and Molecular
Biology
myb

Jean Paul Thiery
Institut Curie
Tumor Cell Motility and Invasion

Gian Paolo Tonini
National Institute for Cancer
Research, Genoa
Pediatric Cancers, Molecular Features

Timothy J. Triche
Keck School of Medicine at the University of
Southern California
Ewing's Sarcoma (Ewing's Family Tumors)

Donald L. Trump
University of Pittsburgh Medical Center
Prostate Cancer

Shigeki Tsuchida
Hirosaki University School of Medicine
Glutathione Transferases

Eugen Uhlmann
Aventis Pharma Deutschland GmbH
Antisense: Medicinal Chemistry

Raul Urrutia
The Mayo Clinic
*Pancreatic Cancer: Cellular and
Molecular Mechanisms*

Marcel R. M. van den Brink
Memorial Sloan-Kettering Cancer Center
*Graft versus Leukemia and Graft versus
Tumor Activity*

Catherine Van Poznak
Memorial Sloan-Kettering Cancer Center
Breast Cancer

Amelia M. Wall
St. Jude Children's Research Hospital
*Genetic Basis for Quantitative and Qualitative
Changes in Drug Targets*

Andrew D. Wallace
National Institute of Environmental Health Sciences
Corticosteroids

Fred Wang
Harvard Medical School
Epstein–Barr Virus and Associated Malignancies

Hwei-Gene Heidi Wang
Bristol Myers Squibb, Wallingford, Connecticut
DNA Tumor Viruses: Adenovirus

Jean Y. J. Wang
University of California, San Diego
Cellular Responses to DNA Damage

Xiao-Fan Wang
Duke University Medical Center
TGFβ Signaling Mechanisms

Carl F. Ware
La Jolla Institute for Allergy and Immunology
Tumor Necrosis Factors

Dennis K. Watson
Medical University of South Carolina
ETS Family of Transcription Factors

Pascal A. Oude Weernink
University Hospital, Utrecht,
The Netherlands
Pyruvate Kinases

Alan B. Weitberg
Boston University School of Medicine
Vinca Alkaloids and Epipodophyllotoxins

Haim Werner
Tel Aviv University, Israel
Insulin-like Growth Factors

Ainsley Weston
National Institute for Occupational Safety and
Health
DNA Damage, DNA Repair, and Mutagenesis

Luke Whitesell
University of Arizona
Neuroblastoma

Peter H. Wiernik
New York Medical College
Acute Myelocytic Leukemia

David W. Will
Avetis Pharma Deutschland GmbH
Antisense: Medicinal Chemistry

David A. Williams
Children's Hospital Medical Center
*Transfer of Drug Resistance Genes to
Hematopoietic Precursors*

Jacqueline Williams
University of Rochester Medical Center
Late Effects of Radiation Therapy

Brian C. Wilson
Ontario Cancer Institute
Photodynamic Therapy: Clinical Applications

D. R. Wilson
Introgen Therapeutics, Inc.
p53 Gene Therapy

Jedd D. Wolchok
Memorial Sloan-Kettering Cancer Center
DNA-Based Cancer Vaccines

Margaret Wrensch
University of California, San Francisco
Brain and Central Nervous System Cancer

Yue Xiong
University of North Carolina at Chapel Hill
p16 and ARF: Crossroads of Tumorigenesis

Yoshiya Yamada
Memorial Sloan-Kettering Cancer Center
Stereotactic Radiosurgery of Intracranial Neoplasms

Chin-Rang Yang
University of Wisconsin–Madison
Radiation Resistance

Wendell G. Yarbrough
University of North Carolina at Chapel Hill
p16 and ARF: Crossroads of Tumorigenesis

James W. Young
Memorial Sloan-Kettering Cancer Center
*Cancer Vaccines: Gene Therapy and Dendritic
Cell-Based Vaccines*

Mimi C. Yu
University of Southern California/Norris
Comprehensive Cancer Center
Bladder Cancer: Epidemiology

Brad Zerler
Locus Discovery Inc., Blue Bell,
Pennsylvania
DNA Tumor Viruses: Adenovirus

Dong-Er Zhang
The Scripps Research Institute
RUNX/CBF Transcription Factors

Foreword

Cancer, a most feared and morbid disease, is the second most common cause of mortality in the United States after cardiovascular disease. Clinical and research information with respect to cancer is expanding at an extraordinary rate. Keeping abreast of information relative to one's field, whether a clinician, researcher, student, or patient, is an increasing challenge. The *Encyclopedia of Cancer, Second Edition* organizes such information in a style that is highly effective and remarkably useful. The encyclopedia will be a source of great assistance to general practitioners, cancer specialists, and researchers and should be available in all institutional and private libraries. The editors and the contributors have been carefully selected for their outstanding credentials and should be congratulated for the excellence of the encyclopedia they produced.

Emil Frei
Director and Physician-in-Chief, Emeritus
Dana-Farber Cancer Institute
Professor of Medicine, Emeritus
Harvard Medical School

Preface

Since the last edition of the *Encyclopedia of Cancer*, there has been an amazing amount of new information published in the cancer research field. This second edition has attempted to capture these advances that have occurred in the etiology, prevention, and treatment of this disease. Accordingly, we have increased the coverage of topics, and the encyclopedia now requires four volumes instead of three volumes to accommodate the increase in articles.

Feedback about and reviews of the first edition have been positive, and this second edition builds on the format of the first edition. Our goal was to cover all aspects of cancer, from basic science to clinical application. A distinguished group of associate editors has provided topics to be covered, suggested authors for those topics, and reviewed the submitted manuscripts. Without them, this compendium would not have been possible. The authors chosen to write the articles are experts in their fields, and we are indebted to them for their contributions.

A major problem in organizing this effort was to avoid overlap of the material presented. While some redundancy is unavoidable, it also may be of interest to the reader to have a subject covered from more than one vantage point. We have limited references to a few key ones listed at the end of each article as a guide for further reading. The intent of the encyclopedia is not to provide a comprehensive, detailed review of each subject, but a concise exposition of the topic, directed toward the reader who would like information on topics outside of his or her expertise. Thus the encyclopedia should be especially useful as a reference for students, fellows in training, and educators.

I thank the many authors who made this second edition possible and the associate editors for their invaluable input. I also thank Craig Panner, Hilary Rowe, and Cindy Minor of Academic Press, who have been instrumental in bringing this effort to fruition.

Joseph R. Bertino

Guide to the Use of the Encyclopedia

The *Encyclopedia of Cancer, Second Edition* is a comprehensive summary of the field of cancer research. This reference work consists of four separate volumes and 220 different articles on various aspects of the disease of cancer, including its epidemiology, its treatment, and its molecular and genetic processes. Each article provides a comprehensive overview of the selected topic to inform a wide range of readers, from research professionals to students.

This *Encyclopedia of Cancer* is the second edition of an award-winning, widely used reference work first published six years ago. Dr. Joseph Bertino has served as Editor-in-Chief for both editions, and the Editorial Board has remained largely the same.

This new version provides a substantial revision of the first edition, reflecting the dynamic nature of cancer research. Of the 220 articles appearing here, more than 60% have been newly commissioned for this edition, and virtually all the others have been significantly rewritten, making this in effect more of an original work than a revision.

ORGANIZATION

The *Encyclopedia of Cancer* is organized to provide the maximum ease of use for its readers. All of the articles are arranged in a single alphabetical sequence by title. Articles whose titles begin with the letters A to Cm are in Volume 1, articles with titles from Co to K are in Volume 2, articles from L to Q to in Volume 3, and R to Z in Volume 4.

So that they can be easily located, article titles generally begin with the key word or phrase indicating the topic, with any descriptive terms following (e.g., "Radiobiology, Principles of" is the article title rather than "Principles of Radiobiology").

TABLE OF CONTENTS

A complete table of contents for the entire encyclopedia appears in the front of each volume. This list of article titles represents topics that have been carefully selected by Dr. Bertino and the members of the Editorial Board (see p. ii for a list of editors).

Following this list of articles by title is a second complete table of contents, in which the articles are listed alphabetically according to subject area. The *Encyclopedia of Cancer* provides coverage of twenty specific subject areas within the overall field of cancer, such as cell proliferation, drug resistance, gene therapy, oncogenes, tumor suppressor genes, and viral carcinogenesis.

INDEX

A subject index is located at the end of Volume 4. Consisting of more than 7,500 entries, this index is the most convenient way to locate a desired topic within the encyclopedia. The subjects in the index are listed alphabetically and indicate the volume and page number where information on this topic can be found.

ARTICLE FORMAT

Each new article in the *Encyclopedia of Cancer* begins at the top of a right-hand page so that it may be quickly located by the reader. The author's name and affiliation are displayed at the beginning of the article.

Each article in the encyclopedia is organized according to a standard format, as follows:

- Title and author
- Outline
- Glossary
- Defining paragraph
- Body of the article
- Cross-references
- Bibliography

OUTLINE

Each article begins with an outline indicating the content of the article to come. This outline provides a brief overview of the article so that the reader can get a sense of what is contained there without having to leaf through the pages. It also serves to highlight

important subtopics that will be discussed within the article (for example, risk factors in the article "Thyroid Cancer"). The outline is intended as an overview and thus it lists only the major headings of the article. In addition, extensive second-level and third-level headings will be found within the article.

GLOSSARY

The glossary contains terms that are important to an understanding of the article and that may be unfamiliar to the reader. Each term is defined in the context of the particular article in which it is used. Thus the same term may be defined in two or more articles, with the details of the definition varying slightly from one article to another. The encyclopedia includes approximately 1,700 glossary entries.

DEFINING PARAGRAPH

The text of each article begins with a single introductory paragraph that defines the topic under discussion and summarizes the content of the article. For example, the article "Camptothecins" begins with the following defining paragraph:

Camptothecin derivatives are a novel group of antitumor agents with clinical utility in the treatment of human malignancies, including colorectal, lung, and ovarian tumors. Camptothecins uniquely target topoisomerase I, an enzyme that catalyzes the relaxation of torsionally strained double-stranded DNA. Camptothecins stabilize the binding of topoisomerase I to DNA and, in the presence of ongoing DNA synthesis, can generate potentially lethal DNA damage.

CROSS-REFERENCES

Many of the articles in the encyclopedia have cross-references to other articles. These cross-references appear at the end of the article, following the article text and preceding the bibliography. The cross-references indicate related articles that can be consulted for further information on the same topic, or for other information on a related topic.

BIBLIOGRAPHY

The bibliography appears as the last element in an article. It lists recent secondary sources to aid the reader in locating more detailed or technical information. Review articles and research papers that are important to an understanding of the topic are also listed.

The bibliographies in this encyclopedia are for the benefit of the reader, to provide references for further research on the given topic. Thus they typically consist of a half-dozen to a dozen entries. They are not intended to represent a complete listing of all materials consulted by the author in preparing the article.

COMPANION WORKS

The *Encyclopedia of Cancer* is one of a series of multivolume references in the life sciences published by Academic Press/Elsevier Science. Other such works include the *Encyclopedia of Human Biology, Encyclopedia of Virology, Encyclopedia of Immunology, Encyclopedia of Microbiology, Encyclopedia of Reproduction, Encyclopedia of Stress,* and *Encyclopedia of Genetics.*

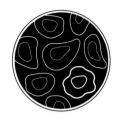

Radiation Resistance

Navneet Sharda
Chin-Rang Yang
Timothy Kinsella
David Boothman
University of Wisconsin–Madison

GLOSSARY

apoptosis Programmed cell death.

DNA promoter A nontranscribed region of DNA located at the 3′ end of a gene, which regulates transcription of that gene in response to various signals, such as the binding of transcription factors.

free radical A reactive chemical species characterized by a free valence shell electron which forms covalent bonds with many different compounds.

M phase The mitotic phase of the cell cycle.

S phase The synthesis phase of the cell cycle, when the genomic DNA is replicated.

transcriptional factor A protein that binds to the promoter region of a gene; this binding either upregulates or downregulates transcription of the gene.

transcription The process of building RNA messenger from the DNA template; the term also applies to duplication of DNA during S phase.

transfection The introduction of foreign DNA into a cell, accomplished via a number of different strategies. Use of Ca_2PO_4, liposomes, electroporation, and dextran sulfate are the most common methods.

translation The process of building protein from mRNA.

Radiation resistance depends on the ability of a cell to recognize DNA or membrane damage caused by ionizing radiation, activate multiple damage sensors which then turn on various signaling cascades that ultimately stop the foreword progression of the cell cycle, specifically in the G_1 and G_2 phases of the cell cycle. Delays in the G phases of the cell cycle are believed to allow the cell extra time for the activation of key proteins which are necessary for DNA rep. Recent data indicate that human cells have the to couple DNA strand break repair and repair of other DNA and membrane-damaged sites by the simultaneous activation of genes and proteins which, in turn, control such cellular responses as apoptosis and cell cycle progression. Such coupling mechanisms allow the cell to simultaneously regulate the cell cycle and DNA repair in a positive feedback loop. In recent years, it has been discovered that most DNA repair proteins also have a dual function in transcription and these two processes are coupled for added regulation of cellular recovery after various cytotoxic insults.

I. INTRODUCTION

Humans are exposed to ionizing and ultraviolet radiation on a daily basis. Cosmic radiation, terrestrial radiation, and medical radiation all contribute to human exposure. As a response to this constant radiation exposure, all organisms have developed methods for coping with the damage caused by radiation. This article discusses the mechanisms by which organisms have developed resistance to such exposures to ionizing and ultraviolet radiation. We will discuss the mechanisms by which organisms have developed cross-resistance to other DNA-damaging and cytotoxic agents, in addition to ionizing radiation.

The extent of cell damage and lethality caused by ionizing radiation is directly proportional to the amount of radiation delivered by the physician or the environment. Lethal damage following ionizing radiation has been directly linked to DNA strand breaks, although membrane damage is implicated in many cellular responses to radiation. Different cells have different inherent sensitivities to radiation. This difference is due to variable abilities in recognizing, responding, and correctly and efficiently repairing DNA damage.

II. CHEMICAL EFFECTS OF IONIZING RADIATION

...ing radiation affects critical cellular molecules _..._ direct and indirect ionization of cellu- _..._ _..ary_ target molecule for ionizing _..._ _..kes_ up 80% of the cell. _..._ it becomes a highly re-

active free radical which contributes to the formation of many other reactive oxygen species, such as OH^-, $OH\cdot$, $O_2\cdot$, and H_2O_2. These reactive oxygen species have very short half-lives, on the order of 10^{-10} to 10^{-5} sec, and diffuse only small distances. The reactive oxygen species caused by the ionization of water molecules then interact with DNA and other cellular targets to cause a variety of chemical bond damage. Damaging events caused by these ionizing events are, therefore, called indirect effects and account for about 80% of the lethal effect of radiation exposure to any given cell.

Direct ionizing radiation effects involve the immediate deposition of energy into DNA or other critical cellular targets. Direct effects occur via Compton scattering, the photoelectric effect, and pair production. The effect of this energy deposition is the ionization of molecules that results in chemical bond damage to critical targets within the cell. The most critical lesions created by these direct ionizations are to the chemical bonds in both the sugar backbone and the purine/pyrimidine bases in DNA. This results in base changes, DNA–protein cross-links, single strand DNA breaks, double strand DNA breaks, and abasic sites. As damaged bases are cleaved by proofreading repair enzymes, additional DNA lesions can be created, e.g., altered bases are quickly converted to abasic sites due to the enzymatic action of DNA glycosylases. Such direct ionization effects account for 20% of cytotoxic responses of cells to radiation.

III. CELLULAR CONTRIBUTIONS TO RADIATION RESISTANCE

Classic radiobiology measures radiation sensitivity and radiation resistance in terms of cell survival. When cultured human or rodent cells are treated with increasing doses of ionizing radiation and survival parameters are then measured, a distinctive dose–response survival curve is observed (Fig. 1). The slope of most radiation survival curves using human cells changes very little with low radiation doses. At some point in the radiation survival curve, as the dose is increased, the percentage of cells remaining viable begins to dramatically decrease, and the slope of the curve begins to increase. The initial portion of the

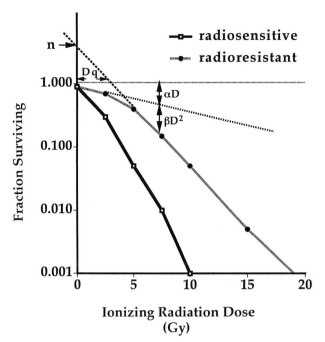

FIGURE 1 A typical dose–response survival curve for human cells. Fraction of cells surviving plotted on a logarithmic scale against radiation dose on a linear scale. At low doses, there is an initial slope. At intermediate doses, the slope changes, creating the "shoulder." At higher doses, the slope once again becomes roughly linear. A mathematical model based on the linear quadratic equation gives a good fit to the experimental results. αD represents the component cell killing that is proportional to dose delivered (D), βD^2 is the component of cell killing proportional to dose squared. n, the extrapolation number, represents with the width of the shoulder. Dq is the dose at which radiation effects become clinically evident. Radioresistant cells are characterized by a large n and Dq.

survival curve is highly variable from cell line to cell line and is commonly called the "shoulder" of the dose–response survival curve. This shoulder (i.e., the Dq measurement) has been used to reflect the radiation resistance or sensitivity of human cells. It is believed that the DNA repair capacity of any given cell plays a major role in the overall shape and size of the shoulder region. Although the DNA repair capacity is probably the most influential factor affecting resistance sensitivity, other factors can affect the killing potency of ionizing radiation. These include the position of the cell in the cell cycle, the dose rate of the ionizing radiation exposure, the number of radiation doses administered to reach the same total exposure (i.e., fractionating the radiation dose), and the oxygen content of the cell at the time of radiation exposure.

A. Cell Cycle Effect

Radioresistance varies in different phases of the cell cycle. Cells are most resistant in G_0, in early G_1, and in the late S phase of the cell cycle. Cells are most radiosensitive in late G_1, G_2, and throughout the M phase of the cell cycle. Radiation resistance in the S phase is thought to be due to an elevated amount of DNA synthesis and repair enzymes, as well as elevations in the intracellular levels of glutathione (a free radical scavenger). Cell cycle blockage in the G_1 phase of the cell cycle after ionizing radiation is believed to allow time for the recognition/repair of DNA damage prior to the initiation of DNA synthesis. Cells are most sensitive in the G_2/M phase of the cell cycle, presumably because there is no time for adequate repair before chromosome segregation takes place. Several gene products have been identified which increase or are posttranslationally altered following DNA damage, and these are thought to participate in halting cell cycle progression. These damage-responsive genes include p53, p21, growth arrest and damage-delay (GADD45), X-ray induced protein (XIP269), the retinoblastoma protein (pRb), and a group of retinoblastoma control proteins (RCPs), which bind to Sp1 sites in DNA promoters and may act to further alter gene transcription in response to DNA damage. As proposed for a damage-responsive G_1 block, halting the cell cycle in G_2/M until DNA damage can be repaired may improve cell survival and impart additional radiation resistance to cells which have the ability to halt at this cell cycle checkpoint.

B. Dose Rate Effects

The rate at which DNA damage is accrued following ionizing radiation also plays a role in radiation resistance/sensitivity. This is called the dose rate effect. When cells are exposed to ionizing radiation at very low dose rates (1–100 cGy/hr), most human cells are able to repair the damage and maintain genomic integrity. At dose rates greater than 100 cGy/hr, the rate of DNA damage accrual is faster than the ability of the cell to repair the damage, and significant lethal effects are noted. Cell cycle effects are also noted and are dependent on the dose rate and length of exposure.

C. Fractionation/Repopulation

Not all human cells are damaged during any given radiation exposure. If cells are dividing quickly, the phenomenon of repopulation becomes clinically evident during multifractionated radiotherapy. Cells have innate abilities to repair, to a certain amount, the damage caused by ionizing radiation, and thus a proportion of cells will survive any given exposure. The cells are not damaged during the initial ionizing radiation exposure give birth to multiple daughter cells. These daughter cells function to keep the tumor supplied with viable cells. Thus, a higher dose or more frequent radiation exposures becomes necessary. Several good clinical studies demonstrate a 10–20% improvement in tumor control with accelerated multifraction radiotherapy.

D. Oxygen Effects

The presence of oxygen markedly affects the potency of ionizing radiation. At tissue oxygen tensions of 30 mmHg or greater, there is a marked decrease in cell survival following ionizing radiation. The difference in lethality is two- to three-fold greater than oxygen-deprived cells. Between 3 and 30 mmHg of oxygen tension, there is a gradual increase in the lethal effects of ionizing radiation. This effect is called the oxygen enhancement ratio and is presumably due to the generation of oxygen-free radicals in the cell following radiation exposure which then causes additional damage to DNA via indirect effects.

E. DNA Repair Capacity

There are two general classes of DNA repair noted in eukaryotic cells following ionizing radiation, potentially lethal damage repair (PLDR) and sublethal damage repair (SLDR). These are operational terms only and are based on cell survival measurements that do not reflect the molecular mechanisms of DNA repair. PLDR represents the effect of environmental conditions on cell survival following ionizing radiation exposure. In general, conditions which cause a delay in the cell cycle (arrest in G_0, G_1, G_1/S, or G_2/M) result in increased cell survival, indicating that cell cycle delay may allow more time for DNA damage repair,

resulting in improved radiation resistance. SLDR is demonstrated during split dose ionizing radiation exposures. A given radiation exposure results in a certain amount of cell death. If the same overall dose of radiation is delivered to a cell culture in two exposures separated by 2 to 4 hr, cell survival is enhanced. Fractionated exposure times under 2 hr do not, generally, result in significant survival enhancement, nor does cell survival further increase when the time between the two doses of ionizing radiation was greater than 6 hr. These results are thought to represent DNA repair kinetics, with a half-time of repair of about 1 hr.

IV. SPECIFIC DATA REPAIR MECHANISMS

Most of the knowledge regarding DNA repair comes from bacteria and yeast, as these organisms have smaller, less complex genomes and are more amenable to experimentation. Since the mid-1980s, a number of very important eukaryotic DNA repair pathways that are active following ionizing radiation exposure have been elucidated, which include:

1. DNA base repair,
2. nucleotide excision (short and long patch) repair (NER),
3. single strand break repair, and
4. double strand break repair.

Repair of base damage after ionizing radiation plays only a small role in prokaryotes and yeast, and many unknown repair mechanisms need to be further clarified. In mammalian cells, the best known class of DNA base repair enzymes are the DNA glycosylases, which participate in base excision repair. Base excision repair is a multistep process which requires the participation of a large number of different proteins/enzymes. The first step is recognizing the damaged base, which is then excised. Base excision repair is mediated by a family of base recognition repair enzymes, including DNA glycosylases and apurinic/apyrimidinic (AP) endonucleases. These enzymes hydrolyze the N-glycosidic bonds between the damaged base and the sugar backbone of DNA, resulting in an AP site. Abasic sites are then recognized by an AP endonuclease which hydrolyzes the phosphodiester bond, causing a single-stranded DNA break and resulting in a 5'-deoxyribose phosphate residue. DNA polymerase, which contains an exonuclease function, then cleaves terminal 5'-deoxyribose residue ends, leaving a 5'-phosphate. DNA polymerase then continues to fill in the repair patch with complementary bases directed by the opposite DNA template. Once completed, the repair patch is then sealed by a DNA ligase to seal the final DNA breaks.

Nucleotide excision repair in human cells is a more specific and complex DNA repair process. Not all of the enzymes which participate in NER have been elucidated. NER detects and repairs single as well as multiply damaged neighboring DNA bases. Certain damage-specific helicases and endonucleases recognize abnormal DNA regions/bases and cleave the phosphodiester backbone on either side of the damaged region. The cleaved DNA patch is then degraded, presumably by DNA polymerase, and the resulting gap in the DNA helix is then filled in by the same DNA polymerase. Unlike DNA replication, which occurs during the synthesis phase of the cell cycle, the DNA polymerase does not require the synthesis of an RNA primer by a DNA-dependent RNA polymerase. The final step in DNA repair is ligation, which acts to seal the single strand break left downstream of the newly synthesized DNA repair patch. Various DNA ligases have been elucidated and all may play a role in DNA repair. It is believed that both NER and base excision repair enzymes are not cell cycle regulated, since these repair processes are active any time during the cell cycle, rather than specifically during S phase. It is interesting to note, however, that at least one DNA base repair enzyme, uracil DNA glycosylase, is expressed only during S phase. It is important to note that the cell cycle regulation of DNA repair enzymes has not been, in general, examined in great detail. In addition, many DNA repair genes have been identified but many more are still unknown.

The bulk of human knowledge regarding the molecular mechanisms of NER comes from the human autosomal recessive disorder, xerodermia pigmentosum (XP). The XP disease is actually a group of seven different genetic mutations, any one of which will result in defective NER. XP patients have high rates of skin cancer, neurologic defects, and marked photo-

sensitivity to ultraviolet radiation and DNA-damaging agents which result in DNA adduct formation. Interestingly, cells from all XP groups are not hypersensitive to agents that create DNA breaks, including neocarzinostatin, bleomycin, or ionizing radiation. Patients exhibiting the XP disease have been classified into eight distinct complementation groups: A, B, C, D, E, F, G, and one variant group called XPV. A complementation group is derived by cell fusion experiments, in which two cell lines with different defects in NER were fused, resulting in a hybrid cell which is able to perform NER at normal levels. The existence of these complementation groups allowed researchers to isolate the specific genes which correct many of the complementation groups. The human XP genes have also been found to be complementary to many of the rodent excision repair cross complementing (ERCC) genes. The XP-A gene expresses a protein that recognizes thymine dimers in DNA created by ultraviolet radiation; the XP-B protein has DNA helicase activity; XP-C encodes a protein which is identical to ERCC1 and also has helicase activity; the XP-D protein is a component of RNA polymerase II-dependent basal transcription factor (TFIIH); and the XP-G protein is an endonuclease. The identities of XP-E, XP-F, and XPV remain unknown. Although long patch NER is not implicated after exposure to ionizing radiation, short patch NER does play a major role in the DNA repair responses to this DNA-damaging agent. The exact role of XP-related genes in ionizing radiation repair responses remains to be elucidated.

NER in mammalian cells is vastly more complex than the systems elucidated for prokaryotic NER. This complexity reflects the increased complexity of the mammalian genome. An average mammalian genome is approximately 3×10^{10} bp. In order to fit the genetic material into the nucleus of a human cell, a greater than 50,000-fold reduction in the size of the genome is necessary. This reduction in size is accomplished through multiple levels of folding, with characteristic chromatin/chromosome topology. This compact folding plays an important, but largely unknown role in NER. Damaged sites caused by ultraviolet and ionizing radiation are not always immediately accessible to repair enzymes, as the majority of the genomic DNA is packaged around histones and tightly coiled, thus leaving no room for repair enzymes to bind the damaged sites.

The enzymes which have been conclusively demonstrated to be necessary for NER in-cell free systems are XPA, XPG, transcription factor II-H, XPC, UV-DDB, ERCC1/XPF, IF7, replication protein A, proliferative cell nuclear antigen, replication factor C, DNA polymerases δ and α, and various DNA ligases. Addition of histones to the cell-free system inhibits NER, thus indicating that additional enzymes are necessary *in vivo* for NER, such as topoisomerases, helicases, and gyrases. Deficiency in any one of these proteins carries significant somatic consequences, as typified by Bloom's syndrome. Bloom's syndrome, like XP, is an autosomal recessive disorder. The molecular defect is believed to be due to deficiency in ligase activity, although no mutation in the DNA ligases themselves has been found.

Since the mid-1980s, it has been discovered that actively transcribing genes are preferentially repaired by the NER system. The same mechanisms that loosen the chromatin structure to allow transcriptional enzymes access to the DNA helix also function to increase the accessibility of damaged DNA to repair enzymes. Additionally, many of the enzymes which are necessary for transcription also play a role in DNA repair. Nontranscriptionally active regions of DNA also undergo NER, but at much slower rates. Interestingly, cells derived from Cockayne's syndrome patients are unable to perform such preferential DNA repair processes. These data have lead many researchers to conclude that NER processes in human cells are truly "transcription coupled."

Double Strand DNA Break Repair Appears to Be the Critical Determinant to Survival Following Ionizing Radiation

Double strand DNA breaks are accepted as the lethal component of DNA damage caused by ionizing radiation. Single strand DNA breaks, if not repaired, can become double strand breaks and therefore their repair is also critical to the survival of human cells after ionizing radiation. Thus, it is of no real surprise that double strand DNA break repair is generally accepted as the primary component of DNA repair which affects radiation resistance/sensitivity.

Biphasic repair kinetics after ionizing radiation exposure have been demonstrated, and a mathematical model of radiation resistance based on the linear quadratic formula has become the standard. The initial, very rapid component of DNA repair is likely due to simple and fast-acting short patch NER, in which the excision of damaged bases and the subsequent ligation of single-stranded DNA breaks are quickly performed. The second component of repair following ionizing radiation is currently under investigation, although a growing body of evidence supports the participation of a series of proteins and enzymes which bind specifically to double-stranded DNA ends. These proteins likely are involved in DNA break repair and serve as double-strand DNA break sensors, which send signals outside of the nucleus to interact with proteins that control the cell cycle, stimulate additional DNA repair processes, and/or induce apoptotic events. These enzymes are also integrally involved in V(D)J recombinational mechanisms in lymphocytes, since double strand DNA breaks are essential intermediates in the process of antibody production.

Cells derived from mice with the inherited severe combined immunodeficiency disorder (SCID) are highly radiosensitive. They also lack the ability to perform V(D)J recombination and have general deficiencies in their immunological responses. These cells, however, are not overly sensitive to UV radiation or monofunctional alkylators but are exquisitely sensitive to low doses of bleomycin, which causes double strand DNA breaks in a "radiomimetic" fashion. Thus, the SCID defect is thought to be due to a deficiency in the repair of double strand DNA breaks. Gene mapping has identified a locus near the centromeric region of human chromosome 8, which is thought to contain the intact gene which is mutated in SCID cells. When this portion of human chromosome 8 is transfected into SCID mouse cells, radiation resistance and V(D)J recombination are both restored to normal levels.

Other experiments have demonstrated that the Ku autoantigen, a heterodimer composed of one 70 kDa (i.e., Ku70) and one 80 kDa (i.e., Ku 80) protein, specifically binds double strand DNA ends. The Ku heterodimer may bind to a wide variety of DNA ends, including 3′-DNA overhangs, 5′-DNA overhangs, blunt DNA ends, replication forks, and stem–loop structures. Interestingly, the Ku 70 and Ku 80 heterodimer does not bind DNA single strand breaks or intact double strand DNA which has little or no complex secondary structure. Thus, the Ku heterodimeric complex is an excellent candidate as a general sensor of double-stranded DNA breaks. Both Ku proteins bind one to one, stoichiometrically, to a 440-kDa protein, called the DNA-PK catalytic subunit (Fig. 2). These three proteins make up the DNA-dependent protein kinase (DNA-PK) holoenzyme. DNA-PK is a serine/threonine kinase located primarily in the nucleus which is active only when bound to DNA. The *in vitro* substrates of DNA-PK include many transcription factors, such as Sp-1, c-fos, c-myc, c-jun, p53, CTR-1/NF-1, Oct-1, Oct-2, RNA polymerase 2, SV40 T antigen, and the Ku 70/80-kDa proteins themselves. Phosphorylation of the Ku proteins is thought to decrease DNA binding, thereby supplying a feedback loop to DNA-PK holoenzyme activity (Fig. 2).

Mutant cells have been identified which are deficient in various proteins of the Ku complex. X-ray sensitive (XRS) 5 and 6 cells are deficient in Ku 80, SXI cells are deficient in Ku 70, and SCID cells are deficient in the DNA-PK$_{cs}$ protein and enzyme activity. As stated before, cells from SCID mice demonstrate marked radiation sensitivity, as measured by survival assays, and are unable to perform V(D)J recombination. When compared to normal cells, the number of double-stranded DNA breaks caused by equivalent doses of radiation is identical in these mutant cells, but the subsequent repair of DNA double strand breaks is deficient. One hour after radiation exposure, there is a two-fold difference in the number of DNA breaks present, and at 2 hr there is a five-fold difference, with normal cells repairing the double-stranded DNA breaks at a greater rate than SCID cells.

Transfection of the Ku 80 cDNA into XRS 5 cells results in a restoration of radiation resistance to near normal levels. Analysis of the number of DNA breaks following ionizing radiation demonstrated that at both 1 and 2 hr there was no significant difference in the total amount of DNA breaks when compared to normal control cells. Similar transfection experiments

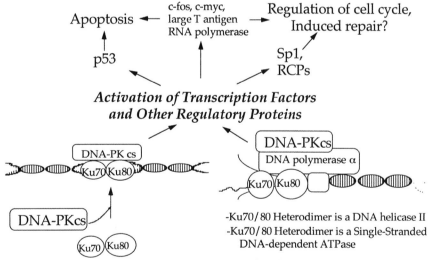

FIGURE 2 Role of DNA-PKcs in DNA break repair. The Ku 70–Ku 80 heterodimeric protein complex binds to each end of a double strand DNA break. The ends of the break are brought in direct juxtaposed position in order for DNA break repair to occur. Once joined, the DNA-PKcs is recruited and the DNA-PK holoenzyme is complete. After association, DNA-PK serine/threonine enzyme activity dramatically increases and several key transcription response factors are then activated through phosphorylation. Activation of DNA-PK, thereby, couples DNA repair to alterations in transcription. Altered transcriptional responses then regulate cell cycle progression and apoptosis processes.

with other mutant cells demonstrate equivalent findings. Analysis of V(D)J recombination following cDNA transfection into these mutant cells showed a return of recombinational ability.

V. TRANSCRIPTIONAL RESPONSES FOLLOWING IONIZING RADIATION

Of the estimated 5×10^4 transcriptionally active genes in the human genome, only about 15 are induced at the level of transcription following ionizing radiation. An additional 15 or so proteins, including p53 protein levels, accumulate independent of new protein synthesis following ionizing radiation (i.e., become transcriptionally active). Many of the genes which are transcriptionally upregulated following ionizing radiation are also induced by a variety of cytotoxic agents, which damage DNA and/or cytoplasmic membranes. Few X-ray inducible genes are specifically induced only by ionizing radiation. There are several broad classes of inducible genes, including (a) enzymes which may play a role in DNA repair; (b) protooncogenes; (c) growth-related/cell cycle regulatory proteins; (d) DNA-binding proteins; and (e) other proteins which have multiple functions in response to ionizing radiation, possibly by acting as signals to couple repair, cell cycle progression, delay division, or initiate apoptosis.

Interestingly, a number of enzymes/proteins involved in cell cycle regulation and DNA repair are markedly induced following ionizing radiation. Thymidine kinase, an essential enzyme in DNA synthesis, was induced 2- to 3-fold in normal human cells following ionization radiation, and up to 10-fold in neoplastic cells. Although this enzyme does not participate directly in double strand DNA break repair or NER, it does supply necessary nucleotides (dTTP) and may be, therefore, indirectly necessary for radiation resistance. Other reported enzymes induced following ionizing radiation include DNA polymerase-β, DNA methyltransferase, DNA glycosylase, and ornithine decarboxylase. Interestingly, the majority of enzymes directly involved in NER do not appear to be induced by ionizing radiation or other DNA-damaging agents. This lack of damage induction following ionizing radiation implicates posttranslational

mechanisms for the induction of enzyme activity. For example, the simultaneous downregulation of topoisomerase I and the upregulation of poly(ADP-ribose)polymerase (PARP) following ionizing radiation occurs by posttranslational modifications within the cell. Activated PARP in turn initiates a cascade of events leading to the activation of a variety of DNA repair enzymes through posttranslational ADP-ribosylation. Cells able to actively upregulate PARP and thereby downregulate topoisomerase I survive better following ionizing radiation exposure.

Certain transcription factor protein binding to their respective DNA consensus sites is also markedly enhanced following ionizing radiation. The DNA-binding activities of proteins to AP-1, CREB, p53, NF-κB, and Sp-1 DNA consensus sites are enhanced following radiation exposure. In addition, the DNA binding of a number of retinoblastoma control proteins (RCPs) is enhanced following ionizing radiation. These DNA consensus sites are present in the promoter elements of a variety of genes that are induced following ionizing radiation. These genes include stromelysin, collagenase, metallothionein, DT diaphorase, tissue plasminogen activator, GADD45, and cyclin D1. The effects of these genes in relation to DNA repair, cell cycle regulation, and/or apoptosis, with resultant effects on radiation resistance/sensitivity, are currently unknown. Considerable research effort is being directed to elucidate these genes and their roles in cell survival.

Recent data indicate the existence of unique intracellular sensors in the cytoplasm and nucleus that act as signaling cascades and are involved in the activation of transcriptional responses following ionizing radiation (Fig. 3). It is likely that many of the specific sensoring pathways are cell and tissue specific, although common pathways have also been elucidated. Many of these same signaling cascades have also been implicated in cellular responses following a wide variety of other DNA-damaging and cytotoxic agents. These universal responses [such as activation of protein kinase C (PKC) and c-jun kinase (JNK)] indicate the involvement of general stress/damage sensors within the membrane and cytoplasm following ionizing radiation. Mitogen-activated protein kinases (MAPKs) act on a very large group of proteins and transcription factors to alter their phosphorylation

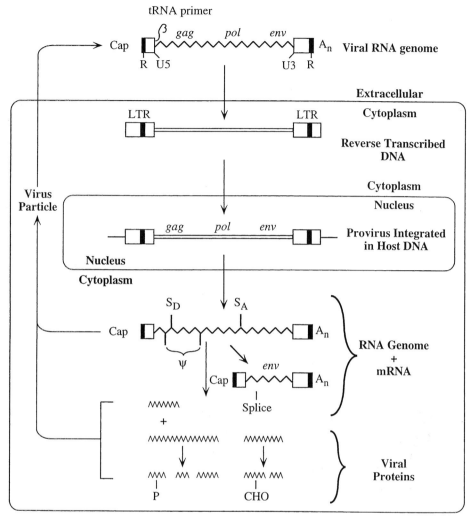

FIGURE 3 Damage transcriptional response sensors. Several key damage-response sensors are present within the nucleus and cytoplasm of any human cell. Known transcriptional response sensors of damage include p53, Sp1, retinoblastoma control proteins (RCPs), NF-κB, and AP1/CREB. Only the Sp1/RCP response has been demonstrated to be directly coupled to DNA damage repair via DNA-PK. Activation of the other transcription response sensors occurs in the cytoplasm. Immediate early genes (IEGs) are noted to be unregulated seconds to minutes following radiation exposure.

states. Phosphorylation and dephosphorylation processes are known to modify/enhance the enzymatic activity of many proteins, as well as affect the DNA-binding avidity and specificity of transcription factors. Many of these protein kinases are, in turn, phosphorylated which results in an induction of their kinase activities. The c-aBl tyrosine kinase is a candidate for an ionizing radiation damage-specific sensor, as is the DNA-dependent protein kinase (DNA-PK) holoen-

zyme. At present the activation of DNA-PKcs is the only known nuclear sensor of DNA damage which also activates a series of transcription factors.

In addition to being the most commonly mutated gene in human cancer, the p53 tumor suppresser acts as a transcription factor which may bind certain regulatory regions of many genes following ionizing radiation, leading to the induction or repression of downstream genes. One hour following ionizing radiation, nuclear levels of p53 increase three- to five-fold, resulting in a variety of cellular effects. The two most relevant cellular responses following radiation are the cell cycle delays and the induction of apoptosis. These responses clearly affect radiation resistance in human cells. Interestingly, cells containing a mutated form of p53 demonstrate increased survival following irradiation. These experiments are, however, complicated by the fact that multiple genomic alterations may have been caused by the mutant p53 phenotype. Although cells with the mutant p53 phenotypes do not demonstrate enhanced nuclear protein levels following ionizing radiation, they normally have elevated nuclear levels of this protein. Thus, it is possible that some of the p53 mutants may retain the ability to augment DNA repair processes, possibly due to an increase in this proteins half-life. Thus, although cells with mutant p53 appear to be unable to alter cell cycle progression or commit cellular suicide via apoptotic events in response to ionizing radiation, the decline in apoptosis enhances survival even in the absence of the G_2 checkpoint.

VI. CELL CYCLE ALTERATIONS THAT AFFECT RADIATION RESISTANCE

Growth inhibition and cell cycle delays are an integral response to ionizing radiation. The two major cell cycle blocks which occur following ionizing radiation are at the G_1/S border and at the G_2/M border. It is believed that the existence of unrepaired double strand DNA breaks during mitosis is almost inevitably fatal. Similarly, unrepaired DNA damage prior to DNA synthesis (i.e., S phase) results in a very high frequency of mutations, which ultimately leads to carcinogenesis or cellular lethality. Thus, many researchers have theorized that a survival advantage is gained if the cell is able to delay in cell cycle progression before the onset of DNA synthesis or mitosis until the DNA damage is repaired.

p53 plays a vital role in cell cycle arrest in G_1/S and possibly also in G_2/M following ionizing radiation exposure. Cells lacking functional p53 do not arrest in G_1. Transfection of wild-type p53 cDNA into these

cells resulted in a regained function of these cells to arrest in G_1 following ionizing radiation exposure. Cellular levels of GADD45, which is regulated by p53, increase following ionizing radiation. As GADD45 has been implicated in cell cycle delays as well as NER, there is a possible coupling among DNA damage, DNA repair, and cell cycle delay. Other p53 substrates which participate in the cell cycle include WAF-1/CIP-1 which inhibits cyclin-dependent kinase complexes that are required for cell cycle progression. In addition, alterations in the phosphorylation status of the retinoblastoma protein (pRb) have been reported following ionizing radiation. Hypophosphorylated pRb binds to and prevents the transcriptional activity of members of the E_2F family of transcription factors. Phosphorylation of pRb results in its dissociation from E_2F. Free E_2F then becomes transcriptionally active and directs the transcription of various genes involved in S phase entry with resultant effects on radiation resistance/sensitivity.

The p53 cellular response following ionizing radiation plays a major role in radiation resistance/sensitivity. Ataxia telangiectasia (AT) is a hereditary condition characterized by hypersensitivity to ionizing radiation, cancer susceptibility, immunologic deficits, and genetic instability. Following exposure to ionizing radiation, the cellular levels of p53, p21, and GADD45 slowly elevate in AT cells, in marked contrast to normal cells where there is a rapid rise in the amount of these proteins. Exposure to ultraviolet radiation results in normal inductions of these proteins, implicating a mutation in sensors specific for ionizing radiation-induced DNA damage in this pathway. The AT cell is unable to halt progression in the cell cycle in response to ionizing radiation exposure, nor is there any delay in S phase noted following ionizing radiation. These findings indicate one possible mechanism for the dramatic radiosensitivity of AT, although it has recently been observed that apoptosis accounts for the major portion of cellular lethality following ionizing radiation exposure. p53 can play a major role in apoptotic processes as well. If AT cells are transfected with the viral oncogene E6 (which binds to and completely inactivates p53), these cells regain near normal survival parameters following ionizing radiation. Transfecting normal cells with E6 has no effect on survival, indicating that AT cells are abnormally responsive to p53-mediated apoptosis following ionizing radiation.

VII. CONCLUSIONS

The major factors affecting sensitivity/resistance to ionizing radiation are cell cycle progression, oxygen tension, DNA repair capacity, dose rates of ionizing radiation used, and whether radiation is fractionated or given as a single dose. Although these factors are interrelated, the manner in which cells respond to various ionizing radiation challenges is to activate various DNA repair processes and nuclear and cytoplasmic transcriptional response sensors. Sensors of damage in the cell include DNA repair and transcriptional responses in the nucleus, as well as the transactivation of transcription factors in both the cytoplasm and the nucleus. The transcriptional response sensors known to date include DNA-PK, p53, Sp1, RCPs, NF-κB, AP-1, and CREB. Further research into the mechanisms by which damaged human cells couple DNA repair and immediate transcriptional responses to cell cycle regulation and apoptosis will be necessary to significantly improve radiotherapy regimens which seek to exploit differences between cancer and normal cells. Clearly, human tumor cells, in general, are altered in many of these very important early responses to DNA damage. In addition, our understanding of how human cells immediately respond to ionizing radiation will aid in our understanding of the initiation of carcinogenesis and aging.

Acknowledgments

We thank Dr. Mark Ritter and the members of the laboratories of Drs. Kinsella and Boothman for their critical reading of this article. This work supported by Grant CA67995-02 to D. A. B. from the National Cancer Institute, National Institutes of Health.

See Also the Following Articles

DOSIMETRY AND TREATMENT PLANNING FOR THREE-DIMENSIONAL RADIATION THERAPY • LATE EFFECTS OF RADIATION THERAPY • MOLECULAR ASPECTS OF RADIATION BIOLOGY • PROTON BEAM RADIATION THERAPY • RADIOBIOLOGY, PRINCIPLES OF

Bibliography

Aboussekhra, A., Biggerstaff, M., Shivji, M. K. K., et al. (1995). Mammalian DNA nucleotide excision repair reconstituted with purified protein components. Cell **80,** 859–868.

Davis, T. W., Meyers, M., Van Patten, C., Sharda, N. N., et al. (1996). Transcriptional responses to damage created by ionizing radiation: Molecular sensors. In "DNA Damage and Repair: Biochemistry, Genetics and Cell Biology" (J. A. Nickoloff and M. F. Hoekstra, eds.), in press.

Friedberg, E. C., Walker, G. C., and Siede, W. (1995). "DNA Repair and Mutagenesis." ASM Press, Washington, DC.

Gottlieb, T. M., and Jackson, S. P. (1993). The DNA-dependent protein kinase: Requirement for DNA ends and association with Ku antigen. Cell **72,** 131–142.

Haffner, R., and Oren, M., (1995). Biochemical properties and biological effects of p53. Curr. Opin. Genet. Dev. **5,** 84–90.

Hall, E. J. (1994). "Radiobiology for the Radiologist," 4th Ed., J. B. Lippincott Company, Philadelphia, Pennsylvania.

Kastan, M. B., Canman, C. E., and Leonard, C. J. (1995). P53, cell cycle control and apoptosis: Implications for cancer. Cancer Metasis Rev. **14,** 3–15.

Ross, G. M., Eady, J. J., Mithal, N. P., et al. (1995). DNA strand break rejoining defect in xrs-6 is complemented by transfection with the human Ku80 gene. Cancer Res. **55,** 1235–1238.

Taccioli, G. E., Gottlieb, T. M., Blunt, T., et al. (1994). Ku 80: Product of the XRCC5 gene and its role in DNA repair and V(D)J recombination. Science **265,** 1442–1445.

Radiobiology, Principles of

Amin Mirhadi
William H. McBride
University of California, Los Angeles

GLOSSARY

DNA repair The processing of DNA damage and restoration of function. Sublethal damage repair is an operational term to describe repair between fractions of radiation. Potentially lethal damage repair is operationally defined as being dependent on signals from the environment of the cells.

Do The dose of radiation that reduces cell survival to e^{-1}, i.e., 37%. It is used as a parameter to describe the slope of a cell survival curve. The effective Do ($_{eff}$Do) describes the slope of a multifraction survival curve.

electrons Negatively charged elementary particles.

free radical Atom or molecule that contains an unpaired electron and is therefore highly reactive.

gray This is the SI unit of absorbed dose and is equivalent to 1 J/kg. It replaces the rad. One gray = 100 rads.

ionizing radiation Radiation that results in the removal of electrons from atoms or molecules causing them to be charged. Radiation is considered ionizing if it has a wave length less than about 10^{-6} cm.

linear energy transfer The rate of loss of energy along an ionization track expressed in kV/μm.

neutrons An uncharged elementary particle. Fast neutrons with an energy in excess of 100,000 electron volts produced in a cyclotron have been used for therapy. They have an RBE value of about 1.6 relative to X rays and a lower oxygen enhancement ratio.

protons Elementary particles with a positive charge and high mass. They have radiobiological properties similar to X rays but the dose is largely deposited in a small area at the end of the particle's range, resulting in a physical advantage, in particular where critical structures need to be avoided.

relative biological effectiveness (RBE) Used to compare the biologic effectiveness of different types of radiation. It is defined as the dose of radiation required for a specific effect, such as a log reduction in cell survival, divided into the dose of X rays needed to result in the same biologic effect.

Radiation therapy has a long history. In 1895 the German physicist, Wilhelm Conrad Roentgen, discovered that electricity passing through a tube of gas at low pressure would emit rays that caused a fluorescent material to glow. At that time, many laboratories were experimenting with electrical discharges from induction coils as they passed through partially evacuated glass tubes, known as a Crooke's tubes. Rontgen was curious as to whether cathode rays could escape the confines of the tube. To avoid interference from the fluorescence of the operating tube, he covered it in black paper and completely darkened his laboratory. During his experimentation, he happened to notice that a fluorescent plate situated elsewhere in the room shone when the apparatus was functioning, even though no light was coming from it and the plate was farther away than cathode rays could travel. His subsequent investigations of the unknown rays, or "X rays," showed that they penetrated objects other than paper, including flesh but not bony structures. This was the birth of diagnostic radiology.

Early X-ray workers soon discovered, to their cost, that large doses of X rays could burn the skin. In 1896, Professor Freund exploited these observations to treat a girl with hirsutes and, subsequently, patients with moles and other skin lesions. Very soon, X rays were being used to treat cancers, as well as a wide variety of benign conditions.

Radiation was further catapulted into the scientific scene by Bequerel's discovery that mineral crusts containing uranium emitted rays that could expose a photographic plate in the dark, showing that naturally occurring substances could emit radioactivity. The Curies confirmed this shortly thereafter by extracting radioactive polonium, uranium, and radium from pitchblende. Within a very short period of time, naturally occurring radioisotopes, as well as X rays, were being used to treat many different clinical conditions.

The scientific community and the general public enthusiastically greeted the discovery of radiation, but within months it became apparent that any benefit to be derived from its application came at a cost. In 1901, Becquerel was prompted to say "I love this radium, but I have a grudge against it." He had left some radium in his vest pocket for 6 h. Ten days later a skin burn appeared that took some weeks to heal. This was one of the first indications of how radiation most often selectively affects clonogenic, as opposed to differentiated, cells, with the delay representing the turnover time of skin tissue. This concept was explored by many workers and became known as the law of Bergonie and Tribondeau. Despite numerous indications, it took many decades for the hazards and advantages of radiation to be fully appreciated, perhaps in part because there is a latent period before the appearance of visible signs of toxicity. Dozens of the first radiation doctors and scientists, including Madame Curie, lost their lives as a direct result of working with radiation. Now, in part as a result of follow-up on the nuclear bomb survivors of Hiroshima and Nagasaki, it is probably the best-understood environmental hazard.

During the first half of the 20th century, radiation was used largely to treat benign disease. Recognition of the associated risks, however, fostered moves away from this use and toward the treatment of cancer. Over the century, the principles governing its therapeutic efficacy have become firmly established. Currently, approximately half of patients with cancer will receive radiation therapy with curative intent and about half of these will be cured as a result of its powerful cytotoxic action. Ironically, improvements in our understanding of radiation and our ability to harness and use it in a controlled way have led to a recent resurgence of interest in its use to treat benign diseases, such as prevention of restenosis after treatment for atherosclerotic plaques in the coronary vasculature and inhibition of growth of heterotopic bone and keloids.

I. PHYSICS AND CHEMISTRY OF RADIOBIOLOGY

A. Ionizing Radiation

Radiation of the ionizing type is chosen for most radiotherapeutic purposes. It has a short wave length and delivers photons in packets that have sufficient energy to expel electrons from atomic orbit. The energy released by the ejection of an outer shell electron (about 33 eV) can break a chemical bond, which has biological consequences. In fact, a chain of physico-chemical reactions is initiated that continues until the energy is dissipated. Various sources can be used to deliver different types of ionizing radiation. These include photons, which are X rays produced when electrons from a linear accelerator are stopped rapidly, γ rays, which are emitted spontaneously by the nuclear decay of radioactive elements, and particles, such as electrons, neutrons, and protons.

Different radiations have distinct properties. One that is important from a radiobiological perspective is the density of ionization events along a track. The average linear energy transfer (LET) is a crude measure of this. Photons and electrons, which are most frequently used in radiation therapy, are characterized by a high energy and low mass. They cause sparse ionization events (low LET), at least until the secondary electrons come to rest at the end of their path. Sparsely ionizing radiation is relatively less effective than densely ionizing radiation at bringing about biological effects. The relative biological efficiency (RBE) of radiation is a measure of this. As would be expected, it varies with LET, although not directly. It reaches a maximum at around an LET of 100 keV/μm (energy/unit distance). RBE is defined as the ratio of the dose required to produce a biologic effect for a given radiation type divided into the dose of 250-kV X rays required to produce the same magnitude of biologic effect. RBE measurements depend on the biological end point, but are useful. The RBE for most conventional therapeutic types of radiation is around one; in other words, they are similar to X rays. However, neutrons and α particles, which have dense ionization tracks, have higher RBEs. Dose for dose, they cause greater biological damage. For example, reduction of cell survival by 90% might require around 2.6 times more X ray than neutron dose (RBE = 2.6).

Ionization events from conventional low LET radiation are spaced at intervals that are large compared to the width of DNA, which is the prime target for radiation-induced cytotoxicity and carcinogenicity. The action of low LET radiation on DNA, and other biological molecules, is in fact largely indirect. Damage results from the generation of free radicals through the ionization of intracellular water, which is the major cellular constituent, rather than by direct action of radiation on biological materials.

The preference in radiation therapy for the use of sparsely ionizing, low LET, radiation, which has a relatively low RBE, might at first sight appear somewhat paradoxical. The reason for its use is that differences in response between tumor and certain normal tissues are exploited, resulting in a greater therapeutic benefit. This contributes significantly to the clinical efficacy of radiation therapy.

B. Generation of Free Radicals

Free radicals resulting from the action of sparsely ionizing radiation on intracellular water that cause most of the cellular damage are hydroxyl radicals, although complex chemical reactions generate a number of different species that play roles. Radicals can also be formed in the biologic materials themselves by direct ionization. About one-third of the damage caused by low LET radiation is direct and two-thirds is indirect. The involvement of reactive oxygen species (ROS) in radiation effects has important mechanistic implications. ROS are short-lived, either reacting rapidly with surrounding molecules or reverting to a stable state. Most of the radical chemistry is over within 10^{-5} s. As a result, only free radicals generated within a few nanometers of DNA will be damaging and the balance of reducing and oxidizing species (redox) close to the DNA will be important in determining the extent of the damage.

Compounds that increase the reactivity or life span of free radicals, such as oxygen and oxygen mimetic drugs like nitroimidazoles, sensitize cells to the cytotoxic effects of radiation. The level of naturally occurring compounds that scavenge free radicals, such as glutathione and other sulfhydryl-containing molecules, present at the time of irradiation will also be important as they can protect against damage. Because densely ionizing, high LET radiation produces more direct than indirect damage, its effects are less influenced by the presence of oxygen and by the redox balance than those of sparsely ionizing, low LET radiation.

C. Role of Oxygen

Molecular oxygen is a very powerful modifier of the biologic effects of ionizing irradiation. The main concept is that oxygen makes radiation-induced free radicals more permanent by interfering with chemical repair processes. This is called the "oxygen fixation" hypothesis. Other mechanisms undoubtedly contribute to the oxygen effect, but the end result is that cells are much better able to resist radiation killing under hypoxic than oxic conditions.

The cause of tumor hypoxic and anoxic regions in tumors is most often that, unlike normal tissues, they outgrow their blood supply. These hypoxic areas may be present either chronically (because of vascular insufficiency) or transiently (because of variable blood flow). Calculations of oxygen diffusion predict that the oxygen tension would decrease to zero at about 150 μm from a capillary. Another possible contributory cause is anemia, which can result in poor oxygen delivery. Anemic patients are generally less responsive to radiation therapy. The concentration of oxygen below which radiation responses are affected is low (less than 10 mm Hg), and hypoxia is generally considered significant in radiotherapy only when it reaches levels less than or equal to 5 mm Hg. These levels are achieved in hypoxic sites in many tumors.

The oxygen enhancement ratio (OER) describes the magnitude of the oxygen effect. This is the ratio of doses required for equivalent cell killing in the absence of oxygen to in its presence. The OER is generally in the range of 2.5 to 3.5, depending on the experimental conditions. This means that three times as much radiation is required under hypoxic as under oxic conditions to produce the same level of effect (e.g., cell killing). This is a large factor. If it were to operate to the same extent daily throughout a course of radiation therapy, hypoxia would be a frequent cause of treatment failure.

Numerous clinical studies have shown a correlation between the hypoxic status of tumors and radiocurability. These studies offer the hope that manipulations that increase tissue oxygenation or that target hypoxic cells will improve the outcome of cancer treatment by radiation. Indeed, one of the justifications for the daily fractionation of dose commonly employed in radiation therapy is that it allows reoxygenation to take place between fractions (see later). Hypoxic cell sensitizers that mimic oxygen in their effects have been tested in the clinic. The best-studied class of agents is nitroimidazoles. By acting in place of oxygen, they can be directly cytotoxic to hypoxic cells, in addition to sensitizing cells to radiation and to those chemotherapeutic agents whose cytotoxicity is oxygen dependent. In general, they have not been proven to be highly successful and their administration is associated with some toxicity. However, this situation might be improved on if they were used only in patients whose tumors have demonstrable hypoxia, which is not the case in most clinical trials to date.

It should be noted that there are dimensions to the cellular influence of hypoxia other than simply deprivation of the radiosensitizing effect of oxygen. At the molecular level, hypoxia induces expression of many genes. Some, such as erythropoietin, vascular endothelial growth factor, and tumor necrosis factor (TNF)-α, are produced in a proangiogenesis response, possibly mimicking a role for hypoxia in driving embryonic growth and development. Others, such as p53, are part of a stress response that encourages apoptosis. A consequence is that there is a selective force for cells in tumors that have mutated toward an anti-apoptotic phenotype, as they will survive better in hypoxic sites. The ability of hypoxia to drive tumors toward a more malignant phenotype might explain why hypoxia has been found in some circumstances to correlate not only with local recurrence after radiation therapy, but also with survival following surgery.

II. RADIATION DOSAGE

The SI unit of absorbed dose in radiation therapy is the gray (Gy). This is the amount of energy imparted per unit mass and is equivalent to 1 J/kg. It equals 100 rads, which is an older measure. One centigray (cGy) is equal to 1 rad. It is important to realize that the gray does not take radiobiological considerations into account. It is a physical dose, and the biological effects of a dose in gray will vary with the quality of the radiation, dose rate, tissue type, end point, redox balance, and other biological parameters. Biological dose is therefore more variable than physical dose.

Radiation therapy plays roles in cancer treatment in three major areas: definitive treatment, palliative treatment, and locoregional control. Radiation is frequently used as sole curative therapy, but it is also used in conjunction with chemotherapy or before or after radical surgery to help decrease the rate of local or regional recurrence and lymph node failure. Regarding palliation, radiation is most importantly used in cases of bone pain due to breast cancer or prostate cancer, but it is also used in many other situations to relieve symptoms. In such cases, higher than normal doses are often given in an abbreviated regimen. However, the most common treatment schedule for definitive treatment administers daily doses of around 2 Gy, five times per week, to a maximum of 50–75 Gy, depending on the clinical circumstances.

III. DNA DAMAGE AND REPAIR FOLLOWING IRRADIATION

A. Radiation-Induced DNA Lesions

Ionization events, whether direct or indirect, can be thought of as occurring randomly throughout the cell. One gray causes several hundred thousand ionization events per cell and in DNA results in thousands of single strand breaks, 30–40 double strand breaks, and numerous DNA–DNA and DNA–protein cross-links. The amount of DNA damage caused by a standard daily clinical dose of 2 Gy does not vary much between different tumor cell lines, however, there is considerable variation in their sensitivity to cytotoxic killing. It follows that the way the damage is processed is important to the outcome. As a rough guide, 2 Gy can be thought of as killing approximately 50% of cells in the field, but over a large number of tumor cell lines the range may be 5 to 80%. Clearly, most radiation-induced DNA damage after 2 Gy is repaired, otherwise all cells would die. The lesion that is lethal is thought to be large, in the order of 15–20 nucleotides in size and the result of multiple events occurring in a cluster within the DNA, giving rise to an unrepairable DNA double strand break.

B. Sublethal Damage Repair/Potentially Lethal Damage Repair

At the cellular level, repair processes are operationally divided into potentially lethal damage repair and sublethal damage repair. Potentially lethal damage is repaired only under certain postirradiation conditions. In general, conditions that suppress cell division favor such repair. Sublethal damage is demonstrated using

divided (split) doses of radiation separated by time and represents reparable lesions that, as dose increases, accumulate and interact with each other to form a lethal lesion. It follows that a single dose of, say 9 Gy, radiation is more cytotoxic than two doses of 4.5 Gy, which is more cytotoxic than three doses of 3 Gy. A proviso is that the interfraction time interval is long enough to allow sublethal damage repair.

Clonogenic assays are commonly used to assess the survival of reproductively viable cells after irradiation. Irradiated and nonirradiated cells are plated at low density, and clones (of >50 cells) are allowed to grow from individual survivors over a period of a few weeks. The resultant survival curve is often relatively flat at low doses (the shoulder of the curve) and the slope increases at higher doses (Fig. 1). This represents a predominance of single lethal hits at a lower dose over accumulated damage from multiple hits, which becomes more important at a higher dose.

If a total dose is divided into smaller doses separated by, say, 6 h, the "shoulder" of the survival curve

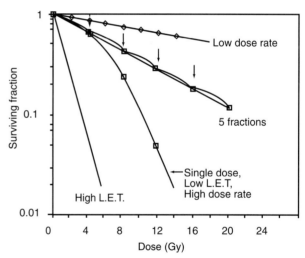

FIGURE 1 The biological effectiveness of ionizing radiation at cell killing varies with the density of the ionization track, dose rate, and fractionation scheme. This stylized figure indicates how high LET radiation is more cytotoxic than low LET radiation and gives a log-linear survival curve. Single doses of low LET radiation result in a survival curve with a "shoulder" region at low dose that increases in slope at higher dose as a result of accumulated sublethal damage. When a single dose of low LET radiation is divided into fractions, in this case of 4 Gy, the shoulder is repeated and the resulting curve is log linear. When delivered at a low-dose rate, low LET radiation is less cytotoxic because of ongoing repair of sublethal damage and also results in a directly log-linear dose–response curve.

is repeated (Fig. 1). Because the half-time for repair of sublethal damage is approximately 1 h, the time interval of 6 h allows most damage to be repaired. In clinical practice, fractionated doses are administered at intervals of at least 4 h and, more usually, of 24 h. This allows repair of sublethal lesions between fractions. The result is that a greater cumulative dose is required to achieve the same level of cell kill as after a single exposure.

Radiation delivered at a low-dose rate is similar to giving a course of very small fractions. The resultant survival curve is linear (Fig. 1). A dose rate of 0.6 Gy/h approximates to the shallowest curve that is generally achieved. Survival decreases up to about 60 Gy/h as interactive damage predominates. Above this dose rate there is little further decrease in cell survival. High LET radiation also gives a flat survival curve, but the slope is steep, consistent with its greater relative biologic effectiveness (Fig. 1).

If all tissues responded to the effects of dose fractionation in the same way, there would be no advantage to be gained from clinical use of low LET radiation. However, this is not the case. Rapidly proliferating tissues, such as bone marrow and gut and most tumors, that respond acutely to irradiation have little shoulder to their survival curve. Consequently, there is little effect of fractionation. In contrast, slowly proliferating tissues, such as in the central nervous system and kidney, that respond late have a broad shoulder and demonstrate a considerable effect of fractionation (Fig. 2). Multiple small-dose fractions of radiation therefore spare late responding tissues more than tumor, resulting in a therapeutic differential. This has important clinical implications, which are discussed later.

C. Molecular Mechanisms of Repair

Single strand breaks in DNA are repaired largely by a base excision repair mechanism. The steps involve removal of damaged bases by glycosylases, formation of an apurinic/apyrimidinic (AP) site by AP endonuclease, and filling in of this site by DNA polymerase β and ligase action. This is a highly efficient and rapid process, most likely because the other DNA strand is used as a template and because thousands of AP sites are produced per cell per day under normal physiologic conditions that have to be repaired by this mech-

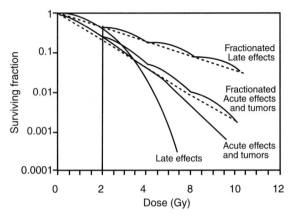

FIGURE 2 The biological effectiveness of ionizing radiation varies with the tissue. Survival curves of acute responding tissues are relatively flat compared to those of late responding tissues, which are "curvier." Fractionation of dose into sizes that are most often used clinically (around 2 Gy) exploits this difference, resulting in a sparing of late responding tissues that is greater than that for acute responding tissues and tumors.

anism. Their removal is important because their persistence can lead to a block in DNA replication, mutation, and increased DNA fragility.

DNA double strand break repair is a more complex process. A sister chromatid or chromosome may be used as a template in a process called homologous recombination (HR). However, mammalian cells repair most DSB lesions by a process of nonhomologous end joining (NHEJ). Physiologically, NHEJ is used both in VDJ recombination, which is required for the formation of immunoglobulin and T-cell receptors, and in meiosis. Insight into the mechanisms involved in NHEJ has come from study of the effects of mutations in molecules involved in DNA repair processes. DSBs in DNA are recognized by a heterodimer of Ku70 and Ku80 proteins. This complex then recruits and activates DNA protein kinase. Two other proteins, XRCC4 and ligase IV, are essential for repair to be completed. Mutations in any of the "sensors" of DNA damage can result in radiosensitivity and, not surprisingly, often in immune deficiency, as is seen in scid mice that have a mutation in DNA-Pk. It has been shown that a protein complex of Rad50, Mre11, and NBS1, which is mutated in Nijmegen breakage syndrome, accumulates at sites of damage and plays a role in HR and NHEJ, but the relationships between these and other multimolecular protein complexes have yet to be defined.

An important aspect of this model is that radiation-induced DNA damage activates molecules in signal transduction pathways that can link DNA repair to other intracellular processes, including cell cycle arrest and apoptotic cell death. DNA-Pk can phosphorylate a number of intracellular downstream molecules *in vitro*, but its *in vivo* substrates have yet to be definitively identified and, until they are, its ability to forge the link must remain somewhat speculative.

In contrast, ATM, the protein mutated in ataxia telangiectasia (A-T), which is the archetypal radiosensitivity syndrome in humans, is also activated following irradiation and appears to play a particularly important role in pathways that result in cell death and cell cycle arrest, especially those involving p53. Although ATM and a related protein ATR are structurally related to DNA-Pk, the relationship of ATM activation to DNA damage and repair and, therefore, the exact cause of radiosensitivity in A-T have still to be defined.

IV. CELL CYCLE EFFECTS OF RADIATION EXPOSURE

A. Cell Cycle and Radiosensitivity

The response to both single and fractionated doses of radiation depends in part on whether cells are traversing the cell cycle. It has been known since the 1950s that cells in different phases of the cell cycle differ in radiosensitivity (Fig. 3). Although considerable variation between cell lines has been reported, the rank order for radioresistance to radiosensitivity for the different cell cycle phases is generally accepted to be late S > early S > G_1 > G_2 > M. It is possible for there to be up to a threefold difference in radiosensitivity across the cell cycle for a given level of biologic effect. Because of this, irradiation causes cycling cells to undergo partial cell cycle synchronization. The proportion of S-phase cells increases after irradiation and they move through the cell cycle together. In a fractionated regimen, it would be of benefit to time the interfraction interval to take account of the movement of cells into the radiosensitive G_2/M phase. Unfortunately, synchronization is rapidly lost with time and variation in the rate of cell cycle progression is too great to make this easily achievable.

B. Cell Cycle Arrest

One of the established consequences of irradiation is cell cycle arrest at the G_1/S, S, and G_2M checkpoints. Cells do not necessarily die if arrested. They can recover to cycle normally. The dose dependency for arrest at the different cell cycle checkpoints varies. G_2 arrest is the most dose sensitive and consistent response. Cells that have mutated the tumor suppressor gene p53, which is approximately half of all human tumors, tend not to arrest at the G_1 checkpoint. This failure to arrest may result in lesions being replicated during the S phase with a resultant increase in DNA mutations and DNA fragility. The same argument can be made for a failure to undergo S-phase arrest, which is one of the features of A-T cells. For cells undergoing mitosis, the integrity of the chromosomes and the replication apparatus is critical. Repair during G_2 arrest may help restore some reproductive viability.

C. Molecular Aspects of Radiation-Induced Cell Cycle Arrest

Progression through cell cycle checkpoints requires the formation of complexes of specific cyclins with cyclin-dependent kinases (CDK). Pathways to radiation-induced cell cycle arrest converge at induction or phosphorylation of CDK inhibitors (CKIs) that block this interaction. CKIs come from three families: Cip (e.g.,

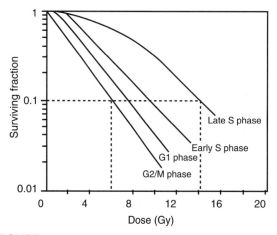

FIGURE 3 The biological effectiveness of ionizing radiation for cell killing varies with cell cycle phase. Cells in the late S phase are 2.5–3 times more radiation resistant than cells in the G_2/M phase. The order and degree of radiosensitivity of different cell cycle phases vary to a certain extent with the cell line, but the consensus is shown in this figure.

p27)/Kip (e.g., p21), Ink4 (e.g., p16), and the pRb pocket protein family. Cell cycle arrest at the G_1/S checkpoint is largely through induction of p21/WAF1, which inhibits CDK2 kinase action. A major pathway leading to p21 expression is through the ATM-dependent up-regulation of wild-type p53 expression and function. At the G_2M checkpoint, induction of the growth arrest DNA damage gene Gadd45, which is another p53-regulated stress protein, appears important.

V. CELL DEATH FOLLOWING IRRADIATION

A. Reproductive Death

The interaction of radiation with cells can influence their participation in normal tissue recovery and tumor cure in several ways. The most important of these is by causing reproductive cell death. Cells are reproductively dead if they leave the cell cycle, even if they retain their viability. Following irradiation they may go into senescence, prolonged G_1 arrest, giant cell formation, or terminal differentiation and remain viable. More often, they die by apoptosis or by mitotic catastrophe (as a result of spindle or chromosome damage) and are removed by phagocytosis.

B. Apoptosis

Apoptosis is a form of suicide that is mechanistically the same as the programmed cell death during development that is required for the formation of body structures. Apoptosis also plays a role in mature tissues removing excess cells produced during proliferation and some senescent cells. Apoptosis following irradiation can be rapid or delayed. Rapid apoptosis normally occurs between 6 and 24 h after irradiation without cell cycle progression and may happen during any cell cycle phase. Delayed apoptosis follows cell cycle progression and attempts at division.

Apoptosis requires activation of genetic programs, including endonucleases that cleave DNA into nucleosomal fragments of multiples of approximately 200 bp. These can be demonstrated by agarose electrophoresis as a "ladder," which is a hallmark of apoptotic death. During the process the nucleus condenses

and apoptotic bodies are formed. Proteolytic caspases are also involved in cellular execution and degradation. Not all cell types in the body express a functional apoptotic machinery. Lymphocytes, spermatogonia, salivary gland epithelial cells, thyroid cells, gut, and oligodendrocytes have a "proapoptotic" tendency that can be triggered by irradiation, but even within these tissues there is considerable variation, depending on the developmental stage and level of functional activation of the cell.

C. Mitotic Death

After irradiation, most cells die by mitotic catastrophe rather than by rapid or delayed apoptosis. This is a result of a failure to reestablish the integrity of the mitotic machinery and a functional complement of chromosomes. This requirement for cell division has important consequences, especially in tissues. One is that most nondividing cells, such as muscle cells and neurons, are relatively radioresistant. Gene expression may be altered following irradiation, but the cells continue to function metabolically as long as they do not attempt to divide.

Cells that do divide may manage one or more postradiation division before dying. The number depends on the dose. After 2 Gy, a cell may go through up to three divisions before dying. After 10 Gy, cells are unlikely to survive even one division cycle. Intermediate outcomes are possible. For example, after a cell divides, one of the progeny may die while the other remains reproductively viable. This is why radiobiologists often consider a reproductively viable clonogenic cell as one that generates at least 50 cells following irradiation, irrespective of the number of progeny that die along the way.

The fact that the mechanism of radiation-induced cell death varies between cell types may have important therapeutic implications, although these have yet to be fully evaluated. The acute parotitis that can develop in the first 24 h after irradiation reflects apoptotic death of serous cells. There is no such acute death in mucous cells, hence the mouth is dry and the saliva is more viscous. There is an apparent correlation between tumors of a histologic lineage whose cells tend to display more spontaneous and radiation-induced apoptosis *in vitro* and control by irradiation or chemotherapy in the clinic. The relationship between apoptosis and radiosensitivity is also suggested by findings that mutations that result in an antiapoptotic phenotype, such as in p53, and that are associated with carcinogenesis and tumor progression, tend to make cells more radioresistant. Gene therapy approaches aimed at negating these mutations generally radiosensitize tumor cells.

However, death by apoptosis in normal tissues can be a mechanism for elimination of surplus cells produced in proliferatively active zones. Tissue recovery may be unaffected by radiation-induced depletion of this reserve. Also, in a tumor, loss of a small percentage of cells by apoptosis would have little effect on cell survival over the many decades of log kill that are required for most cures. A possible explanation for the relationship between apoptosis and radiosensitivity is that there is a link between apoptotic and repair pathways, but this has yet to be proven. Encouraging cells to undergo rapid apoptosis following radiation therapy is, however, a reasonable therapeutic aim, even if the molecular mechanisms responsible for its efficacy have not yet been fully elucidated.

Many clinical and experimental observations on tissue responses can be explained by a requirement for cells to divide to express radiation cytotoxicity. Tissues with slow turnover, such as the central nervous system, lung, liver, bone, and kidney, generally show effects of cell depletion only some considerable time after exposure, often years. In contrast, tissues that require continuous cell proliferation from a stem cell source to maintain function, such as skin, mucosa, and bone marrow, can display damage early after irradiation. The time to expression of radiation-induced injury is therefore related to the turnover kinetics of the tissue. If slowly proliferating tissues are triggered to proliferate by surgical intervention or accidental trauma, cells will die when they attempt to divide. Thus, even though an irradiated tissue looks intact, its healing processes can be compromised.

These differences between tissues in their response to irradiation do not reflect differences in intrinsic cellular radiosensitivity. Rather they are due to differences in proliferative kinetics. The same is true for tumor regression. The rate of regression reflects the cell turnover time. Rapid regression indicates a tumor with a high turnover rate; the tumor can be slow or fast growing. It follows that rapid regression is not necessarily an indicator of a favorable outcome. Similarly, a slow rate of regression may be due to slow proliferation, a low rate of cell loss, a high stromal content, or treatment failure and has little predictive value.

VI. MOLECULAR PATHWAYS IN RADIOBIOLOGY

A. Intrinsic Radiosensitivity

As has already been stated, cells vary in their intrinsic response to irradiation. This is often reflected in the size of the shoulder of the survival curve. The simplest measure of intrinsic tumor radiosensitivity is the fraction of cells that survive exposure to 2 Gy ($S.F._{2Gy}$) in an *in vitro* clonogenic assay. For lymphoma cells or other sensitive cell types, this can be as low as 0.1–0.3. For radioresistant cells, such as melanoma, the $S.F._{2Gy}$ can be as high as 0.8, although the variation between cell lines of a given histology can be large. If differences in $S.F._{2Gy}$ values were to be maintained throughout a clinical fractionated regimen protocol, i.e., there is an equal cytotoxic effect for every 2 Gy, this variation is sufficient to determine tumor radiocurability. For example, around 34 Gy would kill 10^9 tumor cells (approximately a 1-cm tumor) if the $S.F._{2Gy}$ were 0.3, whereas closer to 80 Gy would be needed if the $S.F._{2Gy}$ were 0.6. Eighty gray is the limit of what can be tolerated by any normal tissue and exceeds the limit for many.

The molecular pathways that determine intrinsic radioresponsiveness have yet to be fully elucidated. It has been established that mutations in oncogenes and tumor suppressor genes affect responses, as does overexpression of growth factors and growth factor receptors, such as for epidermal growth factor (EGFR). A concept has developed that is that certain signal transduction pathways that enable cells to survive unfavorable conditions will tend to promote radioresistance. Unfortunately, the presence of any one marker of this type does not always correlate well with the radiocurability of human cancers, most likely because cancer formation requires multiple genetic changes.

However, it is likely that gene array experiments will, in time, indicate patterns of gene expression that are associated with a poor or good response to radiation therapy. In addition to constitutive pathways, intrinsic radiosensitivity of cells and tissues can be modified by radiation-induced signal transduction.

B. Radiation-Induced Molecular Responses

Radiation induces molecular responses through altering transcriptional and posttranscriptional control mechanisms. This is a coordinated response to damage that can affect both cell survival and subsequent responses to radiation and other stimuli. Within minutes of irradiation, cells can upregulate immediate early gene expression, including FOS, JUN, EGR1, and NF-κB. These couple signal transduction to transcriptional activation and phenotypic change. Molecules involved in cell cycle arrest, DNA repair, and apoptosis, such as p53 and p21, are expressed, as are molecules that are important in directing tissue reactions. For example, within hours, cytokines such as TNF-α, platelet-derived growth factor (PDGF), fibroblast growth factor (FGF), and transforming growth factor-β (TGF-β) are elaborated, along with proteinases, cell adhesion molecules, and extracellular matrix materials. This regulated acute tissue reaction triggers and is part of subsequent tissue remodeling.

Radiation-induced gene expression can mediate certain clinically relevant effects of radiation. For example, loss of endothelial cells is one cause of radiation-induced vascular leak, but radiation-induced cytokines, proteases, and cell adhesion molecules can promote a prothrombotic microenvironment that has similar effects. These proinflammatory pathways can also precipitate radiation-induced edema, nausea, and flu-like symptoms. In particular, large doses of whole body irradiation have obvious clinical consequences that are unlike those seen in localized radiation therapy.

C. Molecular Targets and Sensors of Radiation

While DNA is the main target for radiation-induced cytotoxicity and carcinogenesis, there are other targets for pathways that modulate repair, cell cycle pro-

gression, and survival. The extent and nature of these targets have not been fully elucidated. However, evidence shows that EGFR, at least on EGFR-overexpressing cells, can be phosphorylated within minutes of irradiation and this acts through MAP kinase as a survival response for cells that can result in radioresistancy. Other tyrosine kinase receptors may respond similarly. Also, free radicals generated by ionizing radiation appear to be amplified through radical production by mitochondria and within the plasma membrane to influence responses. These free radical pathways triggered by irradiation overlap with other oxidative stress signals so there is some degree of commonality of effects. Radiation is distinguished from these other signals largely by the nature of the damage it causes and its cytotoxic efficacy.

VII. MODELING RADIATION RESPONSES

A. Random Nature of Cell Killing

Our earliest understanding of radiation dose–response relationships came from studies on proteins, bacteria, and phage. For these, equal dose increments cause a constant proportional decrease in survival. When plotted semilogarithmically, the surviving fraction (log) is linearly related to dose, which reflects the random nature of the inactivation process. If a specified number of randomly distributed lethal hits is given to specified number of cells, the probability of a miss is given by $P = e^{-m}$, where m is the average number of hits per cell. If the average is one (one hit on average per cell), the proportion of cells that are missed will be 0.37 or 37%, with some cells being hit two or three times. If the average is 2, the proportion will be $0.37 \times 0.37 = 0.136$. The dose required to reduce the survival fraction to 37% (by one natural logarithm) on the exponential part of the curve is known as the Do (or the mean inactivation dose).

B. Eukaryotic Cell Survival Curves

In 1956, Puck and Marcus reported that survival curves for eukaryotic cells exposed to single doses of X rays, as measured by the ability to form a macroscopic colony, differ from those of bacteria by having a "shoulder" in the low-dose region with the exponential relationship only showing at higher doses (see Fig. 1). In general, the Do for eukaryotic cells does not vary greatly for different cell types, being within 1–2 Gy. It follows that D_{10}, the dose needed to kill one $\log_{10}$, is within 2.3–4.6 Gy (2.3 times Do).

Unlike responses to single doses of X rays, the slopes of survival curves after exposure to X rays delivered in multiple fractions or a low-dose rate, or to high LET radiation, are linear, having no shoulder (Fig. 1). The term "effective" Do ($_{eff}$Do) is sometimes used to define the slope of a multifraction survival curve. $_{eff}$Do values for mammalian cells treated with multiple fractions of radiation in a clinically relevant protocol are in the range 2.5–5 Gy (D_{10} = 5.8–11.5 Gy), considerably larger than Do values, indicative of the shallower slope resulting from the repair of sublethal damage between fractions.

C. Linear Quadratic Model

Because survival curves for eukaryotic cells exposed to single doses of low LET ionizing radiation are not linear, a linear quadratic formulation is often used to mathematically describe the way biological responses change with dose. Commonly, an effect is considered proportional to $\alpha d + \beta d^2$. The S.F. is then equal to $e^{-(\alpha d + \beta d2)}$. The biological interpretation of this mathematical model is that the α component represents a single lethal hit, which is a nonrepairable form of injury, and the β component represents interactions between sublethal repairable lesions that result in the formation of lethal lesions. The linear quadratic curve bends continuously as the dose increases. As a result, the model does not fit data well in the high-dose region and may not in the very low-dose region, but fits well in the region of most clinical interest, which is around 2 Gy.

Importantly, the relative value of α to β determines the shape of the survival curve. If the α component is small relative to β, the curve will bend after a relatively small initial linear region. The α/β ratio, which is the dose (in Gy) where the amount of cell kill from the linear and quadratic components are equal, will be small. This is a characteristic of late responding tissues, which have an α/β ratio of between 1 and 5

Gy. Because of the bendiness of the curve, the effect of dose fractionation will be large (Fig. 2). A high α/β ratio in excess of 6 Gy indicates a relatively long initial linear slope and is a characteristic of acute responding tissues and tumors, which display less of a fractionation effect.

D. Formula for Changing Dose Fractionation Regimens

One of the practical clinical uses of radiobiological models is to equate total doses when the size of dose per fraction in a multifraction regimen is changed. The linear quadratic formula has an advantage over other methods in being able to account for differences in response between late responding tissues and tumors by using estimates of their α/β ratios. Because late responding tissues result in the most serious radiation-induced complications, these tissues most often determine the tolerance dose of the tissue and it is important not to compromise them.

The formula for changing an old dose prescription to a new one is $D_{new} = D_{old} (\alpha/\beta + d_{old})/(\alpha/\beta + d_{new})$, where D_{new} and D_{old} are the new and old total doses, d is the dose per fraction, and α/β is characteristic of the tissue in question. Thus, 68.6 Gy given in 1.5-Gy fractions would be tolerated by late responding normal tissues equally well as 60 Gy in 2-Gy fractions, assuming an α/β ratio of 2 Gy. The lower the α/β ratio, the greater the dose correction. The effect on tumor cell kill of a change in fraction size from 2 to 1.5 Gy, assuming an α/β ratio in excess of 10 Gy, would be minimal. The higher total dose would, however, be more cytotoxic.

The linear quadratic formula has limitations. Small variations in estimates of the values for α/β for late responding tissues can be significant, and uncertainties exist that introduce risks into calculation of new total doses. The model does not fit data very well outside the range of fraction sizes from 2 to 8 Gy. It does not take into account differences in the rate or completeness of repair, proliferation between fractions, or resensitization of cells to the effects of irradiation due to redistribution or reoxygenation. Modifications of the formula can be used to evaluate the influence of these parameters, but estimates of their magnitude are not completely reliable. Despite these numerous caveats, the linear quadratic formula gives a very good guide as to what doses to use and is an improvement on formulae that were previously employed.

VIII. TUMOR CONTROL PROBABILITY

Tumor control requires elimination of the last surviving clonogenic tumor cell. The tumor control probability (TCP) is given by e^{-x}, where x is the number of surviving clonogens (or the number of initial number of clonogens times the S.F.). In other words, if sufficient radiation is given to tumors containing 10^8 clonogens to reduce their survival to 10^{-8}, then 37% of tumors would be cured. For clinically detectable tumors, the TCP curve is sigmoid (Fig. 4) with dose. The slope is steep, at least in theory, an increase from 10 to 90% TCP can be achieved with an increase in dose of 3 $_{eff}$Do's (perhaps 10 Gy). In practice, tumor survival curves derived from clinical data are relatively shallow. This is because of heterogeneity between tumors in volume, intrinsic radiosensitivity, tumor potential doubling times (Tpot), hypoxia, repair,

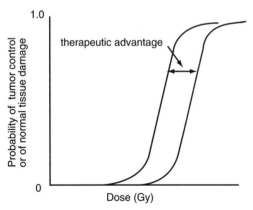

FIGURE 4 The probability of tumor control, at least in theory, increases steeply with dose in a sigmoid fashion above a threshold for clinically detectable cancers. The threshold is determined by the number of clonogenic tumor cells, as well as intrinsic tumor radioresistance, repair, reoxygenation, redistribution, and repopulation. The probability of normal tissue damage has a similar curve shape. A treatment goal is to make sure that the tumor control probability curve is to the left of that for normal tissue damage and to maximize the distance between the two curves (therapeutic advantage). Fractionation is one means of achieving this. The dose that is given depends on the nature of the normal tissue that is in the field and is based on what experience has shown can be tolerated by this tissue.

redistribution, geographical miss, regrowth from underdosed sites (dose inhomogeneity), and other factors.

IX. NORMAL TISSUE TOLERANCE

A. Probability of Complications

The dose that is given in radiation therapy depends on the probability of a normal tissue complication and the seriousness of that complication. The curve for the probability of a normal tissue complication is similar in shape to that for tumor control (Fig. 4). If the threatened complication is myelopathy, the dose that will be administered will be such as to keep the probability of a complication extremely low. If the possible complication is a small area of fibrosis, this can be better tolerated and the tolerance limits can be more closely approached. The art of radiation therapy is to separate the normal tissue and tumor control probability curves so as to maximize the therapeutic advantage. The use of low LET radiation delivered in dose fractions or at a low dose rate is a biological strategy by which to achieve this aim for late responding tissues. In contrast, acute responding normal tissues are spared by proliferation between fractions. Often these tissues are capable of more rapid repopulation than epithelial tumors, resulting in a therapeutic differential that can be exploited. The dose per fraction and time schedule that is used clinically must take all these factors into account (see later).

B. Volume Effects

The volume irradiated is often important in determining the dose that a tissue can tolerate. In reality, there are many different types of volume effects. There is no evidence that increasing the volume that is irradiated influences the intrinsic radiation response of cells within a field. However, a patient may be less able to tolerate a large than a small area of injury. Also, if the tissue is organized as a series of functional subunits, as in a nerve tract, loss of only one link may result in functional damage. In contrast, if the tissue has a large functional reserve, as in the case of the lung, most of the organ can receive a high dose, as long as a portion is left untreated. Irradiation of large volumes also increases the likelihood of an increase in heterogeneity of dose, with resultant "hot spots" of damage.

The opposite of large volume effects is that a small volume may tolerate high doses. This is particularly true if progenitor/stem cells in the tissues have a high migratory capacity, such as in the skin, mucosa, and intestinal tract. Five to 10 surviving stem cells/cm^2 are all that is required to prevent moist desquamation in the skin. However, even if depletion is greater than this, an area of 1–2 cm might still heal by repopulation from surrounding unirradiated tissue and scar contraction. Once a critical migration distance is passed, necrosis may develop and, above a certain dose level, structural damage to connective tissue and the vasculature could prevent regeneration from migrating stem cells. Estimates of this critical distance are uncertain.

C. Remembered Dose

Conventional teaching in radiation oncology has been that a previously irradiated late responding tissue will not tolerate retreatment. In recent years, experimental studies have indicated that, although prior irradiation may limit the tolerance of a tissue, retreatment may be possible. Limitations include the amount of cell depletion caused by prior treatment, the time elapsed since that treatment (and therefore the extent of regeneration), and the tissue at risk. The closer the initial dose is to the tolerance dose and the shorter the time interval between treatments, the less chance there is of recovery. It should be noted that the experimental studies that have been performed are limited in the end points that have been used and progressive very late effects that are seen clinically might not show the same degree of recovery as earlier end points.

X. CLINICAL RADIATION THERAPY

A. Exploiting Physics to Therapeutic Advantage

1. External Beam Irradiation

Until the early 1950s, patients receiving external beam therapy were treated using X-ray machines capable of producing photon beams of limited penetrability. The introduction of orthovoltage X-ray and ^{60}cobalt teletherapy machines that could treat deeper-seated lesions was a major advance. The development of megavoltage electron linear accelerators (linac), which is currently the machine of choice for external beam therapy in most developed countries and which can produce both electrons and photons, was a further advance.

A major advantage of radiation over most other forms of therapy is that the physical dose distribution can be accurately calculated for any type of delivery method. By altering the method of delivery, damage to normal tissue can be minimized and dose to the tumor maximized. This is the purpose of the treatment planning that precedes therapeutic delivery. Advances in imaging and in computer-assisted radiation delivery using multileaf collimators have refined both treatment planning and the physical delivery of radiation. These allow the beam to be shaped to deliver specified doses to defined targets with great precision while minimizing damage to adjacent normal tissues. In this way, a greater therapeutic ratio can be achieved.

Despite these advances in the physical delivery or radiation, the inclusion of normal tissue in the irradiated volume in most cases is unavoidable. In fact, it may even be desirable so as to eliminate tumor deposits extending outside the primary site that are too small to be seen by current imaging modalities. This is why it is currently common practice in radiation therapy to treat a larger volume initially and to deliver a concomitant or sequential boost to the tumor site late in the treatment course. Smaller deposits can be killed by lower doses than are needed for the main tumor.

Other more novel radiation delivery techniques include the use of protons or neutrons. They are available in some radiotherapy centers but the machines are more expensive than standard linacs and are not always considered cost effective or necessarily beneficial except for specific tumor sites and under particular circumstances.

2. Brachytherapy

Radiation can be administered by brachytherapy as well as by external beam teletherapy. This involves placing radioactive sources on or close to the target tissue. The term derives from the Greek word for short distance. Sources may be directly applied to the surface, as in eye plaques for melanoma, or implanted into interstitial or intracavitary sites, as in the treatment of some gynecologic, prostate, and oral tumors. Implants can be permanent or temporary. Intracavitary implants are temporary and are left in place for 1–7 days.

^{226}Radium, which used to be the first choice as isotope, has now largely been replaced by ^{137}cesium, ^{125}iodide, ^{192}iridium, or ^{103}palladium. Different isotopes have different properties and deliver radiation at different rates with different dose distributions. In general, the dose falls off approximately with the square of the distance away from the source, although there are deviations from this rule. This means that the dose is very high close to the source. Low-dose rate implants deliver dose at a rate of 40–200 cGy/hr. Ultralow-dose rates of 0.01–0.3 Gy/h delivered by ^{125}I and ^{103}Pd permanent implants are commonly used to treat prostrate cancer. High-dose rate implants deliver radiation at a rate in excess of 12 Gy/h. High-dose rate delivery is unable to exploit the biological differences between normal tissue and tumor in the same way as the low-dose rate, but in some sites this disadvantage is counterbalanced by the physical advantages of better dose distribution and less safety concerns. These dose rates for brachytherapy contrast with external beam radiotherapy that is normally given at 60–200 Gy/h (2 Gy in about 0.6–2.0 min).

B. Exploiting Biology to Therapeutic Advantage

We have indicated that tumors and normal tissues differ within themselves and from each other with respect to kinetics of cellular proliferation, hypoxic cell content, and their ability to repair and recover from DNA damage and that these differences can be exploited by delivering external beam radiation in small-dose fractions of around 2 Gy given each day, 5 days a week for many weeks, or by using low-dose rate brachytherapy. The fractionation schedule used in radiation therapy is empirically derived and evolved, taking into account financial and logistic pressures, as well as clinical outcome. "Conventional" regimens are not precisely defined or necessarily optimized, but

the general principle that fractionated delivery over a longer time period gives a superior outcome to single high doses has been proven on many occasions over the century. Elucidating the relationship between time and dose in radiotherapy has been a focus of research since its foundation. The principles of radiobiology that determine why fractionated is superior to single-dose treatment reveal fundamental aspects of cell biology, tissue organization, and physiology that are relevant to many different forms of therapy. It is worth restating these radiobiological principles in the context of their relevance to clinical radiation therapy.

1. The 4 R's of Radiobiology Relevant to Clinical Radiotherapy

In 1975, Withers detailed the 4 R's of radiobiology that determine the benefits of dose fractionation during a course of radiation therapy. These encapsulate the radiobiological phenomena described earlier and can be summarized as follows.

a. Repair of Sublethal Damage   Late responding normal tissues are spared at the expense of tumors and acute tissues. Normal tissue complications that appear late (after the course of radiation therapy has been given) are often more difficult to treat than acute complications. In some cases, such as the central nervous system, they may be debilitating or even lethal. The dose that is given in radiation therapy is therefore most often determined by what the late responding tissues in the field should be able to tolerate based on experience.

b. Reassortment/Redistribution of Cells in the Cell Cycle   This will have no effect on late responding tissues, but will help resensitize tumors in radioresistant phases of the cell cycle. Rapidly proliferating normal tissues will also be affected.

c. Reoxygenation   This will not affect normal tissue responses, but reoxygenation between dose fractions will help resensitize hypoxic radioresistant tumor cells.

d. Repopulation   Repopulation in rapidly proliferating normal tissues during fractionated radiation therapy is important for their tolerance. Shortening the overall treatment time, such as by treating for 7 rather than 5 days a week, compromises repopulation in these tissues. In such regimens, the lack of tolerance of acute responding tissues can be the major factor determining the size of the total dose that is given. Before repopulation/regeneration begins, there is a lag period that varies with the tissue. In the mucosa, repopulation starts after 10–12 days and can increase tolerance by at least 1 Gy/day.

Repopulation can, of course, also occur in tumors during a course of radiation therapy. The clinical implication of such repopulation is that any interruption that prolongs the treatment time is likely to decrease the probability of tumor cure. The lag phase before accelerated tumor cell repopulation is initiated in head and neck cancer has been calculated as being around 4 weeks. Thereafter, 0.6 Gy of a 2-Gy fraction of radiation therapy may be lost in combating tumor cell proliferation. In some studies the estimate is as high as 1 Gy. It should be noted that repopulation may be occurring even as the tumor is regressing and that neoadjuvant chemotherapy or surgery may also lead to an accelerated proliferation of surviving tumor cells.

If there were no other considerations, the ideal course of radiation therapy would be completed before tumor repopulation was triggered, perhaps within 4 weeks. However, this would compromise acute responding tissues. Because these can often proliferate faster than tumor tissue, extending the time beyond 4 weeks is still generally advantageous. The dose–time relationship that is chosen is therefore a compromise that seeks to balance cytotoxic effects on tumor and damage to late responding tissues (dose per fraction and total dose) and the possibility of accelerated repopulation of tumor and acute responding normal tissue (time). The rule of thumb is that the dose that is delivered should be the highest that the slowly proliferating/responding tissues can tolerate, that the fraction size should maximize the difference in the level of damage incurred by late responding tissues and tumors, and that the overall time should be the shortest consistent with an acceptable acute response.

2. Altered Fractionation Schedules

Elucidation of these biological principles of radiation therapy has led to consideration of novel and rational ways to deliver radiation so as to optimize the therapeutic ratio. Hyperfractionation or accelerated fractionation schedules have been devised, although a hybrid of the two is more often employed.

Hyperfractionation is defined as the use of smaller than standard radiation doses per fraction without a change in the overall treatment duration. This usually means giving two fractions per day, 5 days a week. Its major aim is to further increase the therapeutic differential between late responding normal tissues and tumors by using smaller sized fractions. The interfraction time interval should be at least 6 h to allow complete repair. In the central nervous system, even this may be too short and additional care has to be exercised. Additional, less well-defined benefits that may result from increasing the number of treatments are that the self-sensitizing effect of cell cycle redistribution and reoxygenation in tumors may be enhanced and that hypoxia is less of a factor at the lower sized fractions that are employed.

Accelerated fractionation is defined as shortening the overall treatment duration without a comparable reduction in total dose. The aim is to minimize the effect of tumor repopulation. The danger is that acutely responding normal tissues are also affected and become dose limiting and consequently the total dose that is administered is often reduced. In practice, accelerated treatment schedules often use conventional or reduced doses per fraction more frequently than normal, resulting in a combined accelerated/hyperfractionated regimen.

XI. CONCLUSIONS

Over the last century, treatment schedules in radiation therapy have evolved empirically to optimize its benefit in different clinical situations. Hand in hand with these developments have come improvements in the physical delivery of the radiation to all sites of the body. The equipment used to deliver this modality has dramatically improved with the advent of computer-controlled machines capable of delivering complex treatment plans in three-dimensions to tumors. This extends our capability to accurately prescribe and deliver dose to the tumor while minimizing the exposure of sensitive normal tissues. At the same time, the basic biological principles responsible for the efficacy of empirically based administration schedules have been elucidated. Experimental observations have opened the door to many clinical investigations in areas such as hypoxic cell sensitizers, radiosensitizers, radioprotectors, and altered fractionation protocols.

In the near future, our understanding of how radiation works at the molecular level will further evolve and generate even more promising clinical approaches. The use of modern biological methodologies to define the molecular mechanisms responsible for radiation sensitivity and resistance is already leading to the development of novel strategies to target pathways of radioresistance. The next major advance in radiation therapy, and cancer therapy in general, is to individualize treatment based on this knowledge for each individual patient. The combination of these new biologic approaches with powerful computer-aided physical delivery systems will increase the therapeutic index of radiotherapy beyond what is presently conceived and will guarantee a promising and exciting future for this treatment modality.

See Also the Following Articles

DNA DAMAGE, DNA REPAIR, AND MUTAGENESIS • DOSIMETRY AND TREATMENT PLANNING FOR THREE-DIMENSIONAL RADIATION THERAPY • LATE EFFECTS OF RADIATION THERAPY • MOLECULAR ASPECTS OF RADIATION BIOLOGY • PROTON BEAM RADIATION THERAPY • RADIATION RESISTANCE • RADIOLABELED ANTIBODIES, OVERVIEW • STEREOTACTIC RADIOSURGERY OF INTRACRANIAL NEOPLASMS

Bibliography

Anno, G. H., Baum, S. J., Withers, H. R., *et al.* (1989). Symptomatology of acute radiation effects in humans after exposure to doses of 0.5-30 Gy. *Health Phys.* **56,** 821.

Bergonie, J., and Tribondeau, L. (1906). Interpretation de quelques resultats de la radiotherapie. *C. R. Acad. Sci.* **143,** 983.

Hall, E. J. (2000). "Radiobiology for the Radiologist." Lippincott, Philadelphia.

Maciejewski, B., Withers, H., Taylor, J., *et al.* (1989). Dose fractionation and regeneration in radiotherapy for cancer of the oral cavity and oropharynx: Tumor dose response and repopulation. *Int. J. Radiat. Oncol. Biol. Phys.* **16,** 831.

McBride, W. H., Daigle, J. L., Tsang, L., Cheng, I., Syljuasen, R., and Raines, M. (1998). Radiation-induced gene expression. *In* "Volume and Kinetics in Tumor Control and Normal Tissue Complications" (B. R. Paliwal, J. F. Fower, D. E. Herbert, and M. P. M. Mehta, eds.), p. 313. Medical Physics Publishing, Madison, WI.

Mould, R. F. (1993). "A Century of X-rays and Radioactivity in Medicine." Institute of Physics Publishing, Bristol.

Puck, T. T., and Marcus, P. I. (1956). Action of x-rays on mammalian cells. *J. Exp. Med.* **103,** 653.

Shackelford, R. E., Kaufmann, W. K., *et al.* (1999). Cell cycle control, checkpoint mechanisms, and genotoxic stress. *Environ. Health Perspect.* **107,** 5.

Withers, H. R. (1975). The 4 R's of radiotherapy. *In* "Advances in Radiation Biology" (J. T. Lett, H. Alder, eds.), Vol. 5, p. 241, Academic Press, New York..

Withers, H. R., and McBride, W. H. (1998). Biologic basis of radiation therapy. *In* "Principles and Practice of Radiation Oncology" (C. A. Perez, and L. W. Brady, eds.), p. 79. Lippincott-Raven, Philadelphia.

Radiolabeled Antibodies, Overview

George Sgouros

Memorial Sloan-Kettering Cancer Center

I. Antibodies
II. Radionuclides
III. Patient Studies and Results
IV. Summary

GLOSSARY

antibodies Multivalent proteins that make up a part of the body's immune system. They are primarily responsible for recognizing foreign molecules and "marking" them for immune attack.

antigen A substance that the body recognizes as "nonself" or "foreign" and against which an immune response is mounted. Antibodies have a complementary chemical structure to a portion of the antigen and bind to the antigen.

chimeric antibody An antibody whose Fc region is human derived and whose Fab regions are murine derived.

half-life The time required for 50% of the atoms of a particular radionuclide to undergo radioactive decay. Each radionuclide has a characteristic half-life, i.e., carbon-14 has a half-life of 5730 years.

human antichimera activity A human immune reaction against a chimeric antibody.

human antihuman activity An immune reaction against a humanized antibody.

human antimouse activity A human immune reaction against a murine-derived protein.

humanized antibody An antibody produced by "grafting" the variable regions (complementarity determining regions) responsible for antigen binding onto a human framework. The resulting protein is predominantly human except for the seven to eight amino acids responsible for antigen binding.

hybridoma technique Kohler and Milstein invented a method for producing antibodies of predetermined specificity against virtually any biologic molecule by creating hybridoma cells capable of growing in a test tube and producing monoclonal antibodies. The hybridoma is a clone of cells derived from the fusion of an immune-competent lymphocyte and a myeloma cell that could proliferate indefinitely in a test tube.

kilo electron volts (keV) A unit of energy used to characterize the energy of radionuclide emissions.

million electron volts (MeV) A unit of energy used to characterize the energy of radionuclide emissions (1 MeV = 1000 keV).

radioactivity The property of certain elements to spontaneously emit energy (photons) and particles associated with the transition to a more stable nuclear state. The term is quantified as the number of such spontaneous transitions occurring per unit time. The CGI and SI units associated with this quantity are curies (Ci) and becquerels (Bq), respectively.

radioimmunoconjugate An antibody that has been labeled (conjugated) with a radionuclide.

radioimmunodiagnosis The use of radiolabeled antibodies to image and thereby detect the antigens that are markers of cancer.

radioimmunotherapy The use of radiolabeled antibodies to deliver cytotoxic radiation to tumor cells or other cells associated with pathologic states.

radionuclide An element that is radioactive.

Radiolabeled antibodies have been used both in the diagnosis (radioimmunodiagnosis) and in the therapy (radioimmunotherapy) of cancer. The approach is founded on the ability to generate antibodies against tumor-associated antigens. Such "tumor-targeting" antibodies are then used to deliver radionuclides specifically to antigen-positive cells. The choice of radionuclide will depend on whether the radiolabeled antibody will be used for diagnosis or therapy. In general, the application of radiolabeled antibodies is a multidisciplinary effort in which expertise in tumor immunology and antibody development must be combined with radiochemistry, nuclear medicine, and physics. This article provides an overview of the development and use of radiolabeled antibodies.

I. ANTIBODIES

A. Overview

Antibodies are multivalent proteins that make up a part of the body's immune system. They are primarily responsible for recognizing foreign molecules and "marking" them for immune attack. Depending on their valency and chemical structure, antibodies have been categorized into a number of classes and types (Table I). The IgG class is most commonly used in clinical applications of radiolabeled antibodies (Fig. 1). The Nobel prize-winning work of Kohler and Milstein in devising the hybridoma technique for obtaining antibodies from a single clone (monoclonal) is perhaps the most important advance toward the de-

TABLE I

Candidate α Particle Emitters for Radioimmunotherapy

Radionuclide Daughters	Half-life	%[a]	Particle	Energy[b]
Bi-213	45.6 min	2	α	6 MeV
		98	β⁻	444 keV
		17	γ	440 keV
Po-213	4.2 μs	98	α	8 MeV
Tl-209	2.2 min	2	β⁻	659 keV
Pb-209	3.25 h	100	β⁻	198 keV
Bi-209	Stable			
Bi-212	1.0 h	36	α	6 MeV
		64	β⁻	492 keV
Po-212	298 ns	64	α	9 MeV
Tl-208	3.05 min	36	β⁻	560 keV
		8	γ	510 keV
		31	γ	580 keV
		36	γ	2.6 MeV
Pb-208	Stable			
At-211	7.21 h	42	α	6 MeV
		19	γ	80 keV
Po-211	516 ms	58	α	7.5 MeV
Bi-207	32 years	24	γ	70 keV
		41	γ	570 keV
		31	γ	1 MeV
Pb-207	Stable			
Ac-225	10 days	100	α	6 MeV
Fr-221	4.9 min	100	α	6 MeV
		10	γ	218 keV
At-217	32.3 ms	100	α	7 MeV
Bi-213	See Bi-123			
Ra-223	11.4 days	100	α	6 MeV
		40	γ	80 keV
		14	γ	270 keV
Rn-219	4 s	100	α	7 MeV
		10	γ	270 keV
Po-215	1.8 ms	100	α	7 MeV
Pb-211	36.1 min	100	β⁻	447 keV
Bi-211	2.1 min	16	α	6 MeV
		84	α	7 MeV
		13	γ	350 keV
Tl-207	4.8 min	100	β⁻	493 keV
Pb-207	Stable			

[a]Percentage emitted per decay of parent radionuclide.
[b]Mean β⁻ energy and approximate α and γ energies are listed.

velopment of radiolabeled antibodies for radioimmunodiagnosis and therapy. The hybridoma technique, in which B cells from a single antibody-producing clone are immortalized by fusion with tumor cells, made it possible to produce large quantities of antibody in which all molecules share the same pharmacologic and tumor-targeting properties. This is in contrast to earlier techniques in which antibodies

Table 28-2. Antibody Fragment Definitions

DESIGNATION	REPRESENTATION	DESCRIPTION
Fabc		Complete IgG
Enzyme-generated products		
Fab	Fd / L	Papain digest; Fd + L
Fab'	Fd' / L	Pepsin digest monomer; Fd' + L
Fab'2	Fab'	Pepsin digest dimer
Fv	V_H / V_L	V region digestion fragment; VH + VL
Fc (or Fc')	CH_2 / CH_3	C region digestion fragment; crystallizable fragment
pFc (or pFc')	CH_2 / CH_3	Smaller fragments of Fc
Genetically engineered products		
delta CH_2	CH_3	Deleted CH_2 domain; dimer of $V - CH_1 - CH_3 + L$
sFv	V_H / V_L	Single-chain Fv; VH and VL joined by peptide linker
Synthetic products		
ABU		Antigen-binding unit; peptide mimic

FIGURE 1　Structure of IgG. From Junghans *et al.* (1996).

were obtained by successive purification from the serum of animals that had been immunized against the antigen of interest (polycolonal antibodies). Other advances, important to the development and application of radiolabeled antibodies, are summarized in Table II.

As shown in Table II, the primary objectives in antibody-targeting developments have been to (1) reduce immunogenicity, (2) reduce molecular weight, (3) increase valency, and (4) alter biodistribution and pharmacokinetics. Each of these objectives is considered individually.

1. Immunogenicity

Antibodies derived using hybridomas are murine in origin and, therefore, elicit an immune reaction when administered to humans. One to 3 weeks after administration of an intact, murine-derived antibody, immunocompetent patients typically develop a human immune reaction against the antibody; this is referred to as a human antimouse antibody (HAMA) reaction. Administration of antibody to HAMA-positive patients leads to near-instantaneous formation of higher molecular weight immune complexes, which are rapidly cleared from the circulation by the spleen and other organs of the reticuloendothelial system (RES). Targeting is consequently abrogated, with radiolabeled antibody circulation half-lives generally reduced to a few minutes compared with the 30- to 40-h half-life typical of most antibodies.

One of the earliest approaches for reducing immunogenicity involved enzymatic cleavage of intact

TABLE II

Advances Relevant to Radiolabeled Antibodies Use

Advance/development	Year
Enzymatic digestion of intact IgG antibodies to yield fragments	1959
Hybridoma technique—method for producing antibodies derived from a single clone	1975
Chimeric mouse (Fab)/human (Fc) antibodies	1984
Multistep targeting using bifunctional hapten	1984
Multistep targeting using avidin–biotin	1987
Humanized antibodies	1988
Production of recombinant constructs: single chain antibody fragments (sFv)	1988
Production of multivalent recombinant constructs; diabody	1993
Fully human antibodies derived from transgenic mouse technology (XenoMouse)	1999

antibodies to smaller and putatively, less-immunogenic fragments (Fig. 2). The resulting lower molecular weight F(ab) and F(ab')$_2$ fragments lacked the F$_c$ region, which is involved in the immune recognition functions of the antibody. More sophisticated approaches to reducing immunogenicity without compromising function have been implemented using genetic engineering techniques. One such approach involves "grafting" the gene sequence for the complementarity-determining regions (CDRs) of a murine-derived antibody onto a gene sequence coding for the human IgG framework. The resulting "humanized" antibody is mostly human and, therefore, nonimmunogenic, except for the 10–15 amino acid sequences present in the CDRs, which are murine derived and are involved in antigen binding (Fig. 3). More recently, transgenic mice have been developed that promise to provide fully human high-affinity antibodies against any human protein. In these mice, the complement of genes associated with human an-

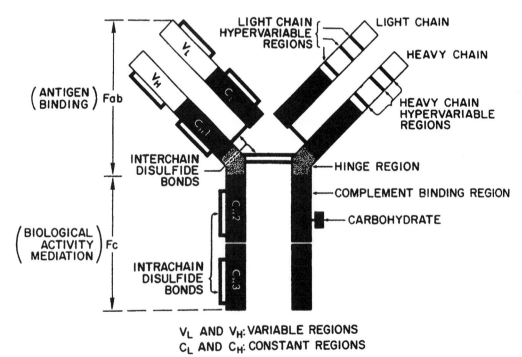

FIGURE 2 Antibody fragment definitions. From Junghans *et al.* (1996).

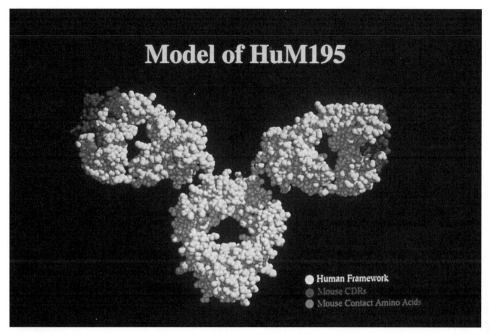

FIGURE 3 Structure of the humanized antibody, HuM195. Courtesy of David Scheinberg, Memorial Sloan-Kettering Cancer Center, New York.

tibody production has been inserted into the mouse genome, while those associated with murine antibody production are suppressed.

2. Molecular Weight

Antibody targeting has been described using terms such as "guided missile," "magic bullet," and "smart bomb." Such terms suggest that upon administration, antibodies localize directly to the tumor. The actual physical process by which antibodies "target" requires (1) that an intravenously administered antibody distributes throughout the extravascular space. Assuming that tumor cells are located within this volume, the antibody must then (2) encounter a tumor cell and bind to the antigen. Finally, (3) the antibody must remain bound to the tumor cell antigen while (4) the unattached antibody clears from the extravascular space and eventually from the circulation.

Table III lists the molecular mass of intact antibodies and antibody fragments. More recently developed multivalent constructs generally have a molecular mass that is a multiple of the sFv fragment. The time required for the completion of steps 1 through 4 is of the order of 24 to 48 h for intact, 150,000 molecular weight antibodies. Diagnostic imaging using intact radiolabeled antibodies is usually performed after such a time period. Prior to this, tumor localization is generally obscured by radioactivity in the circulation. In radiolabeled antibody therapy, the long circulation times required for targeting of intact antibodies increase the absorbed dose to the red marrow, the dose-limiting organ in radioimmunotherapy. Although tumor vascular endothelium is characterized by a greater permeability, tumor vessels introduce a barrier to transcapillary flow of higher molecular weight proteins. Animal studies have shown that lower molecular weight constructs localize to the tumor more rapidly and are also cleared more rapidly from the circulation, primarily by renal excretion. The increase in the kinetics of tumor localization and

TABLE III
Molecular Mass of Ab Constructs

Construct or fragment	Molecular mass (kDa)
Intact IgG (Fabc)	150
sFv	25
Fab'	50
F(ab')$_2$	100

clearance has yielded tumor-to-blood and tumor-to-red marrow activity concentration ratios that are substantially (2- to 10-fold) greater than those obtained for intact antibodies. In most cases, however, the absolute amount of activity localized to the tumor is very low. If cancer therapy is the objective, the low absolute uptake requires administered radioactivity levels that are substantially higher than those typically used in most clinical settings. If, however, the objective is diagnosis, then the higher ratios serve to increase the diagnostic value of lower molecular agents.

3. Valency

As shown in Fig. 2, intact antibodies are bivalent and can, therefore, bind to two antigen sites simultaneously. Valency is a critical determinant of antibody retention at the tumor site. A number of multivalent immune constructs engineered to a low molecular weight have been generated. These constructs exhibit greater tumor penetration and more rapid targeting while retaining tumor retention. Such constructs are still in the development stage and preclinical testing is still ongoing.

4. Pharmacologic/physiologic Interventions

The approaches just described have centered on modifications made to the antibody. Approaches that involve pharmacologic or physiologic interventions include (a) extracorporal immunoadsorption (ECIA), (b) multistep targeting, (c) pre- or coinjection of unlabeled antibody, and (d) external beam irradiation.

The objective of ECIA or plasmapheresis, a related approach, is to remove unbound, radiolabeled antibody from the circulation and thereby reduce the absorbed dose to normal organs; in most cases, the bone marrow. In ECIA, this is accomplished by establishing a connection between the patient's circulatory system and an external blood circuit; following separation from whole blood, the plasma is carried through an affinity column that removes antibody from the circulation. The connection with the column is typically established 10 to 20 h after injection of the radiolabeled antibody. Based on experience gained in the treatment of autoimmune diseases, such an approach can reduce the concentration of circulating

antibody by three- to fivefold. In plasmapheresis, on-line, continuous separation of plasma from whole blood is implemented. The red blood cells are reintroduced to the patient, whereas the antibody-containing plasma is not. In part, because it is highly invasive and may involve radiation safety concerns associated with the radioactivity that will be contained in the external circuit, column, or discarded plasma, this approach has not gained wide clinical acceptance.

Multistep targeting techniques are essentially noninvasive analogs of ECIA and plasmapheresis. The general features of multistep targeting are as follows. In the first step, an agent that localizes to the tumor but that is not radiolabeled is administered. Depending on the number of steps in the approach, the tumor-targeting agent may be followed by a clearing agent to remove excess material from the circulation. A smaller radiolabeled ligand is then administered that binds the initial, tumor-targeting agent. Again, depending on the details of the implementation, the radiolabeled ligand may be followed by a clearing agent to remove circulating radioactivity. The general strategy is founded upon the idea that the smaller, radiolabeled ligand will target and clear from the circulation much faster than if the tumor-targeting agent were radiolabeled. By dissociating the time required for tumor targeting from radionuclide exposure time, it becomes possible to deliver a greater amount of radiation dose to the target while substantially diminishing the absorbed dose delivered to the red marrow. The most widely investigated implementation of multistep targeting has used avidin or streptavidin in combination with biotin. Avidin (found in egg white) and streptavidin (produced by *Streptomyces avidini*) are 66- and 60-kDa proteins, respectively, that have an affinity constant for biotin of 10^{15} M^{-1} ($k_D = 10^{-15}$ M). Both molecules have four biotin-binding sites. They differ in that the former is a glycoprotein, bearing a single-branched oligosaccharide unit per subunit, whereas the latter is not a glycoprotein. Biotin (vitamin H) is a 244-Da compound with a valeric side chain. This system has been chosen because of the very tight binding between avidin/streptavidin and biotin. Because avidin is the larger molecule, this is usually conjugated to the tumor-associated antibody, and the nonradioactive avidin (or streptavidin)–antibody conjugate is injected as the first step in the approach. After enough time has elapsed so that the antibody has localized to the tumor, radiolabeled biotin is injected, which because of its low molecular weight, rapidly distributes in a volume that includes the avidin (or streptavidin)-tagged tumor. After the radiolabeled biotin has localized to the tumor, streptavidin (or avidin) may be administered as a third step to remove excess biotin from the circulation. The avidin–biotin approach has made it possible to administer levels of radioactivity that far exceed the maximum tolerated dose defined by direct radiolabeled antibody injection. The complications and drawbacks of this approach include the very high immunogenicity of avidin and biotin and the high kidney uptake of the radiolabeled biotin. Clinical trials of this approach are briefly described later. Another multistep targeting approach that has yielded promising results in animal studies and clinical trials uses a bifunctional antibody in which one arm binds to tumor antigen and the other to a radiolabeled ligand. In some implementations, the radiolabeled ligand is designed to be multivalent and therefore capable of attaching to the ligand-binding arms of two different bifunctional antibodies.

II. RADIONUCLIDES

A. Overview

Once an appropriate antibody is identified for tumor targeting, selection of the radionuclide conjugate will depend on the anticipated use of the radioimmunoconjugate. Because the largest body of clinical and preclinical experience with radiolabeled antibodies has been obtained using intact IgGs, the discussion relative to radionuclides will focuses on intact antibodies rather than the lower molecular weight constructs described in the previous section.

Radionuclides chosen for diagnostic use generally require half-lives in the range of 2 to 8 days. Ideally, they should decay by emission of low to intermediate energy photons (80 to 250 keV), such photon energies are optimal for nuclear medicine imaging by a gamma camera. There should be little or no energetic particulate emissions (e.g., β particles), as these would increase the radiation dose associated with the diagnostic procedure. A half-life of several days is desired to match the kinetics of antibody targeting and to be compatible with logistical considerations inherent in patient imaging (i.e., the radionuclide should not be eliminated by physical decay prior to imaging). Positron emitters have been used for antibody imaging using positron emission tomography (PET) cameras. Positron-emitting radionuclides developed for PET imaging are generally analogs of therapeutic radionuclides (e.g., I-124 for I-131; Y-86 for Y-90).

The radionuclide properties required for radioimmunotherapy should generally be matched with the disease architecture and stage of disease being targeted. For example, β particle emitters such as ^{131}I and ^{90}Y are preferred for bulky tumor targeting. The rationale for this is that the range of β particles (0.8 to 2 mm) in tissue is sufficient to irradiate tumor cells that are not specifically targeted by the antibody, thereby overcoming the nonuniform distribution of antibody seen in solid tumors thought to arise due to poor antibody penetration. If the antibody distribution is uniform and the antibody–antigen complex is internalized, then shorter ranged conversion or Auger electron-emitting radionuclides would be appropriate. Beyond the emission type, internalization also impacts upon radionuclide selection in terms of the chemistry of the radionuclide. In most cases, halogens such as I-131 or I-125 clear rapidly from tumor cells and are excreted via the kidneys. Radiometals such as Y-90 or In-111 are retained within tumor cells and are, therefore, generally preferred for both diagnosis and therapy because they provide a longer residence time in tumor cells.

Radionuclides that emit α particles have been gaining considerable attention for therapy; the first two trials were initiated in 1999 and are still ongoing. α particle emitters are seen as particularly promising because α particles are several thousandfold more efficient at tumor cell killing than β or electron emitters.

B. Linear Energy Transfer (LET)

An important aspect in characterizing the biological effects of different emission types (β vs Auger vs α) is the amount of energy transferred to the cell as the particle traverses the cell. This is characterized by LET, which is the energy transferred per unit distance traveled by the particle. LET will influence the likely biological effect for a given amount of energy deposition to a cell. For example, high LET emissions (e.g., α particles, low-energy Auger electrons) yield a very dense track of ionization-induced damage that is capable of causing irreparable double strand DNA damage. The same amount of total energy deposition by low LET emissions (β particles) has a very low probability of yielding irreparable double strand DNA damage, as the track is much less dense and double-stranded DNA breaks are infrequent. In cell culture experiments, the absorbed dose (energy per unit mass) required to achieve a particular level of cell kill is approximately five to eight times greater for low LET emissions relative to that required for high LET emissions.

C. Dosimetry

The energy deposited per unit mass of tissue is defined as the absorbed dose. The absorbed dose is a measure of potential therapeutic efficacy and toxicity, in this sense it is analogous to "dose" as applied to chemotherapy. Absorbed dose is calculated as the total number of radionuclide transformations (also referred to as decays or disintegrations) occurring in a particular tissue (i.e., the source), multiplied by the energy emitted per transformation and by a factor that represents the fraction of energy emitted by the source that is absorbed by a target tissue. The total energy absorbed by a target tissue from all source tissues is then divided by the mass of the target tissue to give the absorbed dose. Although all radioactivity-containing tissues will contribute dose to a particular target, the dominant contribution arises from the self-dose, i.e., the fraction of energy emitted by the target (assuming it has taken up radioactivity) that is absorbed within the target. Mathematically, this may be represented by

$$D = \frac{\tilde{A} \cdot \Delta \cdot \varphi}{M}$$

where $\tilde{A}$, Δ, and φ are the total number of transformations, the energy emitted per transformation, and the fraction of that energy that is absorbed in the tissue, respectively; M is the mass of the target tissue; and D is the target tissue self-dose. The energy emit-

ted per transformation and fraction absorbed are listed by radionuclide and source target organ combination in compilations provided by the Medical Internal Radionuclide Dose Committee. The mass must generally be determined by CT or other imaging modality. The number of transformations, $\tilde{A}$, is generally obtained by imaging or sampling at different times after injection of the radiolabeled antibody.

D. β Emitters

Table IV lists β emitters that have been used in radiolabeled antibody therapy. β particles may be thought of as electrons that originate from the nucleus. Unlike orbital shell electron emissions, they do not have a single value for the initial energy, rather the emitted energy is selected from a range of possible initial energies according to a probability function that provides the likelihood that a particle with a chosen energy will be emitted in a given decay. Tabulated values of the energy or range of β particle emissions, therefore, typically list the most likely (mean) energy emitted or the maximum possible (end point) energy. Because the range of a particle depends on its initial energy, the range of β particle emissions is correspondingly represented by a probability distribution of possible ranges with the mean or maximum ranges typically provided in tabulations. The two most popular radionuclides for radioimmunotherapy, ^{131}I and ^{90}Y, are β emitters. Iodine-131 was used almost exclusively in initial trials of radioimmunotherapy because the behavior of I-131 (as a free radionuclide) in humans had been well established in the treatment of thyroid cancer and also because of the ease with which antibodies may be labeled with this radionuclide.

TABLE IV
β Electron Emitters

Radionuclide	Half-life (h)	Mean energy (keV)
I-131	193	182
Y-90	64	934
Re-188	17	765
Re-186	91	323
Cu-67	62	142
Lu-177	161	133

Yttrium-90 has gained in popularity recently because it provides the following advantages over ^{131}I: (1) No γ-particle (photon) emissions, thereby eliminating the need to keep patients in radiation isolation; (2) longer range of β particle emissions, an advantage in overcoming a nonuniform distribution of antibody within tumors; (3) it is a metal that is retained within the cytosol of cells following internalization of the radiolabeled antibody. A drawback related to the second advantage of this radionuclide is that it is not possible to obtain imaging-based biodistribution information directly from ^{90}Y because it does not emit photons. This problem has been overcome by using ^{111}In as a surrogate for its biodistribution.

E. Positron Emitters

Table V lists positron emitters that have either been used or are being considered for use with antibodies. The description provided earlier for β emitters also applies to positron emitters with the exception that positrons are the antimatter of electrons and are, therefore, positively charged. When positrons encounter electrons, the two particles annihilate each other, leading to the release of energy in the form of high-energy photons. High-energy photons are emitted in the opposite direction, and this aspect of positron emitters is used for imaging with positron emission tomography (PET).

F. Auger Emitters

In contrast to β particles, Auger electrons are emitted from the orbital shells of atoms. They are characterized by a single energy (they are monoenergetic) and, therefore, by a single range. Table VI lists Auger emitters that have been used or considered for use in

TABLE V
Positron (+) Emitters

Radionuclide	Half-life (h)	Mean energy (keV) (%)
I-124	100	188 (25)
Y-86	15	219 (34)
Br-76	16	642 (57)
Ga-66	10	986 (57)

TABLE VI
Auger or Conversion Electron Emitters

Radionuclide	Half-life (h)	Mean energy (keV)
I-125	1440	18
In-111	67	34
I-123	13	28

radioimmunotherapy; the best studied of these is ^{125}I. The range of Auger electrons ranges from a few nanometers to several micrometers. Emissions in the nanometer range are therapeutically effective only if the radionuclide is incorporated into the DNA, and micrometer-ranged emissions, if of sufficient abundance, may be effective in tumor cell killing even if the radiolabeled antibody remains on the surface. In general, however, radionuclides with such emissions demonstrate enhanced cell killing if the radionuclide–antibody complex is internalized and remains within the cell and in close proximity to the cell nucleus.

G. α Particle Emitters

Table VII lists α particle emitters that have been used or considered for use in radioimmunotherapy. The range of α particles in tissues is on the order of 40 to 90 μm; the LET is 50- to 500-fold greater than that of β particles. In most cases, one to three α particle tracks through the cell nucleus are sufficient to sterilize the cell. This is in contrast to the thousands to tens of thousands required of β particles. The two α particle emitters that have been used clinically, ^{211}At and ^{213}Bi, have relatively short half-lives and are, therefore, best suited for locoregional injection or in targeting rapidly accessible disease such as micrometastases.

III. PATIENT STUDIES AND RESULTS

A. Leukemia/Lymphoma

A list of the highlights in radioimmunotherapy over the past several years would begin with the impact that this treatment modality has had on the therapy

TABLE VII
α Particle Emitters

Radionuclide Daughters	Half-life	Emissions		
		%[a]	Particle	Energy[b]
Bi-213	45.6 min	2	α	6 MeV
		98	β⁻	444 keV
		17	γ	440 keV
Po-213	4.2 μs	98	α	8 MeV
Tl-209	2.2 min	2	β⁻	659 keV
Pb-209	3.25 h	100	β⁻	198 keV
Bi-209	Stable			
Bi-212	1.0 h	36	α	6 MeV
		64	β⁻	492 keV
Po-212	298 ns	64	α	9 MeV
Tl-208	3.05 min	36	β⁻	560 keV
		8	γ	510 keV
		31	γ	580 keV
		36	γ	2.6 MeV
Pb-208	Stable			
At-211	7.21 h	42	α	6 MeV
		19	γ	80 keV
Po-211	516 ms	58	α	7.5 MeV
Bi-207	32 years	24	γ	70 keV
		41	γ	570 keV
		31	γ	1 MeV
Pb-207	Stable			
Ac-225	10 days	100	α	6 MeV
Fr-221	4.9 min	100	α	6 MeV
		10	γ	218 keV
At-217	32.3 ms	100	α	7 MeV
Bi-213	See Bi-123			
Ra-223	11.4 days	100	α	6 MeV
		40	γ	80 keV
		14	γ	270 keV
Rn-219	4 s	100	α	7 MeV
		10	γ	270 keV
Po-215	1.8 ms	100	α	7 MeV
Pb-211	36.1 min	100	β⁻	447 keV
Bi-211	2.1 min	16	α	6 MeV
		84	α	7 MeV
		13	γ	350 keV
Tl-207	4.8 min	100	β⁻	493 keV
Pb-207	Stable			

[a]Percentage emitted per decay of parent radionuclide.
[b]Mean β⁻ energy and approximate α and γ energies are listed.

of non-Hodgkin's lymphoma (NHL). At an advanced stage, when conventional therapy is ineffective, radioimmunotherapy, using the anti-B1 antibody labeled with either [131]I (Bexxar, Coulter Pharmaceuticals) or [90]Y (Zevalin, IDEC Pharmaceuticals), has been consistently and reproducibly effective against this disease; recent investigations suggest that these agents will have an even greater efficacy as first-line treatment. These agents are on their way to being the first radiolabeled antibodies to enter the armamentarium of available agents for NHL treatment.

In leukemia, radioimmunotherapy has played a significant role as a preparative regimen for bone marrow ablation. Much of the initial work was carried out with ^{131}I-labeled anti-CD45 or anti-CD33 antibodies. Recently, ^{131}I is being replaced by [90]Y. Yttrium-90 emits a longer range β particle and does not emit γ rays, thereby eliminating the need to keep patients in radiation isolation. This work is ongoing and holds the promise that radioimmunotherapy will allow for the intensification of myeloablative preparative regimens while reducing toxicity to normal organs. Unequivocal assessment of the clinical benefit of such an approach versus total body irradiation will require randomized clinical trials.

Unlike solid disease, leukemia is rapidly accessible to an intravenously administered antibody. Because of this and because the only α-emitting radionuclide/antibody combination ready for clinical use at the time was the anti-CD33 antibody, HuM195, labeled with Bi-213 (45.6 min half-life), the first trial using an α particle emitter was carried out in leukemia patients. This trial demonstrated the feasibility and safety of α emitter radioimmunotherapy.

B. Solid Tumors

Radioimmunotherapy against solid disease has not yielded the positive results seen in the leukemias and lymphomas. The results have not been as favorable in part because antibody access to solid tumors is substantially reduced relative to the hematologic cancers. A review of radioimmunotherapy trials against solid tumors yields the following common themes. With a few exceptions, which are discussed later, the amount of intravenously injected radiolabeled antibody that localizes to tumor tissue is generally between 0.001 and 0.02% of the injected dose per gram tumor. Values in the upper portion of the range are usually seen in smaller volume disease and there is an inverse relationship between tumor mass and percentage uptake per gram. The amount of radiolabeled antibody administered cannot be increased to overcome the low uptake because of hematologic toxicity, which is dose limiting in almost all implementations of radioimmunotherapy, including intrathecal and intraperitoneal administrations. A number of studies have included autologous marrow rescue to increase the administered activity. These studies have shown some promise, but randomized trials have not been conducted.

Intracavitary or intratumor injections have also been examined in an effort to increase tumor concentration while avoiding marrow toxicity. These studies have been the most successful in the treatment of high-grade glioblastomas. In particular, antibodies against tenascin, a tumor-associated extracellular matrix glycoprotein present in human gliomas but not in normal brain, have been used by a number of investigators with different administration strategies. Promising results have been obtained by injection of a radiolabeled antitenascin antibody into surgically created cavities following surgical removal of the lesion. These studies have been carried out using I-131 and, more recently, the α particle emitter At-211. Dose-limiting toxicity has been limited to the brain.

The most promising approach to increasing tumor radioactivity concentration while reducing red marrow exposure is the streptavidin–biotin-based multistep targeting approach (see earlier discussion). Clinical trials using this technique have demonstrated tumor-to-marrow-absorbed dose ratios of 63:1 compared to 6:1 for conventional radioimmunotherapy. As expected, given the high immunogenicity of avidin/streptavidin, all patients developed an immune response against the antibody–streptavidin conjugate 4 weeks after injection. The dose-limiting toxicity seen in these trials has not been hematologic, but rather related to the gastrointestinal tract. This is because the initial antibody selected for use in this strategy was found to cross-react with the bowel epithelium. The unfortunate selection of a cross-reactive antibody notwithstanding, this approach holds significant promise for improving responses in radioimmunotherapy of solid disease.

The availability of genetically engineered humanized antibodies has made possible fractionated administration of radiolabeled antibodies. Early trials using less immunogic chimeric antibodies have suggested that this approach may allow for greater total radioactivity administration because marrow toxicity is reduced. There is also the possible advantage of increased tumor accessibility with a prolonged treatment schedule. Comparative studies of single vs fractionated radioimmunotherapy have only recently begun and it is still too early to define the potential advantages of this approach, if any.

IV. SUMMARY

Radioimmunotherapy and radioimmunodiagnosis have been evolving since the 1970s. Because these approaches to treatment and diagnosis draw upon a diversity of disciplines, advances in each of these areas have fueled ongoing developments. In particular, the high initial enthusiasm associated with the promise of radioimmunotherapy of a "magic bullet" was replaced by disillusionment at the disappointing early clinical results. This disillusionment has, in turn, been replaced by a cautious optimism that has been fostered by the introduction of engineered proteins, by a better understanding of tumor targeting and normal organ toxicity, and by the availability of promising new antigenic targets and radionuclides.

See Also the Following Articles

ANTIBODIES IN THE GENE THERAPY OF CANCER • ANTIBODY-TOXIN AND GROWTH FACTOR-TOXIN FUSION PROTEINS • ANTI-IDIOTYPIC ANTIBODY VACCINES • MONOCLONAL ANTIBODIES: LEUKEMIA AND LYMPHOMA • RADIOBIOLOGY, PRINCIPLES OF • RESISTANCE TO ANTIBODY THERAPY • TARGETED TOXINS

Bibliography

Boulianne, G. L., Hozumi, N., and Shulman, M. J. (1984). Production of functional chimaeric mouse/human antibody. *Nature* **312,** 643–646.

Caron, P. C., Co, M.S., Bull, M.K., Avdalovic, N.M., Queen, C., *et al.* (1992). Biological and immunological features of humanized M195 (anti-Cd33) monoclonal antibodies. *Cancer Res.* **52,** 6761–6767.

Chatal, J. F. (ed.) (1989). "Monoclonal Antibodies in Immunoscintigraphy." CRC Press, Boca Raton, FL.

Goldenberg, D. M. (ed.) (1990). "Cancer Imaging with Radiolabeled Antibodies." Kluwer Academic, Boston.

Goldenberg, D. M. (ed.) (1995). "Cancer Therapy with Radiolabeled Antibodies." CRC Press, Boca Raton, FL.

Goldenberg, D. M., Deland, F., Kim, E., Bennett, S., Primus, F.J., *et al.* (1978). Use of radiolabeled antibodies to carcinoembryonic antigen for the detection and localization of diverse cancers by external photoscanning. *N. Engl. J. Med.* **298,** 1384–1386.

Green, L. L. (1999). Antibody engineering via genetic engineering of the mouse: Xenomouse strains are a vehicle for the facile generation of therapeutic human monoclonal antibodies. *J. Immunol. Methods* **231,** 11–23.

Hale, G., Dyer, M. J., Clark, M. R., Phillips, J. M., Marcus, R., *et al.* (1988). Remission induction in non-Hodgkin lymphoma with reshaped human monoclonal antibody Campath-1h. *Lancet* **2,** 1394–1399.

Hnatowich, D. J., Virzi, F., and Rusckowski, M. (1987). Investigations of avidin and biotin for imaging applications. *J. Nuclear Med.* **28,** 1294–1302.

Huston, J. S., Levinson, D., Mudgett-Hunter, M., Tai, M. S., Novotny, J., *et al.* (1988). Protein engineering of antibody binding sites: Recovery of specific activity in an anti-digoxin single-chain Fv analogue produced in *Escherichia coli. Proc. Natl. Acad. Sci. USA* **85,** 5879–5883.

Junghans, R. P., Sgouros, G., and Scheinberg, D. A. (1996). Antibody-based immunotherapies of cancer. *In* "Cancer Chemother. Biother." (B. A. Chabner and D. L. Longo, eds.), 2nd Ed., pp. 655–689. Lippincott-Raven, Philadelphia, PA.

Kaminski, M. S., Zasadny, K., Francis, I. R., Milik, A. W., Ross, C. W., *et al.* (1993). Radioimmunotherapy of B-cell lymphoma with [131i]anti-B1 (anti-Cd20) antibody. *N. Engl. J. Med.* **329,** 459–465.

Khaw, B. A., Beller, G. A., and Haber, E. (1978). Experimental myocardial infarct imaging following intravenous administration of iodine-131 labeled antibody (Fab')2 fragments specific for cardiac myosin. *Circulation* **57,** 743–750.

Kohler, G., and Milstein, C. (1975). Continuous cultures of fused cells secreting antibody of predefined specificity. *Nature* **256,** 495–497.

Larson, S. M., Carrasquillo, J. A., Krohn, K. A., Brown, J. P., McGuffin, R. W., *et al.* (1983). Localization of 131i-labeled P97-specific Fab fragments in human melanoma as a basis for radiotherapy. *J. Clin. Invest.* **72,** 2101–2114.

Larson, S. M., Divgi, C. R., Sgouros, G., Cheung, N.-K. V., Scheinberg, D. A., *et al.* (2000). Radioisotope conjugates. *In* "Principles and Practice of the Biological Therapy of Cancer" (S. A. Rosenberg, ed.), 3rd Ed., pp. 396–412. Lippincott Williams & Wilkins, Philadelphia, PA.

Le Doussal, J. M., Martin, M., Gautherot, E., Delaage, M., Barbet, J., *et al.* (1989). In vitro and in vivo targeting of radiolabeled monovalent and divalent haptens with dual specificity monoclonal antibody conjugates: Enhanced divalent hapten affinity for cell-bound antibody conjugate. *J. Nuclear Med.* **30,** 1358–1366.

LoBuglio, A. F., Wheeler, R. H., Trang, J., Haynes, A., Rogers, K., *et al.* (1989). Mouse/human chimeric monoclonal antibody in man: Kinetics and immune response. *Proc. Natl. Acad. Sci. USA* **86,** 4220–4224.

Loevinger, R., Budinger, T. F., and Watson, E. E. (1991). "Mird Primer for Absorbed Dose Calculations." The Society of Nuclear Medicine, Inc., New York.

Macklis, R. M., Kinsey, B. M., Kassis, A. I., Ferrara, J. L., Atcher, R. W., *et al.* (1988). Radioimmunotherapy with alpha-particle-emitting immunoconjugates. *Science* **240,** 1024–1026.

McDevitt, M. R., Sgouros, G., Finn, R. D., Humm, J. L., Jurcic, J. G., *et al.* (1998). Radioimmunotherapy with alpha-emitting nuclides. *Eur. J. Nuclear Med.* **25,** 1341–1351.

Morrison, S. L., Johnson, M. J., Herzenberg, L. A., and Oi, V. T. (1984). Chimeric human antibody molecules: Mouse antigen-binding domains with human constant region domains. *Proc. Natl. Acad. Sci. USA* **81,** 6851–6855.

Pluckthun, A., and Pack, P. (1997). New protein engineering approaches to multivalent and bispecific antibody fragments. *Immunotechnology* **3,** 83–105.

Porter, R. R. (1959). The hydrolysis of rabbit gamma-globulin and antibodies with crystalline papain. *Biochem. J.* **73,** 119–126.

Sgouros, G., Ballangrud, A. M., Jurcic, J. G., McDevitt, M. R., Humm, J. L., *et al.* (1999). Pharmacokinetics and dosimetry of an alpha-particle emitter labeled antibody: ^{213}Bi-Hum195 (anti-CD33) in patients with leukemia. *J. Nuclear Med.* **40,** 1935–1946.

Wiseman, G. A., White, C. A., Witzig, T. E., Gordon, L. I., Emmanouilides, C., *et al.* (1999). Radioimmunotherapy of relapsed non-Hodgkin's lymphoma with zevalin, a 90y-labeled anti-Cd20 monoclonal antibody. *Clin. Cancer Res.* **5**(Suppl.), 3281s–3286s.

Zalutsky, M. R., and Vaidyanathan, G. (2000). Astatine-211-labeled radiotherapeutics: An emerging approach to targeted alpha-particle radiotherapy. *Curr. Pharm. Des.* **6,** 1433–1455.

Ras Proteins

Wendy Morse Pruitt
Channing J. Der
University of North Carolina at Chapel Hill

GLOSSARY

CAAX motif A carboxyl-terminal tetrapeptide sequence, where C = cysteine, A = aliphatic amino acid, and X = serine or methionine, that is recognized by farnesyltransferase to catalyze the addition of a farnesol group to the cysteine residue.

effector Downstream mediator of Ras function, shows preferential binding to the activated, GTP-bound form of Ras. Association with Ras requires an intact core effector domain corresponding to Ras residues 32 to 40.

farnesol C15 isoprenoid that is a product of the mevalonate biosynthetic pathway and is a substrate for the farnesyltransferase-catalyzed covalent addition to the cysteine residue of carboxyl-terminal CAAX tetrapeptide sequences that terminate with X = serine or methionine.

farnesyltransferase Enzyme that catalyzes the covalent addition of the farnesol group from farnesyl pyrophosphate to the cysteine residue of the carboxyl-terminal CAAX motif of Ras proteins.

GTPase Guanine nucleotide binding protein that possesses intrinsic GTP hydrolysis and GDP/GTP exchange activity. Contains consensus amino acid sequence motifs shared with other GTPases.

GTPase-activating protein A negative regulator of Ras, stimulates the intrinsic GTP hydrolytic activity of Ras to promote the formation of inactive Ras-GDP.

guanine nucleotide exchange factor A positive regulator of Ras, stimulates the intrinsic GDP/GTP exchange activity of Ras to promote the formation of active Ras-GTP.

Research findings since the mid-1970s have revealed that cancer is a genetic disease characterized by the mutation of specific oncogenes and tumor suppressor genes. It is this stepwise accumulation of changes that promotes the complex malignant growth properties of cancerous cells. Among the many genes implicated in human carcinogenesis, *ras* protooncogenes have been found to be the most frequently mutated oncogenes (30% in all human cancers) and have been the subject of intense research scrutiny. Mutations in *ras* genes are associated with the development of a wide spectrum of hematopoietic and solid cancers. Thus, understanding how Ras proteins function in normal cell physiology is critical to our understanding of what goes awry in cancerous cells.

In addition to their involvement in cancer development, Ras proteins also have been found to be key regulators of diverse signaling pathways that relay extracellular stimuli-mediated signals to cytoplasmic signaling pathways. Moreover, Ras proteins are the founding members and prototype of a large and continually expanding superfamily of Ras-related proteins. This article provides an overview of Ras protein structure and biochemistry, highlights its role in signal transduction, and introduces other important members of this family of functionally diverse small GTPases. Finally, it ends with a brief discussion of the therapeutic potential of specifically targeting Ras proteins and their aberrant signaling pathways in the development of novel antineoplastic drugs for cancer treatment.

I. Ras PROTEIN STRUCTURE AND BIOCHEMISTRY

A. Protein Structure

ras genes were discovered initially as genes responsible for the potent cancer-causing activity of the Harvey and Kirsten murine sarcoma viruses (Ha-MSV and Ki-MSV). Viral H-*ras* and K-*ras* genes represent genes that were transduced into the viral genome from normal rat cellular sequences. A third mammalian *ras* gene was identified subsequently as a transforming gene isolated from a human neuroblastoma cell line, hence designated N-*ras*.

The three human *ras* genes encode four different Ras proteins (H-Ras, K-Ras4A, K-Ras4B, and N-Ras) that are remarkably similar in sequence identity (85%) and biochemical and biological properties. Genes encoding homologous proteins have been found in diverse invertebrate species that include flies (*Drosophila melanogaster*), worms (*Caenorhabditis elegans*), and yeast (*Saccharomyces cerevisiae* and *Schizosaccha-*

romyces pombe). The high sequence and functional identity among this gene family suggest that they serve important functions in fundamental cellular processes. Accordingly, *ras* gene transcription is ubiquitous and detectable in all tissues and cell types.

Figure 1 depicts the human *ras* gene product, a 188 to189 amino acid protein of approximately 21 kDa in size. The K-*ras* gene encodes two different proteins by use of alternative fourth exons that differ only in their carboxyl-terminal 25 amino acids (designated K-Ras4A and K-Ras4B). The amino terminal 84 residues are identical among the four Ras proteins. The significance of sequence identity in this region is highlighted by the fact that it includes the effector domain (residues 25 to 45), as well as switch I (residues 30 to 38) and II (residues 59 to 76) regions. The effector domain is involved in the binding of activated Ras with its downstream effector targets (see later). Identity among effector domains and flanking sequences suggests that the different Ras proteins are capable of binding to and/or activating the same targets, a point that will be discussed in greater detail later.

The next 80 residues of the four Ras proteins also share strong sequence identity (85%). However, the carboxyl-terminal 25 residues of Ras proteins are

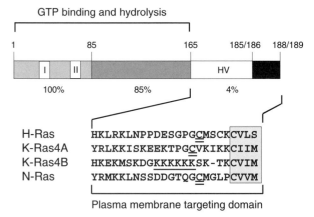

FIGURE 1 Functional domains of Ras. The amino-terminal 165 amino acids of Ras proteins possess GDP/GTP binding and GTPase activities. The amino-terminal 85 amino acids are identical in all Ras proteins and contain the core effector domain (residues 25–45) and the switch I and II sequences. The carboxyl-terminal 25 amino acids constitute the plasma membrane targeting sequence of Ras proteins, which consists of the CAAX tetrapeptide sequence and the hypervariable (HV) domain.

highly variable (4% identity) and therefore comprise the "hypervariable" region. In concert with post-translational modifications signaled by the carboxyl-terminal CAAX tetrapeptide motif (where C = cysteine, A = aliphatic amino acid, and X = methionine or serine; H-Ras residues 186 to 189), the hypervariable region contains sequence determinants that specify Ras protein association with the inner surface of the plasma membrane.

B. Ras Proteins Function as GDP/GTP-Regulated Switches

Ras protein function is regulated by its association with the guanine nucleotides guanosine triphosphate (GTP) and guanosine diphosphate (GDP). Thus, Ras functions as a binary molecular switch that cycles between an active GTP-bound and an inactive GDP-bound state (Fig. 2). Although Ras possesses an intrinsic GTPase activity that catalyzes the hydrolysis of the bound GTP to GDP, and an intrinsic GDP/GTP exchange activity to cycle back to the active state, these activities are too low to allow Ras proteins to be rapidly controlled in its GDP/GTP cycling. Instead, GDP/GTP cycling is controlled by guanine nucleotide exchange factors (GEFs; Sos1/2, RasGRF1/2,

and RasGRP) that act as positive regulators to promote the formation of Ras-GTP. GDP/GTP cycling is also controlled by GTPase activating proteins (GAPs; p120 GAP and neurofibromatosis type 1 protein, NF1) that act as negative regulators to cycle Ras back to its inactive GDP-bound state.

In quiescent, nondividing cells, Ras is found predominantly in the GDP-bound form (greater than 95%). Following an extracellular growth stimulus, GDP/GTP exchange induces a rapid and transient cycling to the GTP-bound state. GDP/GTP cycling causes a change in the structural conformation of Ras, corresponding to the switch I and II regions, which greatly increases its binding affinity for downstream cytoplasmic effector targets, thus initiating various signaling pathways. Upon hydrolysis to GDP, the activated effector protein dissociates from the GTPase and the relay of the signal is terminated. In tumors, mutated *ras* genes encode Ras proteins with single amino acid substitutions at position 12, 13, or 61. These mutated Ras proteins are insensitive to the negative regulation of GAPs and therefore are constitutively GTP bound and activated in a stimulus-independent fashion. Consequently, the Ras signaling pathway is under persistent stimulation, which is a primary mechanism whereby activated Ras contributes to cell proliferation.

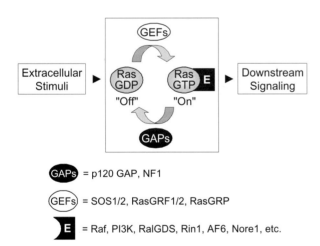

FIGURE 2 Ras is regulated by GDP/GTP cycling. Guanine nucleotide exchange factors (GEFs) promote the formation of active Ras-GTP, and GTPase-activating proteins (GAPs) stimulate the intrinsic GTPase activity of Ras to promote the formation of inactive Ras-GDP. Ras-GTP has increased affinity for its downstream effector (E) targets and promotes effector activation and activation of various cytoplasmic signaling pathways.

C. Posttranslational Processing and Plasma Membrane Localization

Fully functional Ras proteins require attachment to the inner surface of the plasma membrane, which is brought about by a series of closely linked posttranslational modifications of the nascent protein. As depicted in Fig. 3, immediately following the synthesis of Ras proteins in the cytoplasm, the farnesyltransferase (FTase) enzyme catalyzes the covalent addition of the 15 carbon farnesyl isoprenoid lipid to the invariant cysteine residue of the CAAX motif. Endoplasmic reticulum-resident enzymes then catalyze the proteolytic cleavage of the AAX peptide sequence and carboxylmethylation of the now farnesylated cysteine.

The modifications signaled by the CAAX motif increase the hydrophobic nature of the carboxyl terminus of Ras proteins, increasing the affinity for membranes. However, a "second signal" within the

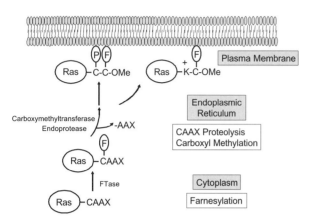

FIGURE 3 Ras processing and membrane localization. The carboxyl-terminal CAAX motif is necessary and sufficient to signal for three posttranslational modifications that are necessary, but not sufficient, for targeting Ras to the inner surface of the plasma membrane. The cytosolic farnesyltransferase (FTase) catalyzes the addition of a farnesyl isoprenoid (F) to the cysteine residue of the CAAX motif. This is rapidly followed by endosome-associated enzymes that cleave the AAX residues (endoprotease) and catalyze the transfer of a methyl group (Ome) to the farnesylated cysteine residue (carboxylmethyltransferase). A second signal present in the hypervariable region, either a lysine-rich sequence (K-Ras4B) or a palmitylated (P) cysteine (H-Ras, N-Ras, and K-Ras4A), is essential to promote the targeting and stable association of Ras with the plasma membrane.

hypervariable region is needed to promote the stable and selective binding of Ras proteins to the plasma membrane. For K-Ras4B, the polylysine sequence between residues 175 and 180 provides the second signal for targeting to the plasma membrane. This small stretch of positively charged amino acids maintains electrostatic interactions with the negatively charged membrane phospholipids to enhance membrane binding. For H-Ras, N-Ras, and K-Ras4A, the second signal for enhanced binding is provided by cysteine residue 181 and/or 184 upstream of the CAAX motif that undergoes posttranslational modification by the covalent addition of the palmitate fatty acid. This lipid modification is a dynamic, reversible modification, which may allow for regulated association with the plasma membrane.

II. Ras AND SIGNAL TRANSDUCTION

Ras proteins function as key regulators of cytoplasmic signaling networks initiated by the binding of various

ligands to their cognate cell surface receptors. These include receptor tyrosine kinases, tyrosine kinase-associated receptors, G protein-coupled receptors, and integrins. Once activated, Ras can interact with a spectrum of functionally diverse effectors, thus stimulating a multitude of cytoplasmic signaling cascades. Therefore, Ras proteins function as a point of convergence of different signaling pathways to then facilitate the stimulation of divergent pathways.

A. Ras Regulation of the Epidermal Growth Factor Receptor Pathway

The best characterized signaling pathway utilizing Ras involves activation of the epidermal growth factor receptor (EGFR) tyrosine protein kinase. Shown in Figure 4, this pathway is present in mammalian cells as well as in *Drosophila* and *C. elegans*. The EGF peptide growth factor binds to and activates the EGFR tyrosine kinase activity, which then causes autophosphorylation of tyrosine residues in its cytoplasmic domain. Phosphorylated tyrosines serve as recognition sequences for Src homology 2 (SH2) domain-containing proteins that include the Grb2 adapter protein. Grb2 also contains a second protein–protein interaction domain, the Src homology 3 (SH3) domain, which recognizes specific proline-rich sequences. In addition to Grb2, SH2 and SH3 domains are found in many other proteins involved in signal transduction. Tandem SH3 domains within Grb2 promote its association with Sos, a Ras GEF. Thus, EGFR association with Grb2 recruits the cytosolic Grb2:Sos complex to the plasma membrane where it then activates membrane-bound Ras.

Once activated, Ras binds to the normally cytoplasmic Raf-1 serine/threonine kinase to recruit it to the plasma membrane to facilitate the activation of its kinase activity. Activated Raf-1 then associates with and activates MEK1/2 dual specificity protein kinases, which in turn associate with and activate p42 and p44 ERK mitogen-activated serine/threonine protein kinases. Subsequently, activated ERKs traverse from the cytoplasm into the nucleus where they phosphorylate various substrates, including the Elk-1 nuclear transcription factor. Thus, this cytoplasmic kinase cascade relays the signal from activated Ras to the nucleus to initiate changes in gene expression that facilitate Ras function.

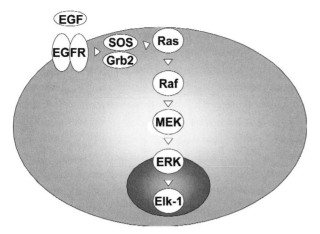

FIGURE 4 Ras and epidermal growth factor signal transduction. EGF binding to the EGFR causes activation of the intrinsic tyrosine kinase activity of the receptor. This causes phosphorylation of tyrosine residues in the cytoplasmic domain, which are then recognized by the SH2 domain of the Grb2 adaptor protein. Grb2 forms a stable complex with Sos, a Ras GEF, via the tandem SH3 domains of Grb2. The association of the Grb2:Sos complex with the activated EGFR allows Sos to activate Ras. Activated Ras then binds and promotes the plasma membrane translocation of Raf, where additional membrane-associated events are required to promote the activation of Raf kinase function. Activated Raf phosphorylates and activates MEK1 and MEK2 dual specificity kinases, and activated MEKs then phosphorylate and activate ERK mitogen-activated protein kinases. Activated ERKs translocate to the nucleus where they phosphorylate the Elk-1 transcription factor.

In *Drosophila*, Ras (Dras) is a downstream component of a related receptor tyrosine kinase (Sevenless) signaling pathway that regulates eye development, whereas in *C. elegans*, Ras (Let-60) is activated by a related receptor tyrosine kinase (Let-23) signaling pathway that promotes vulva development. In contrast, in the yeast *S. cerevisiae*, Ras (RAS1/RAS2) interacts with and activates the adenyl cyclase to mediate the production of cAMP.

B. Ras Activation of Multiple Downstream Effectors

Although Raf kinases have been established as key effectors of Ras function, it is clear that Ras function depends upon interaction with a broad spectrum of additional downstream effectors. The functions of Ras effectors are diverse and include lipid kinases (phosphatidylinositol 3-phosphate kinases; PI3K), GEFs for the Ral Ras-related proteins (Ral GEFs), Ras GAPs,

and proteins of unknown function (e.g., Nore-1). All effectors bind preferentially to the GTP-bound form of Ras by interaction with the effector domain.

PI3K lipid kinases represent the second best characterized effectors of Ras function. As with Raf, their association with activated Ras promotes their recruitment to the plasma membrane to facilitate the activation of PI3K catalytic function. PI3K controls phosphoinositide metabolism, including the conversion of phosphoinositide-4,5-phosphate (PIP2) to phosphoinositide-3,4,5-phosphate (PIP3). PIP3 in turn can regulate the function of a multitude of proteins that include the Akt/PKB serine/threonine kinase. Activated Akt/PKB then phosphorylates a variety of substrates that serve antiapoptotic functions. Thus, Ras activation of the PI3K/Akt pathway promotes cell survival. A family of GEFs for Ral proteins (RalGDS, Rgl, Rgl2/Rlf) represents the third best characterized effectors of Ras and these proteins act as positive regulators of the Ral Ras-related proteins.

III. THE Ras SUPERFAMILY: REGULATORS OF DIVERSE CELLULAR PROCESSES

Ras is the founding member and prototype of a continually expanding superfamily of small GTPases with biological functions that are as diverse as the proteins are numerous (Fig. 5). This superfamily is classified into large subfamilies based on structural and functional similarities. The currently known Ras superfamily subgroups include Ras, Rho, Rab, Arf, Ran, Rad/Gem, and Rit/Rin families. Generally, members of the Ras superfamily are characterized by their primary amino acid sequence identity with Ras (approximately 25% or greater), their small size (20 to 25 kDa), and their ability to serve as GDP/GTP-regulated molecular switches. Their divergent functions are dictated by the nature of the stimuli that promote their GDP/GTP cycling and by the proteins that they interact with when GTP bound.

A. The Ras Family

In addition to the four Ras proteins, this branch of the Ras superfamily consists of small GTPases that

Ras	Rab	Rho	Arf	Rad	Ran	Rheb	Rit	κB-Ras
H-Ras	Rab1A	RhoA	Arf1	Rad	Ran	Rheb	Rit	κB-Ras1
K-Ras	Rab1B	RhoB	Arf2	Gem			Rin	κB-Ras2
N-Ras	Rab2	RhoC	Arf3	Kir			Ric	
R-Ras	Rab3A	RhoD	Arf4	Rem1				
TC21	Rab3B	RhoE	Arf5	Rem2				
M-Ras	Rab4	RhoG	Arf6					
Rap1A	Rab5A	Rnd1	Arf7					
Rap1B	Rab5B	Rnd2						
Rap2A	Rab6	Rac1						
Rap2B	Rab7	Rac2						
RalA	Rab8	Rac3						
RalB	Rab9	Cdc42						
	Rab10	TC10						
	Etc.	TCL						
		TTF						
		Chp						
		Rif						

FIGURE 5 Ras superfamily of small GTPases. Members of the Ras superfamily of small GTPases share significant primary sequence identity with Ras (25 to 55%) and are regulated by GDP/GTP association. The sequence and functional similarities define at least nine distinct families. The three largest branches are the Ras, Rho, and Rab families.

share the strongest amino acid identity (~50%) with Ras proteins. Included in this branch are the three R-Ras proteins (R-Ras, R-Ras2/TC21, and R-Ras3/M-Ras) that, like Ras, exhibit transforming activity. However, to date, only mutated TC21 proteins have been identified in human cancers. Other members of this branch are linked to Ras signaling, with Rap proteins activated concurrently with Ras via shared GEFs, and with Ral proteins activated via the Ras effectors that function as Ral GEFs.

B. The Rho Family

Rho proteins are generally recognized for their ability to coordinately organize the actin cytoskeleton and to regulate cell growth. To date, 15 distinct Rho family proteins have been identified, with RhoA, Rac1, and Cdc42 being the best characterized. Like Ras, Rho family GTPases are also intermediates in signal transduction pathways initiated by extracellular signals that stimulate G protein-coupled receptors, receptor tyrosine kinases, and integrins. Rho-specific GEFs and GAPs regulate the cycling of these proteins between active GTP-bound and inactive GDP-bound states.

RhoA, Rac1, and Cdc42 were originally distinguished by their specific effects on the actin cytoskeleton in response to extracellular stimuli. RhoA controls the formation of stress fibers and the assembly of focal adhesion complexes, Rac1 regulates actin dynamics for membrane ruffles and lamellipodia, and Cdc42 controls the formation of actin microspikes and filopodia. The coordinate regulation of cellular morphology and motility by these GTPases can greatly influence normal cell–cell and cell–matrix interactions. Moreover, the aberrant activation of Rho GTPases has been found to promote tumor cell invasion and metastasis. Two additional functions associated with Rho GTPases involve regulation of the activity of a variety of transcription factors (e.g., serum response factor, NF-κB, c-Fos, c-Jun, ternary complex factors) and the regulation of progression through the G1 phase of the cell cycle.

There is growing evidence for the importance of Rho family GTPases in oncogenesis. First, specific Rho family GTPases (e.g., RhoA, Rac1, and Cdc42) have been shown to be required for the transforming activity of Ras and other oncoproteins. Second, aberrant activation of Rho GTPases can promote the uncontrolled proliferation and the invasive and metastatic properties of tumor cells. Third, many Rho GEFs were identified initially as transforming proteins and some have been found to be rearranged in human cancers (e.g., BCR and LARG).

C. The Rab Family

Rab proteins comprise the largest subgroup within the Ras superfamily and consist of over 60 mammalian members. Unlike Ras, which is always bound to the plasma membrane, Rab GDP/GTP cycling regulates their dynamic association with distinct plasma and endomembrane compartments. Many of the Rab family members have been localized to various functional compartments on specific biosynthetic/secretory as well as endocytic pathways. Specifically, numerous studies done in yeast and mammalian cells have demonstrated their involvement in processes underlying the docking and fusion of transport vesicles to target membranes. Like Ras proteins, Rab proteins also are posttranslationally modified. However, another prenyl protein transferase, geranylgeranyltransferase II, catalyzes the covalent addition of the more hydrophobic C20 geranylgeranyl isoprenoid to carboxyl-terminal cysteine residues found in CC, CXC, or CXXX motifs (C = cysteine, X = any amino acid).

D. The Ran Family

The Ran subgroup is represented by its lone member, Ran, which is distinguished from Ras GTPases by its lipid modification and atypical subcellular localization. Unlike most other Ras-related proteins, Ran is not modified to bind to cell membranes. Instead, Ran protein is localized throughout the cell, where it is concentrated primarily in the nucleus. Ran-GDP has been shown to shuttle from the cytoplasm to the nucleus, where Ran becomes GTP bound and active. Accordingly, the strongest direct evidence of Ran function is its role in nuclear protein import and export. However, Ran function also has been implicated in numerous cellular processes, including cell cycle progression, DNA replication, RNA processing, and mitotic spindle assembly.

IV. TARGETING Ras FOR CANCER TREATMENT: THE FUTURE OF ANTICANCER DRUG DEVELOPMENT

A. Ras Mutations in Human Cancer

The frequency of Ras mutations varies according to tumor type, with rates as high as 90, 50, and 30% for pancreatic, colorectal, and lung carcinoma, respectively. Thus, aberrant Ras function is believed to contribute to the development of a significant portion of these neoplasms. However, activating mutations in *ras* genes are rarely found in neoplasms developed in the breast, ovaries, or cervix. However, another common defect in tumor cells is the upregulated function of receptor tyrosine kinase function (e.g., Her2/Neu in breast and ovarian cancer). Because Her2 and other receptor tyrosine kinases cause transformation, in part, by causing Ras activation, the importance of Ras activation in human cancers may well be quite higher than the 30% frequency of *ras* mutations.

The presence of *ras* mutations alone does not provide complete validation of the importance of aberrant Ras function in cancer development. However, the considerable body of experimental studies in cell culture and animal model systems argues strongly that aberrant Ras function contributes significantly to malignancy and that therapeutic approaches to correct defects in Ras function may have an important impact on tumor progression. Moreover, because *ras* mutations are especially frequent in human cancers that are ineffectively cured by current therapeutic approaches, the development of anti-Ras drugs as novel anticancer agents has been a very active pursuit by the pharmaceutical and biotechnology industries.

B. Farnesyltransferase Inhibitors

Two main approaches have been considered and pursued for the development of anti-Ras drugs. First, much attention has been focused on the development of inhibitors of FTase, the enzyme that catalyzes Ras processing and attachment to the plasma membrane. A key advantage of FTase inhibitors (FTIs) as anti-Ras drugs is the fact that Ras biological function is dependent absolutely on farnesylation-mediated membrane association. However, because farnesylation is also required for the function of normal Ras proteins, as well as other proteins, FTIs will not specifically block the function of mutated Ras proteins. Despite this concern for selectivity, FTIs have shown remarkable antitumor activity in cell-based and animal model studies, with surprisingly limited toxicity to normal cells. A number of FTIs are now under evaluation in phase II clinical trials for antitumor activity in cancer patients. Interestingly, one unexpected complexity in the development of FTIs as anti-Ras drugs is the widely held belief that the antitumor activity of FTIs may not be due to the inhibition of Ras function at all. Instead, while FTase is still the likely target for these inhibitors, whether a farnesylated Ras-related protein (e.g., RhoB) or another FTase substrate is the real target is currently under investigation.

C. Targeting Ras Effector Signaling

A second approach for the development of anti-Ras drugs has been to target the downstream signaling pathways that are activated by Ras. In particular, inhibitors of MEK have been developed that prevent Ras activation of the ERK cascade. Both cell culture and animal studies have documented the potent antitumor activity of these kinase inhibitors. However, in light of the fact that Ras must activate a multitude of effector signaling pathways for oncogenesis, the effectiveness of blocking only the Raf>MEK>ERK pathway as a means of abrogating Ras-mediated tumor cell proliferation is not clear.

V. SUMMARY

In light of the involvement of Ras proteins in a multitude of signaling pathways that regulate normal cell physiology, it is not surprising that the aberrant activation of Ras can contribute significantly to the growth properties of cancerous cells. Whether anti-Ras drugs will become effective anticancer drugs is presently uncertain. Nevertheless, the rational design of pharmacologic inhibitors of Ras and other specific signal transduction molecules is widely believed to be the direction of drug development. It is generally acknowledged that the current arsenal of cytotoxic compounds that are in use today in the clinic have reached their limits in efficacy for cancer treatment. Therefore, it is hoped that anti-Ras and other target-based inhibitors will make a significant impact in drug development for the cure or palliative treatment of cancer.

See Also the Following Articles

FOS ONCOGENE • LUNG CANCER: MOLECULAR AND CELLULAR ABNORMALITIES • MAP KINASE MODULES IN SIGNALING • MOLECULAR ASPECTS OF RADIATION BIOLOGY • MYB • PANCREATIC CANCER: CELLULAR AND MOLECULAR MECHANISMS • RIBOZYMES AND THEIR APPLICATIONS • SIGNAL TRANSDUCTION MECHANISMS INITIATED BY RECEPTOR TYROSINE KINASES

Bibiography

Barbacid, M. (1987). *ras* genes. *Annu. Rev. Biochem.* **56,** 779–827.

Bos, J. L. (1989). *ras* oncogenes in human cancer: A review. *Cancer Res.* **49,** 4682–4689.

Bourne, H. R., Sanders, D. A., and McCormick, F. (1990). The GTPase superfamily: A conserved switch for diverse cell functions. *Nature* **348,** 125–132.

Bourne, H. R., Sanders, D. A., and McCormick, F. (1990). The GTPase superfamily: Conserved structure and molecular mechanism. *Nature* **349,** 117–126.

Chardin, P. (1993). Structural conservation of ras-related proteins and its functional implications. *GTPases Biol. I* **108,** 159–176.

Clark, G. J., and Der, C. J. (1993). Oncogenic activation of *Ras* proteins. *In* "GTPases in Biology I" (B. F. Dickey and L. Birnbaumer, eds.), pp. 259–288. Springer Verlag, Berlin.

Cox, A. D., and Der, C. J. (1997). Farnesyltransferase inhibitors and cancer treatment: Targeting simply Ras? *Biochem. Biophys. Acta* **1333,** F51–F71.

Malumbres, M., and Pellicer, A. (1998). Ras pathways to cell cycle control and cell transformation. *Front. Biosci.* **3,** 887–912.

Reuther, G. W., and Der, C. J. (2000). The Ras branch of small GTPases: Ras family members don't fall far from the tree. *Curr. Opin. Cell Biol.* **12,** 157–165.

Shields, J. M., Pruitt, K., McFall, A., Shaub, A., and Der, C. J. (2000). Understanding Ras: "it ain't over 'til it's over." *Trends Cell Biol.* **10,** 147–153.

Van Aelst, L., and D'Souza-Schorey, G. (1997). Rho GTPases and signaling networks. *Genes Dev.* **11,** 2295–2322.

Recombination: Mechanisms and Roles in Tumorigenesis

Jac A. Nickoloff
University of New Mexico School of Medicine

GLOSSARY

allelic recombination Exchange between alleles on homologous chromosomes.

crossover Precise exchange between two DNA molecules (reciprocal exchange).

ectopic recombination Recombination between nonallelic homologous sequences.

extrachromosomal recombination Exchange between plasmids introduced into cells; often followed by integration into host chromosomal DNA.

gene conversion Nonreciprocal transfer of information between homologous loci. Sequence information in recipient allele is replaced by information from donor allele; donor allele is not changed.

heteroduplex DNA (hDNA) Mismatched base-pair(s) in hybrid DNA created during strand exchange between two homologous DNAs containing one or more heterologies.

homeologous recombination Exchange between diverged DNA sequences.

homologous recombination Exchange between two regions of DNA sharing substantial sequence identity.

illegitimate recombination Exchanges between DNAs sharing little or no sequence homology (also called nonhomologous recombination).

intrachromosomal recombination Exchange or transfer of information between direct or inverted repeated regions on a single chromosome; a type of ectopic recombination.

loss of heterozygosity (LOH) Allele loss by deletion, reciprocal recombination and segregation of like alleles, or gene conversion.

nonhomologous end-joining (NHEJ) Joining of two DNA ends sharing little or no homology.

sister chromatid exchange (SCE) Reciprocal recombination between sister chromatids.

site-specific recombination Exchanges catalyzed by specialized enzymatic machinery operating at a single site or few sites in a genome; usually produces a single product or a limited spectrum of products by reciprocal recombination.

Recombination is defined as the exchange of information between DNA molecules. Recombination describes a wide variety of DNA interactions with diverse genetic outcomes, such as gene conversion, duplication/amplification, deletion, inversion, and chromosome translocation. In addition to its well-known role in the generation of genetic diversity, recombination is involved in DNA replication, chromosome segregation, DNA repair, gene regulation, antibody gene assembly, and development. Recombination is regulated at several levels, and defects in these regulatory systems are associated with defective DNA repair and genomic instability, which are common characteristics of cancer cells.

I. INTRODUCTION

Recombination can occur between homologous or nonhomologous DNA molecules. Homologous recombination during meiosis generates genetic diversity across generations, ensures proper chromosome disjunction, and appears to improve fitness independently of its role in generating genetic diversity. Antibody diversity is generated by nonhomologous recombination and by somatic hypermutation, which may involve homologous recombination. Homologous and nonhomologous recombination play important roles in DNA repair. DNA double-strand damage, including double-strand breaks (DSBs) and interstrand crosslinks, can be repaired with high fidelity by homologous recombination, although such repair sometimes results in chromosomal rearrangements. Homologous recombination intermediates may include DNA mismatches (heteroduplex DNA; hDNA) that can be processed by the mismatch repair (MMR) system. The MMR system also regulates the frequency of homologous recombination. Little or no homology is required for nonhomologous recombination, which includes nonhomologous end-joining

(NHEJ) and illegitimate recombination. Many proteins are now known to be involved in recombination; most act either in homologous or in nonhomologous pathways, but some influence both pathways. Consistent with fundamental roles for recombination in DNA dynamics, many recombination proteins have been highly conserved through evolution. The genetic consequences of recombination are well understood, but recombination mechanisms, enzymology, and regulation are still largely a mystery. Recombination has several key roles in carcinogenesis, including inactivation of tumor suppressor genes as a result of loss of heterozygosity (LOH) and oncogene activation by gene amplification or translocation. Recombination underlies genomic instability seen in tumor cells, and the resulting mutagenic effects of such instability may be an important determinant of tumor progression. Several diseases that predispose to cancer show altered DNA repair and recombination phenotypes.

II. TYPES OF RECOMBINATION EVENTS

Recombination may occur between any two DNA molecules or regions of a single molecule. Interactions between regions sharing significant homology (>200 bp) is termed homologous recombination; nonhomologous events involve little or no homology. Recombination creates new DNA arrangements characteristic of the type of event and the original arrangement of the interacting DNAs. For homologous events, interacting regions can be arranged in several ways. Allelic recombination occurs between allelic loci on homologous chromosomes. Ectopic recombination describes all nonallelic interactions, including those between repeats on nonhomologous chromosomes, nonallelic loci on homologous chromosomes, and linked repeats (Fig. 1A). Homologous recombination may be reciprocal (crossover) or nonreciprocal (gene conversion).

Gene conversion involves information transfer from a donor locus to a recipient; the donor locus is unchanged, but information in the recipient is converted (lost) because it is precisely replaced with donor information. DSBs strongly enhance gene con-

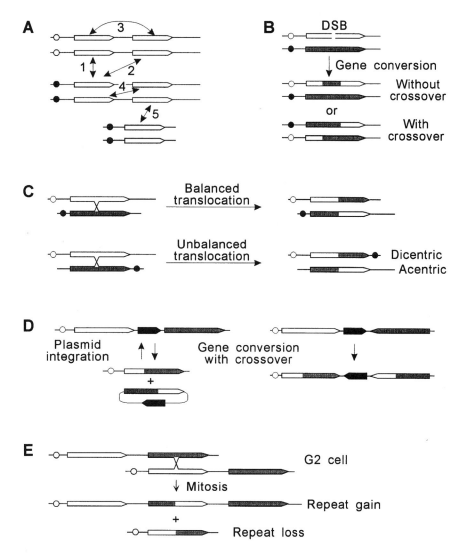

FIGURE 1 Types of recombination events. (A) Five types of interactions between repeated regions. Sister chromatids are shown for homologous chromosomes (G2 cell) with centromeres indicated by white and black circles. Repeats are shown as open boxes; in this case in direct orientation. A heterologous chromosome is shown as a single pair of sister chromatids (gray centromeres), also carrying a copy of the repeated DNA. 1, Allelic recombination; 2, recombination between nonallelic repeats on homologs; 3, intrachromosomal recombination; 4, unequal sister chromatid recombination; 5, recombination between repeats on heterologous chromosomes. All events except #4 are possible in G1 and G2 cells. Inverted repeats are shown in (D). (B) Gene conversion initiated by DSB (repeats are distinguished by shading). Conversion may or may not be associated with a crossover. (C) Translocations result from crossovers between heterologous chromosomes, with balanced and unbalanced events dependent on the relative orientations of repeats and centromeres. Unbalanced translocations create dicentric chromosomes that often break during mitosis, and acentric fragments that are usually lost. (D) Crossovers between direct repeats excises a repeat and DNA between repeat as a circular molecule. The reverse reaction integrates plasmid DNA into a chromosome (a type of gene targeting), creating direct repeats. Crossovers between inverted repeats inverts DNA between repeats. These inversions can also occur by sister chromatid conversion (not shown). (E) Unequal sister chromatid exchange produces repeat gain and loss in daughter cells.

version, and alleles suffering a DSB are almost always recipients. Gene conversion does not cause gross alteration of chromosomal structures, but it is often associated with crossovers (Fig. 1B). Crossovers are precise exchanges that involve no gain or loss of DNA at the junction, but can result in gross chromosome rearrangements including translocations, deletions, and inversions (Figs. 1C and 1D). Deletion of DNA between linked repeats can occur during sister chromatid recombination. In G2 cells, most recombination occurs between sister chromatids, and because sister chromatids are essentially identical, such events usually have no genetic consequence. However, unequal reciprocal exchange in direct repeats causes repeat loss in one daughter cell and repeat gain in the other (Fig. 1E).

Crossing over between allelic loci has no immediate genetic effect since it results only in flanking marker exchange between homologous chromosomes. However, allelic crossovers lead to LOH for all heterozygous markers that are centromere-distal to the crossover point in 50% of subsequent mitotic divisions (Fig. 2). In contrast, gene conversion results in localized LOH (Fig. 1B). Gene conversion and crossing over are conservative events, but homologous recombination between direct repeats can also occur by a nonconservative mechanism termed single-strand annealing (SSA) (Fig. 3). SSA may be initiated by

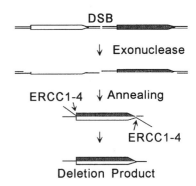

FIGURE 3 Single-strand annealing. Annealing occurs after processing of DSB ends exposes complementary strands in direct repeats. 3′ tails in the intermediate are cleaved by ERCC1/ERCC4 endonuclease. Annealing can form mismatches that are subject to repair (paired open/shaded regions). SSA always produces a deletion product.

DSBs located within or between repeated DNA. In SSA, broken ends are processed to expose single-stranded tails within the repeats. These tails anneal to form a deletion product similar to that formed by a crossover. However, unlike direct repeat crossovers in which DNA between repeats is excised as a circular molecule, SSA is nonconservative because DNA between repeats is not recoverable. In yeast, SSA is common for both extrachromosomal and chromosomal direct repeats. In contrast, in mammalian cells SSA events are predominant in extrachromosomal direct repeats, but gene conversions (without associated crossovers) are predominant in chromosomal direct repeats.

Nonhomologous recombination includes both simple end-rejoining of DSBs (NHEJ) and illegitimate recombination, which includes end-joining of different broken chromosomes (or different regions of a single chromosome) and integration of exogenous DNA into a nonhomologous locus. NHEJ is an important pathway for repairing DSBs, such as those caused by ionizing radiation. However, unlike homologous recombination, NHEJ is often imprecise. Before ends are rejoined, they may be degraded by an exonuclease or lengthened in a nontemplated fashion by terminal deoxynucleotidyl transferase, yielding junctions with deletions or insertions. This imprecision during V(D)J recombination generates antibody diversity. Because NHEJ can join any two regions of DNA, it can cause translocations, insertions, inversions, and deletions.

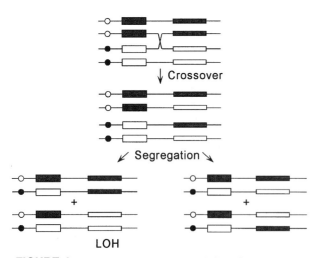

FIGURE 2 Crossing over causes LOH of all markers centromere distal the crossover point in 50% of subsequent mitoses. Symbols as in Fig. 1.

Site-specific recombination involves the joining of specific DNA sequences by specialized enzymatic machinery. Often, site-specific recombination is conservative with DNA inserted precisely into a target site (e.g., phage λ integration into the *E. coli* chromosome mediated by the Int protein), precise DNA sequence inversion (e.g., Flp mediated recombination of 2-μm circle sequences in yeast), or site-specific gene conversion (e.g., yeast mating-type switching initiated by HO nuclease). V(D)J recombination is an example of an imprecise, nonconservative site-specific recombination event since it is initiated at specific sites that are cleaved by RAG1/RAG2 endonuclease.

III. RECOMBINATION MECHANISMS AND ENZYMOLOGY

Despite the widespread occurrence of homologous recombination, our understanding of recombination mechanisms has lagged behind that of other DNA metabolic processes such as replication and transcription. This is because recombination involves little or no DNA synthesis or degradation, but only rearranges existing DNA, and because recombination is a relatively infrequent event. Homologous recombination involves initiation, end-processing, strand transfer to produce hDNA, and resolution of intermediates. Resolution includes repair of mismatches in hDNA and resolution of Holliday junctions. These steps are common to a variety of models proposed to explain homologous recombination, such as those shown in Figure 4.

It is not known how spontaneous homologous recombination is initiated, but it is possible that DSBs are involved. Spontaneous DSBs may form when replication forks encounter natural "pause" sites or DNA lesions such as oxidative damage or single-strand breaks. Recombination is thought to play an important role in restart of stalled replication complexes. Many types of single-strand DNA damage are highly recombinogenic, such as that caused by chemical agents and UV, and this may reflect replication-dependent conversion of single-strand damage to DSBs. Broken ends are processed by a 5′ → 3′ exonuclease, exposing 3′ single-stranded tails; in mammals this step probably requires the RAD50/MRE11/NBS1 complex. This complex is also involved

in DSB induction in meiosis, telomere length maintenance, damage sensing for the G2/M cell cycle checkpoint, and NHEJ. Strand transfer is effected by RAD51, a homolog of *Escherichia coli* RecA. RAD51 interacts directly or indirectly with many proteins known or presumed to be involved in homologous recombination, including at least five RAD51 paralogs (RAD51B, RAD51C, RAD51D, XRCC2 and XRCC3), RAD52, RAD54, RAD54B, UBL1, UBC9, replication protein A (RPA), the c-Abl oncoprotein, the tumor suppressor protein p53, and the breast cancer suppressor proteins BRCA1 and BRCA2 (Fig. 5). RAD51 is a DNA-dependent ATPase and is able to pair or transfer complementary strands. RAD51 binds to processed ends (3′ single-stranded tails), forming nucleoprotein filaments. RAD51 nuclear foci have been detected in S phase, and after exposure to ionizing radiation, RAD51 foci coincide with single-stranded DNA, presumably reflecting regions of DNA repair. Human RAD52 binds to DSBs, promotes strand annealing, enhances RAD51 strand-exchange activity, and forms nuclear foci in response to ionizing radiation. RAD54 is a DNA-dependent ATPase and a putative helicase based on sequence similarity to other known helicases. However, RAD54 helicase activity has not been demonstrated, and the ATPase activity appears to be dispensable for some aspects of RAD54 function *in vivo*. RAD54B is a RAD54 homolog of unknown function. XRCC2, XRCC3, and BRCA1 all are required for efficient DSB-induced homologous recombination in mammalian cells. BRCA2 has many RAD51-interaction domains, suggesting that BRCA2 might interact with RAD51 nucleoprotein filaments (i.e., at processed ends of damaged DNA). Recent evidence indicates that BRCA2 has important roles in the repair of DSBs by homologous recombination in mouse and human cells. *XRCC2, XRCC3, BRCA1,* and *BRCA2* mutants all show reduced cellular viability, a specific spectrum of sensitivities to DNA-damaging agents, and chromosomal instability. Replication protein A (RPA) binds single-stranded DNA, is involved in DNA replication and recombination, interacts and colocalizes with RAD51 and RAD52, and stimulates RAD52 strand annealing activity. UBL1 and UBC9 interact with RAD51, RAD52, and with each other, and UBL1 inhibits homologous recombination. Both p53 and c-Abl

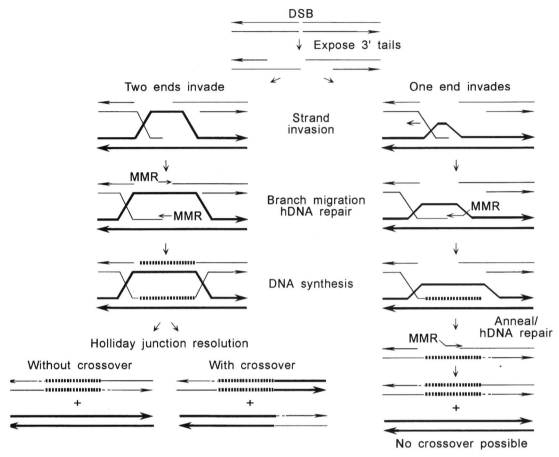

FIGURE 4 Gene conversion models. A DSB is processed to 3′ tails, of which either one or both can invade a homologous duplex (thick lines). hDNA shown by paired thin and thick lines is created by strand invasion and/or branch migration. DNA synthesis (dashed lines) copies information from the donor duplex, and MMR of hDNA results in conversion. On the left, two Holliday junctions are formed; these can be resolved to give crossover or noncrossover products. On the right, no Holliday junctions form and crossovers are not possible. In this model, break repair is effected when newly synthesized DNA separates from the donor duplex and anneals to the non-invading strand. Conversion again reflects MMR of hDNA.

interact with RAD51. c-Abl phosphorylates RAD51, which is required for the formation of DNA damage-induced RAD51 foci. Recombination may be mediated by multiple RAD51-containing protein complexes.

In mammals, NHEJ requires the heterotrimeric DNA-dependent protein kinase (DNA-PK), consisting of Ku70, Ku80, and the DNA-PK catalytic subunit (DNA-PKcs). Ku70 and Ku80 form a dimer with DNA end-binding activity. DNA-PKcs is a kinase that is activated when bound to single-stranded DNA ends of processed DSBs. Defects in Ku or DNA-PKcs confer sensitivity to ionizing radiation and prevent V(D)J recombination. NHEJ requires DNA ligase IV and its associated XRCC4 protein. The RAD50/

MRE11/NBS1 complex is also important for NHEJ; this complex has DNA unwinding and nucleolytic activities, and it forms nuclear foci in irradiated cells that appear to be distinct from RAD51 foci.

Evidence indicates that there are complex relationships among several DNA repair pathways. DNA-PK is a key enzyme in NHEJ, yet it phosphorylates several proteins involved in homologous recombination, including RPA, p53, and ATM, the protein defective in ataxia telangiectasia (AT). p53 and ATM have important roles in checkpoint responses and apoptosis; it is unclear whether DNA-PK phosphorylation of these proteins influences their roles in recombination or other processes. BRCA1 is part of a

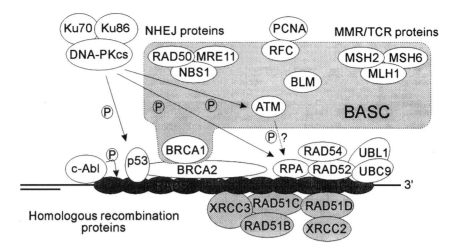

FIGURE 5 Recombination proteins. Homologous recombination proteins are shown clustered around RAD51, which forms a nucleoprotein filament on 3′ tails of processed ends of DSBs. Overlapping symbols represent known protein–protein interactions. Most of the proteins that interact directly or indirectly with RAD51 are known to be involved in homologous recombination. RAD51 paralogs are shown by shaded ovals below. BRCA1 interacts indirectly with RAD51 through BRCA2. BRCA1 is part of the BASC complex (light shading) that includes proteins involved in NHEJ (top left), MMR/TCR (top right, plus BRCA1), DNA replication (RFC), and other aspects of DNA dynamics (ATM, BLM). DNA-PK, a key player in NHEJ, phosphorylates several proteins involved in recombination (arrows). RAD51 is phosphorylated by c-Abl. It is unlikely that RAD51 and its interacting proteins form a single complex; different groups of proteins may associate during different cell-cycle stages, in different cell types, and in response to DNA damage.

large protein complex termed BASC (BRCA1-associated genome surveillance complex) composed of proteins with roles in homologous recombination, NHEJ, and DNA replication, including RAD50, MRE11, NBS1, ATM, BLM (a helicase mutated in Bloom's syndrome), and replication factor C (RFC) which loads PCNA onto DNA. BASC also includes MSH2, MSH6, and MLH1, which are involved in MMR, and in the enhancement of nucleotide excision repair by transcription (transcription coupled repair; TCR). It has been suggested that BASC functions in maintaining genomic integrity during DNA replication and repair of a wide range of DNA damage.

IV. REGULATION OF RECOMBINATION

Recombination levels must be regulated to provide appropriate levels of repair and genome stability. Meiotic and V(D)J recombination are regulated at the level of initiation due to tissue-specific expression of

SPO11 and RAG1/RAG2 endonucleases, respectively. Some recombination genes are expressed at different levels during the cell cycle and/or in response to DNA damage. *RAD51* mRNA is present from late G1 to M, and RAD51 is present in the nucleus from late G1 through G2. RAD51 is most abundant in actively proliferating tissues and during meiosis and is essential for cell viability and genome stability in higher eukaryotes. Together, these results suggest that RAD51 has important roles in replication and DNA repair. BRCA1 and BRCA2 expression patterns are similar to RAD51, and these proteins colocalize with RAD51 in the nucleus. RAD54B is highly expressed in tissues active in meiotic and mitotic recombination, including testis and spleen. *RAD51, RAD52,* and *RAD54* are induced by DNA damage, but it is unclear whether this enhances recombinational repair. *RAD51* or *RAD52* overexpression in mammalian cells increases homologous recombination, but there are no known examples of overexpressed recombination genes causing genomic instability and/or cancer.

p53 suppresses recombination and this might depend on its interaction with RAD51. An alternative (but not mutually exclusive) explanation is that the checkpoint defect in *p53* mutants increases replication-dependent conversion of spontaneous damage to recombinogenic DSBs. The latter idea is consistent with the finding that recombination is also increased in *ATM* mutants, since ATM functions in the p53 checkpoint pathway. The *XRCC9/FANCG* gene is another negative regulator of homologous recombination. Defects in *FANCG* cause the cancer-prone syndrome Fanconi's anemia (FA) and enhance SCE and chromosome instability.

The MMR system suppresses recombination between similar but not identical sequences (termed homeologous recombination). Crossovers also appear to be actively suppressed, perhaps to minimize chromosomal rearrangements and large-scale LOH (Fig. 2). Crossovers are thought to reflect resolution of Holliday junctions (Fig. 4). The paucity of crossovers during ectopic recombination may reflect biased resolution of Holliday junctions or simply the absence of Holliday junctions, as proposed in one-end invasion models (Fig. 4). Crossover interference refers to the observation that a crossover at one locus reduces the probability that a second crossover will occur nearby. The regulation of crossover interference is not well understood but apparently involves the MMR proteins MLH1 and PMS2.

V. RELATIONSHIPS AMONG DNA DAMAGE AND REPAIR, TRANSCRIPTION, AND RECOMBINATION

Numerous studies in bacteria, yeast, and mammalian cells have documented the association of altered recombination phenotypes with altered sensitivities to DNA damaging agents, including X-rays, UV, radiomimetic chemicals, and other DNA-reactive chemicals such as alkylating and crosslinking agents. Many types of single-strand DNA damage, including UV dimers, strongly enhance recombination. Transcription enhances nucleotide excision repair of UV damage (TCR), and transcription also enhances recombination. Since nucleotide excision repair creates strand breaks and exposes short single-stranded regions, it was reasonable to suppose that this repair pathway might stimulate recombination. However, even though both transcription and UV individually enhance recombination, transcription reduces levels of UV-induced recombination, suggesting that TCR removes recombinogenic UV lesions. Similarly, mutant cells with defects in UV repair display increased levels of recombination. These results indicate that UV damage, not its repair, is recombinogenic.

Double-strand damage including DSBs and gaps present the cell with a different repair problem than single-strand damage since there is no immediately available repair template. Homologous recombination provides a high-fidelity system for repairing double-strand damage. In contrast to the results with UV, recombination is usually reduced or absent in cells hypersensitive to ionizing radiation, underscoring the importance of recombinational mechanisms for repairing double-strand damage.

MMR helps maintain genomic integrity by correcting replication errors and by inhibiting homeologous recombination. This inhibition may involve scanning hDNA to determine the number of mismatches and aborting recombination if too many are detected. By inhibiting homeologous recombination, the MMR system maintains differences between members of gene families and minimizes chromosomal rearrangements. Thus, in addition to increasing mutation rates, MMR defects may increase cancer risk by enhancing recombination between diverged, repetitive elements (revealed as chromosome instability).

VI. LOSS OF HETEROZYGOSITY

LOH at several target genes is now well documented in tumors. First identified at the *RB* locus in retinoblastoma, many tumors display LOH at any of a number of tumor suppressor genes, including *p53*, *WT1* (Wilm's tumor), the neurofibromatosis type 1 gene, and the human nonpolyposis colon cancer MMR genes. Because mutant p53 proteins can be dominant negative, LOH is not required at the *p53* locus to lose tumor suppressor activity. However, LOH at *p53* is quite common in many tumor types. Both copies of *RB* must be inactivated to lose *RB* activity. LOH at

RB has been confirmed or is suspected in many cancers besides retinoblastoma, including breast cancer, small and large cell lung, and squamous cell lung cancers, osteosarcoma, and hepatocellular cancer. Individuals with a heterozygous tumor suppressor gene, such as *RB*, are strongly predisposed to cancer. Loss of function by LOH can occur by simple deletion, reciprocal recombination, or gene conversion. Although it is also possible for LOH to arise by nondisjunction or replication error-mediated mutagenesis, these processes occur at lower rates than recombination. As might be expected, recombination-dependent LOH is more prevalent in rapidly growing cells. This observation provides at least a partial explanation as to why persons heterozygous for a tumor suppressor develop variable but somewhat localized cancers. It has been suggested that many human cancers may be initiated by loss of tumor suppressor function (except lymphomas and leukemias, which are often initiated by oncogene activation). Alternatively, LOH may occur during tumor progression as a consequence of genomic instability.

VII. CANCER PREDISPOSITION AND DEFECTS IN DNA REPAIR AND RECOMBINATION

Several inherited human diseases that predispose to cancer exhibit hallmarks of DNA repair deficiencies and show altered recombination phenotypes. These include xeroderma pigmentosum (XP), FA, Bloom's syndrome (BS), and AT. XP is comprised of at least 7 complementation groups (termed A–G), all of which are hypersensitive to UV and show increased sister chromatid exchange (SCE) upon UV exposure. XP patients are extremely photosensitive and usually develop multiple skin cancers. Another UV repair disorder, Cockayne's syndrome (CS), shows some overlap with XP group G, both being defective in preferential repair of UV damage in transcribed DNA. However, CS patients do not show an increased incidence of cancer. CS cells are hypersensitive to ionizing radiation due to defective preferential repair of ionizing radiation damage; none of the XP groups show this sensitivity, although XP group G is very deficient in overall genomic repair. Thus, the increased

cancer incidence in XP is not simply a consequence of increased mutagenesis due to defective repair. Instead, the XP defect, but not that in CS, may lead to increased genome instability.

BS cells exhibit several abnormal phenotypes, including increased mutation rates, increased cytogenetic abnormalities including SCE, and elevated recombination levels. FA cells are hypersensitive to crosslinking agents and show increased SCE. AT cells are markedly hypersensitive to the cytotoxic but not the mutagenic effects of ionizing radiation. This sensitivity is associated with a lack of the normal G1-S checkpoint following irradiation. However, the G2 checkpoint is intact in AT cells, and they are not defective in DSB repair. AT cells show 100-fold higher mitotic recombination rates than normal cells. Increased recombination-mediated mutagenesis, revealed by marked genomic instability, may account for the increased cancer incidence in BS, FA, and AT patients.

Defects in RAD51 have not been correlated with cancer, perhaps reflecting the essential role of RAD51 in DNA replication. However, several proteins that interact with RAD51 are associated with cancer, including BRCA1 and BRCA2 (but not RAD52). Defects in RAD54 and RAD54B are associated with several tumor types. *RAD54* shows frequent LOH in breast tumors, although no coding sequence mutations have been found. The *RAD54B* locus is associated with chromosomal abnormalities in cancer cells, and homozygous mutations have been demonstrated in colon tumors and lymphoma. LOH at *RAD51*, *RAD52*, *RAD54*, *BRCA1*, and *BRCA2* is seen in breast cancer, and LOH at more than one of these loci predicts a poor prognosis.

VIII. CHROMOSOME TRANSLOCATIONS

Early cytogenetic studies showed that specific translocations are common in particular cancers. Subsequent molecular analyses showed that translocations in some tumors involve transfer of an oncogene from a transcriptionally inactive locus to an active locus, or inactivation of a tumor suppressor gene. A classic example of oncogene activation is seen in Burkitt's lymphoma, in which *myc* is translocated from chromosome 8 to an expressed locus within the chromosome 14 immunoglobulin genes. These translocations probably result from errors during recombination of immunoglobulin genes in T and B cells, since they are usually seen in lymphoid tissues. In other cases, translocation mechanisms are unclear, but they may involve site-specific recombination errors, homologous recombination between DNA repeats, or nonhomologous recombination. Translocation breakpoints in tumor cells have been used to identified new oncogenes and tumor suppressor genes.

IX. GENE AMPLIFICATION AND TUMORIGENESIS

Amplifications of oncogenes such as *myc*, *myb*, *ras*, *ets*, and *erb2* are common in cancer cells. Amplified genes often occur on small, circular copies of autonomous chromatin bodies (double-minutes; DMs), but also may occur in chromosomal DNA (termed heterogenously staining regions; HSR). Amplification is greatly enhanced in cells mutant for *p53*. Increased expression of growth-promoting oncogenes by amplification provides a growth advantage to transformed cells both *in vitro* and *in vivo*. Amplification can reduce the efficacy of chemotherapeutic treatment, one example being the amplification of *DHFR* in cells treated with the anticancer folate inhibitor, methotrexate.

Mechanistic details of gene amplification are beginning to be elucidated, primarily due to studies of *DHFR*. Amplified regions (amplicons) seen in HSRs are very large (30 to 450 Mbp), and are often >10-fold larger than the amplified gene. Amplicons occur in large arrays of head-to-head/tail-to-tail repeats with perfect junctions. Arrays are usually present on the same chromosome as the original gene (which remains intact), but at distant sites and often are near telomeres. DM structure has been more difficult to characterize, although DMs usually have one or a few amplicons that are ≥1 Mbp. In DMs with multiple amplicons, repeat organization is usually different from that seen in HSRs. Amplified DNA is generated experimentally by incremental increases in drug concentration. However, even at the earliest stages of

amplification in low drug concentrations, extremely large regions of DNA are amplified (up to 15 Mbp). Amplification is enhanced in cells pretreated with a variety of DNA damaging agents, which may explain the limited success of chemotherapy after radiotherapy with some tumors (e.g., head and neck).

These features, especially perfect repeat structures and enhancement by DNA damage, though not incompatible with an early hypothesis suggesting that amplification involves over-replication and reintegration, are more easily explained by recombinational pathways. One model for HSR genesis suggests that amplification initiates when a chromosome is broken (perhaps during an aborted topoisomerase exchange) leading to sister chromatid fusion. The resulting dicentric chromosome is likely to break in the next mitosis. Amplification would then result from repeated rounds of chromosome breakage and fusion. One possibility is that DMs are intermediates in HSR formation, but an alternative model suggests that they arise by interstitial deletion. Selection of a gene carried by a DM that confers a growth advantage can increase DM copy number due to missegregation during mitosis.

Bibliography

Barton, N. H., and Charlesworth, B. (1998). Why sex and recombination? *Science* **281**, 1986–1990.

Benson, F. E., Baumann, P., and West, S. C. (1998). Synergistic actions of Rad51 and Rad52 in recombination and DNA repair. *Nature* **391**, 401–404.

Bhattacharyya, N. P., Maher, V. M., and McCormick, J. J. (1990). Effect of nucleotide excision repair in human cells on intrachromosomal homologous recombination induced by UV and 1-nitrosopyrene. *Mol. Cell. Biol.* **10**, 3945–3951.

Critchlow, S. E., and Jackson, S. P. (1998). DNA end-joining: From yeast to man. *Trends Biochem. Sci.* **23**, 394–398.

Deng, W. P., and Nickoloff, J. A. (1994). Preferential repair of UV damage in highly transcribed DNA diminishes UV-induced intrachromosomal recombination in mammalian cells. *Mol. Cell. Biol.* **14**, 391–399.

Gonzalez, R., Silva, J. M., Dominguez, G., Garcia, J. M., Martinez, G., Vargas, J., Provencio, M., Espana, P., and Bonilla, F. (1999). Detection of loss of heterozygosity at *RAD51*, *RAD52*, *RAD54* and *BRCA1* and *BRCA2* loci in breast cancer: Pathological correlations. *Brit. J. Cancer* **81**, 503–509.

Hanawalt, P. C. (1994). Evolution of concepts in DNA repair. *Environ. Mol. Mutagens* **23(Suppl. 24)**, 78–85.

Knudson, A. G. (1993). Antioncogenes and human cancer. *Proc. Natl. Acad. Sci. USA* **90**, 10914–10921.

Kong, Q. Z., Harris, R. S., and Maizels, N. (1998). Recombination-based mechanisms for somatic hypermutation. *Immunol. Rev.* **162,** 67–76.

Ramsden, D. A., van Gent, D. C., and Gellert, M. (1997). Specificity in V(D)J recombination: New lessons from biochemistry and genetics. *Curr. Opin. Immunol.* **9,** 114–120.

Rothstein, R., Michel, B., and Gangloff, S. (2000). Replication fork pausing and recombination or "gimme a break." *Genes Dev.* **14,** 1–10.

Schwab, M. (1998). Amplification of oncogenes in human cancer cells. *Bioessays* **20,** 473–479.

Steen, S. B., Zhu, C. M., and Roth, D. B. (1996). Double-strand breaks, DNA hairpins, and the mechanism of V(D)J recombination. *Curr. Topics Microbiol. Immunol.* **217,** 61–77.

Swagemakers, S. M. A., Essers, J., de Wit, J., Hoeijmakers, J. H. J., and Kanaar, R. (1998). The human Rad54 recombinational DNA repair protein is a double-stranded DNA-dependent ATPase. *J. Biol. Chem.* **273,** 28292–28297.

Taghian, D. G., and Nickoloff, J. A. (1997). Chromosomal double-strand breaks induce gene conversion at high frequency in mammalian cells. *Mol. Cell. Biol.* **17,** 6386–6393.

Thacker, J. (1999). A surfeit of RAD51-like genes? *Trends Genet.* **15,** 166–168.

Tlsty, T. D. (1997). Genomic instability and its role in neoplasia. *Curr. Topics Microbiol. Immunol.* **221,** 37–46.

Wang, Y., Cortez, D., Yazdi, Y., Neff, N., Elledge, S. J., and Qin, J. (2000). BASC, a super complex of BRCA1-associated proteins involved in the recognition and repair of aberrant DNA structures. *Genes Dev.* **14,** 927–939.

Renal Cell Cancer

Joseph P. Grande
Mary E. Fidler

Mayo Foundation, Rochester, Minnesota

I. Introduction
II. Clinical Epidemiology of Renal Cancer
III. Pathologic Features of Renal Tumors
IV. Prognostic Features
V. Clinical Correlations
VI. Diagnosis
VII. Management

GLOSSARY

adenocarcinoma A malignant tumor arising from glandular epithelium. The vast majority of renal tumors are adenocarcinomas. These tumors have a capacity to metastasize.

adenoma A benign tumor arising from glandular epithelium. By definition, adenomas lack the capacity to metastasize.

grade The pathologic assessment of a tumor based on the degree of cytologic and architectural differentiation and the number of mitoses.

metastasis A tumor implant in a site that is discontinuous with the primary tumor.

papillary A pattern of tumor growth characterized by finger-like projections lined by a single layer of neoplastic epithelial cells.

stage The clinical pathologic assessment of a tumor based on the size of the primary lesion, the extent of spread to regional structures, and the presence or absence of distant metastases.

A variety of tumors may arise in the kidneys, which vary widely in clinical significance. In adults, the most common form of malignant renal tumor is the adenocarcinoma, which arises from tubular epithelium. In part because the kidneys are located in the retroperitoneum, renal cell adenocarcinomas are characterized by a lack of early clinical warning signs; a substantial proportion of patients with renal cancer present with disseminated metastases. At present, surgical removal of renal cell adenocarcinomas is the only effective means of curing the disease, as these tumors are resistant to standard chemotherapy and radiation therapy. A potential role for immunotherapy in treating advanced renal cell cancer is being evaluated. Increased utilization of radiologic imaging techniques has led to the identification of small renal lesions in asymptomatic patients.

Early detection of renal tumors has prompted the development of objective criteria for the classification of renal tumors of low and high metastatic potential and the establishment of uniformly accepted pathologic features of prognostic significance. Studies of patients with inherited predisposition to developing renal cell cancer have greatly contributed to our understanding of the pathogenesis of renal cell carcinoma. Inherited mutations in different genes predispose to the development of histologically distinct types of renal cancer. These studies provide support for the inclusion of genetic alterations in the histopathologic classification of renal tumors.

I. INTRODUCTION

Most renal parenchymal neoplasms in adults are renal cell adenocarcinomas. Over 30,600 new cases of renal cell carcinoma are diagnosed and approximately 12,000 people die from this disease per year. Renal cell carcinoma accounts for 1 to 3% of all visceral cancers reported annually and approximately 2% of cancer deaths per year. The incidence of renal cell cancer in the United States has increased by about 2% per year since 1970. Although renal cell carcinoma may affect individuals of any age, this tumor most commonly presents in individuals in the fifth to seventh decades of life. Renal cell carcinoma is more common in males than in females (ratio 2–3:1). Because small renal cell carcinomas do not typically produce any significant clinical signs or symptoms, many patients with newly diagnosed renal cell carcinoma present with metastatic disease. Because complete surgical resection of these tumors is the only effective means of curing this disease and it is not cost-effective to perform radiologic screening studies on the entire population, recent efforts at cancer prevention have focused on the identification of patients who are at increased risk of developing renal cell carcinoma.

II. CLINICAL EPIDEMIOLOGY OF RENAL CANCER

The most important known environmental risk factor for the development of renal cell carcinoma is to-bacco. Cigarette smokers have twice the incidence of renal cell carcinoma as nonsmokers. Cigarette smoking may contribute to as many as one-third of all cases of renal cancer. It should be noted that this risk far exceeds that attributable to inherited forms of renal cell carcinoma. Other risk factors include obesity, hypertension, unopposed estrogen therapy, and exposure to asbestos, petroleum products, dry cleaning solvents, and heavy metals. Patients with chronic renal failure and acquired cystic disease also have an increased risk of developing renal cell carcinoma. Half of patients on long-term dialysis develop acquired cystic disease, and 10% of these develop renal cell carcinoma. Papillary hyperplasia is a consistent finding in patients with acquired cystic disease, which may be a precursor of renal cell carcinomas. Dietary factors (a high-fat, low fruit and vegetable diet) have been associated with an increased risk of developing renal cell carcinoma. Citrus fruits, vitamin C, β-carotene, and α-tocopherol have demonstrated a protective effect against renal cell cancer.

Studies of patients with an inherited predisposition to developing renal cell carcinoma have led to the identification of several critical genes involved in renal carcinogenesis. These familial forms of renal cancer are thought to account for approximately 4% of all renal cancers. In general, these syndromes are inherited in an autosomal-dominant manner, with incomplete penetrance. Renal tumors in affected family members often occur at a young age and are often multicentric and bilateral.

III. PATHOLOGIC FEATURES OF RENAL TUMORS

The most clinically relevant criterion for the classification of renal tumors is based on the potential to develop disseminated metastases. Application of molecular cytogenetics to the study of renal tumors has prompted a reevaluation and reclassification of these tumors based on the correlation of histologic appearance with characteristic cytogenetic alterations. By definition, renal adenomas are benign tumors with no capacity to metastasize. The clear cell variant is the most common form of renal cell carcinoma. This histologic variance is characteristically associated with abnormalities in the short arm of chromosome 3 (3p). Several other histologic forms of renal cell carcinoma are associated with different risks of metastatic dissemination and are briefly discussed.

A. Renal Adenoma

Renal adenomas are the most common neoplasms of renal tubular epithelium and are frequent incidental findings in adult kidneys. Although renal adenomas are easily distinguished from fluid-filled simple cysts (which are also commonly found in adults) by ultrasonography, it may be difficult to differentiate large renal adenomas from renal cell carcinoma. These neoplasms are found within the cortex as pale yellow-gray discrete nodules. Microscopically, renal cortical adenomas consist of complex, branching tubular and papillary structures lined by a single layer of cells. These cells are bland appearing, with small, regular nuclei and scanty cytoplasm (Fig. 1). The cytologic appearance of renal adenomas may be indistinguishable from that of low-grade papillary renal cell carcinomas. Size

alone does not determine whether a renal tumor is a benign adenoma or a renal cell carcinoma. Although lesions less than 3 cm in diameter rarely metastasize, metastatic lesions have been associated with primary tumors as small as 1 cm in diameter. The presence of clear cells, mitotic activity, cell stratification, or necrosis in a lesion of any size should prompt a diagnosis of a renal cell carcinoma. Papillary renal adenomas contain cytogenetic abnormalities (trisomy 7 and 17, loss of the Y chromosome in males) that are similar to, but less extensive than, abnormalities found in papillary renal cell carcinomas.

B. Oncocytoma

Oncocytomas are relatively uncommon tumors, comprising approximately 5% of all renal tubular neoplasms. Oncocytomas are well-circumscribed, mahogany brown, solid lesions that characteristically have a central stellate scar. These tumors are usually solitary, although they may be large (greater than 12 cm in diameter). Hemorrhage and necrosis are rarely

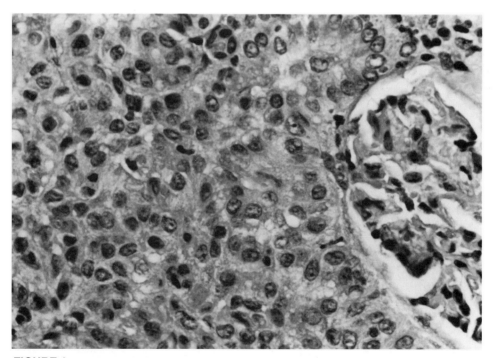

FIGURE 1 Renal cortical adenoma. This tumor was identified as an incidental lesion in a nephrectomy specimen obtained from a patient with a renal cell carcinoma involving another region of the kidney. The tumor cells are small, with scanty cytoplasm and small nuclei; nucleoli are not apparent. A normal glomerulus (right) is adjacent to the tumor.

observed. Histologically, oncocytomas are composed of nests, cords, and tubular structures made up of large polygonal cells with a brightly eosinophilic, granular cytoplasm (Fig. 2). Nuclei are usually small and uniform; mitotic figures are rare or absent. The cells are rich in mitochondria. This tumor is derived from intercalated cells of the collecting ducts. Cytogenetic studies have shown several characteristic alterations in patients with oncocytomas. One alteration is characterized by the loss of chromosome 1p (the short arm of chromosome 1); another type is characterized by somatic chromosome translocations with 11q13 as the common breakpoint. Loss of the Y chromosome in males is also frequently observed. However, abnormalities in chromosome 3p, which are frequently observed in renal cell carcinoma, have not been identified in oncocytomas. Abnormalities in mitochondrial DNA have been observed in some oncocytomas. There have been several case reports of patients with bilateral, multiple renal oncocytomas. These families appear to have an inherited predisposition to developing renal oncocytomas. Renal oncocytomas are considered to have low malignant potential; recurrence or metastasis is rare.

C. Clear Cell Carcinoma

The most common histologic type of renal cell carcinoma is the clear cell variant, which is seen in approximately 70% of cases. Renal cell carcinomas are generally well-defined, spherical masses with irregular margins (Fig. 3). These lesions have a variable appearance, with colors ranging from pale or bright yellow to orange, gray, or tan. Regions of hemorrhage or necrosis are commonly observed. Normal renal parenchyma at the edges of these tumors is frequently compressed, giving rise to the impression that the tumor is surrounded by a capsule. However, there is invariably microscopic evidence of invasion. Renal cell carcinomas have a propensity to invade the renal vein. Infrequently, this tumor may grow from the renal vein to the vena cava and may present clinically with symptoms attributable to tumor invasion of the right atrium.

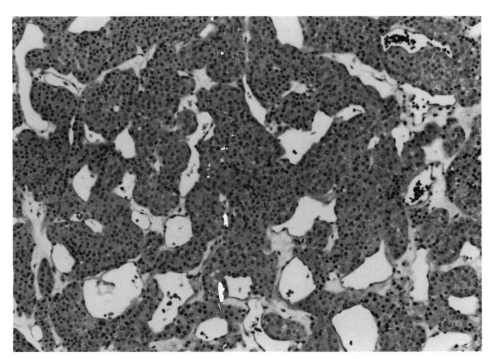

FIGURE 2 Renal oncocytoma. The tumor is composed of nests of cells with an abundant granular cytoplasm. Nuclei are small, round, and regular.

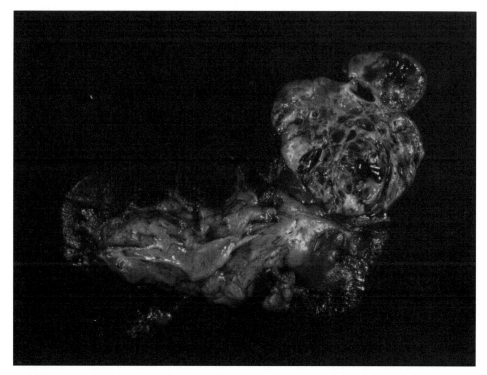

FIGURE 3 Renal cell carcinoma, gross appearance. This 7-cm neoplasm arises from the upper pole of the left kidney. Central areas of hemorrhage and small foci of necrosis are identified.

Clear cell carcinomas are characterized by sheets or acini of round cells with abundant clear cytoplasm (Fig. 4). The clear cell appearance is due to the presence of abundant quantities of glycogen and fat, which can be identified by appropriate histochemical stains. Clear cell carcinomas arise from proximal tubular epithelium. These tumors stain for epithelial markers such as keratin, epithelial membrane antigen, and carcinoembryonic antigen. Renal cell carcinomas, but not normal renal tubular epithelium, are vimentin positive. Both sporadic and familial renal cell carcinomas of this histologic subtype are frequently associated with abnormalities in the short arm of chromosome 3 (chromosome 3p); a variety of other cytogenetic alterations have been identified. Clinical stage is the most important prognostic determinate in patients with clear cell carcinoma, although pathologic grading of these lesions appears to provide additional information. Sarcomatoid changes can be seen in approximately 5% of patients with renal cell carcinoma; this finding is associated with a poor prognosis.

D. Papillary Renal Cell Carcinoma

Papillary renal cell carcinomas are the second most common carcinoma of renal tubular epithelium, comprising approximately 10–15% of cases. These tumors are thought to arise from distal tubular epithelium. Papillary carcinomas are soft, tan, well-circumscribed lesions that may contain large areas of necrosis (Fig. 5). By light microscopy, the tumor forms complex tubules and papillary structures lined by a single layer of cuboidal cells with a delicate fibrous core. This core is highly vascular and often contains lipid-laden macrophages (Fig. 6). Papillary renal cell carcinomas do not have abnormalities of chromosome 3p, which is characteristic of the clear cell forms of renal cell carcinoma. Other cytogenetic abnormalities include trisomy 7, trisomy 16, trisomy 17, and loss of the Y chromosome in males. Other trisomies, involving chromosomes 3q, 12, and 20, have also been reported. The clinical outcome of patients with papillary renal cell carcinoma tends to be better than that of patients with other forms of renal cell carcinoma.

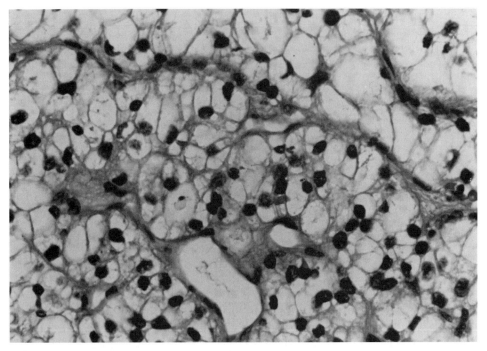

FIGURE 4 Renal cell carcinoma, clear cell variant. Large clusters of cells with abundant clear cytoplasm are separated by a highly vascular stroma.

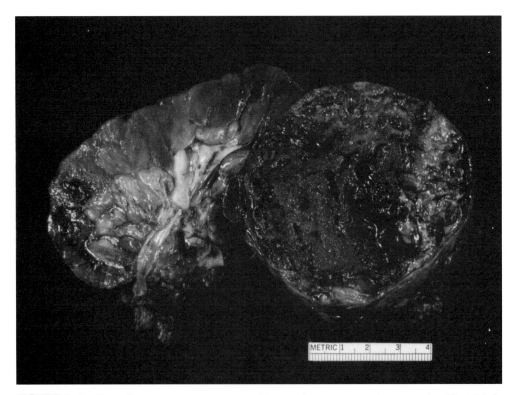

FIGURE 5 Papillary cell carcinoma, gross appearance. This neoplasm arises from the upper pole of the left kidney and grossly appears to be well encapsulated. On cut section, the tumor contains a large area of central necrosis and hemorrhage.

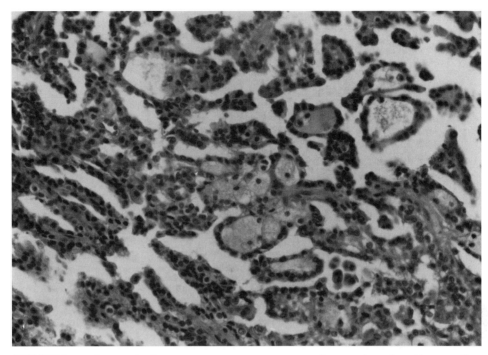

FIGURE 6 Papillary renal cell carcinoma, microscopic appearance. The tumor forms finger-like or papillary projections lined by a single layer of cuboidal cells with a delicate fibrovascular core. The large cells within the fibrous core are lipid-laden macrophages.

E. Chromophobe Renal Cell Carcinoma

The chromophobe renal cell carcinoma is the third most common cancer involving renal tubular epithelium, accounting for approximately 5% of cases. This tumor consists of cells arranged in solid and tubular patterns. Unlike the clear cell variant of renal cell carcinoma, chromophobe tumors lack abundant lipid or glycogen and contain numerous cytoplasmic vesicles, approximately 150–300 nm in diameter. The cytoplasm tends to condense near the cell membrane, producing a perinuclear halo (Fig. 7). The cells vary widely in size. Chromophobe renal cell carcinoma is characterized by monosomy of multiple chromosomes, including 1, 2, 6, 10, 13, 17, and 21, and hypodiploidy. In general, patients with these tumors have a good prognosis.

F. Other Variants of Renal Cell Carcinoma

A few additional histologic variants of renal cell carcinoma have been identified. In general, these variants are rare, accounting for less than 1% of renal cell carcinomas. Collecting duct carcinomas are located within the medullary portion of the kidney. These carcinomas are firm, gray-white lesions with infiltrating borders. The tumor cells are arranged as infiltrating tumors and papillary structures with a dense stromal desmoplastic response. Cells are large and cuboidal, with a moderately high nuclear grade. Unlike conventional renal cell carcinoma, collecting duct carcinoma cells produce mucin. Clinically, these lesions tend to present with gross hematuria. It is important to distinguish collecting duct carcinomas from other variants because these tumors tend to be aggressive, with early metastases a characteristic feature. Medullary carcinoma of the kidney is an aggressive tumor arising from collecting ducts and is associated with sickle cell trait. A number of cytogenetic abnormalities have been reported, including monosomy 11.

IV. PROGNOSTIC FEATURES

A. Pathologic Stage

Prognostic determinants of patients with renal cell carcinoma include stage, grade, cell type, and histologic

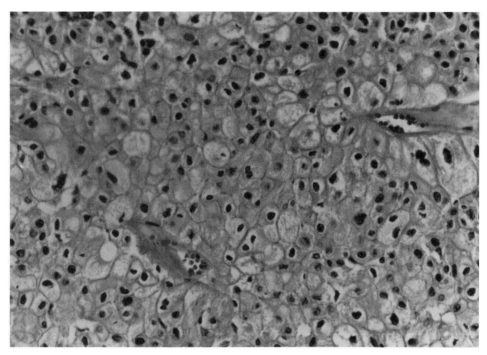

FIGURE 7 Chromophobe renal cell carcinoma, microscopic appearance. Tumor consists of cells of variable size containing prominent perinuclear "halos."

pattern. Because surgical removal is the only effective means of curing the disease, the pathologic stage, which defines the anatomic spread of the tumor at time of surgery, is the single most important factor that predicts outcome in patients with renal cell carcinoma. The two most commonly used staging systems for renal cell carcinoma are the Robson classification and the Union Internationale Contre Cancer (UICC). A summary of the two classification schemes is shown in Table I. The Robson classification is a four-stage system. The UICC employs a TNM system for tumor staging, where T refers to primary tumor size, N to regional lymph nodes, and M to metastasis. Using either system, 5-year survival is inversely correlated with the pathologic stage. Invasion of perinephric fat or regional lymph nodes adversely affects prognosis; less than one-third of patients with regional lymph node metastasis survive 5 years. Renal cell carcinomas have a propensity to invade the renal vein, the inferior vena cava, and even the right atrium. In patients without perinephric fat or lymph node invasion, several studies have suggested that involvement of the renal vein or inferior vena cava does not

adversely affect survival, provided that the tumor is completely resected; 5-year survival approaches 50% in these cases. Patients with distant metastasis (stage IV) have a poor prognosis, with 5-year survival rates of less than 10%. Following radical nephrectomy, 10–30% of patients with localized tumors relapse. Less than 5% have local recurrence, whereas lung metastases are the most common sites of distant relapse, occurring in over half of patients. The median time to relapse is 15–18 months; 85% of relapses occur within 3 years. No recognized systemic therapy reduces the likelihood of relapse.

B. Pathologic Grade

Several schemes have been developed to correlate morphologic features of renal cell carcinoma with clinical outcome. The most widely employed grading schemes emphasize nuclear architecture. Low-grade neoplasms tend to have small (10 μm), regular nuclei with a fine, delicate chromatin pattern and inconspicuous nucleoli; mitoses are rare. Large nuclei, nucleoli pleomorphism, prominent nuclei, and abun-

TABLE I
Staging of Renal Cell Carcinoma by the
Robson and UICC Classification[a]

	Robson	UICC
Small tumor, confined to capsule	I	T1
Large tumor, confined to capsule, distortion of calices	I	T2
Extension to perirenal fat or ipsilateral adrenal gland	II	T3a
Renal vein involvement	IIIa	T3b
Renal vein + vena cava involvement	IIIa	T3c
Vena cava involved above diaphragm	IIIa	T4b
Single ipsilateral lymph node involved	IIIb	N1
Multiple regional, contralateral lymph nodes involved	IIIb	N2
Fixed regional nodes	IIIb	N3
Juxtaregional lymph nodes	IIIb	N4
Spread to contiguous organs except ipsilateral adrenal gland	IVa	T4a
Distant metastases	IVb	M1

[a]Adapted from Thrasher and Paulson (1993).

dant mitotic activity are associated with high-grade renal cell carcinomas. Using various grading schemes, it has been possible to group patients into those with a favorable prognosis and those with an unfavorable prognosis, even after correcting for pathologic stage. Many of the differences in survival observed in patients with different histologic subtypes of renal cell carcinoma may be attributed to differences in pathologic grade. For example, papillary renal cell carcinomas, which are associated with a good prognosis, typically are grade 1 lesions, whereas sarcomatoid renal carcinomas, which are associated with a poor prognosis, are almost always grade 4 lesions.

C. DNA Content

Several clinical pathologic studies have demonstrated that DNA content may be useful in predicting patient outcome. Analysis of tumors by DNA flow cytometry may be performed to categorize lesions as diploid (normal DNA content) or aneuploid (abnormal DNA content). Aneuploid lesions have been associated with decreased survival, whereas diploid tumors indicate a favorable prognosis. However, it is not clear that DNA content is an independent prognostic determinant of survival. DNA content tends to correlate with tumor grade and stage.

V. CLINICAL CORRELATIONS

The classic triad of urologic symptoms (costovertebral pain, palpable mass, and hematuria) is only found in approximately 15% of patients with renal cell carcinoma. Hematuria is the most common clinical manifestation of renal cell carcinoma, followed by abdominal mass, pain, and weight loss. Hematuria may be absent in over half of patients with renal cell carcinoma. These tumors may be associated with a constant, dull, aching pain arising in the flank or abdomen. Renal colic may be present, secondary to the passage of blood clots into the urine. Systemic symptoms of weight loss, fever, or hypertension may also be seen. Renal cell carcinoma is associated with a number of paraneoplastic syndromes due to peptide production by the tumor cells. Paraneoplastic syndromes are observed in up to 25% of patients with renal cell carcinoma. Frequent associations include hypertension, Cushing's syndrome, polycythemia, hypercalcemia, and hepatic dysfunction.

As many as 25% of patients with renal cell carcinoma present clinically with distant metastases. Renal cell carcinoma metastasizes by both lymphatic and hematogenous routes. Renal cell carcinoma most frequently metastasizes to the lung (50% of cases); metastases to regional and distant liver nodes, liver, and bone are also frequently observed. Metastatic renal cell carcinoma has been identified in almost every organ, including those rarely involved by metastatic tumors.

VI. DIAGNOSIS

The increased use of imaging techniques such as ultrasonography and computerized tomographic (CT) scanning has led to earlier diagnosis of renal tumors. Because clinical stage is the most important prognostic determinant, it would be expected that earlier diagnosis would lead to increased survival in patients with this tumor. Because it is not economically feasible to employ current radiologic imaging techniques to screen the general population for the presence of incidental renal cell carcinomas, it is important to identify individuals who are at increased risk of developing this tumor. Many of these patients can be identified through a careful family history and evaluation for extrarenal manifestations of an inherited cancer syndrome such as von Hippel–Lindau disease. In asymptomatic patients evaluated for other conditions, radiologic imaging techniques are frequently employed to distinguish renal cell carcinoma from other lesions that do not require surgical intervention. One important diagnostic feature of renal cancers is that the image intensity is enhanced following the administration of intravenous contrast material, which reflects the increased vascularity of these tumors. Ultrasonography is useful in distinguishing fluid-filled simple cysts from solid renal neoplasms. Although oncocytomas characteristically have a central stellate scar, it may be difficult to distinguish oncocytomas from renal cell carcinomas by routine radiologic imaging studies.

VII. MANAGEMENT

Surgical excision is the only effective treatment of renal cell carcinoma. In patients with a solitary metastasis, surgical intervention may improve survival. Renal cell carcinomas are resistant to radiation therapy and to standard chemotherapy. Immunotherapy has been employed in treating advanced renal cell carcinoma. Interleukin (IL)-2 has been approved by the U.S. Food and Drug Administration for the treatment of advanced renal cell carcinoma. Response rates to IL-2 are on the order of 15%, with a complete response rate of only 5%. High-dose IL-2 therapy is associated with severe and potentially life-threatening toxicity (pulmonary edema, hypotension, renal insufficiency, multiorgan system failure). IL-2 affects tumor growth by activating lymphoid cells *in vivo* without affecting tumor proliferation directly. Concomitant administration of lymphocytes primed *ex vivo* with IL-2 has not improved survival. Interferon-α has also been employed as an immunotherapeutic agent. Interferons have a direct antiproliferative effect on renal tumor cells *in vitro*, stimulate host mononuclear cells, and enhance the expression of major histocompatibility complex molecules. The overall response to interferon-α is on the order of 10%, with only a 1% complete response. Combination therapies employing interferon-α plus 13-*cis* retinoic acid have shown somewhat increased response rates. Experimental protocols using gene therapy are in their initial phases.

The management of small (less than 3 cm) incidental renal lesions detected by radiologic studies often performed for other reasons is not without controversy. Clinical observations indicate that most of these lesions grow slowly and do not seem to metastasize until they obtain a size greater than 3–4 cm. However, disseminated metastases have been found in patients with primary lesions as small as 1 cm. Other factors, such as age, ability to undergo surgery, and presence of other significant diseases, will play an important role in the optimal management of patients with small incidental renal lesions.

See Also the Following Articles

Bladder Cancer: Epidemiology • Kidney, Epidemiology • Liver Cancer: Etiology and Prevention • Pancreatic Cancer: Cellular and Molecular Mechanisms • Prostate Cancer • Thyroid Cancer • Tobacco Carcinogenesis

Bibliography

Gelb, A. (1997). Renal cell carcinoma: Current prognostic factors. *Cancer* **80,** 981–986.

Godley, P., and Escobar, M. (1998). Renal cell carcinoma. *Curr. Opin. Oncol.* **10,** 261–265.

Kovacs, G., Akhtar, M., Beckwith, B., *et al.* (1997). The Heidelberg classification of renal cell tumours. *J. Pathol.* **183,** 131–133.

Lanigan, D., Conroy, R., Barry-Walsh, C., Loftus, B., Royston, D., and Leader, M. (1994). A comparative analysis of grading systems in renal adenocarcinoma. *Histopathology* **24,** 473–476.

Motzer, R., Bander, N., and Nanus, D. (1996). Medical progress: Renal cell carcinoma. *N. Engl. J. Med.* **335,** 865–875.

Savage, P. (1996). Renal cell carcinoma. *Curr. Opin. Oncol.* **8,** 247–251.

Thrasher, J., and Paulson, D. (1993). Prognostic factors in renal cancer. *Urol. Clin. North Am.* **20,** 247–262.

Vogelzang, N., and Stadler, W. (1998). Kidney cancer. *Lancet* **352,** 1691–1696.

Replication-Selective Viruses for Cancer Treatment

Lynda K. Hawkins
David Kirn
Cancer Research UK

T his article reviews the discovery and development of replication-selective oncolytic viruses, with an emphasis on recently acquired data from phase I and II clinical trials with an attenuated adenovirus. The goal is to summarize (1) the genetic targets and mechanisms of selectivity for these agents; (2) clinical trial data and what it has taught us to date about the promise but also the potential hurdles to be over-come with this approach; and (3) future approaches to overcome these hurdles.

I. INTRODUCTION

The clinical utility of any cancer treatment is defined by both its antitumoral potency and its therapeutic index between cancerous and normal cells. Most currently available therapies for metastatic solid tumors fail on one or both of these counts. Countless changes in dose, frequency, and/or combinations of standard cytotoxic chemotherapies or radiotherapy have not overcome the inherent resistance to these approaches. Although standard chemotherapies and radiotherapy target a variety of different structures within cancer cells, almost all of them kill cancer cells through the induction of apoptosis. Not surprisingly, therefore, apoptosis-resistant clones almost universally develop following standard therapy for metastatic solid epithelial cancers (e.g., nonsmall cell lung, colon, breast, prostate, and pancreatic), even if numerous high-dose chemotherapeutic agents are used in combination. The overall survival rates for most metastatic solid tumors have changed relatively little despite decades of work with this approach (adjuvant therapy in contrast, applied by definition when tumor burden is low, has resulted in clinically significant improvements in mortality). Novel therapeutic approaches must therefore have not only greater potency and greater selectivity than currently available treatments, they should also have novel mechanisms of action that will not lead to cross-resistance with existing approaches (i.e., do not rely exclusively on apoptosis induction in cancer cells).

Tumor-targeted oncolytic viruses (virotherapy with replication-selective viruses) have the potential to fulfill these criteria. Viruses have evolved over millions of years to infect target cells, multiply, cause cell death and release of viral particles, and finally to spread in human tissues. Their ability to replicate in tumor tissue allows for amplification of the input dose (e.g., 1000- to 10,000-fold increases) at the tumor site, while their lack of replication in normal tissues results in efficient clearance and reduced toxicity (Fig. 1A). This selective replication within tumor tissue can theoretically increase the therapeutic index of these agents dramatically over standard replication-incompetent approaches. In addition, viruses lead to infected cell death through a number of unique and distinct mechanisms. In addition to direct lysis at the conclusion of the replicative cycle, viruses can kill cells through expression of toxic proteins, induction of both inflammatory cytokines and T-cell-mediated immunity, and enhancement of cellular sensitivity to their effects. Therefore, because activation of classical apoptosis pathways in the cancer cell is not the exclusive mode of killing, cross-resistance with standard chemotherapeutics or radiotherapy is much less likely to occur.

Clinicians have treated hundreds of cancer patients with a wide variety of wild-type, replication-competent viruses over the last century; these include viruses as varied as Newcastle disease virus, mumps, vaccinia, western Nile, autonomous parvoviruses, and others. Due to intolerable toxicities and/or only transient efficacy with wild-type viruses, however, this virotherapy approach has been alternately pursued and then temporarily abandoned. Revolutionary advances in molecular biology and genetics have led to a fundamental understanding of both (1) the replication and patho-

genicity of viruses and (2) carcinogenesis. These advances have allowed novel agents to be engineered to enhance their safety and/or their antitumoral potency. Over the past decade, genetically engineered viruses in development have included adenoviruses, herpesviruses, and vaccinia. Inherently tumor-selective viruses such as reovirus, autonomous parvoviruses, Newcastle disease virus, measles virus strains, and vesicular stomatitis virus have each been characterized. Each of these agents has shown tumor selectivity *in vitro* and/or *in vivo*, and efficacy has been demonstrated in murine tumor models with many of these agents following intratumoral, intraperitoneal, and/or intravenous routes of administration.

II. FAVORABLE ATTRIBUTES OF REPLICATION-SELECTIVE VIRUSES FOR CANCER TREATMENT

A number of efficacy, safety, and manufacturing issues need to be assessed when considering a virus species for development as an oncolytic therapy. First, by definition, the virus must replicate in and destroy human tumor cells. An understanding of the genes modulating infection, replication, or pathogenesis is necessary if rational engineering of the virus is to be possible. Because most solid human tumors have relatively low growth fractions, the virus should ideally infect noncycling cells. In addition, receptors for viral entry must be expressed on the target tumor(s) in patients. From a safety standpoint, the parental wild-type virus should ideally cause only a mild, well-characterized human disease(s). Nonintegrating viruses have potential safety advantages as well. A genetically stable virus is desirable from both safety and manufacturing standpoints. Finally, the virus must be amenable to high-titer production and purification under good manufacturing practice (GMP) guidelines for clinical studies.

III. APPROACHES TO OPTIMIZING TUMOR-SELECTIVE VIRAL REPLICATION

Five broad approaches are currently being used for tumor-selective virus replication (Table I). These

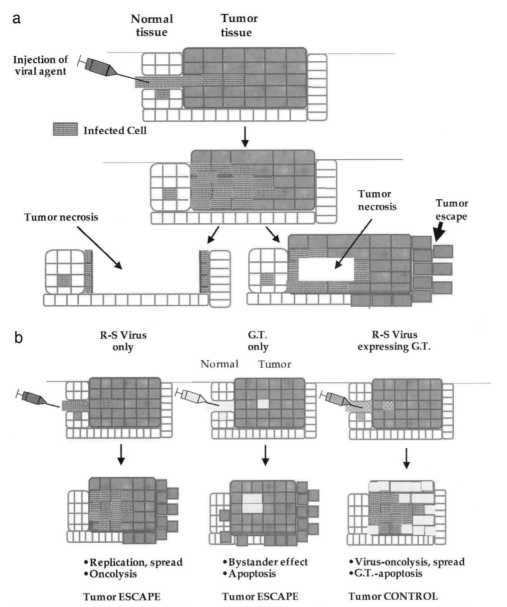

FIGURE 1 Tumor-selective viral replication and cell killing (A) and tumor-selective tissue necrosis (B). (A) Viral replication and spread within a tumor mass can lead to tumor eradication or, if viral killing and spread are not efficient enough, localized tumor necrosis with tumor escape at the margins. (B) Potential advantages of combining replication-selective viruses (R-S Virus) and standard gene therapy (G.T.) to allow spread and bystander effect killing of tumor cells. See color insert in Volume 1.

include (1) the use of viruses with inherent tumor selectivity (e.g., NDV, reovirus, VSV, autonomous parvovirus) (2) engineering of tumor/tissue-specific promoters into viruses to limit expression of the gene(s) necessary for replication to cancer cells (e.g., HSV, adenovirus) (3) deletion of entire genes that are necessary for efficient replication and/or toxicity in normal cells but are expendable in tumor cells (e.g., HSV,

adenovirus, vaccinia, poliovirus) (4) deletion of functional gene regions that are necessary for efficient replication and/or toxicity in normal cells but are expendable in tumor cells (e.g., adenovirus, poliovirus) and (5) modification of the viral coat to target uptake selectively to tumor cells (e.g., adenovirus, poliovirus).

Each of these approaches has potential advantages and disadvantages. The use of inherently selective

TABLE I

Mechanisms of Tumor-Specific Viral Replication[a]

Approach to selectivity	Agent example(s)	Genetic alterations within virus resulting in selectivity	Genetic phenotypic target within tumors
Deletion of entire viral gene that is		Deletion of	
(a) *necessary* for replication in normal cells, but	G207 (HSV-1)	Ribonucleotide reductase subunit disruption (ICP6 gene)	Proliferation
(b) *expendable* in tumor cells	1716 (HSV-1)	Gamma34.5 deletion	Loss of neurovirulence
	*dl*1520 (Ad)	E1B-55kD deletion	Loss of p53 function; proliferation
Deletion of functional region within viral gene that is		Deletion of	
(a) *necessary* for replication in normal cells, but	*dl*922-947 (Ad)	E1A CR2 (pRB protein family member binding region)	Loss of G1–S phase checkpoint control; loss of pRB function
(b) *expendable* in tumor cells	AdDelta24 (Ad)	Same	Same
	KD1, KD3 (Ad) *dl*1101/1107	E1A CR1 and CR2 (p300, pRB binding regions)	Same
	PV1 (RIPO) (PV)	Same 5′ IRES—replace with IRES from HRV2	Loss of neurovirulence
Engineer tumor-/tissue-specific promoter/enhancer elements to drive expression of early viral genes	CN706 (Ad)	E1A under PSE element	Prostate tissue
	CN787 (Ad)	E1A under rat probasin promoter, E1B under PSA promoter/enhancer	Same
	AvE1a041 (Ad)	E1A under AFP promoter	HCC, testicular carcinomas
	MUC-1 (Ad)	E1A under MUC-1 promoter	Breast, ovarian carcinomas
	G92A (HSV-1)	ICP4 under albumin enhancer/promoter	Liver tissue, HCC
Engineer ligand for tumor-selective receptor into virus coat	Adenovirus	Delete CAR/integrin binding, replace with tumor-targeting ligand	Tumor-specific receptor
Use of inherently tumor-selective viruses	NDV (73-T)	None identified (serial passage on tumor cells)	Unknown
	Reovirus	None	Ras pathway activation
	VSV	None	Interferon resistance
	Autonomous parvovirus (H1)	None	unknown

[a]HSV, herpes simplex virus; Ad, adenovirus; CR, conserved region; PV, poliovirus; IRES, internal ribosomal entry site; HRV, human rhinovirus; PSE, prostate-specific enhancer; PSA, prostate-specific antigen; AFP, α-fetoprotein; HCC, hepatocellular carcinoma; NDV, Newcastle disease virus; VSV, vesicular stomatitis virus.

agents is attractive because of its ease, but optimization of these agents may be difficult if the molecular mechanisms responsible for selectivity are unknown. The gene deletion approach can augment safety but also has the potential to reduce antitumoral potency, particularly if the deleted viral gene is multifunctional. For example, because the adenovirus EIB-55kD gene product inhibits p53, deletion of this gene in the adenovirus *dl*1520 (Onyx-015) appears to make this virus more sensitive to suppression by a functional p53 pathway in most (but not all) *in vitro* cell systems. However, this safety advantage comes at the price of significantly reduced potency versus wild-type adenovirus in most tumor cells, even those lacking p53;

this may be due to the loss of other EIB-55kD gene functions (e.g., viral mRNA transport). HSV-1 mutants with deletions in the thymidine kinase or ribonucleotide reductase genes appear to share a similar phenotype. One approach to maintain antitumoral potency is to make partial rather than complete deletions in target genes. In this way, functional subunits of proteins can be inactivated while leaving other protein functions intact. For example, an adenoviral mutant with a targeted partial deletion within the E1A gene of adenovirus does not have the attenuated phenotype but does demonstrate tumor selectivity.

The clinical utility of the tumor/tissue-specific promoter approach is dependent on other factors, including the promoter activity in target tumors and in normal tissues exposed to the virus. Engineering tumor-selective viral uptake requires ablation of the natural viral uptake mechanism, identification of tumor-specific "receptor" targets on cancer cells, and engineering of new "ligands" into the viral coat without disrupting viral integrity.

IV. EXAMPLES OF REPLICATION-SELECTIVE ONCOLYTIC VIRUSES IN PRECLINICAL OR CLINICAL DEVELOPMENT

A. Adenoviruses

Human adenoviruses are nonenveloped, double-stranded DNA viruses of approximately 38 kb; roughly 50 serotypes have been identified to date (Fig. 2). Adenoviruses can induce cancer cell death by several distinct mechanisms (Table II). Two general approaches to engineering adenovirus selectivity have been pursued to date. The first approach was to com-plement loss-of-function mutations in cancers with loss-of-function mutations within the adenovirus genome. Many of the same critical regulatory proteins that are inactivated by viral gene products during adenovirus replication are also inactivated during carcinogenesis. Because of this convergence, the deletion of viral genes that inactivate these cellular regulatory proteins can be complemented by genetic inactivation of these proteins within cancer cells. This pioneering approach was first described with herpesvirus. Martuza and colleagues deleted the thymidine kinase gene (*dlsptk*). Subsequently, it was hypothesized that an adenovirus with a deletion of the gene encoding a p53-inhibitory protein E1B-55kD (*dl1520*, or Onyx-015) would be selective for tumors that already had inhibited or lost p53 function. p53 function is lost in the majority of human cancers through mechanisms including gene mutation, overexpression of p53-binding inhibitors (e.g., mdm2, human papillomavirus E6) and loss of the p53-inhibitory pathway modulated by p14^{ARF}. However, the precise role of p53 in the inhibition of adenoviral replication has not been defined to date. In addition, other adenoviral proteins also

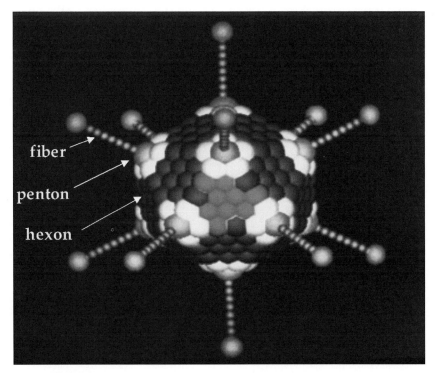

FIGURE 2 Human adenovirus coat structure. See color insert in Volume 1.

TABLE II
Potential Mechanisms of Antitumoral Efficacy
with Replication-Selective Adenoviruses

Mechanism[a]	Example of adenoviral genes modulating effect
I. Direct cytotoxicity due to viral proteins	E3 11.6kD E4ORF4
II. Augmentation of antitumoral immunity	
CTL infiltration, killing	E3 gp19kD[b]
Tumor cell death, antigen release	E3 11.6kD
Immunostimulatory cytokine induction	E3 10.4/14.5, 14.7kD[b]
Antitumoral cytokine induction (e.g., TNF)	E3 10.4/14.5, 14.7kD[b]
Enhanced sensitivity to cytokines (e.g., TNF)	E1A
III. Sensitization to chemotherapy	Unknown (? E1A, others)
IV. Expression of exogenous therapeutic genes	Not applicable

[a]CTL, cytotoxic T lymphocyte; TNF, tumor necrosis factor.
[b]Viral protein inhibits antitumoral mechanism.

have direct or indirect effects on p53 function (e.g., E4orf6, E1B 19kD, E1A). Finally, E1B-55kD itself has important viral functions that are unrelated to p53 inhibition (e.g., viral mRNA transport, host cell protein synthesis shutoff) (Fig. 3). Not surprisingly, therefore, the role of p53 in determining the replication selectivity of *dl*1520 has varied in magnitude depending on the cell system studied. Clinical trials were ultimately necessary to determine the selectivity and clinical utility of *dl*1520; approximately 250 patients have been treated to date with *dl*1520 (see later).

A second class of E1 region deletion mutants have now been described. Mutants in E1A conserved region 2 are defective in pRB binding. These viruses are

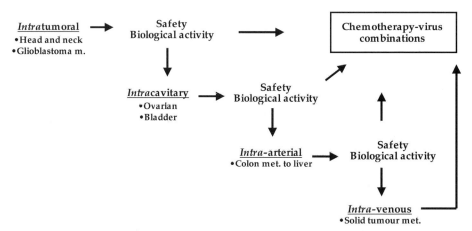

FIGURE 3 A staged clinical research and development approach for a replication-selective agent in cancer patients. Following demonstration of safety and biological activity by the intratumoral route, trials were sequentially initiated to study intracavitary instillation (initially intraperitoneal), intraarterial infusion (initially hepatic artery), and eventually intravenous administration. In addition, only patients with advanced and incurable cancers were initially enrolled in trials. Only after safety had been demonstrated in terminal cancer patients were trials initiated for patients with premalignant conditions. Finally, clinical trials of combinations with chemotherapy were initiated only after the saety of *dl*1520 as a single agent had been documented by the relevant route of administration.

being evaluated for use against tumors with pRB pathway abnormalities and the resultant loss in G1–S checkpoint control; this checkpoint is lost in over 90% of all human tumors. With *dl*922/947, for example, S-phase induction and viral replication are significantly reduced in quiescent normal cells, whereas replication and cytopathic effects are not reduced in tumor cells; interestingly, *dl*922/947 demonstrates significantly greater potency than *dl*1520 both *in vitro* and *in vivo*, and in a nude mouse–human tumor xenograft model, intravenously administered *dl*922/947 had significantly superior efficacy to even wild-type adenovirus. Unlike the complete deletion of E1B-55kD in *dl*1520, these mutations in E1A are targeted to a single conserved region and may therefore leave other important functions of the gene product intact.

A second approach has been to limit the expression of the E1A gene product, and therefore replication, to tumor tissues through the use of tumor- and/or tissue-specific promoters. For example, the prostate-specific antigen (PSA), MUC-1, and α-fetoprotein promoter/enhancer elements have been utilized to target prostate, breast, and hepatocellular carcinomas, respectively. Phase I clinical trials of the prostate-targeted adenovirus are underway.

B. Herpesvirus

Herpes virus (HSV) is an enveloped double-stranded DNA virus of approximately 152 kb. It contains a number of genes with identified essential and nonessential functions (*in vitro*) whose expression is regulated in a complex manner. HSV has a natural tropism for neuronal and mucosal cells. Techniques have been developed for genetic engineering and it is possible to replace some genes. It has a built-in safety mechanism through its tk gene; antiviral agents such as acyclovir and gancyclovir can be administered to halt the spread of the virus. Conversely, the deletion of this gene leads to attenuation of the virus in nondividing cells, which may give it some selectivity for replication in cycling cancer cells.

It was then discovered that deletion of the gene for ICP34.5 attenuates HSV in nondividing cells (such as neurons) but allows replication in cycling cells (such as tumor cells). This approach leaves the tk

gene intact, thereby retaining a potential safety mechanism. ICP34.5 gives the virus the ability to replicate in central nervous system (CNS) cells for unknown reasons and therefore the deletion abrogates this ability. Deletion of both copies of this gene attenuates propagation in normal cells. One version of this ICP34.5-deleted virus is known as HSV-1716 (originally made by M. Brown, Glasgow, Scotland). In malignant mesothelioma tumors grown ip in SCID mice, ip virus injections reduced tumor burden and prolonged survival. Although there did not appear to be any cytopathic changes in normal tissues, there were still some unexplained animal deaths. This virus is now in phase I clinical trials for patients with recurrent glioblastoma (see later).

In addition to ICP34.5, another HSV-1 gene has been deleted to enhance safety and selectivity. This gene encodes the protein ICP6, the large subunit of ribonucleotide reductase (RR), and this doubly deleted virus is known as G207. In this instance the ICP6 gene was disrupted by insertion of the lacZ marker gene. Loss of the RR subunit further decreases the ability of G207 to replicate in nondividing cells and therefore increases specificity for tumor cells. The favorable attributes of G207 include (1) its replication-competence in dividing cells, (2) attenuated neurovirulence, (3) temperature sensitivity, (4) enhanced sensitivity to gancyclovir or acyclovir, (5) multiple deletions (making reversion to wild-type virus less likely), and (6) presence of the lacZ marker. Animal models in which G207 has been tested for antitumoral efficacy and toxicity include head and neck cancer, colorectal cancer with liver metastasis, neuroblastoma and epithelial ovarian cancer; safety has been tested with intracerebral inoculations in *Aotus* owl monkeys. In all of these examples, the virus was nontoxic at therapeutic doses, and tumor selectivity and efficacy were observed. Therefore, this vector was demonstrated to have significantly reduced toxicity in two animal models, while being efficacious in nude mice with gliomas. G207 has now moved forward into phase I trials.

The role of preexisting immunity to HSV-1 has been assessed in rodent tumor models of direct intratumoral injection of the mutant hrR3 (RR-LacZ$^+$). Preexisting antibodies to HSV did not ablate gene expression from the virus or its efficacy, although gene expression was reduced 80%. In order to induce antitumoral immunity, HSV has been used in combination with antitumoral cytokines. The IL-12 gene was added to the genome of a replication-defective HSV, and this virus was used in combination with G207. IL-12 has multifunctional roles, including promotion of a TH1 cellular immune response. Another group engineered the HSV-1 mutant R3659 to express the IL-12 gene. This virus, known as M002, was used to treat experimental murine brain tumors in syngeneic models. It was demonstrated that (1) physiological levels of IL-12 were produced, (2) there was an increase in median survival as compared to R3659, and (3) there was infiltration of inflammatory mediators into the tumor.

Combinations of standard therapies with HSV have been explored. HSV-1716 plus various chemotherapeutic drugs were used together *in vitro* to look at the effect on viral replication. Most seem to augment oncolytic activity at relevant concentrations, implying that use of these agents together could lead to increased efficacy. The combination of HSV plus radiation was also tested. R3616 was shown to have enhanced replication as a result of radiation in U-87 malignant glioma xenografts, which resulted in greater tumor reduction. This same phenomenon was also true when using HSV mutants with other deletions and thus does not appear to be specific for the ICP34.5 mutation.

Two phase I clinical trials have been completed with replication-selective HSV mutants in patients with glioblastoma multiforme (GBM) or anaplastic astrocytomas (AA). In one trial of 1716, an HSV with a deletion in the ICP34.5 gene, 9 patients were injected with up to 10^5 pfu of virus. No significant toxicity was reported. Unfortunately, viral replication and antitumoral efficacy could not be assessed on this phase I trial. Similar results were found in the phase I study of G207 (described earlier) ($n = 21$ patients). The virus was injected at doses up to 3×10^9 pfu at five sites. Additional studies are needed to determine the maximum tolerated doses, the extent of viral replication, and the antitumoral efficacy.

The use of HSV-1 viral mutants is continuing in preclinical models and clinical trials. Other mutations that have improved selectivity for tumor cells versus normal tissue are being explored. The inclusion of additional therapeutic genes, including multiple genes from different classes, should further enhance the oncolytic function of this replicating agent.

C. Vaccinia Virus

Vaccinia virus (VV) is an enveloped, double-stranded DNA virus of approximately 200 kb. This virus replicates in the cytoplasm, bringing with its infectious particle the enzymes required for DNA replication and transcription of its genes. VV has a broad host range. Its advantages as an oncolytic virus are its large genome size with the capacity to accommodate multiple foreign genes, its wide tropism, rapid replication, and ease of recombination for making viral mutants. Its safety record has been well established with its use as a smallpox vaccine. Only in rare cases involving severely immunocompromised patients can wild-type VV be lethal. Most VV recombinants have inserted transgenes into the VV's own tk gene; this gene deletion may help give the virus selectivity in dividing cells, although it does remove a potential safety valve.

VV has been used both as a tool to induce an antitumoral immune response and as a means of lysing tumor cells directly following virus replication. A number of genes have been inserted into VV, including the costimulatory molecules ICAM-1 (intercellular adhesion molecule) and CD70; EMAP-II (endothelial monocyte-activating factor); cytokines such as IL-2 and GM-CSF; viral antigens such as HPV-16 viral proteins and HIV-1 envelope protein; tumor-associated antigens (TAA), such as Mart-1, tyrosinase, CEA, PSA, and Melan A peptide gene; markers such as lacZ or luciferase; and finally the prodrug converting enzyme cytosine deaminase (CD). Many of these constructs have been tested in both nude and immunocompetent mouse models and the results have been encouraging. Injected tumors usually undergo growth inhibition or regression, survival of the animal is prolonged, and, in many cases, a protective immune response against rechallenge is elicited.

Wild-type VV was used in a clinical trial of patients with recurrent superficial melanoma (intratumoral injection) and intravesicle treatment of bladder cancer ($n = 4$). No significant toxicity was reported, and a humoral immune response to VV developed. However, even with multiple injections, virus replication occurred, indicating that the immune response did not totally inhibit virus replication.

A subsequent phase I trial tested VV containing the GM-CSF gene in patients with surgically incurable cutaneous melanoma ($n = 7$); GM-CSF is a potent immune enhancing agent in murine tumor models. The agent was injected into superficial lesions twice weekly for 6 weeks. All patients developed an anti-VV response. GM-CSF expression was detectable for as long as 31 weeks following treatment initiation. Toxicity was minimal, consisting primarily of flu-like symptoms of ≤ 24 h duration. All patients had local inflammation at higher doses, dense infiltration by $CD4^+$ and $CD8^+$ lymphocytes, and anti-VV humoral immune responses above baseline levels (all patients had been vaccinated against smallpox as children). The local responses for the seven patients in this study were as follows: one complete response, one partial response, three mixed responses, and two had no response. Unlike studies with autologous tumor cell preparations infected with retroviral GM-CSF, responses were not demonstrated at distant sites. This study showed that VV could be administered safely with potential for a local antitumoral response, but the ability to induce effective systemic antitumoral immunity was not demonstrated.

VV encoding the IL-2 gene was administered intratumorally weekly for 12 weeks to 6 patients with refractory malignant mesothelioma. A T lymphocyte infiltrate was observed and VV IgG rose in all patients. Nevertheless, the expression of IL-12 continued up to 3 weeks postinjection. There was no significant toxicity; however, no tumor regressions were observed.

In another phase I study, VV carrying the CEA gene was administered to 20 patients with metastatic adenocarcinoma, either intradermally or subcutaneously. CEA is a TAA expressed in a range of tumors, including a majority of colorectal, gastric, and pancreatic cancers. Both routes of injections were equivalent for the development of cellular and humoral immune responses to the vector. Although there was only minimal toxicity in less than 20% of the patients, there were no objective responses.

A phase I trial was also performed with VV encoding PSA via intradermal inoculation in 33 patients with prostate cancer and who had elevated PSA levels despite previous treatment. There were three doses administered per patient at three escalating dose lev-

els. This treatment was in the presence or absence of exogenously administered GM-CSF. A specific T-cell response to PSA was induced in some patients. Nine patients had no apparent clinical progression for 11–25 months, although no objective responses occurred. Thus, repeated vaccination with VV-PSA was safe (grade 1 toxicity only) and resulted in a specific tumor antigen response.

In summary, VV-expressing TAAs, IL-2, or GM-CSF were well tolerated in a number of phase I trials using sc, intradermal, or intratumoral inoculation. Not surprisingly, no objective systemic antitumoral responses were seen in these patients with advanced disease on phase I trials. Phase II testing in patients with minimal disease will be necessary to assess the usefulness of VVs as cancer vaccines.

D. Reovirus

Reovirus is a highly stable, nonenveloped double-stranded RNA virus that results in either an asymptomatic, nonpathogenic infection or mild gastroenteritis in humans. Approximately 50% of the population possess antibodies to reovirus. A wide variety of mammalian cells can be infected via its receptor, sialic acid. Early work had shown that reovirus could productively infect transformed cells but not normal cells (such as primary human and primate, rat kidney, and baby hamster kidney cells).

Intratumoral injection of xenografts in immunodeficient mice has resulted in tumor regressions in several models. Importantly, however, toxicity was seen in immunodeficient mice that was not seen in an immunocompetent mouse model. In immunocompetent models, significant tumor regressions resulted following multiple intratumoral injections. Therefore, the selectivity of reovirus for tumors *in vivo* is questionable, and selectivity may be dependent on T cell-mediated clearance from normal tissues. More testing needs to be done.

E. Poliovirus

Attenuated poliovirus is one of the most recently described oncolytic viruses for the treatment of cancer. Poliovirus is a nonenveloped, positive-strand RNA virus and the agent that causes paralytic poliomyelitis.

Cell tropism is to lower motor neurons within the spinal cord and brain stem, and infection results in the clinical syndrome dominated by flaccid paralysis. The neuropathogenicity of poliovirus has been mapped to the 5′ IRES (internal ribosome entry site). Deletion of this sequence and replacement with an IRES from HRV2 (human rhinovirus type 2), as in PV1 (RIPO), eliminated the neurovirulent phenotype and allowed the virus to replicate in other cell lines (e.g., HeLa cells). This mutant was no longer pathogenic in the mouse model for poliomyelitis and after intraspinal inoculation into *Cynomolgus* monkeys. In addition to demonstrating poor growth in neuronal-derived cell lines in tissue culture and lack of virulence in a mouse model, PV1 (RIPO) has been shown to infect and propagate in cell lines derived from malignant gliomas. Additionally, treatment of sc or intracerebral tumors in nude mice inhibited tumor growth and resulted in tumor elimination. This research points to the potential use of attenuated poliovirus as an anticancer therapeutic.

F. Vesicular Stomatitis Virus

Vesicular stomatitis virus (VSV) is an enveloped, negative-sense RNA virus that infects a wide variety of mammalian and insect cells. Infections in humans are asymptomatic or result in a mild febrile illness. This virus is also exquisitely sensitive to interferons (IFN). Its advantages as an oncolytic virus include that it can be grown to high titers (up to 10^9 pfu/ml in some tumor cell lines), has a short replication cycle (1 to 2 h in tumor cells), and is not endemic to North America, implying that preexisting antibodies in patients will not interfere with its infection process. Its sensitivity to IFN might potentially be used as a safety measure.

In vitro experiments demonstrated that VSV replicated better in tumor cells than in normal cells; this difference was even more striking in the presence of IFN-α. Treatment of xenografts with VSV (intratumoral injection of VSV or VSV-infected cells) in nude mice resulted in regression or growth inhibition. When VSV administration was coupled with administration of exogenous IFN-α (ip), all of the mice survived, whereas in the absence of IFN, mice died after about 10 days. Whether the amount of IFN adminis-

tered is similar to physiologic levels is unclear from this report. Although the recently discovered oncolytic potential of this agent is intriguing, much more research is required, including research into its selectivity mechanism, toxicity, mechanism(s) of selective cell killing, optimal route of administration, and manufacturing issues.

V. A NOVEL STAGED APPROACH TO CLINICAL RESEARCH WITH REPLICATION-SELECTIVE VIRUSES: THE EXAMPLE OF *dl*1520 (ONYX-015)

A. Clinical Trial Results with Replication-Competent Adenoviruses in Cancer Patients

1. Clinical Trial Results with Wild-Type Adenovirus: Flawed Study Design

Over the last century a diverse array of viruses were injected into cancer patients by various routes, including adenovirus, Bunyamwara, coxsackie, dengue, feline panleukemia, Ilheus, mumps, Newcastle disease virus, vaccinia, and west Nile. These studies illustrated both the promise and the hurdles to overcome with oncolytic viral therapy. Unfortunately, these previous clinical studies were not performed to current clinical research standards, and therefore none give interpretable and definitive results. At best, these studies are useful in generating hypotheses that can be tested in future trials.

Although suffering from many of the trial design flaws that are listed later, a trial with wild-type adenovirus is one of the most useful for hypothesis generation but also for illustrating how clinical trial design flaws severely curtail the utility of the study results. The knowledge that adenoviruses could eradicate a variety of tumor cells *in vitro* led to a clinical trial in the 1950s with wild-type adenovirus. Ten different serotypes were used to treat 30 cervical cancer patients. Forty total treatments were administered by direct intratumoral injection ($n = 23$), injection into the artery perfusing the tumor ($n = 10$), treatment by both routes ($n = 6$), or intravenous administration ($n = 1$). Characterization of the material injected into patients was minimal. The volume of viral supernatant injected is reported, but actual viral titers/doses are not; injection volumes (and by extension doses) varied greatly. When possible, the patients were treated with a serotype to which they had no neutralizing antibodies present. Corticosteroids were administered as nonspecific immunosuppressive agents in roughly half of the cases. Therefore, no two patients were treated in identical fashion.

Nevertheless, the results are intriguing. No significant local or systemic toxicity was reported. This relative safety is notable given the lack of preexisting immunity to the serotype used and concomitant corticosteroid use in many patients. Some patients reported a relatively mild viral syndrome lasting 2–7 days (severity not defined); this viral syndrome resolved spontaneously. Infectious adenovirus was recovered from the tumor in two-thirds of the patients for up to 17 days postinoculation.

Two-thirds of the patients had a "marked to moderate local tumor response" with necrosis and ulceration of the tumor (definition of "response" not reported). None of the seven control patients treated with either virus-free tissue culture fluid or heat-inactivated virus had a local tumor response (statistical significance not reported). Therefore, clinically evident tumor necrosis was only reported with viable virus. Neutralizing antibodies increased within 7 days after administration. Although the clinical benefit to these patients is unclear, and all patients eventually had tumor progression and died, this study did demonstrate that wild-type adenoviruses can be safely administered to patients and that these viruses can replicate and cause necrosis in solid tumors despite a humoral immune response. The maximally tolerated dose, dose-limiting toxicity, objective response rate, and time to tumor progression, however, remain unknown for any of these serotypes by any route of administration.

2. A Novel Staged Approach to Clinical Research with Replication-Selective Viruses: The Example of dl1520 (Onyx-015)

For the first time since viruses were first conceived as agents to treat cancer over a century ago, we now have definitive data from numerous phase I and II clinical trials with a well-characterized and well-quantitated virus. dl1520 (Onyx-015, now CI-1042, Pfizer, Inc.) is a novel agent with a novel mechanism of action. This virus was to become the first virus to be used in humans that had been genetically engineered for replication selectivity. We predicted that both toxicity and efficacy would be dependent on multiple factors, including (1) the inherent ability of a given tumor to replicate and shed the virus, (2) the location of the tumor to be treated (e.g., intracranial vs peripheral), and (3) the route of administration of the virus. In addition, we felt it would be critical to obtain biological data on viral replication, antiviral immune responses, and their relationship to antitumoral efficacy in the earliest phases of clinical research.

We therefore designed and implemented a novel staged clinical research and development approach with this virus (Fig. 3). The goal of this approach was to sequentially increase systemic exposure to the virus only after safety with more localized delivery had been demonstrated. Following demonstration of safety and biological activity by the intratumoral route, trials were sequentially initiated to study intracavitary instillation (initially intraperitoneal), intraarterial infusion (initially hepatic artery), and eventually intravenous administration. In addition, only patients with advanced and incurable cancers were initially enrolled on trials. Only after safety had been demonstrated in terminal cancer patients were trials initiated for patients with premalignant conditions. Finally, clinical trials of combinations with chemotherapy were initiated only after the safety of dl1520 as a single agent had been documented by the relevant route of administration.

3. Results from Clinical Trials with dl1520 (Onyx-015, or CI-1042): Toxicity

No maximally tolerated dose or dose-limiting toxicities were identified at doses up to 2×10^{12} particles administered by intratumoral injection. Flu-like symptoms and injection-site pain were the most common associated toxicities. This safety is remarkable given the daily or even twice-daily dosing that was repeated every 1–3 weeks in the head and neck region or pancreas.

Intraperitoneal, intraarterial, and intravenous administrations were also remarkably well tolerated, in general. Intraperitoneal administration was feasible at doses up to 10^{13} particles divided over 5 days. The most common toxicites included fever, abdominal pain, nausea/vomiting, and bowel motility changes (diarrhea, constipation). The severity of the symptoms appeared to correlate with tumor burden. Patients with heavy tumor burdens reached a maximally tolerated dose at 10^{12} particles (dose-limiting toxicities were abdominal pain and diarrhea), whereas patients with a low tumor burden tolerated 10^{13} without significant toxicity.

No dose-limiting toxicities were reported following repeated intravascular injection at doses up to 2×10^{12} particles (hepatic artery) or 2×10^{13} particles (intravenous) (Table III). Fever, chills, and asthenia following intravascular injection were more common and more severe than after intratumoral injections (grade 2–3 fever and chills vs grade 1). Dose-related transaminitis was reported infrequently. The transaminitis was typically transient (<10 days) and low grade (grade 1–2) and was not clinically relevant. Further dose escalation was limited by supply of the virus.

4. Results from Clinical Trials with dl1520: Viral Replication

Viral replication has been documented at early time points after intratumoral injection in head and neck cancer patients. Roughly 70% of patients had evidence of replication on days 1–3 after their last treatment. In contrast, day 14–17 samples were uniformly negative. Intratumoral injection of liver metastases (primarily colorectal) led to similar results at the highest doses of a phase I trial. Patients with injected pancreatic tumors, in contrast, showed no evidence of viral replication by plasma polymerase chain reaction (PCR) or fine needle aspiration. Similarly, intraperitoneal dl1520 could not be shown to reproducibly infect ovarian carcinoma cells within the peritoneum. Therefore, different tumor types can vary dramatically in their permissiveness for viral infection and replication.

Proof of concept for tumor infection following intraarterial or intravenous administration with human adenovirus has also been achieved. Approximately half of the roughly 25 patients receiving hepatic artery infusions of 2×10^{12} particles were positive by PCR 3–5 following treatment. Patients with elevated neutralizing antibody titers prior to treatment were substantially less likely to have evidence of viral replication 3–5 days posttreatment. Three of 4 patients with metastatic carcinoma to the lung treated intravenously with $\geq 2 \times 10^{12}$ particles were positive for replication by PCR on day 3 (± 1). Therefore, it is

---

TABLE III

Toxicity Data from Phase I and I/II Trials of dl1520 (Onyx-015): Intraperitoneal, Intraarterial or Intravenous Injection

Route of administration	n	Tumor type	Dose/cycle (particles)	Regimen/ cycle frequency	Maximally tolerated dose/ dose-limiting toxicity	Most frequent adverse events (% of patients with event)
Intraperitoneal Phase I	16	Ovarian	10^{11}–10^{13}	Daily × 5/ every 3 weeks	Bulky tumors (≥ 2 cm)— DLT at 10^{12}: abdominal pain, diarrhea, nausea/ vomiting Nonbulky tumors (< 2 cm)— no DLT at 10^{13}	Fever (75) Abdominal pain (60) Nausea/vomiting (60)
Intraarterial (hepatic artery) Phase I/II	33	Gastrointestinal; primarily colorectal	2×10^{9}–10^{12}	Single dose/every 1 week (2 weeks on, 2 off)	None	Fever (90) Chills (68) Nausea (42)
Intravenous Phase I	10	Metastatic carcinoma	2×10^{8}–10^{12}	Single dose/every 1 week (3 weeks on, 1 off)	None	Fever (100) Chills (100) Transaminitis (67) grades 1–2 (mild-moderate) transient (< 10 days)

feasible to infect distant tumor nodules following intravenous or intraarterial administration.

5. Results from Clinical Trials with dl1520: Immune Response

Neutralizing antibody titers to the coat (Ad5) of dl1520 were positive but relatively low in roughly 50–60% of all clinical trial patients at baseline. Antibody titers increased uniformly following the administration of dl1520 by any of the routes tested, in some cases to levels >1:80,000. Antibody increases occurred regardless of evidence for replication or shedding into the bloodstream. Acute inflammatory cytokine levels were determined prior to treatment (by hepatic artery infusion), 3 h post-,

and 18 h posttreatment: IL-1, IL-6, IL-10, interferon-γ, tumor necrosis factor. Significant increases were demonstrated within 3 h for IL-1, IL-6, tumor necrosis factor, and, to a lesser extent, interferon-γ; all cytokines were back down to pretreatment levels by 18 h. In contrast, IL-10 did not increase until 18 h.

6. Results from Clinical Trials with dl1520: Efficacy with dl1520 as a Single Agent (Table IV)

Two phase II trials enrolled a total of 40 patients with recurrent head and neck cancer. Tumors were treated very aggressively with 6–8 daily needle passes for 5 consecutive days (30–40 needle passes per 5 day cy-

TABLE IV

Antitumoral Efficacy Data of dl1520 (Onyx-015) as a Single Agent:
Intratumoral, Intraperitoneal, Intraarterial, or Intravenous Injection

Route of administration	Tumor type	Phase	Dose/cycle (particles)	Regimen/ cycle frequencey	≥50% tumor regression[a] No. responders/total (%)
Intratumoral	Head and neck	I	2×10^8–10^{12}	Single dose/every 4 weeks	3/22 (14)
Intratumoral	Head and neck	II	10^{12}	Daily × 5/every 3 weeks	Intent to treat: 4/30 (13) Confirmed, intent to treat[b]: 2/30 (7) Unconfirmed, evaluable: 4/19 (20)
Intratumoral	Gastrointestinal liver metastases— colorectal, gastric pancreatic	I	2×10^9–10^{12}	Single dose/every 4 weeks	0/19 (0)
Intratumoral	Pancreatic (CT guided)	I	2×10^8–10^{12}	Single dose/every 4 weeks	0/22 (0)
Intratumoral	Pancreatic	I	2×10^{10} (n=3)	Single dose/ days 1, 5, 8, 15	0/3 (0)
	(endoscopic US)	II	2×10^{11} (n=18)		0/18 (0)[c]
Intraperitoneal	Ovarian	I	10^{11}–10^{13}	Daily × 5/every 3 weeks	0/16 (0)
Intravenous	Carcinoma metastatic to lung	I	2×10^8–10^{12}	Single dose/every 1 week (3 weeks on, 1 off)	0/9 (0)

[a]Nonnecrotic cross-sectional area used for response assessment (i.e., necrotic area subtracted from total cross-sectional area). All responses refer to shrinkage of the injected tumor mass only (i.e., distant, noninjected tumors not included). All responses were in tumors with a p53 gene mutation.

[b]Evaluable patients defined as those receiving >1 cycle of therapy and measurable tumor at baseline and at least one occasion >6 weeks after treatment initially (i.e., patients without follow-up tumor measurements after 1+ cycles of treatment were excluded). Intent-to-treat analysis includes all patients receiving at least one dose of ONYX-015. Confirmed responses reflect those that were confirmed to be durable for ≥4 weeks on an intent-to-treat basis.

[c]Responses of single agent ONYX-015 determined after four cycles (on day 35) on the pancreatic EUS phase I/II trial. Subsequent cycles given with chemotherapy.

cle; $n = 30$) and 10–15 per day on a second trial (50–75 needle passes per cycle; $n = 10$). The median tumor volume on these studies was approximately 25 cm^3; an average cubic centimeters of tumor therefore received an estimated 4–5 needle passes per cycle. Despite the intensity of this local treatment, the unconfirmed response rate at the injected site was only 14% and the confirmed local response rate was <10% (Table V). Interestingly, there was no correlation between evidence of antitumoral activity and neutralizing antibody levels at baseline or posttreatment. No objective responses were demonstrated in patients with tumor types that could not be so aggressively injected (due to their deep locations), although some evidence of minor shrinkage or necrosis was obtained (Table V). In summary, single agent responses across all studies were rare, and therefore combinations with chemotherapy were explored.

TABLE V

Evidence for Potential Synergy between *dl*1520 (Onyx-015) and Chemotherapy from Clinical Trials

Route of administration	Tumor type	Phase	Dose/cycle (particles)	Regimen/ cycle frequency[a]	Evidence for potential synergy[b]
Intratumoral	Head and neck	II	10^{12}	ONYX-015 daily × 5 + cisplatin day 1 i.v.b. 5-FU days 1-5 c.i. every 3 weeks	ONYX-015-injected tumors significantly more likely to respond than matched, noninjected control tumors ($p=0.017$; McNemar's test) ONYX-015-injected tumors less likely to progress than matched, noninjected control tumors ($p=0.06$; long rank test) Two of four tumors progressing on chemotherapy responded to same chemotherapy plus ONYX-015 Uncontrolled: response rate 63% vs historical 30–40% with chemotherapy and 14% with ONYX-015 alone
Intratumoral (endoscopic US)	Pancreatic	I / II	2×10^{10} ($n=3$) / 2×10^{11} ($n=3$)	ONYX-015 single dose + gemcitabine i.v.b. every 1 week	None—2 of 21 patients responded to combination
Intraperitoneal	Ovarian	I	10^{11}–10^{13}	ONYX-015 daily × 5/ every 3 weeks	One patient had tumor responses (>50% reduction in CA-125) on platinum-based chemotherapy following ONYX-015, despite previous tumor progression on platinum-based chemotherapy alone and on ONYX-015 alone
Intraarterial (hepatic artery)	Gastrointestinal liver metastases— primarily colorectal	I / II	2×10^{9}–6×10^{11} / 2×10^{12}	ONYX-015 single dose + 5-FU/leucovorin i.v.b. every 4 weeks	One partial response, 10 stable disease 2–7+ months) to combination ONYX-015 plus 5-FU/leucovorin in patients with tumor progression on both single agent ONYX-015 and 5-FU/leucovorin alone Three of three chemotherapy-naïve patients responded to combination therapy
Intravenous	Metastatic carcinoma	I	2×10^{10}–10^{13}	Single dose/ every 1 week (3 weeks on, 1 off), then with weekly carboplatin/paclitaxel	Stable disease for 6.5+ months in a patient with carboplatin/paclitaxel-refractory disease

[a] i.v.b., intravenous bolus; c.i., continuous infusion; 5-FU, 5-fluorouracil.
[b] Although synergy cannot be definitively proven in phase II clinical trials, these clinical trial results are consistent with synergy and/or a positive interaction between ONYX-015 and chemotherapy with cisplatin and 5-FU.

7. Results from Clinical Trials with dl1520: Potential Synergy in Combination with Chemotherapy (Table V)

Evidence for a potentially synergistic interaction between adenoviral therapy and chemotherapy has been obtained on multiple trials. Encouraging clinical data have been obtained in patients with recurrent head and neck cancer treated with intratumoral dl1520 in combination with intravenous cispaltin and 5-fluorouracil. Thirty-seven patients were treated and 19 responded (54%, intent to treat; 63%, evaluable); this compares favorably with response rates to chemotherapy alone in previous trials (30–40%, generally). The time-to-tumor progression was also superior to previously reported studies. However, comparisons to historical controls are unreliable. We therefore used patients as their own controls whenever possible ($n = 11$ patients). Patients with more than one tumor mass had a single tumor injected with dl1520, whereas the other mass(es) was left uninjected. Because both masses were exposed to chemotherapy, the effect of the addition of viral therapy to chemotherapy could be assessed. dl1520-injected tumors were significantly more likely to respond ($p = 0.017$) and less likely to progress ($p = 0.06$) than noninjected tumors. Noninjected control tumors that progressed on chemotherapy alone were subsequently treated with Onyx-015 in some cases; two of the four injected tumors underwent complete regressions. This datum illustrates the potential of viral and chemotherapy combinations. The clinical utility of dl1520 in this indication will be definitively determined in a phase III randomized trial.

A phase I/II trial of dl1520 administered by hepatic artery infusion in combination with intravenous 5-fluorouracil and leukovorin was carried out ($n = 33$ total). Following phase I dose escalation, 15 patients with colorectal carcinoma who had previously failed the same chemotherapy were treated with combination therapy after failing to respond to dl1520 alone; 1 patient underwent a partial response and 10 had stable disease (2–7+ months). Chemosensitization of colorectal liver metastases is therefore possible via hepatic artery infusions, although the magnitude and frequency of this effect remain to be determined. In contrast, data from a phase I/II trial studying the combination of dl1520 and gemcitabine chemotherapy were disappointing ($n = 21$); the combination resulted in only two responses, and these patients had not received prior gemcitabine. Therefore, potential synergy was demonstrated with dl1520 and chemotherapy in two tumor types that supported viral replication (head and neck, colorectal), but not in a tumor type that was resistant to viral replication (pancreatic).

B. Results from Clinical Trials with dl1520 (Onyx-015): Summary

dl1520 has been well tolerated at the highest practical doses that could be administered (2×10^{12}–10^{13} particles) by intratumoral, intraperitoneal, intraarterial, and intravenous routes. The lack of clinically significant toxicity in the liver or other organs was notable. Flu-like symptoms (fever, rigors, and asthenia) were the most common toxicities and were increased in patients receiving intravascular treatment. Acute inflammatory cytokines (especially IL-1 and IL-6) increased within 3 h following intraarterial infusion. Neutralizing antibodies increased in all patients, regardless of dose, route, or tumor type. Viral replication was documented in head and neck and colorectal tumors following intratumoral or intraarterial administration. Neutralizing antibodies did not block antitumoral activity in head and neck cancer trials of intratumoral injection. However, viral replication/shedding into the blood was inhibited by neutralizing antibodies; the intraarterial virus was more sensitive to antibody inhibition than the intratumorally injected virus. Single-agent antitumoral activity was minimal (approximately 15%) in head and neck cancers that could be repeatedly and aggressively injected. No objective responses were documented with single-agent therapy in phase I or I/II trials in patients with pancreatic, colorectal, or ovarian carcinomas. A favorable and potentially synergistic interaction with chemotherapy was discovered in some tumor types and by different routes of administration.

C. Future Directions: Why Has *dl*1520 (Onyx-015) Failed to Date as a Single Agent for Refractory Solid Tumors?

Future improvements with this approach will be possible if the reasons for *dl*1520 failure as a single agent, and success in combination with chemotherapy, are uncovered. Factors that are specific to this adenoviral mutant, as well as factors that may be generalizable to other viruses, should be considered. Regarding this particular adenoviral mutant, it is important to remember that this virus is attenuated relative to wild-type adenovirus in most tumor cell lines *in vitro* and *in vivo*, including even p53 mutant tumors. This is not an unexpected phenotype because this virus has lost critical E1B-55kD functions that are unrelated to p53, including viral mRNA transport. This attenuated potency is not apparent with other adenovirus mutants, such as *dl*922/947.

In addition, a second deletion in the E3 gene region (10.4/14.5 complex) may make this virus more sensitive to the antiviral effects of tumor necrosis factor; an immunocompetent animal model will need to be identified in order to resolve this issue. Factors likely to be an issue with any virus include barriers to intratumoral spread, antiviral immune responses, and inadequate viral receptor expression (e.g., CAR, integrins). Viral coat modifications may be beneficial if inadequate CAR expression plays a role in the resistance of particular tumor types.

VI. FUTURE DIRECTIONS: APPROACHES TO IMPROVING THE EFFICACY OF REPLICATION-SELECTIVE VIRAL AGENTS

Second-generation viruses are being engineered for greater potency while maintaining safety. For example, a promising adenoviral E1A CR-2 mutant (*dl*922/947) has been described that demonstrates not only tumor selectivity (based on the G_1–S checkpoint status of the cell) but also significantly greater antitumoral efficacy *in vivo* compared to the first-generation virus *dl*1520, and even wild-type adenovirus in one model. Deletion of antiapoptotic genes or overexpression of death proteins may result in more rapid tumor cell killing *in vitro*; it remains to be seen whether these *in vitro* observations are followed by evidence for improved efficacy *in vivo* over wild-type adenovirus (Table VI).

Potency can also be improved by arming viruses with therapeutic genes (e.g., prodrug-activating enzymes and cytokines) (Fig. 1B). Viral coat modifications may be beneficial if inadequate CAR expression plays a role in the resistance of particular tumor types. Improved systemic delivery may require novel formulations or coat modifications, as well as suppression of the humoral immune response. Finally, the identification of mechanisms leading to the favorable interaction between replicating viral therapy and chemotherapy may allow augmentation of this interaction.

VII. SUMMARY

Replication-selective oncolytic viruses have a number of attractive features as novel cancer treatments. A number of these agents have or will soon enter clinical trials. Clinical studies have demonstrated that viral treatment can be well tolerated and that tumor necrosis can result. The feasibility of virus delivery to tumors through the bloodstream has also been demonstrated. The inherent ability of replication-competent adenoviruses to sensitize tumor cells to chemotherapy was a novel discovery that has led to chemosensitization strategies. These data will support the further development of viral agents, including second-generation constructs containing exogenous therapeutic genes to enhance both local and systemic antitumoral activity. Given the limited ability of *in vitro* cell-based assays and murine tumor model systems to accurately predict the efficacy and therapeutic index of replication-selective viruses in patients, we believe that the timely translation of encouraging viral agents into well-designed clinical trials with relevant biological end points is critical. Only then can the true therapeutic potential of these agents be realized.

Acknowledgments

The following individuals have been instrumental in making this manuscript possible: John Nemunaitis, Stan Kaye, Tony Reid, Fadlo Khuri, James Abruzzese, Eva Galanis, Joseph Rubin, Antonio Grillo-Lopez, Carla Heise, Larry Romel, Chris Maack, Sherry Toney, Nick Lemoine, Britta Randlev, Patrick Trown, Fran Kahane, Frank McCormick, and Margaret Uprichard.

TABLE VI
Examples of Replication-Selective Viruses in Clinical Trials for Cancer Patients[a]

Parental strain	Agent	Clinical phase	Tumor targets in clinical trials	Genetic alterations	Cell phenotype allowing selective replication
Engineered					
Adenovirus (2/5 chimera)	*dl*1520 (Onyx-015	I–III	SCCHN Colorectal Ovarian Pancreatic	E1B-55kD gene deletion	Cells lacking p53 function (e.g., deletion, mutation, HPV infection)
Adenovirus (serotype 5)	CN706 CN787	I I	Prostate	E1A expression driven by PSE element E1A driven by rat probasin promoter/E1B by PSE/ promoter	Prostate cells (malignant, normal)
Adenovirus (2/5 chimera)	Ad5-CD/ tk-rep	I	Prostate	E1B-55kD gene deletion Insertion of HSV-*tk*/CD fusion gene	Cells lacking p53 function (e.g., deletion, mutation, HPB infection)
Herpes simplex virus-1	G207 1716	I–II	GBM	Ribonucleotide reductase disruption (lac-Z insertion into ICP6 gene) Neuropathogenesis gene mutation (γ34.5 gene)	Proliferating cells
Vaccinia virus	Wild type +/− GM-CSF	I	Melanoma	For selectivity: none or tk deletion Immunostimulatory gene (GM-CSF) insertion	Unknown
Nonengineered					
Newcastle disease virus	73-T	I		Unknown (serial passage on tumor cells)	Unknown
Autonomous parvoviruses	H-1	I–II		None	Transformed cells ↑proliferation ↓differentiation ras, p53 mutation
Reovirus	Reolysin	I	SCCHN	None	Ras pathway activation (e.g., ras mutation, EGFR signaling)

[a]SCCHN, squamous cell carcinoma of head and neck; GBM, glioblastoma multiforme; HPV, human papillomavirus; PSE, prostate-specific enhancer; LPS, lipopolysaccharide; EGFR, epidermal growth factor receptor; tk, thymidine kinase.

See Also the Following Articles

ADENO-ASSOCIATED VIRUS • TARGETED VECTORS FOR CANCER GENE THERAPY • VIRAL AGENTS

Bibliography

Advani, S. J., Sibley, G. S., Song, P. Y., Hallahan, D. E., Kataoka, Y., Roizman, B., and Weichselbaum, R. R. (1998). Enhancement of replication of genetically engineered herpes simplex viruses by ionizing radiation: a new paradigm for destruction of therapeutically intractable tumors. *Gene Ther.* **5**, 160–165.

Agha-Mohammadi, S., and Lotze, M. (2000). Immunomodulation of cancer: Potential use of replication-selective agents. *J. Clin. Invest.* **105**, 1173–1176.

Asada, T., Treatment of human cancer with mumps virus. *Cancer* **34**, 1907–1928.

Barker, D. D., and Berk, A. J. (1987). Adenovirus proteins from both E1B reading frames are required for transformation of rodent cells by viral infection and DNA transfection. *Virology* **156**, 107–121.

Bischoff, J. R., Kirn, D. H., Williams, A., Heise, C., Horn, S., Muna, M., Ng, L., Nye, J. A., Sampson-Johannes, A., Fattaey, A., and McCormick, F. (1996). An adenovirus mutant that replicates selectively in p53-deficient human tumor cells. *Science* **274**, 373–376.

Carew, J. F., Kooby, D. A., Halterman, M. W., Federoff, H. J., and Fong, Y. (1999). Selective infection and cytolysis of human head and neck squamous cell carcinoma with sparing of normal mucosa by a cytotoxic herpes simplex virus type 1 (G207). *Hum. Gene Ther.* **10,** 1599–1606.

Chinnadurai, G. (1983). Adenovirus 2 Ip+ locus codes for a 19 kd tumor antigen that plays an essential role in cell transformation. *Cell* **33,** 759–766.

Coffey, M., Strong, J., Forsyth, P., and Lee, P. (1998). Reovirus therapy of tumors with activated ras pathway. *Science* **282,** 1332–1334.

Colella, T. A., Bullock, T. N., Russell, L. B., Mullins, D. W., Overwijk, W. W., Luckey, C. J., Pierce, R. A., Restifo, N. P., and Engelhard, V. H. (2000). Self-tolerance to the murine homologue of a tyrosinase-derived melanoma antigen: Implications for tumor immunotherapy. *J. Exp. Med.* **191,** 1221–1232.

Conry, R. M., Khazaeli, M. B., Saleh, M. N., Allen, K. O., Barlow, D. L., Moore, S. E., Craig, D., Arani, R. B., Schlom, J., and LoBuglio, A. F. (1999). Phase I trial of a recombinant vaccinia virus encoding carcinoembryonic antigen in metastatic adenocarcinoma: Comparison of intradermal versus subcutaneous administration. *Clin. Cancer Res.* **5,** 2330–2337.

Coukos, G., Makrigiannakis, A., Montas, S., Kaiser, L. R., Toyozumi, T., Benjamin, I., Albelda, S. M., Rubin, S. C., and Molnar-Kimber, K. L. (2000). Multiattenuated herpes simplex virus-1 mutant G207 exerts cytotoxicity against epithelial ovarian cancer but not normal mesothelium and is suitable for intraperitoneal oncolytic therapy. *Cancer Gene Ther.* **7,** 275–283.

Dietzschold, B., Rupprecht, C. E., Fu, Z. F., and Koprowski, D. (1996). Rhabdoviruses. *In* "Fields Virology" (B. N. Fields, ed.), Lippincott-Raven, Philadelphia.

Dobner, T., Horikoshi, N., Rubenwolf, S., and Shenk, T. (1996). Blockage by adenovirus E4orf6 of transcriptional activation by the p53 tumor suppressor. *Science* **272,** 1470–1473.

Doronin, K., Toth, K., Kuppuswamy, M., Ward, P., Tollefson, A., and Wold, W. (2000). Tumor-specific, replication-competent adenovirus vectors overexpressing the adenovirus death protein. *J. Virol.* **74,** 6147–6155.

Douglas, J. T., Rogers, B. E., Rosenfeld, M. E., Michael, S. I., Feng, M., and Curiel, D. T. (1996). Targeted gene delivery by tropism-modified adenoviral vectors. *Nature Biotechnol.* **14,** 1574–1578.

Drexler, I., Antunes, E., Schmitz, M., Wolfel, T., Huber, C., Erfle, V., Rieber, P., Theobald, M., and Sutter, G. (1999). Modified vaccinia virus Ankara for delivery of human tyrosinase as melanoma-associated antigen: Induction of tyrosinase- and melanoma-specific human leukocyte antigen A*0201-restricted cytotoxic T cells in vitro and in vivo. *Cancer Res.* **59,** 4955–4963.

Dupressoir, T., Vanacker, J. M., Cornelis, J. J., Duponchel, N., and Rommelaere, J. (1989). Inhibition by parvovirus H-1 of the formation of tumors in nude mice and colonies in vitro by transformed human mammary epithelial cells. *Cancer Res.* **49,** 3203–3208.

Eder, J. P., Kantoff, P. W., Roper, K., Xu, G. X., Bubley, G. J., Boyden, J., Gritz, L., Mazzara, G., Oh, W. K., Arlen, P., Tsang, K. Y., Panicali, D., Schlom, J., and Kufe, D. W. (2000). A phase I trial of a recombinant vaccinia virus expressing prostate-specific antigen in advanced prostate cancer. *Clin. Cancer Res.* **6,** 1632–1638.

Freytag, S. O., Rogulski, K. R., Paielli, D. L., Gilbert, J. D., and Kim, J. H. (1998). A novel three-pronged approach to kill cancer cells selectively: concomitant viral, double suicide gene, and radiotherapy. *Hum. Gene Ther.* **9,** 1323–1333.

Fueyo, J., Gomez-Manzano, C., Alemany, R., Lee, P., McDonnell, T., Mitlianga, P., Shi, Y., Levin, V., Yung, W., and Kyritsis, A. (2000). A mutant oncolytic adenovirus targeting the Rb pathway produces anti-glioma effect in vivo. *Oncogene* **19,** 2–12.

Ganly, I., Kirn, D., Eckhardt, S., Rodriguez, G., Souter, D., Von Hoff, D., and Kaye, S. (2000). A phase I study of Onyx-015, an E1B attenuated adenovirus, administered intratumorally to patients with recurrent head and neck cancer. *Clin. Cancer Res.* **6,** 798–806.

Gnant, M. F., Berger, A. C., Huang, J., Puhlmann, M., Wu, P. C., Merino, M. J., Bartlett, D. L., Alexander, H. R., Jr., and Libutti, S. K. (1999). Sensitization of tumor necrosis factor alpha-resistant human melanoma by tumor-specific in vivo transfer of the gene encoding endothelial monocyte-activating polypeptide II using recombinant vaccinia virus. *Cancer Res.* **59,** 4668–4674.

Goodrum, F. D., and Ornelles, D. A. (1997). The early region 1B 55-kilodalton oncoprotein of adenovirus relieves growth restrictions imposed on viral replication by the cell cycle. *J. Virol.* **71,** 548–561.

Gromeier, M., Alexander, L., and Wimmer, E. (1996). Internal ribosomal entry site substitution eliminates neurovirulence in intergeneric poliovirus recombinants. *Proc. Natl. Acad. Sci. USA* **93,** 2370–2375.

Gromeier, M., Bossert, B., Arita, M., Nomoto, A., and Wimmer, E. (1999). Dual stem loops within the poliovirus internal ribosomal entry site control neurovirulence. *J. Virol.* **73,** 958–964.

Gromeier, M., Lachmann, S., Rosenfeld, M. R., Gutin, P. H., and Wimmer, E. (2000). Intergeneric poliovirus recombinants for the treatment of malignant glioma. *Proc. Natl. Acad. Sci. USA* **97,** 6803–6808.

Hallenbeck, P. (1999). A novel tumor-specific replication-restricted adenoviral vector for gene therapy of hepatocellular carcinoma. *Human Gene Ther.* **10,** 1721–1733.

Harada, J., and Berk, A. (1999). p53-independent and -dependent requirements for E1B-55kD in adenovirus type 5 replication. *J. Virol.* **73,** 5333–5344.

Hawkins, L., Nye, J., Castro, D., Johnson, L., Kirn, D., and Hermiston, T. (1999). Replicating adenoviral gene therapy. *Proc. Am. Assoc. Cancer Res.* **40,** 3145. [Abstract]

He, Z., Wlazlo, A. P., Kowalczyk, D. W., Cheng, J., Xiang, Z. Q., Giles-Davis, W., and Ertl, H. C. (2000). Viral recombinant vaccines to the E6 and E7 antigens of HPV-16. *Virology* **270,** 146–161.

Hecht, R., Abbruzzese, J., Bedford, R., Randlev, B., Romel, L., Lahodi, S., and Kirn, D. (2000). A phase I/II trial of intratumoral endoscopic injection of Onyx-015 with intravenous gemcitabine in unresectable pancreatic carcinoma. *Proc. Am. Soc. Clin. Oncol.* **19**, 1039. [Abstract]

Heise, C., Hermiston, T., Johnson, L., Brooks, G., Sampson-Johannes, A., Williams, A., Hawkins, L., and Kirn, D. (2000). An adenovirus E1A mutant that demonstrates potent and selective antitumoral efficacy. *Nature Medicine* **6**, 1134–1139.

Heise, C., and Kirn, D. (2000). Replication-selective adenviruses as oncolytic agents. *J. Clin. Invest.* **105**, 847–851.

Heise, C., Sampson, J. A., Williams, A., McCormick, F., Von, H. D., and Kirn, D. H. (1997). ONYX-015, an E1B gene-attenuated adenovirus, causes tumor-specific cytolysis and antitumoral efficacy that can be augmented by standard chemotherapeutic agents. *Nat. Med.* **3**, 639–645.

Heise, C., Williams, A., Xue, S., Propst, M., and Kirn, D. (1999). Intravenous administration of ONYX-015, a selectively-replicating adenovirus, induces antitumoral efficacy. *Cancer Res.* **59**, 2623–2628.

Hermiston, T. (2000). Gene delivery from replication-selective viruses: arming guided missiles in the war against cancer. *J. Clin. Invest.* **105**, 1169–1172.

Herrlinger, U., Kramm, C. M., Aboody-Guterman, K. S., Silver, J. S., Ikeda, K., Johnston, K. M., Pechan, P. A., Barth, R. F., Finkelstein, D., Chiocca, E. A., Louis, D. N., and Breakefield, X. O. (1998). Pre-existing herpes simplex virus 1 (HSV-1) immunity decreases, but does not abolish, gene transfer to experimental brain tumors by a HSV-1 vector. *Gene Ther.* **5**, 809–819.

Hollstein, M., Sidransky, D., Vogelstein, B., and Harris, C. C. (1991). p53 mutations in human cancers. *Science* **253**, 49–53.

Hunter, W. D., Martuza, R. L., Feigenbaum, F., Todo, T., Mineta, T., Yazaki, T., Toda, M., Newsome, J. T., Platenberg, R. C., Manz, H. J., and Rabkin, S. D. (1999). Attenuated, replication-competent herpes simplex virus type 1 mutant G207: Safety evaluation of intracerebral injection in nonhuman primates. *J. Virol.* **73**, 6319–6326.

Khuri, F., Nemunaitis, J., Ganly, I., Gore, M., MacDougal, M., Tannock, I., Kaye, S., Hong, W., and Kirn, D. (2000). A controlled trial of Onyx-015, an E1B gene-deleted adenovirus, in combination with chemotherapy in patients with recurrent head and neck cancer. *Nat. Med.* **6**, 879–885.

Kim, M., Wright, M., Deshane, J., Accavitti, M. A., Tilden, A., Saleh, M., Vaughan, W. P., Carabasi, M. H., Rogers, M. D., Hockett, R. J., Grizzle, W. E., and Curiel, D. T. (1997). A novel gene therapy strategy for elimination of prostate carcinoma cells from human bone marrow. *Hum. Gene Ther.* **8**, 157–170.

Kirn, D. (2000). A tale of two trials: Selectively replicating herpesviruses for brain tumors. *Gene Ther.* **7**, 815–816.

Kirn, D. (2000). Replication-selective micro-organisms: Fighting cancer with targeted germ warfare. *J. Clin. Invest.* **105**, 836–838.

Kirn, D., Heise, C., Williams, M., Propst, M., and Hermiston, T. (1998). Adenovirus E1A CR2 mutants as selectively-replicating agents for cancer. *In* "Cancer Gene Therapy." Academic Press, San Diego.

Kirn, D., Hermiston, T., and McCormick, F. (1998). ONYX-015: Clinical data are encouraging. *Nature Med.* **4**, 1341–1342.

Kooby, D. A., Carew, J. F., Halterman, M. W., Mack, J. E., Bertino, J. R., Blumgart, L. H., Federoff, H. J., and Fong, Y. (1999). Oncolytic viral therapy for human colorectal cancer and liver metastases using a multi-mutated herpes simplex virus type-1 (G207). *FASEB J.* **13**, 1325–1334.

Kucharczuk, J. C., Randazzo, B., Chang, M. Y., Amin, K. M., Elshami, A. A., Sterman, D. H., Rizk, N. P., Molnar-Kimber, K. L., Brown, S. M., MacLean, A. R., Litzky, L. A., Fraser, N. W., Albelda, S. M., and Kaiser, L. R. (1997). Use of a "replication-restricted" herpes virus to treat experimental human malignant mesothelioma. *Cancer Res.* **57**, 466–471.

Lorenz, M. G., Kantor, J. A., Schlom, J., and Hodge, J. W. (1999). Anti-tumor immunity elicited by a recombinant vaccinia virus expressing CD70 (CD27L). *Hum. Gene Ther.* **10**, 1095–1103.

Markert, J., Medlock, M., Rabkin, S., Gillespie, G., Todo, T., Hunter, W., Palmer, C., Feigenbaum, F., Tornatore, C., Tufaro, F., and Martuza, R. (2000). Conditionally replicating herpes simplex virus mutant, G207 for the treatment of malignant glioma: results of a phase I trial. *Gene Ther.* **7**, 867–874.

Martuza, R. (2000). Conditionally replicating herpes viruses for cancer therapy. *J. Clin. Invest.* **105**, 841–846.

Martuza, R. L., Malick, A., Markert, J. M., Ruffner, K. L., and Coen, D. M. (1991). Experimental therapy of human glioma by means of a genetically engineered virus mutant. *Science* **252**, 854–856.

Mastrangelo, M., Eisenlohr, L., Gomella, L., and Lattime, E. (2000). Poxvirus vectors: Orphaned and underappreciated. *J. Clin. Invest.* **105**, 1031–1034.

Mastrangelo, M. J., Maguire, H. C., Jr., Eisenlohr, L. C., Laughlin, C. E., Monken, C. E., McCue, P. A., Kovatich, A. J., and Lattime, E. C. (1999). Intratumoral recombinant GM-CSF-encoding virus as gene therapy in patients with cutaneous melanoma. *Cancer Gene Ther.* **6**, 409–422.

McCart, J. A., Puhlmann, M., Lee, J., Hu, Y., Libutti, S. K., Alexander, H. R., and Bartlett, D. L. (2000). Complex interactions between the replicating oncolytic effect and the enzyme/prodrug effect of vaccinia-mediated tumor regression. *Gene Ther.* **7**, 1217–1223.

Medina, D. J., Sheay, W., Goodell, L., Kidd, P., White, E., Rabson, A. B., and Strair, R. K. (1999). Adenovirus-mediated cytotoxicity of chronic lymphocytic leukemia cells. *Blood* **94**, 3499–3508.

Mineta, T., Rabkin, S. D., Yazaki, T., Hunter, W. D., and Martuza, R. L. (1995). Attenuated multi-mutated herpes simplex virus-1 for the treatment of malignant gliomas. *Nat. Med.* **1**, 938–943.

Moss, B. (1996). Poxiviridae: The viruses and their replication. In "Fields Virology" (B. N. Fields, ed.), 3rd Ed. Lippincott-Raven, Philadelphia.

Moss, B. (1996). Genetically engineered poxviruses for recombinant gene expression, vaccination, and safety. *Proc. Natl. Acad. Sci. USA* **93,** 11341–11348.

Mukherjee, S., Haenel, T., Himbeck, R., Scott, B., Ramshaw, I., Lake, R. A., Harnett, G., Phillips, P., Morey, S., Smith, D., Davidson, J. A., Musk, A. W., and Robinson, B. (2000). Replication-restricted vaccinia as a cytokine gene therapy vector in cancer: persistent transgene expression despite antibody generation. *Cancer Gene Ther.* **7,** 663–670.

Nemunaitis, J., Cunningham, C., Edelman, G., Berman, B., and Kirn, D. (1999). Phase I dose-escalation trial of intravenous ONYX-015 in patients with refractory cancer. Proceedings of the Cancer Gene Therapy Meeting.

Nemunaitis, J., Cunningham, C., Randlev, B., and Kirn, D. (2000). A phase I dose escalation trial of intravenous infusion with a replication-selective adenovirus, dl 1520, in patients with refractory cancer. *Proc. Am. Soc. Clin. Oncol.* **19,** 724. [Abstract]

Nemunaitis, J., Ganly, I., Khuri, F., Arsenau, J., Kuhn, J., McCarty, T., Landers, S., Maples, P., Romel, L., Randlev, B., Reid, T., Kaye, S., and Kirn, D. (2000). Selective replication and oncolysis in p53 mutant tumors with Onyx-015, an E1B-55kD gene-deleted adenovirus, in patients with advanced head and neck cancer: A phase II trial. *Cancer Res.* **60,** 6359–6366.

Nielsch, U., Fognani, C., and Babiss, L. E. (1991). Adenovirus E1A-p105(Rb) protein interactions play a direct role in the initiation but not the maintenance of the rodent cell transformed phenotype. *Oncogene* **6,** 1031–1036.

Norman, K., and Lee, P. (2000). Reovirus as a novel oncolytic agent. *J. Clin. Invest.* **105,** 1035–1038.

Olson, D. C., and Levine, A. J. (1994). The properties of p53 proteins selected for the loss of suppression of transformation. *Cell Growth Differ.* **5,** 61–71.

Parker, J., Gillespie, G., Love, C., Randall, S., Whitley, R., and Markert, J. (2000). Engineered herpes simplex virus expressing IL-12 in the treatment of experimental murine brain tumors. *Proc. Natl. Acad. Sci. USA* **97,** 2208–2213.

Puhlmann, M., Brown, C. K., Gnant, M., Huang, J., Libutti, S. K., Alexander, H. R., and Bartlett, D. L. (2000). Vaccinia as a vector for tumor-directed gene therapy: Biodistribution of a thymidine kinase-deleted mutant. *Cancer Gene Ther.* **7,** 66–73.

Rampling, R., Cruickchank, G., Papanastassiou, V., Nicoll, J., Hadley, D., Brennan, D., Petty, R., Maclean, A., Harland, J., McKie, E., Mabbs, R., and Brown, M. (2000). Toxicity evaluation of replication-competent herpes simplex virus (ICP 34.5 null mutant 1716) in patients with recurrent malignant glioma. *Gene Ther.* **7,** 1–4.

Reid, T., Galanis, E., Abbruzzese, J., Randlev, B., Romel, L., Rubin, J., and Kirn, D. (2000). Hepatic artery infusion of Onyx-015, a replication-selective adenovirus, in combination with 5-FU/leucovorin for gastrointestinal carcinoma metastatic to the liver: A phase I/ II clinical trial. *Proc. Am. Soc. Clin. Oncol.* **19,** 953. [Abstract]

Reid, A., Galanis, E., Abbruzzese, J., Romel, L., Rubin, J., and Kirn, D. (1999). A phase I/II trial of ONYX-015 administered by hepatic artery infusion to patients with colorectal carcinoma. EORTC-NCI-AACR Meeting on Molecular Therapeutics of Cancer.

Rodriguez, R., Schuur, E. R., Lim, H. Y., Henderson, G. A., Simons, J. W., and Henderson, D. R. (1997). Prostate attenuated replication competent adenovirus (ARCA) CN706: A selective cytotoxic for prostate-specific antigen-positive prostate cancer cells. *Cancer Res.* **57,** 2559–2563.

Roelvink, P., Mi, G., Einfeld, D., Kovesdi, I., and Wickham, T. (1999). Identification of a conserved reseptor-binding site on the fiber proteins of CAR-recognizing adenoviridae. *Science* **286,** 1568–1571.

Roizman, B. (1996). The function of herpes simplex virus genes: A primer for genetic engineering of novel vectors. *Proc. Natl. Acad. Sci. USA* **93,** 11307–11312.

Rothmann, T., Hengstermann, A., Whitaker, N. J., Scheffner, M., and zur Hausen, H. (1998). Replication of ONYX-015, a potential anticancer adenovirus, is independent of p53 status in tumor cells. *J. Virol.* **72,** 9470–9478.

Sauthoff, H., Heitner, S., Rom, W., and Hay, J. (2000). Deletion of the adenoviral E1B-19kD gene enhances tumor cell killing of a replicating adenoviral vector. *Hum. Gene Ther.* **11,** 379–388.

Scheffner, M., Munger, K., Byrne, J. C., and Howley, P. M. (1991). The state of the p53 and retinoblastoma genes in human cervical carcinoma cell lines. *Proc. Natl. Acad. Sci. USA* **88,** 5523–5527.

Sherr, C. J. (1996). Cancer cell cycles. *Science* **274,** 1672–1677.

Smith, R., Huebner, R. J., Rowe, W. P., Schatten, W. E., and Thomas, L. B. (1956). Studies on the use of viruses in the treatment of carcinoma of the cervix. *Cancer* **9,** 1211–1218.

Southam, C. M., and Moore, A. E. (1952). Clinical studies of viruses as antineoplastic agents, with particular reference to Egypt 101 virus. *Cancer* **5,** 1025–1034.

Stojdl, D. F., Lichty, B., Knowles, S., Marius, R., Atkins, H., Sonenberg, N., and Bell, J. C. (2000). Exploiting tumor-specific defects in the interferon pathway with a previously unknown oncolytic virus. *Nat. Med.* **6,** 821–825.

Toda, M., Martuza, R. L., Kojima, H., and Rabkin, S. D. (1998). In situ cancer vaccination: An IL-12 defective vector/replication-competent herpes simplex virus combination induces local and systemic antitumor activity. *J. Immunol.* **160,** 4457–4464.

Todo, T., Rabkin, S. D., Sundaresan, P., Wu, A., Meehan, K. R., Herscowitz, H. B., and Martuza, R. L. (1999). Systemic antitumor immunity in experimental brain tumor therapy using a multimutated, replication-competent herpes simplex virus, *Hum. Gene Ther.* **10,** 2741–2755.

Toyoizumi, T., Mick, R., Abbas, A. E., Kang, E. H., Kaiser, L. R., and Molnar-Kimber, K. L. (1999). Combined therapy with chemotherapeutic agents and herpes simplex virus type 1 ICP34.5 mutant (HSV-1716) in human non-small cell lung cancer. *Hum Gene Ther.* **10,** 3013–3029.

Tyler, K. L., and Fields, B. N. (1996). Reoviruses. *In* "Fields Virology" (B. N. Fields, ed.), 3rd Ed. Lippincott-Raven, Philadelphia.

Uzendoski, K., Kantor, J. A., Abrams, S. I., Schlom, J., and Hodge, J. W. (1997). Construction and characterization of a recombinant vaccinia virus expressing murine intercellular adhesion molecule-1: Induction and potentiation of antitumor responses. *Hum. Gene Ther.* **8,** 851–860.

Valmori, D., Levy, F., Miconnet, I., Zajac, P., Spagnoli, G. C., Rimoldi, D., Lienard, D., Cerundolo, V., Cerottini, J. C., and Romero, P. (2000). Induction of potent antitumor CTL responses by recombinant vaccinia encoding a melan-A peptide analogue. *J. Immunol.* **164,** 1125–1131.

Vasey, P., Shulman, L., Gore, M., Kirn, D., and Kaye, S. (2000). Phase I trial of intraperitoneal Onyx-015 adenovirus in patients with recurrent ovarian carcinoma. *Proc. Am. Soc. Clin. Oncol.* **19,** 1512. [Abstract]

Wickham, T. J., Segal, D. M., Roelvink, P. W., Carrion, M. E., Lizonova, A., Lee, G. M., and Kovesdi, I. (1996). Targeted adenovirus gene transfer to endothelial and smooth muscle cells by using bispecific antibodies. *J. Virol.* **70,** 6831–6838.

Wildner, O., Blaese, R. M., and Morris, J. M. (1999). Therapy of colon cancer with oncolytic adenovirus is enhanced by the addition of herpes simplex virus-thymidine kinase. *Cancer Res.* **59,** 410–413.

Yew, P. R., Liu, X., and Berk, A. J. (1994). Adenovirus E1B oncoprotein tethers a transcriptional repression domain to p53. *Genes Dev.* **8,** 190–202.

Zajac, P., Oertli, D., Spagnoli, G. C., Noppen, C., Schaefer, C., Heberer, M., and Marti, W. R. (1997). Generation of tumoricidal cytotoxic T lymphocytes from healthy donors after in vitro stimulation with a replication-incompetent vaccinia virus encoding MART-1/Melan-A 27-35 epitope. *Int. J. Cancer* **71,** 491–496.

Zhang, Y., Xiong, Y., and Yarbrough, W. G. (1998). ARF promotes MDM2 degradation and stabilizes p53: ARF-INK4a locus deletion impairs both the Rb and p53 tumor suppression pathways. *Cell* **92,** 725–734.

Resistance to Antibody Therapy

Melissa S. McGrath
David A. Scheinberg
Memorial Sloan-Kettering Cancer Center

GLOSSARY

antibody modulation Internalization or redistribution of the cell surface antigen–antibody complex after binding of a monoclonal antibody.

anti-idiotype An antibody specific for the unique amino acid sequence of the immunoglobulin variable region or idiotype.

complement cascade Pathway of complement activation mediated by antibody binding to antigen on the surface of a cell. This binding initiates a series of events, which culminates in the formation of a membrane attack complex within the cell membrane, resulting in cell lysis.

complement inhibitory proteins Proteins expressed on the surface of the cell that proteolytically inactivate or disassemble complement components to regulate or prevent the complement cascade and lysis.

immunoconjugate A class of hybrid proteins consisting of a monoclonal antibody and a cytotoxic molecule, including toxins, chemotherapuetic drugs, and radioisotopes.

immunotoxin A class of hybrid proteins that consists of a monoclonal antibody covalently or genetically linked to plant or bacterial-derived toxic molecules. Examples of toxins used are gelonin, ricin, and diptheria toxin.

multidrug resistance (MDR) A phenomenon describing the ability of a cell to survive lethal concentrations of a broad range of structurally and pharmacologically distinct cytotoxic compounds. MDR is associated with a decrease in intracellular accumulation of drug and changes in intracellular pH.

P-glycoprotein (P-gp) A 170-kDa plasma membrane-associated glycoprotein encoded by the MDR1 gene. P-gp is a member of the ATP-binding cassette transporter superfamily. Overexpression of P-gp can mediate MDR.

radioimmunotherapy Therapy with a radioactive immunoconjugate.

The role of monoclonal antibody therapy in the treatment of cancer has become more widely recognized as five monoclonal antibodies have been approved by the FDA for the treatment of cancer. The utilization of monoclonal antibodies is ideal for cancer therapy due to their ability to selectively target tumor cells while sparing normal tissue from their cytotoxic effects. Native monoclonal antibodies are effective instruments in the elimination of tumor cells by recruiting the host effector functions of complement-mediated cytotoxicity and antibody-dependent cell-mediated cytotoxicity.

I. INTRODUCTION

Resistance to antibody therapy may be host derived (as in the development of neutralizing anti-antibody responses), pharmacological (as in poor delivery to the target site), or intrinsic to the tumor cell (as in antigenic modulation or MDR). Initial clinical trials using murine monoclonal antibodies resulted in a human antimouse antibody response (HAMA) in many cases. This immune response against the foreign antibodies increased their clearance from the circulation and therefore decreased efficacy. Hence, the first form of resistance was host derived, rather then tumor derived. Later clinical trials using human or humanized monoclonal antibodies reduced the incidence of HAMA, but highlighted additional mechanisms by which tumor cells could resist immunological attack. These tumor-based mechanisms of resistance included antigenic heterogeneity, antigen shedding, antigen modulation, and mutation. Additional pharmacologic hurdles were discovered, such as the issue of poor antibody diffusion into areas of large tumor burden and high levels of infusional toxicity. Finally, most antibodies were not effective at initiating or recruiting CMC or ADCC and failed due to lack of potency.

One solution to inadequately potent native antibodies was the utilization of cytotoxic antibody immunoconjugates. The antibodies would serve solely to selectively deliver cytotoxic agents such as bacterial or plant toxins, synthetic small molecule drug substances, or radioisotopes to the site of tumor. In principle, these cytotoxic immunoconjugates would be both highly specific for the tumor cells and extremely potent, while not relying on the activation of the immune system. Despite their increased effectiveness as compared to native antibodies, resistance to immunoconjugates has been observed as well.

The development of nonnative antibody forms was also attempted in an effort to increase potency. Bispecific antibodies were manufactured with one Fab specific for the tumor cell surface antigen and a second Fab directed to an activating receptor on an effector cell. These constructs served to deliver the effector cell activity more directly to the target.

II. MULTIDRUG RESISTANCE

Although the major cause of failure in antibody therapy stemmed from the inability of the antibody to reach the tumor cells or to inadequately activate host effectors, evidence of intrinsic resistance of the tumor cell to antibody attack was observed. The development of drug resistance has been a major obstacle to effective chemotherapy. One subtype of drug resistance known as multidrug resistance is characterized by broad resistance to several structurally, chemically, and pharmacologically distinct cytotoxic compounds. MDR expression correlates with intracellular changes of pH, altered accumulation of drug, and overexpression of proteins belonging to the ATP-binding cassette transmembrane transporter superfamily.

Proteins thought to contribute to this resistance include the MDR 1 gene product P-glycoprotein (P-gp). P-gp can be induced by many antitumor agents, and its expression on the surface of the cell correlates with decreased responses to chemotherapeutic drugs. Also associated with MDR is multidrug resistance related protein (MRP). Structurally similar to MDR1, MRP is also a member of the ABC transporter superfamily and causes a pattern of drug resistance similar to that of P-gp.

An increase in the major vault protein (MVP; sometimes known as the lung resistance protein, LRP) corresponds with the development of drug resistance in multiple myeloma. Unlike the other proteins associated with MDR, these are ribonuceloproteins, which congregate in the nuclear pore complex and in vesicle junctions in the cytoplasm. MVP is thought to contribute to drug resistance by the transport of xenobiotic toxins out of the cell. Other proteins, such as the newly discovered breast cancer resistance protein (BCRP), have been shown to contribute to the MDR phenotype. Surprisingly, it has been shown that MDR cells are also resistant to antibody-mediated cytotoxicity, including complement-mediated cytotoxicity, radioimmunotherapy, and immunotoxin attack.

III. MECHANISMS OF RESISTANCE TO ANTIBODY THERAPY

A. Native (Unmodified) Antibodies

Native antibodies are often limited in their capacity to kill cancer cells due to their inability to potently activate the effector mechanisms of the immune system at the tumor cell surface. This failure is multifactorial: first, the antibody must reach the site of tumor. Antibodies have molecular masses of approximately 150 and 900 kDa for IgG and IgM, respectively, and even in the case of modest sized tumors are unable to diffuse quickly to the cells. As a consequence, these Ig are unable to accumulate at the site of disease in adequate concentrations to achieve a response. In the case of IgG, two or more antibodies must bind to the surface of the cell in close proximity to initiate and fix complement or to recruit cellular mediators of ADCC. On some tumor cells there is insufficient antigen density on the surface of the cell for the minimum threshold of activation by antibody to occur, even if the antibody can reach the cells. With high-affinity antibodies, a binding site barrier caused by initial binding at the outer edges of the tumor can further limit diffusion into cells deeper within the tumor. Antibodies themselves may be immunogenic, limiting the number of infusions possible and therefore the efficacy of antibody therapy. Finally, circulating antigen (shed or secreted by tumors) may block the delivery of the antibody to its target.

Once at the cell surface, an additional frequently observed obstacle is modulation of the antigen/antibody complex, resulting in loss of the antibody from the cell surface, thus abrogating the effector response. Exposure of the cell to high-affinity antibodies may also cause the redistribution and prolonged downregulation of that antigen. Such modulation is seen with many protein antigens, and several clinical trials have demonstrated antigenic modulation occurring in patients *in vivo*.

An additional mechanism of resistance to antibody therapy is selection of antigen-negative tumor cell variants (Fig. 1). These tumor clones will thus become completely resistant to the effects of the antigen-specific monoclonal therapy. The development of mutant idiotype variants has been observed in trials of anti-idiotypic monoclonal antibodies in the treatment B-cell lymphoma. This phenomenon is not due to modulation of the target immunoglobulin antigen, but rather to a somatic mutation in the idiotype of the immunoglobulin antigen itself. A simple structural (amino acid) change in the idiotype target can prevent the binding of the idiotype-specific therapeutic monoclonal antibody, allowing the outgrowth of idiotype-negative clones. Another example of this is antibody therapy directed to disialoganglioside GD2. When GD2 is targeted by a monoclonal antibody in models of neuroblastoma, antigen-negative clones arise, which escape immune detection. Similar mechanisms may rarely occur with protein targets such as CD20. CD20-negative lymphomas have been observed with the anti-CD20 monoclonal antibody. Antigenic heterogeneity of the tumor cells may cause a similar outcome following monoclonal antibody therapy (Fig. 1). If the target antigen is not present at the same level of expression on all tumor cells, residual tumor cells will remain following therapy, allowing resistant tumor outgrowth.

B. Complement-Mediated Cytotoxicity

Another mechanism of tumor cell escape from immune destruction is resistance to complement-mediated cytotoxicity. This is a significant escape outlet because complement killing may be critical for immunotherapy with both native (unconjugated) antibodies and immunoconjugates. Activation of the complement cascade via antibody binding to the cell surface results in the formation of the membrane attack complex (MAC), which creates a pore within the cell membrane mediating cell lysis. As described earlier, the initiation of complement-mediated lysis requires a minimum number of target antigens on the cell surface and stability of the complex. Thus, antigen–antibody modulation will reduce complement-mediated killing. To prevent nonspecific lysis of normal cells by complement, its activation is regulated through membrane-bound regulatory proteins known as complement resistance proteins. These protein regulators may be overexpressed in tumor cells. Table I lists protein regulators of complement and the role

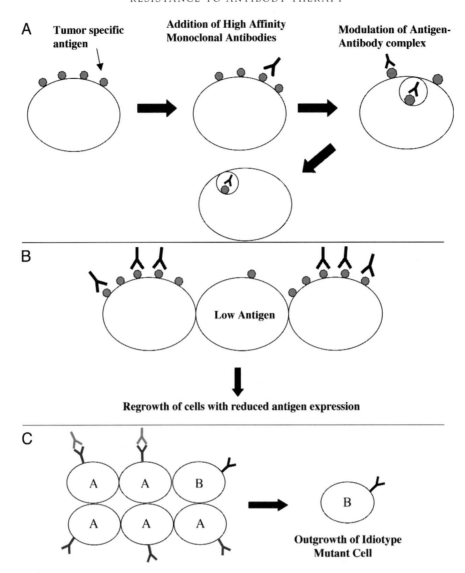

FIGURE 1 Three mechanisms of resistance resulting from monoclonal antibody therapy. (A) Modulation of tumor antigen–antibody complex from the cell surface prevents antibody from binding to the tumor cell, resulting in the emergence of antigen-negative clones. (B) Antigenic heterogeneity may allow outgrowth of cells that do not express sufficient antigen. (C) Emergence of idiotype variants "B" following treatment of tumor expressing "A" with monoclonal antibody.

each plays in protecting the cell from complement mediated cell lysis. Elevated levels of decay accelerating factor (CD55), membrane cofactor protein (CD46), and homologous restriction factor (CD59) contribute to tumor cell resistance to complement.

A second contributing factor to escape is shedding of these regulatory proteins from the surface of tumor cells. A soluble form of both CD46 and CD55 may serve to further inhibit complement-mediated lysis in regions where the proteins are found. In addition to the highly characterized complement regulatory proteins, other proteins, including the ecto-proteases p69 and p41, may also serve to protect tumor cells by cleaving complement activators. These proteases are reported to protect against C3 deposition.

Less well characterized pathways of resistance involve the removal of the MAC (by internalization or exocytosis) from the surface of the cell or possibly shedding of proteins on the surface of the cell, which are covalently bound to targeted complement (i.e., C3b and C4b). It

TABLE I
Complement Resistance Proteins or Membrane-Bound Complement Regulatory Proteins
Inhibit Activation of the Complement Cascade

Protein	Function
CD46 (membrane cofactor protein)	Activates factors H and I, which result in the inhibition of C3/C5 convertase formation
CD55 (decay accelerating factor)	Accelerates decay or dissociation of C3 and C5 convertases from complement proteins
CD59 (homologous restriction factor)	Binds C8 and prevents C9 polymerization and MAC formation

has also been suggested that tumor cells have the ability to repair complement damage in their cell membrane.

Another protective mechanism functions by altering the amount of activated complement on the surface of the cell. Complement-induced protection can occur when tumor (leukemia) cells are exposed to doses of complement that are insufficient to lyse the cell. Consequently, the cell becomes desensitized against further complement assaults.

Interestingly, evidence *in vitro* has demonstrated that MDR cells that overexpress P-gp (either via selection in drug or retroviral transfection) are resistant to complement-mediated cytotoxicity. This resistance is thought to involve an increase in intracellular pH, which results in a decrease in the deposition of membrane attack complexes on the surface of the cell.

C. Immunotoxins

Immunotoxins are a class of proteins that consist of a monoclonal antibody covalently linked to a toxic molecule. The toxic protein may be of plant origin, including ribosome-inactivating proteins ricin and gelonin. Other toxins widely used include diptheria toxin, pseudomonas exotoxin, and calicheamicin. The FDA-approved immunoconjugate CMA-676, used in the treatment of myeloid leukemia, incorporates calicheamicin, which works by creating double-stranded DNA breaks. The antibody in this construct is specific for CD33, which is expressed on 85% of acute myeloid leukemias. HuM195-gelonin is another immunotoxin specific for CD33. Gelonin is a ribosome-inactivating protein that works by irreversibly inactivating the large 60S ribosomal subunit. Some cells that exhibit the MDR phenotype are resistant to the effects of both of these immunotoxins as compared with parental cell lines. The mechanism for this is currently unclear.

Immunotoxins are directed to target antigen in the same manner as native antibodies, which consequently makes immunotoxins susceptible to some of the same mechanisms of resistance affecting unconjugated antibodies. Immunotoxins must be specifically targeted to the surface via monoclonal antibody. Once bound, the immunotoxin will be internalized via receptor-mediated endocytosis and delivered into an endosomal compartment. The immunotoxin will then be trafficked and processed within the cell until the enzymatically active domain is translocated into the cytosol before finally reaching its target. Therefore, mutation, heterogeneity of expression, or shedding of the target antigen may contribute to resistance. Shedding of the antigen target from the surface of the cell or structural changes in the epitope will prevent antigen recognition and inhibit immunotoxin binding.

D. Radioimmunconjugates

Another commonly used form of antibody therapy is radioimmunotherapy (RIT) in which a monoclonal antibody is linked to a radioisotope. Similar to other immunoconjugates, radioimmunoconjugates may be relatively specific for tumor cells and can potently deliver radiation to the tumor cell with less cytotoxicity to the surrounding normal tissues. β-emitting isotopes have moderate energy levels (300–2000 KeV) and a long particle range (0.5–10 mm). α-emitting isotopes have high energy (5000–10,000 KeV) and a short range (0.04–0.1 mm), thus traversing only one or two cell lengths, thereby increasing the specificity of the radiation dramatically. One advantage of RIT is that cytotoxicity does not require either internalization of the radioimmunoconjugate or the recruitment of immune effector cells so that antigen modulation is less likely to cause resistance. Tumor cells that shed antigen from the surface of the tumor cell may preclude the efficacy of RIT, however. Intrinsic resistance pathways to the radiation will also abrogate the effects of RIT.

IV. FUTURE DIRECTIONS TO OVERCOME RESISTANCE

Although monoclonal antibody therapies have made large recent advances, many obstacles of resistance to antibody therapy remain. A major goal of antibody therapy is to understand and surmount these obstacles. To combat host-derived and pharmacological resistance to antibody therapy, human monoclonal antibody fragments have been utilized to prevent both HAMA and HAHA. Antibody fragments including Fv, Fab, and F(ab′)₂ have been substituted for intact immunoglobulin to increase the diffusion of native and conjugated antibodies to sites of tumor in an effort to prevent pharmacological resistance. These fragments typically display binding specificity and affinity similar to that of the intact Ig. To ensure that the immune system will be activated and the appropriate effector cells recruited, bispecific antibodies directed against both the effector and the target have been utilized.

One of the most common mechanisms of resistance intrinsic to the tumor cell, MDR, remains a barrier for both chemotherapy and antibody therapy. Attempts to reverse MDR pharmacologically using chemosensitizers such as verapamil or trifluoperazin have met with limited success. Monoclonal antibodies directed against P-gp, which inhibit its biological function, have been used to block its activity while administering therapy. Thus far, these reversal agents have been shown to add little improvement to efficacy. Investigations of novel approaches to reverse MDR in the clinical setting are under study.

The emergence of antigen-negative variants after high-affinity monoclonal antibody therapy remains a problem in terms of the efficacy of therapy. The development of monoclonal antibody cocktails to multiple target antigens may prevent outgrowth of tumors that do not express the single target antigen. Using more then one antibody will also increase the likelihood of sufficient antibodies binding to the cell to activate CMC and ADCC. Targeting of multiple antibodies to the tumor cells may also prevent cells with antigenic modulation and heterogeneity from escaping immune destruction. It is likely that future antibody therapies will be conducted in combination with other forms of therapy to reduce the possibility of escape.

See Also the Following Articles

ANTIBODIES IN THE GENE THERAPY OF CANCER • ANTIBODY-TOXIN AND GROWTH FACTOR-TOXIN FUSION PROTEINS • ANTIIDIOTYPIC ANTIBODY VACCINES • MONOCLONAL ANTIBODIES: LEUKEMIA AND LYMPHOMA • MULTIDRUG RESISTANCE I: P-GLYCOPROTEIN • MULTIDRUG RESISTANCE II: MRP AND RELATED PROTEINS • RADIOLABELED ANTIBODIES, OVERVIEW • RESISTANCE TO DNA-DAMAGING AGENTS

Bibliography

Germann, U. A. (1996). P-glycoprotein—A mediator of multidrug resistance in tumour cells. *Eur. J. Cancer* **32A,** 927–944.

Gorter, A., and Meri, S. (1999). Immune evasion of tumor cells using membrane-bound complement regulatory proteins. *Immunol. Tod.* **20,** 576–581.

Janeway, C. A., and Travers, P. (1997). "Immunobiology: The Immune System in Health and Disease." Garland Publishing, New York.

Loe, D. W., Deeley, R. G., and Cole, S. P. C. (1996). Biology of the multidrug resistance-associated protein, MRP. *Eur. J. Cancer* **32A,** 945–957.

Meeker, T., Lowder, J., Cleary, M. L., Stewart, S., Warnke, R., Sklar, J., and Levy, R. (1985). Emergence of idiotype variants during treatment of B-cell lymphoma with anti-idiotype antibodies. *N. Engl. J. Med.* **312,** 1658–1665.

Paul, W. E. (Ed.) (1996). "Fundamental Immunology." Raven Press, New York.

Reiter, Y., Ciobotariu, A., and Fishelson, Z. (1992). Sublytic complement attack protects tumor cells from lytic doses of antibody and complement. *Eur. J. Immunol.* **22,** 1207–1213.

Segal, D. M., Weiner, G. J., and Weiner, L. M. (1999). Bispecific antibodies in cancer therapy. *Curr. Opin. Immunol.* **11,** 558–562.

Thrush, G. R., Lark, L. R., Clinchy, B. C., and Vitteta, E. S. (1996). Immunotoxins: An update. *Annu. Rev. Immunol.* **14,** 49–71.

Weiner, L. M. (1999). Monoclonal antibody therapy of cancer. *Sem. Oncol.* **26,** 43–51.

Weisberg, J. H., Curcio, M., Caron, P. C., Raghi, G., Mechetner, E. B., Roepe, P. D., and Scheinberg, D. A. (1996). The multidrug resistance phenotype confers immunological resistance. *J. Exp. Med.* **183,** 2699–2704.

Weisberg, J. H., Roepe, P. D., Dzekunov, S., and Scheinberg, D. A. (1999). Intracellular pH and multidrug resistance regulates complement-mediated cytotoxicity of nucleated human cells. *J. Biol. Chem.* **274,** 10877–10888.

Resistance to DNA-Damaging Agents

M. Eileen Dolan

University of Chicago

GLOSSARY

alkylating agents In chemotherapy, a drug that generates covalent adducts on DNA-containing alkyl groups.

DNA repair The enzymatic or nonenzymatic removal from DNA of adducts and lesions that can lead to mutation or cell death.

drug resistance The ability of cells to withstand challenges by therapeutic compounds that were lethal to previous generations.

A large number of cancer treatment regimens incorporate DNA-damaging agents. Chemotherapeutic agents that damage DNA directly include, but are not limited to, alkylating agents (nitrogen mustards, alkyl-nitrosoureas, alkyltriazenes), platinum-containing compounds (*cis*-platinum, carboplatin), and anthracyclines (doxorubicin). All are distinct moieties sharing only the property of having an electrophilic function. A major limitation of effective chemotherapeutic DNA-damaging therapy is the innate presence and/or subsequent development of resistance. Cellular protection can involve endogenous nucleophilic thiols, decreased drug entry into the cell, decreased drug-activating enzymes, increased enzymatic detoxification pathways, or repair of damaged DNA. It is likely that multiple mechanisms of cellular resistance occur in a given tumor cell population and are responsible for clinically evident drug resistance. Knowledge of mechanisms of alkylating agent resistance serves as the foundation for the clinical development of alkylating agent modulation strategies. Biochemical modulation is an attempt to favorably alter the interaction of conventional chemotherapeutic agents with their targets in malignant cells. This article focuses on mechanisms of resistance to DNA-damaging agents and specific strategies for preventing or overcoming resistance to improve clinical outcome.

I. INTRODUCTION

Eucaryotic cells have evolved several mechanisms to protect key cellular constituents, especially DNA, from highly reactive molecules generated from anti-cancer therapy. There are two forms of resistance: (1) tumors that are intrinsically resistant to therapy and (2) tumors that are initially sensitive to therapy, but after an initial response become resistant to the drugs (i.e., acquired resistance). Acquired resistance represents selection of a subpopulation of resistant cells. There are several mechanisms by which tumor cells become resistant to DNA-damaging agents. As a class, the activity of most DNA-damaging agents is decreased in the presence of high levels of glutathione (GSH). However, they differ in toxicity profiles and antitumor activity and the differences may be related to transport properties, detoxification reactions, and specific enzymatic reactions capable of repairing damaged sites on DNA. For example, varying degrees of cross-resistance between alkylating agents are seen, but a tumor that is resistant to one alkylating agent may remain significantly sensitive to another. This article provides an overview of mechanisms of resistance responsible for the ineffectiveness or eventual failure of DNA-damaging chemotherapeutic agents. Strategies to overcome resistance will be examined. The more well-studied mechanisms, including nonprotein thiol (GSH and related enzymes) and DNA repair [O^6-alkylguanine-DNA alkyltransferase (AGT) and mismatch repair (MMR)], are discussed.

II. GLUTATHIONE (GSH) AND GSH-RELATED ENZYMES

The association of elevated levels of GSH and glutathione S-transferases (GSTs) with the development of resistance to DNA-damaging agents was established several decades ago. The greater affinity of electrophiles for thiol groups than for hydroxyl or amine groups provides the basis for GSH as a pivotal nonprotein thiol in the protection of cells from electrophiles created during exposure to DNA-damaging agents. The ability to form glutathione conjugates, a reaction involving GSH, GST, and related enzymes, such as peroxidases, is a ubiquitous function of drug detoxification. The process is the formation of more polar and water-soluble derivatives that result in the reduction of the chemical reactivity of a drug and its rapid excretion. As a result, reactive species are unavailable to damage cellular constituents, particularly DNA. There has been a revival of interest in the study of GSH and GSH-utilizing enzymes driven by discoveries that have implicated redox balance as an important regulator of cell death and transmembrane drug transport. The available intracellular GSH content is determined in part by the redox state of the cell. Under conditions of redox stress, GSH dimerizes to oxidized glutathione (GSSG), making available reducing equivalents to neutralize reactive oxygen species.

A. GSH in Drug Resistance

GSH is highly abundant (up to 10 mM) in normal cells, although tumor cell content varies widely. The standard clinically useful anticancer drugs known to interact with GSH include alkylating agents (primarily melphalan and cyclophosphamide), "platinating drugs" (cisplatin), and anthracylines (doxorubicin). Human tumor cell lines made resistant to alkylating agents had increased GSH, and depletion of GSH increased sensitivity to these agents. Precise mechanisms of how GSH protects tumor cells from various cytotoxic agents include (1) detoxifying DNA-damaging agents by conjugation reactions catalyzed by GSTs; (2) quenching drug–DNA adducts; (3) redox reactions (i.e., reducing hydroxyl radicals); and (4) as a component of drug resistance secondary to decreased intracellular drug accumulation.

B. GSH-Associated Enzymes

Three groups of enzymes are associated with GSH. Altered expression of each of these has been implicated in the drug resistance phenotype in laboratory models and/or in patient tumors. They are γ-glutamylcysteine synthetase (γ-GCS), which is the rate-limiting enzyme in GSH synthesis; GSH reductase responsible for maintaining reduced GSH levels; and GSTs responsible for conjugation of GSH and reactive intermediates. GSTs form a group of multigene isoenzymes and have been divided into a number of subclasses: α, μ, pi, and theta. GSTs show a high level of specificity toward GSH, but the electrophilic second substrate can vary significantly both between and within the classes, despite their sequence similarity. Catalysis by conjugation with GSH and excretion of the less toxic and more hydrophilic products is an invaluable service to rid the body of toxins, but is disadvantageous during chemotherapy where GSTs have been associated with multidrug resistance of tumor cells. Levels of expression of different isoforms of GSTs are tissue specific. The variations in expression between normal and tumor cells are of interest and, in most cases, the GST levels are increased, especially GST-pi. Studies have indicated that GST-pi may play an important role in the resistance of cancer cells to alkylating agents, including cisplatin compounds. GST expression correlates well with response to platinum-based chemotherapy in head and neck cancer and in nonsmall lung cancer. The use of isozyme-specific GSH analogs as inhibitors to modulate GST activity during chemotherapy is a promising modulation strategy.

C. Manipulation of GSH Levels to Sensitize Tumors to DNA-Damaging Agents

Depletion of GSH to gain a therapeutic advantage for DNA-damaging agents has been studied extensively. A number of oxidizing agents, including diethylmaleate and phorone, have been tried; however, although these were successful in achieving tumor cell GSH depletion, they proved to be too toxic for clinical use. The toxicities and complications associated with the use of nonspecific depletors of GSH were circumvented by the design and synthesis of agents that acted as inhibitors of certain enzymes involved in the synthesis of GSH. By far the most effective approach to reducing the GSH biosynthetic capacity of a cell has been achieved by amino acid sulfoximines, which inhibit γ-GCS. The lead compound to emerge from these studies has been L-buthionine(SR)-sulfoximine (BSO). The R-stereoisomer is the active inhibitor. In parallel with GSH depletion, *in vitro* and *in vivo* studies demonstrate that resistant cells exhibited restored sensitivity to platinum compounds and alkylating agents following BSO pretreatment. Studies in mice indicate some selectivity for tumor cells,

as the combination of BSO and melphalan enhances the survival of ovarian tumor-bearing mice over that of mice treated with melphalan alone. There was an increase in bone marrow toxicity. The use of BSO has spurred evaluation of this inhibitor in clinical studies. Phase I clinical trials of BSO plus melphalan observed little toxicity with BSO alone and increased myelosuppression with the combination. Consistent and profound GSH depletion was observed in serial determinations of tumor GSH levels in patients receiving BSO. The clinical effectiveness of the combination has not been fully elucidated.

An alternative approach to depleting GSH is to inhibit enzymes that utilize GSH as a cofactor. The plant phenolic acid, ethacrynic acid (EA), was the first to be developed to the stage of clinical trials. EA conjugates GSH through a nucleophilic attack at the α,β-unsaturated ketone of the drug in a mechanism similar to that described for acrolein. Preclinical studies demonstrate that EA is effective at improving the efficacy of alkylating agent treatment in human tumor xenografts. EA is presently in clinical trials.

III. DNA REPAIR AS A MECHANISM OF RESISTANCE TO DNA-DAMAGING AGENTS

Studies have now implicated DNA repair processes as likely to be involved in the multifactorial phenomenon of drug resistance to DNA-damaging drugs. The repair of damaged DNA is an essential cellular function involving a large, and ever increasing, number of gene products. Some pathways for DNA repair are able to deal with a variety of types of DNA lesions, whereas others are highly specific. Such mechanisms include an increased activity of AGT in cells exhibiting resistance to chloroethylnitrosoureas or methylating agents; increased activity of poly(ADP-ribose)-polymerase, a DNA-binding protein protecting cells against drugs such as *cis*-platin or bleomycin; and an increased nucleotide excision repair system in cells resistant to several DNA cross-linking agents, such as *cis*-platin, 1,3-bis(2-chloroethyl)-3-nitrosourea (BCNU), cyclophosphamide, L-phenylalanine mustard, and mechlorethamine. More recently, base excision repair, which removes a wide variety of alkylated bases from DNA, has been found to be important in drug resistance to mitomycin C, BCNU, and the nitrogen mustards. In contrast to resistance resulting from overexpression of DNA repair proteins, a deficiency in MMR can cause resistance to various DNA-damaging agents, including busulfan, methylating agents, doxorubicin, and platinum compounds. DNA repair mechanisms provide useful pharmacological targets with the aim of reducing and/or sensitizing tumor cells to anticancer drugs that damage DNA. Both AGT and MMR are discussed in detail.

A. AGT

The AGT repair protein plays a major role in the resistance to alkylnitrosourea therapy, including methylating (procarbazine, dacarbazine, temozolomide) and chloroethylating (BCNU, CCNU, meCCNU, SarCNU) agents. AGT is a unique DNA repair protein that is able to remove adducts formed at the O^6 position of guanine in DNA and to restore the original DNA in a single step. Production of adducts at the O^6-position of guanine is a major contributor to the toxic and mutagenic effects of alkylating agents. Their repair is, therefore, of critical importance in limiting the production of mutations and/or toxic lesions in response to carcinogenic and chemotherapeutic alkylating agents. Methylating agents are known to produce O^6-methylguanine, a toxic lesion on DNA. Persistence of the O^6-methylguanine lesion introduced by methylating agents has been correlated with cytotoxicity. Chloroethylating agents form a number of adducts on DNA, including a toxic interstrand cross-link between guanine and cytosine on the opposite strand of DNA. This lesion is formed by an initial attack at the O^6-position of guanine by the chloroethylnitrosourea to produce 2-chloroethylguanine followed by an intramolecular rearrangement to form 1, O^6-ethanoguanine. Within about 10–12 h this adduct reacts with the opposite cytosine to form the 1-(3-cytosinyl)-2-(1-guanyl)ethane cross-link. There is a strong correlation between the number of cross-links formed and cell kill.

The AGT protein protects cells from alkylation damage by removing lesions from the O^6 position of guanine in a reaction that leaves guanine intact in DNA. Cross-links are prevented from forming following exposure to chloroethylating agents by two reactions with the AGT protein: (1) removal of the chloroethyl lesion from the O^6 position prior to rearrangement or (2) reaction with the intermediate, 1-O^6-ethanoguanine to form a cross-link between DNA and the repair protein. There are no other proteins or cofactors involved in this reaction and the protein is inactivated in the repair process. The high degree of correlation that exists between AGT activity and sensitivity to nitrosoureas *in vitro* and in animal models suggests that the elimination of this protein may reverse resistance.

1. Clinical Evidence Implicating AGT as a Mechanism of Resistance

Using human tumor xenografts, evidence shows that AGT expression influences both intrinsic and acquired colon tumor resistance to chloroethylnitrosoureas and that selective expansion of colon tumor cells expressing AGT commonly occurs after exposure to BCNU. Studies evaluating AGT levels in patients receiving BCNU therapy have supported this concept as well. Following an evaluation of 226 high-grade astrocytoma patients receiving BCNU therapy, Belanich and co-workers reported that the AGT content in tumors correlates with a high response to treatment and greater survival. Conversely, the presence of a subpopulation of cells in a tumor with elevated AGT is correlated with poor prognosis. These results have been found in retrospective and prospective studies.

2. Inactivation of AGT to Enhance Alkylating Agent Effectiveness

It was believed that because the mechanism of repair involves inactivation of the protein and lower levels of AGT correlate with increased sensitivity to alkylnitrosoureas, then efforts to design potent AGT substrates would have considerable therapeutic potential in combination with chemotherapy. The first modulation experiments utilized a combination of methylating and chloroethylating agents. The rationale for this combination is that pretreatment of cells with methylating agents decreases AGT levels by introducing O^6-methylguanine residues in DNA, which are then repaired by the AGT. Exposure of tumor cells in culture to N-methyl-N-nitro-N-nitrosoguanidine or streptozotocin results in the depletion of AGT activity, an increase in BCNU-induced interstrand cross-linking, and an enhancement of BCNU cytotoxicity *in vitro*.

Unfortunately, human tumor xenograft studies in mice did not result in an increase in the therapeutic index of BCNU. Nonetheless, because several methylating agents are already FDA approved, clinical trials were initiated. Phase I and II studies indicate that the dose-limiting toxicity was hematologic, although there are also reports of significant hepatic and pulmonary toxicity. Most studies using this approach indicate an absence of clinical activity of the combination. Some of the factors contributing to the lack of effectiveness of this combination include enhanced toxicity by addition of the methylating agent and the possibility that depletion in the tumor was not significant to overcome clinical resistance to BCNU.

Over the past decade, direct substrates for the AGT protein have been designed and tested for their ability to effectively inactivate the protein. First-generation direct substrates, including O^6-methylguanine, required high concentrations for adequate loss of AGT activity and subsequent increase in tumor cell sensitivity to alkylating agents. Although preliminary results in cells looked promising, there was no enhancement of the therapeutic index of BCNU when combined with O^6-methylguanine to treat mice carrying human tumor xenografts and, as a result, this modulator never entered clinical trials. A more effective agent, O^6-benzylguanine, was designed based on an understanding of the bimolecular displacement reaction between the AGT protein and the leaving group at the O^6 position of guanine. Benzyl groups are known to enter more readily into bimolecular reactions compared to alkyl groups because the electron charge stabilizes the benzyl group in the transition state. Depletion of AGT by O^6-benzylguanine led to a marked enhancement of the sensitivity of cells to the cytotoxic effects of chloroethylating and methylating agents. Treatment of nude mice carrying human tumor xenografts with O^6-benzylguanine prior to chloroethylating agents leads to a significant inhibition of tumor growth as compared to chloroethylating agents alone. Although the toxicity of BCNU was enhanced with O^6-benzylguanine, thus requiring the administration of a lower dose of BCNU, the combination was clearly better than the maximally tolerated dose of BCNU alone. O^6-Benzylguanine is effective in sensitizing tumors to BCNU, even when only a small fraction of the cells in a heterogeneous tumor express AGT. Phase I clinical trials of the combination of O^6-benzylguanine and BCNU have been completed and phase II trials are ongoing. Phase I trials indicated enhanced myelosuppression resulting in a four- to fivefold lower dose of BCNU administered when combined with O^6-benzylguanine. Clinical efficacy of the combination has yet to be established. A considerable number of additional compounds have been tested for AGT inactivation potential and, in some cases, for the ability to sensitize cells to the effects of chloroethylating agents.

B. MMR as a Mechanism of Resistance to DNA-Damaging Agents

The primary role of the DNA MMR system is to correct DNA polymerase errors produced during replication by recognizing and repairing mismatches in the DNA double helix. MMR machinery also prevents recombination between highly divergent DNA sequences. The most extensively characterized general MMR system is the *Escherichia coli* MutHLS system, which repairs a broad spectrum of mispaired bases. Mismatch recognition is accomplished by a MutS dimer. MutL binds the MutS–DNA complex, and the resulting complex stimulates MutH to generate a nick on the unmethylated strand. The MMR system is not only able to detect and repair mismatches derived from spontaneous base modification and replication, but can also process chemically induced DNA damage. Increasing evidence suggests that tumors could acquire resistance to DNA-damaging drugs by loss of DNA–MMR activity. These agents include alkylating agents busulfan, procarbazine, and temozolomide, the antimetabolites, mercaptopurine and 6-thioguanine, the platinum compounds carboplatin and *cis*-platin, the anthracycline doxorubicin through their direct or indirect interaction with DNA.

1. Clinical Evidence of MMR Drug Resistance

Reports indicate that ovarian cancer is biologically altered after chemotherapy consistent with treatment-induced selection for cells expressing lower hMLH1 and hMSH2 levels. There are two general mechanisms by which MMR results in drug resistance. A deficiency in MMR could result in drug resistance directly by impairing the ability of the cells to detect damage and indirectly by increasing the rate of mutation in the coding or regulatory loci that mediate resistance to other classes of drugs. The MMR system recognizes the damaged bases or the mismatch that results in attempted replication across the damaged base. Recognition is followed by events, not yet well defined, that generate a signal capable of activating apoptosis. If MMR is defective, the cell cannot sense the damage present on its DNA, the apoptotic cascade is not activated, and the cell is phenotypically resistant.

2. Resistance to DNA-Methylating Agents

Methylating agents, such as temozolomide and procarbazine, form a variety of methylated adducts on DNA, one of which is O^6-methylguanine. Although MMR does not recognize the alkylated guanine, it does recognize the O^6-methylguanine–thymine mismatch that occurs after erroneous incorporation of a thymine rather than a cytosine opposite the O^6-methylguanine during the next cycle of DNA replication. One hypothesis is that having recognized the mismatch, the MMR system incises the thymine-containing strand, excises the thymine and surrounding bases, creating a gap, and then fills in the gap via repair synthesis. However, because a thymine is again incorporated opposite the persisting O^6-methylguanine, the site is once again recognized by the MMR system and a new round of attempted repair is triggered. This futile cycle either increases the risk of double strand breaks during the next S phase that could trigger apoptosis or signals apoptotic functions due to faulty MMR activity. Because O^6-methylguanine is a highly mutagenic and cytotoxic lesion, there is an interplay between AGT repair as described earlier and MMR. AGT is the major route by which these types of lesions are repaired. For cells with normal MMR and high AGT activity, sensitivity can be reversed by O^6-benzylguanine. In MMR-deficient lines, inactivation of AGT does not sensitize to killing by temozolomide. Thus, MMR deficiency can override the AGT mechanism.

3. Resistance to Platinum-Containing Compounds

Several studies have suggested a relationship between MMR status and sensitivity to platinum-containing compounds. MMR-deficient cells are resistant to the platinum-containing drugs cisplatin and carboplatin, both of which produce similar adducts in DNA and are particularly important because of their widespread clinical use. The MMR-deficient HCT-116 colon cancer and HEC59 endometrial cancer lines both exhibit low-level resistance to cisplatin compared to their MMR-proficient counterparts. A possible explanation for involvement of the MMR system in repair of this DNA damage is that the MMR proteins try to excise these adducts. However, the MMR system is not able to repair DNA damage caused by platinum compounds. These continuous attempts to repair lead to futile cycles of DNA synthesis past the DNA lesion, followed by recognition and removal of the newly synthesized strand by an active MMR system. This event results in the generation of gaps or strand breaks that induce programmed cell death. The binding of MMR compounds to platinum-dependent DNA damage is also proposed to render the DNA adducts refractory to alternative repair mechanisms. A third hypothesis is that resistance to platinum drugs because of decreased MMR results from the inability of MMR-deficient tumor cells to detect DNA damage and activate apoptosis or cell cycle arrest.

IV. SUMMARY

In clinical situations, drug resistance is too often the cause of treatment failure. It is thought that clinically occurring types of drug resistance are caused by complex mechanisms consisting of different pathways, perhaps working in concert. GSH levels and DNA repair systems are mechanisms of resistance known to be important clinically; however, they only represent individual pathways. The challenge is to develop new strategies to overcome resistance without compromising efficacy.

See Also the Following Articles

Akylating Agents • Cellular Responses to DNA Damage • DNA Methylation and Cancer • Hereditary Colon Cancer and DNA Mismatch Repair • Mismatch Repair: Biochemistry and Genetics • Recombination: Mechanisms and Roles in Tumorigenesis • Resistance to Antibody Therapy

Bibliography

Alper, T. (1956). The modification of damage caused by primary ionization of biological targets. *Radiat. Res.* **5,** 573–586.

Anderson, M. E. (1998). Glutathione: An overview of biosynthesis and modulation. *Chem. Biol. Interact.* **111-112,** 1–14.

Arai, T., Yasuda, Y., *et al.* (2000). Immunohistochemical expression of glutathione transferase-pi in untreated primary non-small-cell lung cancer. *Cancer Detect Prev.* **24**(3), 252–257.

Bailey, H. H. (1998). L-S,R-buthionine sulfoximine: Historical development and clinical issues. *Chem. Biol. Interact.* **111-112,** 239–254.

Bailey, H. H., Ripple, G., *et al.* (1997). Phase I study of continuous-infusion L-S, R-buthionine sulfoximine with intravenous melphalan. *J. Natl. Cancer Inst.* **89**(23), 1789–1796.

Belanich, M., Pastor, M., *et al.* (1996). Retrospective study of the correlation between the DNA repair protein alkyltransferase and survival of brain tumor patients treated with carmustine. *Cancer Res.* **56**(4), 783–788.

Beneke, R., Geisen, C., *et al.* (2000). DNA excision repair and DNA damage-induced apoptosis are linked to Poly(ADP-Ribosyl)ation but have different requirements for p53. *Mol. Cell Biol.* **20**(18), 6695–6703.

Bignami, M., O'Driscoll, M., *et al.* (2000). Unmasking a killer: DNA O(6)-methylguanine and the cytotoxicity of methylating agents. *Mutat. Res.* **462**(2-3), 71–82.

Dolan, M. E. (1997). Inhibition of DNA repair as a means of increasing the antitumor activity of DNA reactive agents. *Adv. Drug Deliv. Rev.* **26**(2-3), 105–118.

Dolan, M. E., Larkin, G. L., *et al.* (1989). Depletion of O^6-alkylguanine-DNA alkyltransferase activity in mammalian tissues and human tumor xenografts in nude mice by treatment with O^6-methylguanine. *Cancer Chemother. Pharmacol.* **25**(2), 103–108.

Dolan, M. E., Moschel, R. C., *et al.* (1990). Depletion of mammalian O^6-alkylguanine-DNA alkyltransferase activity by O^6-benzylguanine provides a means to evaluate the role of this protein in protection against carcinogenic and therapeutic alkylating agents. *Proc. Natl. Acad. Sci. USA* **87**(14), 5368–5372.

Dolan, M. E., and Pegg, A. E. (1997). O^6-Benzylguanine and its role in chemotherapy. *Clin. Cancer Res.* **3**(6), 837–847.

Fink, D., Aebi, S., *et al.* (1998). The role of DNA mismatch repair in drug resistance. *Clin. Cancer Res.* **4**(4), 1–6.

Gamcsik, M. P., Dolan, M. E., *et al.* (1999). Mechanisms of resistance to the toxicity of cyclophosphamide. *Curr. Pharm. Des.* **5**(8), 587–605.

Gonzaga, P. E., Potter, P. M., *et al.* (1992). Identification of the cross-link between human O^6-methylguanine-DNA methyltransferase and chloroethylnitrosourea-treated DNA. *Cancer Res.* **52**(21), 6052–6058.

Green, J. A., Vistica, D. T., *et al.* (1984). Potentiation of melphalan cytotoxicity in human ovarian cancer cell lines by glutathione depletion. *Cancer Res.* **44**(11), 5427–5431.

Griffin, S., Branch, P., *et al.* (1994). DNA mismatch binding and incision at modified guanine bases by extracts of mammalian cells: Implications for tolerance to DNA methylation damage. *Biochemistry* **33**(16), 4787–4893.

Hall, A. G. (1999). Glutathione and the regulation of cell death. *Adv. Exp. Med. Biol.* **457,** 199–203.

Jiricny, J. (1998). Eukaryotic mismatch repair: An update. *Mutat. Res.* **409**(3), 107–121.

Kohn, K. W. (1977). Interstrand cross-linking of DNA by 1,3-bis(2-chloroethyl)-1-nitrosourea and other 1-(2-haloethyl)-1-nitrosoureas. *Cancer Res.* **37**(5), 1450–1454.

Kohn, K. W. (1996). Beyond DNA cross-linking: History and prospects of DNA-targeted cancer treatment—fifteenth Bruce F. Cain Memorial Award Lecture. *Cancer Res.* **567**(24), 5533–5546.

Lage, H., and Dietel, M. (1999). Involvement of the DNA mismatch repair system in antineoplastic drug resistance. *J. Cancer Res. Clin. Oncol.* **125**(3-4), 156–165.

Liu, L., Markowitz, S., *et al.* (1996). Mismatch repair mutations override alkyltransferase in conferring resistance to temozolomide but not to 1,3-bis(2-chloroethyl)nitrosourea. *Cancer Res.* **56**(23), 5375–5379.

Ludlum, D. B. (1997). The chloroethylnitrosourea: Sensitivity and resistance to cancer chemotherapy at the molecular level. *Cancer Invest.* **15**(6), 588–598.

Mechanic, L. E., Frankel, B. A., *et al.* (2000). *Escherichia coli* MutL loads DNA helicase II onto DNA. *J. Biol. Chem.* **275,** 38337–38346.

Modrich, P. (1994). Mismatch repair, genetic stability, and cancer. *Science* **266**(5193), 1959–1960.

Nishimura, T., Newkirk, K., *et al.* (1998). Association between expression of glutathione-associated enzymes and response to platinum-based chemotherapy in head and neck cancer. *Chem. Biol. Interact.* **111-112,** 187–198.

Oakley, A. J., Lo Bello, M., *et al.* (1997). The glutathione conjugate of ethacrynic acid can bind to human pi class glutathione transferase P1-1 in two different modes. *FEBS Lett.* **419**(1), 32–36.

O'Dwyer, P. J., Hamilton, T. C., *et al.* (1996). Phase I trial of buthionine sulfoximine in combination with melphalan in patients with cancer. *J. Clin. Oncol.* **14**(1), 249–256.

Pegg, A. E. (2000). Repair of O(6)-alkylguanine by alkyltransferases. *Mutat. Res.* **462**(2-3), 83–100.

Pegg, A. E., Dolan, M. E., *et al.* (1995). Structure, function, and inhibition of O^6-alkylguanine-DNA alkyltransferase. *Prog. Nucleic Acid Res. Mol. Biol.* **51,** 167–223.

Phillips, W. P., Jr., Willson, J. K., *et al.* (1997). O^6-methylguanine-DNA methyltransferase (MGMT) transfectants of a 1,3-bis(2-chloroethyl)-1-nitrosourea (BCNU)-sensitive colon cancer cell line selectively repopulate heterogenous MGMT+/MGMT− xenografts after BCNU and O^6-benzylguanine plus BCNU. *Cancer Res.* **57**(21), 4817–4823.

Salinas, A. E., and Wong, M. G. (1999). Glutathione S-transferases: A review. *Curr. Med. Chem.* **6**(4), 279–309.

Samimi, G., Fink, D., *et al.* (2000). Analysis of MLH1 and MSH2 expression in ovarian cancer before and after platinum drug-based chemotherapy. *Clin. Cancer Res.* **6**(4), 1415–1421.

Sangrajrang, S., Calvo, F., *et al.* (1999). Estramustine resistance. *Gen. Pharmacol.* **33**(2), 107–113.

Su, S. S., and Modrich, P. (1986). *Escherichia coli* mutS-encoded protein binds to mismatched DNA base pairs. *Proc. Natl. Acad. Sci. USA* **83**(14), 5057–5061.

Trimmer, E. E., and Essigmann, J. M. (1999). Cisplatin. *Essays Biochem.* **34,** 191–211.

Worth, L., Jr., Clark, S., *et al.* (1994). Mismatch repair pro-teins MutS and MutL inhibit RecA-catalyzed strand trans-fer between diverged DNAs. *Proc. Natl. Acad. Sci. USA* **91**(8), 3238–3241.

Wyatt, M. D., Allan, J. M., *et al.* (1999). 3-methyladenine DNA glycosylases: Structure, function, and biological im-portance. *Bioessays* **21**(8), 668–676.

Resistance to Inhibitor Compounds of Thymidylate Synthase

Edward Chu
Ashwin Gollerkeri

Yale University School of Medicine and
VA Connecticut Healthcare System

GLOSSARY

drug resistance The resistance to structurally and functionally distinct anticancer drugs.

5-fluorouracil A characterized and most widely used TS inhibitor compound.

thymidylate synthase A folate-dependent enzyme that plays a major role in DNA biosynthesis and, as such, is an important target in cancer chemotherapy.

Thymidylate synthase (TS) is a folate-dependent enzyme that plays a major role in DNA biosynthesis and, as such, is an important target in cancer chemotherapy. The best characterized and most widely used TS inhibitor compound in the clinic is the fluoropyrimidine 5-fluorouracil (5-FU). Several antifolate analogs have been developed that directly inhibit TS. Although all of these compounds have demonstrated broad-spectrum antineoplastic activity against a variety of human cancers, the development of cellular resistance to these agents represents an important factor significantly limiting their clinical efficacy. Studies to investigate the underlying mechanisms involved in this process are of critical importance, as they may identify novel strategies to prevent and/or overcome cellular resistance.

I. INTRODUCTION

Thymidylate synthase is a folate-dependent enzyme that catalyzes the reductive methylation of 2'-deoxyuridine-5'-monophosphate (dUMP) by the reduced folate 5,10-methylenetetrahydrofolate (CH$_2$THF) to 2'-deoxythymidine-5'-monophosphate (dTMP, thymidylate) and dihydrofolate. Once synthesized, dTMP is then metabolized intracellularly to the dTTP triphosphate form, an essential precursor for DNA biosynthesis. While dTMP is also formed through the salvage pathway using thymidine kinase, the TS-catalyzed reaction provides the sole intracellular *de novo* source of dTMP. Given its central role in dTMP and DNA biosynthesis, TS represents an important target for cancer chemotherapy.

II. THYMIDYLATE SYNTHASE AS A CHEMOTHERAPEUTIC TARGET

Several lines of evidence provide further support for the concept that TS is an important chemotherapeutic target. Various *in vitro*, *in vivo*, and clinical studies have demonstrated a strong association between the level of intracellular expression of TS enzyme activity and fluoropyrimidine sensitivity. Thus, human cell lines and human solid tumors with increased TS enzyme activity and expression of TS protein are relatively more resistant to the cytotoxic effects of fluoropyrimidines. Clinical studies have shown a strong correlation between the level of TS enzyme inhibition within patient tumor samples after 5-fluorouracil-based chemotherapy and eventual response to treatment. Further evidence for the role of TS as a chemotherapeutic target includes the significantly enhanced clinical activity of 5-FU when combined with the reduced folate leucovorin. The rationale for this approach was to provide the necessary reduced folate sub-

strates that will interact with the 5-FU metabolite FdUMP to form a ternary complex resulting in enhanced inhibition of TS. Finally, the clinical activity of the antifolate analog ZD1694 (Tomudex, Raltitrexed), which specifically targets TS, further validates TS as an important target in advanced colorectal cancer.

III. THYMIDYLATE SYNTHASE INHIBITORS

A. 5-Fluorouracil

The best characterized inhibitor of TS is the fluoropyrimidine 5-FU, which has been used in the treatment of human malignancies since the early 1960s. Clinically, 5-FU has shown efficacy in the treatment of a wide variety of solid tumors, including breast, head and neck, ovary, and gastrointestinal malignancies. It remains the single most active agent for the treatment of patients with colorectal cancer. In its parent form, 5-FU is inactive, and it must be converted intracellularly to various cytotoxic nucleotide metabolites, including 5-fluoro-2'-deoxyuridylate (FdUMP), 5-fluorouridine-5'-triphosphate (FUTP), and 5-fluoro-2'-deoxyuridine-5'-triphosphate (FdUTP). In the presence of the reduced folate, CH$_2$THF, FdUMP forms a stable covalent ternary complex with TS, allowing for optimal inhibition of enzyme activity. While inhibition of TS is considered to be a critical event determining 5-FU cytotoxicy, other cytotoxic effects of 5-FU have been described. These include incorporation of FUTP into RNA, resulting in interference with RNA processing and translation, and incorporation of FdUTP into DNA, resulting in inhibition of DNA synthesis and function. To date, it remains unclear which of these mechanisms is relevant in the clinical setting.

B. Antifolate Analogs

The quinazoline analog, ZD1694 (Tomudex, Raltitrexed), and the pyrrolopyrimidine analog, LY231514, are two antifolate analog inhibitors of TS with documented clinical activity. ZD1694 is an antifolate analog with activity in breast, pancreas, and colorectal cancers. LY231514 primarily inhibits TS but also targets dihydrofolate reductase (DHFR) and glycinamide ribonucleotide formyltransferase (GARFT); for this reason, it is also known as multitargeted antifolate (MTA). It has activity in a variety of human tumors, including mesothelioma and colorectal, breast, head and neck, bladder, cervix, and non-small cell lung cancer.

Several other TS inhibitors are currently being tested in the clinic. One such compound is the non-polyglutamylatable, antifolate analog ZD9331. This compound was originally designed for use against tumors that are resistant to ZD1694 based on defects in polyglutamation. The most potent inhibitor of TS, identified to date, is the benzoquinazoline compound GW1843U89. While polyglutamation to the higher polyglutamate forms is not required for enzyme inhibition, this compound is metabolized rapidly to the diglutamate form by FPGS. Polyglutamation to the diglutamate level appears to be necessary for optimal activity of GW1843U89, presumably by enhancing intracellular retention and allowing for maximal inhibition of TS.

Finally, a rational drug design approach was used in the development of two compounds with "nonclassical" structures. AG337 and AG331 were synthesized based on the X-ray crystallographic modeling of the interaction among TS, FdUMP, and the folate analog CB3717. Both of these compounds are less potent inhibitors of TS when compared to the classic antifolate analogs. However, the advantages of these designer inhibitors of TS are twofold: (1) they do not rely on polyglutamation for their cytotoxic activity and (2) they enter the cell via passive diffusion rather than use the RFC for transmembrane transport.

IV. REGULATION OF THYMIDYLATE SYNTHASE EXPRESSION

Given its role in DNA biosynthesis, the regulation of expression of TS has been extensively studied with regard to cell cycle-directed events. Maximal TS enzyme levels occur during periods of active DNA synthesis, and many of the earlier studies suggested that this increased enzyme activity was primarily regulated at the transcriptional level. In addition, studies investigating the regulation of TS in synchronized normal human mammary epithelial cells and human breast cancer MCF-7 cells revealed a sharp (40-fold) increase in TS enzyme levels during the S phase of the cell cycle with no accompanying change in the

level of TS mRNA expression. Thus, transcriptional as well as posttranscriptional and translational events appear to be involved in mediating the regulation of TS expression during the cell cycle.

V. RESISTANCE TO THYMIDYLATE SYNTHASE INHIBITORS

One of the major limitations in the clinical efficacy of chemotherapy is the development of primary and/or acquired drug resistance. The concept of primary drug resistance has its roots in the seminal studies of Luria and Delbruck, who, in 1943, observed that the bacterium *Escherichia coli* developed resistance to bacterial viruses by expanding clones of bacteria that had spontaneously mutated to a type inherently resistant to phage infection. Goldie and Coldman later applied this principle to the development of intrinsic resistance by cancer cells. They proposed that the inherent cytogenetic instability of human cancers was tightly associated with mutations that would select for cells that had developed the capacity to resist the action of certain types of anticancer drugs. Their mathematical model suggested that tumor cells mutate to drug resistance at a rate intrinsic to the genetic instability of a particular tumor and that the development of resistance is independent of prior drug exposure. Acquired drug resistance refers to the process of cellular resistance, which develops in response to exposure, either short or long term, to a cytotoxic agent.

A. 5-Fluorouracil

Characterization of the resistance mechanisms to TS inhibitor compounds has been an active area of investigation. The mechanisms of drug resistance to 5-FU have been most extensively characterized. Given the multiple sites of 5-FU action, it is not surprising that various resistance mechanisms have been identified in a host of *in vitro* and *in vivo* experimental model systems. These mechanisms include increased levels of the target enzyme TS, alterations in the binding affinity of TS for the 5-FU metabolite FdUMP, decreased incorporation of 5-FU into cellular RNA, decreased incorporation of 5-FU into cellular DNA, decreased intracellular pools of the reduced folate substrate 5,10-methylenetetrahydrofolate, increased levels of dUTPase preventing accumulation of dUTP and FdUTP into cellular DNA, decreased levels of anabolic enzymes resulting in decreased formation of active 5-FU metabolites, and increased activity of catabolic enzymes, such as acid and alkaline phosphatases, leading to the decreased formation of active 5-FU metabolites.

The regulation of TS expression following treatment with a TS inhibitor compound is a complex process. Several mechanisms of TS regulation have been characterized in cells following treatment with fluoropyrimidines. Some of these mechanisms include gene amplification, transcriptional, translational, and posttranslational regulatory events. The predominant mechanism of regulation may depend on the particular cell type as well as the specific TS inhibitor compound being used. In addition, other factors, such as drug dosage, schedule of administration, route of administration, and cellular environment of the tumor, may affect the final expression of TS.

Gene amplification has been identified as an important mechanism of regulation of TS expression following chronic treatment with a TS inhibitor. Jenh and co-workers demonstrated a 50- to 100-fold amplification of the TS gene in fluorodeoxyuridine (FdUrd)-resistant mouse fibroblast LU3-7 and FdUrd-resistant mouse neuroblastoma FUdR-R cell lines. Berger and colleagues also observed TS gene amplification as the predominant mechanism of resistance in FdUrd-resistant human laryngeal carcinoma Hep-2 cells. Similarly, Copur and co-workers showed that increased TS expression was the result of TS gene amplification in human colon carcinoma H630-R$_{10}$ cells that had been made resistant to 5-FU following long-term exposure to the drug.

While amplification of the TS gene is a well-documented mechanism for the increased expression of TS, other regulatory processes have been described that involve transcriptional control. Studies by Scanlon and colleagues demonstrated that selection of human ovarian cancer cells in cisplatin led to the development of cross-resistance to 5-FU. They found that cisplatin-resistant cells expressed three- to four-fold higher levels of TS when compared to wild-type parental cells. Moreover, the increased level of expression of TS was not associated with TS gene am-

plification, but rather was the direct result of an increased transcriptional rate. A series of adriamycin-resistant human breast cancer MCF-7 and human colon cancer DLD-1 cells were found to be cross-resistant to both 5-FU and FdUrd. Of note, these resistant cell lines had not previously been exposed to either of the fluoropyrimidines. Further evaluation revealed that the development of fluoropyrimidine resistance was directly associated with an increased expression of TS protein. Moreover, maintenance of the selective pressure of adriamycin within the growth medium of these cells was essential in establishing the enhanced expression of TS and consequent cross-resistance to 5-FU. As in the case of the cisplatin-resistant human ovarian cancer cell line described by Scanlon and co-workers, the increased expression of TS was not the result of gene amplification of the TS gene, but rather was directly regulated at the transcriptional level.

In addition to transcriptional control of TS expression, there is growing evidence that translational and posttranslational mechanisms are involved in response to treatment with TS inhibitors. In various experimental systems, rapid increases in TS enzyme levels have been observed following short-term exposure (12–48 h) to 5-FU. Based on these observations, it was proposed that the increase in TS enzyme activity in response to fluoropyrimidine exposure might represent a mechanism by which malignant cells rapidly developed cellular resistance to the drug. Swain and colleagues measured TS enzyme levels in the cutaneous tumor specimens of female patients with advanced breast cancer pre- and 24 h-posttreatment with 5-FU and leucovorin. They observed an approximately threefold increase in total levels of TS enzyme in tumor samples taken 24 h post 5-FU exposure when compared to pretreatment levels. Moreover, patients with unresponsive disease had a significantly lower fraction of TS enzyme bound in the form of the ternary complex when compared to those patients with responsive disease. Thus, findings from this clinical study suggested that the acute induction of TS enzyme may represent a biologically and clinically relevant mechanism of fluoropyrimidine resistance. Chu and co-workers observed that the increased level of expression of TS following exposure to 5-FU was not accompanied by a corresponding increase in the level of expression of TS mRNA. Their studies revealed that the increased intracellular synthesis of TS was directly mediated by an enhanced translational efficiency of TS mRNA. Thus, the acute induction of TS in human colon cancer cells following 5-FU exposure was regulated at the translational level. These findings, taken together, provided further evidence for the critical role of translation regulatory mechanisms in controlling the expression of TS.

The role of posttranslational control in the induction of TS following drug exposure was investigated by Berger and colleagues. Treatment of human colon cancer HCT15 cells in the absence and presence of fluoropyrimidine FdUrd revealed a significant prolongation (threefold) in the half-life of TS following drug treatment. Thus, stabilization of the TS enzyme was the primary mechanism of TS induction in response to fluoropyrimidine exposure using this particular model system.

B. Antifolate Analogs

Resistance to the antifolate analog ZD1694 has been characterized in a number of human cancer cell lines. As a structural analog of the physiologic folate CH_2THF, ZD1694 requires active transport into the cell. It is then metabolized by folypolyglutamate synthase (FPGS) to its higher polyglutamate forms, which are cytotoxic. Several mechanisms have now been described with regard to the development of cellular resistance to ZD1694.

Two studies investigated the mechanisms of acquired ZD1694 resistance in the murine L1210 leukemia, human W1L2 lymphoblastoid, and two human ovarian (CH1 and 41M) cell lines. The primary mechanism of resistance in W1L2:R cells appeared to be increased TS enzyme activity along with increased expression of TS protein levels. In human ovarian cancer CH1:R cells, a 14-fold resistance to ZD1694 was largely accounted for by a 4.2-fold increase in TS enzyme activity and a 2-fold increase in TS protein levels. In contrast, resistance to ZD1694 in the 41M:R human ovarian cell line was mediated by impaired transport of the drug via the RFC. Finally, in murine L1210 leukemia cells, resistance to ZD1694 was associated with decreased polyglutamation due to reduced FPGS enzyme activity. The development of resistance to ZD1694 as a result of decreased FPGS enzyme ac-

tivity was also documented in the human ileocecal adenocarcinoma HCT-8 cell line.

Drake and colleagues used human breast cancer MCF-7 and human colon cancer H630 cell lines to study ZD1694 drug resistance. Of note, the development of resistance was dependent on the duration of exposure to the drug. The predominant mechanism of resistance to ZD1694 in early passage (passage number, $p < 10$) H630 cells was overexpression of TS. These cells expressed increased levels of TS mRNA, TS protein, and TS enzyme activity. In late passage H630 cells, however, the levels of TS mRNA, TS protein, and TS enzyme activity had decreased to those expressed in ZD1694-sensitive H630 cells. Further analysis of these late passage H630 cells suggested that altered ZD1694 transport along with decreased FPGS activity were the major mechanisms of resistance. In ZD1694-resistant, MCF-7 cells, overexpression of TS with increases in TS mRNA, TS protein, and enzyme activity accounted for drug resistance. Finally, the increased expression of TS was due to a 20-fold amplification of the TS gene with no evidence for translocation or mutation. Moreover, both early and late-passage MCF-7-resistant cells expressed this TS-mediated mechanism.

Schultz and co-workers investigated the mechanisms of resistance to LY231514 in several human cancer cell lines, including colon carcinoma GC3, ileocecal adenocarcinoma HCT-8, leukemia CCRF-CEM, breast MCF-7, and colon H630. LY231514-resistant cell lines were established by gradual exposure to stepwise increases in the concentration of LY231514. LY231514-resistant GC3 cells expressed a 40-fold increase in TS enzyme activity that was due to TS gene amplification. In some resistant clones not displaying TS gene amplification, the predominant resistance mechanism involved a decrease in intracellular drug accumulation. Although LY231514 activation requires transport via the RFC and subsequent polyglutamation, these LY231514-resistant cells were only moderately cross-resistant to LY390887, an agent that requires polyglutamation, and methotrexate, which requires transport by RFC and polyglutamation. Thus, these findings suggest that the development of resistance to LY231514 is a complex process and may be dependent on unique mechanisms of transport and activation.

The development of cellular resistance to other TS inhibitors, including ZD9331, has also been investigated. ZD9331 is a quinazoline-based inhibitor of TS, which is transported into the cell via the RFC. In contrast to ZD1694, this analog is not a substrate for FPGS and thus does not require polyglutamation for its activation. Kobayashi and colleagues observed that resistance to ZD9331 in a human acute lymphoblastic leukemia MOLT-3 cell line was the direct result of TS gene amplification combined with decreased cellular uptake. Analysis of RFC expression revealed a 30% decrease in RFC mRNA levels in the absence of a change in gene copy number and gross gene rearrangements. Although further studies are needed, these initial findings suggest that the decreased cellular uptake of ZD9331 in MOLT-3 cells was due to transcriptional downregulation of RFC.

VI. CONCLUSION

TS has served as an important target in cancer chemotherapy since the early 1960s. Inhibitor compounds of TS have demonstrated broad-spectrum antineoplastic activity in a variety of human cancers. However, the development of cellular resistance to these agents represents an important factor significantly limiting their clinical efficacy. It is now clear that cancer cells have the ability to develop inherent, primary, and acquired mechanisms of resistance. Studies to investigate the underlying mechanisms involved in this process are of critical importance as they may identify novel strategies to prevent and/or overcome cellular resistance.

See Also the Following Articles

CHEMOTHERAPY: SYNERGISM AND ANTAGONISM • FOLATE ANTAGONISTS • RESISTANCE TO ANTIBODY THERAPY • RESISTANCE TO DNA-DAMAGING AGENTS • RESISTANCE TO INHIBITORS OF DIHYDROFOLATE REDUCTASE • RESISTANCE TO TOPOISOMERASE-TARGETING AGENTS

Bibliography

Appelt, K., Bacquet, R. J., Bartlett, C. A., *et al.* (1991). Design of enzyme inhibitors using iterative protein crystallographic analysis. *J. Med. Chem.* **34,** 904–917.

Berger, S. H., Jenh, C. H., Johnson, L. F., and Berger, F. (1985). Thymidylate synthase overproduction and gene amplification in fluorodeoxyuridine-resistant human cells. *Mol. Pharmacol.* **28,** 461–467.

Berne, M. H., Gustavsson, B. G., Almersjo, O., Spears, P. C., and Frosing, R. (1986). Sequential methotrexate/5-FU:FdUMP formation and TS inhibition in a transplantable rodent colon adenocarcinoma. *Cancer Chemother. Pharmacol.* **16,** 237–242.

Carreras, C. W., and Santi, D. V. (1995). The catalytic mechanism and structure of thymidylate synthase. *Annu. Rev. Biochem.* **64,** 721–762.

Chu, E., and Allegra, C. J. (1996). Mechanisms of clinical resistance to 5-fluorouracil chemotherapy. *In* "Drug Resistance" (W. N. Hait, ed.), pp. 175–196. Kluwer Academic, Boston.

Chu, E., and DeVita, V. T., Jr. (2000). Principles of chemotherapy. *In* "Cancer: Principles and Practice of Oncology" (V. T. DeVita Jr., S. Hellman, and S. A. Rosenberg, eds.). Lippincott, Philadelphia.

Chu, E., Drake, J. C., Koeller, D. M., Zinn, S., Jamis-Dow, C. A., Yeh, G. C., and Allegra, C. J. (1991). Induction of thymidylate synthase associated with multidrug resistance in human breast and colon cancer cell lines. *Mol. Pharmacol.* **39,** 136–143.

Chu, E., Ju, J., and Schmitz, J. C. (1998). Molecular regulation of expression of thymidylate synthase. *In* "Anticancer Drug Development Guide: Antifolate Drugs in Cancer Therapy" (A. L. Jackman, ed.), pp. 397–408. Humana Press, Totowa, NJ.

Chu, E., Koeller, D. M., Johnston, P. G., Zinn, S., and Allegra, C. J. (1993). Regulation of thymidylate synthase in human colon cancer cells treated with 5-fluorouracil and interferon-gamma. *Mol. Pharmacol.* **43,** 527–533.

Copur, S., Aiba, K., Drake, J. C., Allegra, C. J., and Chu, E. (1995). Thymidylate synthase gene amplification in human colon cancer cell lines resistant to 5-fluorouracil. *Biochem. Pharmacol.* **49,** 1419–1426.

Danenberg, P. V., Malli, H., and Swenson, S. (1999). Thymidylate synthase inhibitors. *Semin. Oncol.* **26,** 621–631.

Drake, J. C., Allegra, C. J., Moran, R. G., and Johnston, P. G. (1996). Resistance to Tomudex (ZD1649): Multifactorial in human breast and colon carcinoma cell lines. *Biochem. Pharmacol.* **51,** 1349–1355.

Freemantle, S. J., Jackman, A. L., Kelland, L. R., Calvert, A. H., and Lunec, J. (1995). Molecular characterization of two cell lines selected for resistance to the folate-based thymidylate synthase inhibitor, ZD1649. *Br. J. Cancer* **71,** 925–930.

Goldie, J. H., and Coldman, A. J. (1979). A mathematic model for relating the drug sensitivity of tumors to the spontaneous mutation rate. *Cancer Treat. Rep.* **63,** 1727.

Jackman, A. L, Kelland, L. R., Kimbell, R., Brown, M., Gibson, W., Aherne, G. W., Hardcastle, A., and Boyle, F. T. (1995). Mechanisms of acquired resistance to the quinazoline thymidylate synthase inhibitor ZD1649 (Tomudex) in one mouse and three human cell lines. *Br. J. Cancer* **71,** 914–924.

Jenh, C. H., Geyer, P. K., and Johnson, L. F. (1985). Control of thymidylate synthase mRNA content and gene transcription in an overproducing mouse cell line. *Mol. Cell. Biol.* **5,** 2527–2532.

Keyomarsi, K., Samet, J., Moinar, G., and Pardee, A. B. (1993). The thymidylate synthase inhibitor, ICI ID 1694, overcomes translational detainment of the enzyme. *J. Biol. Chem.* **268,** 15142–15149.

Kitchens, M. E., Forsthoefel, A. M., Barbour, K. W., Spencer, H. T., and Berger, F. G. (1999). Mechanisms of acquired resistance to thymidylate synthase inhibitors: The role of enzyme stability. *Mol. Pharm.* **56,** 1063–1070.

Kobayashi, H., Takemura, Y., and Miyachi, H. (1998). Molecular characterization of human acute leukemia cell line resistant to ZD9331, a non-polyglutamatable thymidylate synthase inhibitor. *Cancer Chemother. Pharmacol.* **42,** 105–110.

Lu, K., Yin, M.-B., McGuire, J. J., Bonmassar, E., and Rustum, Y. M. (1995). Mechanisms of resistance to N-[5-[N-(3,4-dihydro-2-methyl-4-oxoquinazolin-6-ylmethyl)-N-methlyamino]-2-thenoyl]-L-glutamic acid (ZD1649), a folate-based thymidylate synthase inhibitor, in the HCT-8 human ileocecal adenocarcinoma cell line. *Biochem. Pharmacol.* **50,** 391–398.

O'Dwyer, P. J., Nelson, K., and Thornton, D. E. (1999). Overview of phase II trials of MTA in solid tumors. *Semin. Oncol.* **26,** 99–104.

Scanlon, K. J., and Kashani-Saabet, M. (1988). Elevated expression of thymidylate synthase cycle genes in cisplatin-resistant human ovarian carcinoma A2780 cells. *Proc. Natl. Acad. Sci. USA* **85,** 650–653.

Schultz, R. M., Chen, V. J., Bewley, J. R., Roberts, E. F., Shih, C., and Dempsey, J. A. (1999). Biological activity of the multitargeted antifolate, MTA (LY231514), in human cell lines with different resistance mechanisms to antifolate drugs. *Semin. Oncol.* **26,** 68–73.

Shoichet, B. K., Stroud, R. M., Santi, D. V., Kuntz, I. D., and Perry, K. M. (1993). Structure-based discovery of inhibitors of thymidylate synthase. *Science* **259,** 1445–1450.

Swain S. M., Lippman, M. E., Egan, E. F., Drake, J. C., Steinberg, S. M., and Allegra, C. J. (1989). 5-Fluorouracil and high-dose leucovorin in previously treated patients with metastatic breast cancer. *J. Clin. Oncol.* **7,** 890–899.

Resistance to Inhibitors of Dihydrofolate Reductase

Peter W. Melera

University of Maryland School of Medicine

homogeneously staining region Expanded chromosomal areas that stain with a uniform shade rather than with the irregularity of color and banding generally seen with Giemsa.

PteGlu Shorthand designation for pteroylglutamate, i.e., folic acid.

GLOSSARY

allelic polymorphism Nucleotide sequence differences between two genes at the same locus on homologous chromosomes, occurring in at least 2% of the population.

antimetabolite A synthetic compound designed to interfere with the normal utilization of a specific metabolite (substrate) for which the compound is usually a structural analog.

double minute chromosomes Small paired chromatin bodies seen in metaphase preparations. They generally stain poorly with Giemsa and other chromatin stains as well. They do not contain centromeres and are considered to be euchromatic.

gene amplification An increase in the number of copies of a specific gene in a single cell.

Resistance to the cytotoxic effects of antitumor drugs is a major cause for lack of a favorable outcome in patients undergoing cancer chemotherapy. Such resistance may manifest itself as a normal, i.e., intrinsic, component of the original tumor phenotype or it may emerge during treatment as an acquired characteristic. Mechanisms responsible vary widely and can involve virtually any aspect of a drug's metabolism, from its entry into the cell to its modification, detoxification, degradation, sequestration, and efflux. In many cases, more than one mechanism is operative at any given time, making the task of circumvention extremely difficult. This article considers resistance as it applies to antifolates, specifically those that target the enzyme dihydrofolate reductase (E.C. 1.5.1.3). These drugs have been the subjects of investigation since their inception in the 1950s, and one of them, methotrexate (MTX), is still widely used for the treatment of cancer. Indeed, it is largely from the wealth of information that has been directly and indirectly obtained as a result of its study that newer generation antifolates and other drugs have been developed and an appreciation for the complexity of drug resistance has evolved.

I. INTRODUCTION

Antimetabolites represent one of several classes of antitumor agents including alkylators (nitrosoureas, melphalan, etc.), certain antibiotics (actinomycin D, daunomycin, etc.), biological agents (growth factors, hormones, or antibodies), and plant alkaloids (vincristine, etoposide, etc.). Generally speaking, each class exhibits a different mode of action, and in the case of antimetabolites, it is the inhibition of specific enzyme function. That such an approach might be an effective means for therapy was suggested by the early observations of D. D. Woods, who, in the early 1940s, recognized the structural similarity between the antibacterial agent sulfanilamide and p-aminobenzoic acid (PABA), a bacterial growth factor, and speculated that the reason for the effectiveness of the drug was that it interfered with the normal metabolism of PABA. Subsequently, this was proven to be the case when it was learned that sulfanilamide inhibits the bacterial enzyme responsible for the incorporation of PABA into the structure of folic acid.

While sulfanilamide is a naturally occurring compound, these early observations suggested that synthetic structural analogs of other important compounds might serve as therapeutic agents for the treatment of human diseases, including cancer. Hence aminopterin was synthesized as an analog of folic acid, which had been recognized previously as being required for cell growth. Subsequently it was used by Sidney Farber's group for the treatment of acute leukemia in children and was shown to induce temporary remission. These results were taken as a proof of principle and led to the production of additional folate analogs of which amethopterin (methotrexate) became the most popular.

Aminopterin and MTX are referred to as antifolates, so called because they disrupt metabolism via direct interference with folate substrates, and by doing so, prevent the synthesis of compounds required for cell replication and growth. Both serve as competitive inhibitors of the enzyme dihydrofolate reductase, whereas others are specific for additional folate requiring enzymes. Regardless of their target, however, all antifolates act in essentially the same manner in that they are designed as analogs that compete with natural folates for the active site of specific enzymes. While these characteristics greatly enhance drug specificity, they also subject these agents to many of the same biochemical modifications that affect the normal substrates and, in addition, allow them to be susceptible to other genetic changes that alter substrate transport and target enzyme structure as well. As a result, any one of these may serve as an avenue for the development of resistance because of the selective pressure generated by the presence of the drug. Hence, when one begins to consider the possible mechanisms that may compromise drug efficacy, one must not only include those changes that may occur in the target enzyme or to the drug itself, but must also add the additional interactions that can occur between the drug and other cellular components. Largely because of the complex nature of folate biochemistry, virtually all of these factors have been found to be of importance in efforts to understand the mechanisms of antifolate resistance.

II. OVERVIEW OF FOLATE METABOLISM

Folate vitamins serve as cofactors for a number of biochemical reactions that are pivotal for the maintenance of metabolic stasis. The major ones of these are involved with one carbon transfers and mediate the synthesis of key compounds, including thymidine, purines, and the amino acids glycine, serine and methionine (Fig. 1). Perhaps the most well-known reaction and one of the most interesting biochemically is the formation of thymidine monophosphate (TMP) from deoxyuridine monophosphate (dUMP) by thymidylate synthase (TS) in which 5,10-methylene tetrahydrofolic acid (H_4PteGlu) serves as the cofac-

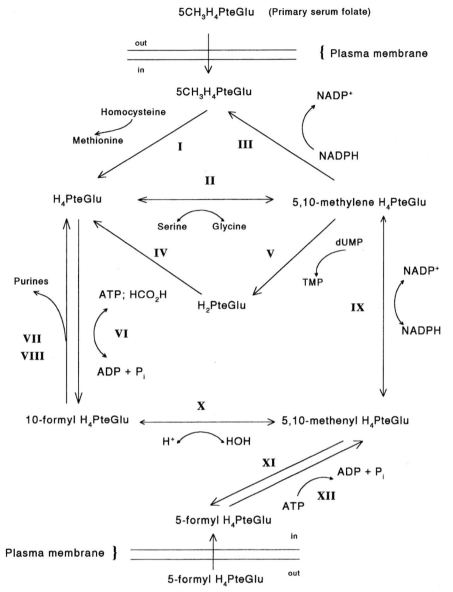

FIGURE 1 Diagram of the folate cycle. Major enzymes include (I) methionine synthetase; (II) serine hydroxymethyl transferase; (III) methylene tetrahydrofolate reductase; (IV) dihydrofolate reductase; (V) thymidylate synthase; (VI) 10-formyl tetrahydrofolate synthetase; (VII) glycinamide ribonucleotide transformylase; (VIII) aminoimidazolecarboxamide ribonucleotide transformylase; (IX) methylene tetrahydrofolate dehydrogenase; (X) methenyl tetrahydrofolate cyclohydrolase; (XI) serine hydroxymethyl transferase (secondary activity); and (XII) methenyl tetrahydrofolate synthetase.

tor. The enzyme actually catalyzes both a 1 carbon transfer and a reduction of dUMP to form TMP and the folate cofactor supplies both the carbon atom and two electrons. As a result, dihydrofolic acid ($H_2PteGlu$) is generated as a product of the reaction and is rapidly converted to $H_4PteGlu$ by the enzyme

dihydrofolate reductase (DHFR). This step is critical not only for maintaining appropriate intracellular concentrations of $H_4PteGlu$, the parent molecule upon which synthesis of the various folate cofactors depends, but also for meeting the cellular demand for the production of thymidylate. Consequently, it places the enzymtic activity of DHFR at the center of the folate cycle and provides the rational for why it has been a primary target for chemotherapy.

As a group, dietary folates exist as polyglutamates and must be converted to the monoglutamate form before efficiently being transported inward. A small family of enzymes called γ-glutamyl hydrolases or conjugases, some of which reside on the cell surface or are secreted and as a result carry out their enzymatic activity extracellularly, display peptidase-like activity and hydrolyze the peptide bonds that exist between glutamate residues, reducing polyglutamates to the monoglutamate. Ironically, after the monoglutamates are internalized, they are rapidly converted to polyglutamates, as are the classical antifolates, by the enzyme folypolyglutamate synthetase (FPGS). Mammalian cells more readily retain polyglutamated as opposed to monoglutamated forms of folates and antifolates, and these often display an enhanced affinity not only for their specific target enzymes but also in some cases for other folate-requiring enzymes as well. Interestingly, one of the secreted forms of conjugase, glutamyl hydrolase (GH), is also localized internally in lysosomes. Given their respective functions, the relative activities of conjugase and FPGS play an important role in maintaining cellular folate equilibrium.

Another important aspect of folate metabolism concerns the manner in which these components enter and exit cells. There are at least three mechanisms responsible for folate uptake in mammals. One is active transport via the classical high-affinity, low-capacity reduced folate carrier (RFC); the second by use of cell surface folate-binding proteins (FBP), also referred to as folate receptors (FR); and the third by a low pH-activated transporter, the molecular characterization of which has not yet been elucidated. Each of these displays specific biochemical characteristics, suggesting that specific cell types may differentially utilize them under different biological conditions. Additional "novel" folate transport systems have been biochemically described in hepatocytes, small intestine, lysosomes, and mitochondria, but it is not clear whether they, in fact, represent separate entities or are modified forms of the other known types.

The classical reduced folate transporter displays a much higher affinity ($k_t \approx$ 1–5 μM) for compounds such as 5-methyl-H4PteGlu and 5-formyl-H4PteGlu than it does for PteGlu ($k_t \approx$ 200–400 μM) and func-tions as an anion transporter. Given that the serum concentration of reduced folate is in the nanomoler range and the carrier displays micromolar k_t values for these compounds, its normal biological function once seemed obscure. However, it has been calculated that this carrier alone mediates sufficient folate uptake to support cell growth in L1210 (mouse) and CCRF-CEM (human) leukemia cells. Moreover, in L1210 cells and in many tumor cell lines, it is the major folate transport system present.

Folate-binding proteins, however, function via an endocytosis-like mechanism that has been referred to as potocytosis, which utilizes caveolae on the cell surface to concentrate and internalize ligand-bound receptors. Whether in fact potocytosis is the correct mechanism remains controversial. Receptor-mediated uptake of folates does occur, however, through the internalization of surface-bound receptors into membrane-bound compartments that, once acidified, permit disassociation of the folate ligands and their transfer to the cytoplasm, after which empty receptors are returned to the surface. FBPs are glycosyl-phosphatidylinositol (GPI)-anchored membrane proteins that display higher affinities for PteGlu ($k_d \approx$ 1 nM) than for reduced folate ($k_d >$ 100 nM). Nevertheless, they are able to effectively mediate the uptake of reduced folate and MTX present in media at physiologic concentrations, i.e., within the nanomolar range. Three receptor isoforms, i.e., FRα, FRβ, and FRγ, have been identified to date. They display tissue-specific patterns of expression. The function of FRβ and FRγ remains uncertain, although the former is widely expressed among normal tissues. FRα, however, does mediate the uptake of folates and antifolates alike and is overexpresed in many tumors, particulary carcinomas. Moreover, its presence on the cell surface is inversely correlated with media folate levels, which are known to directly affect internal folate pool sizes. Hence both internal and external levels of folates, coupled with the functional needs of the cell, likely play a role in determining which transport mechanism or combination thereof is utilized by a given cell at a given time.

Less is known concerning the mechanisms of folate efflux from mammalian cells, although studies with MTX indicate that multiple pathways exist, including use of the reduced folate carrier itself and separate ATP-dependent transporters including multidrug resistance protein-1 (MRP1), canalicular multispecific organic anion transporter (cMOAT/MRP2), and MRP3 as well. These three members of the ATP-binding cassette family of gylcosylated membrane proteins are organic anion transporters. MRP1 is ubiquitously expressed in animals, MRP2 is found specifically expressed in the canalicular membrane of hepatocytes, and MRP3 is more broadly expressed in liver, colon, intestine, and adrenal gland. Additionally, in the human leukemia cell line CEM/MTX R1-R3, in which the RFC is inactivated, P-glycoprotein (Pgp-1), another member of the ABC family, can mediate MTX efflux.

III. EXAMPLES OF ANTIFOLATE DRUGS THAT TARGET DIHYDROFOLATE REDUCTASE

Given the key role played by DHFR in maintenance of the folate cycle, antifolates were originally designed to inhibit the activity of this enzyme. Hence, classi-

cal antifolates are structural analogs of folic acid and, as such, are composed of a pteridine ring and a *p*-aminobenzoic acid moiety (or derivatives of these groups), coupled to a terminal glutamate residue (Fig. 2A). Such compounds are hydrophilic and are transported across the plasma membrane by the RFC, folate receptors, or possibly the low pH transporter. They are also subject to polyglutamylation by FPGS and deglutamylation by GH. Although the target enzyme for these drugs may be DHFR, as in the case of MTX and 10-EDAM, newer generation compounds, such as MTA (LY231514), are actually multitargeted and inhibit more than one folate requiring enzyme, in this case TS, GARFT, and DHFR (Table I). Attempts to escape the requirments for polyglutamylation have led to the development of antifolates that, while classical in their transport properties, are not substrates for FPGS. An example is the drug PT523 (Table I), which contains a hemiphthaloyl-L-ornithine side chain, rather than glutamic acid. The compound is transported by the RFC, but is not polyglutamylated.

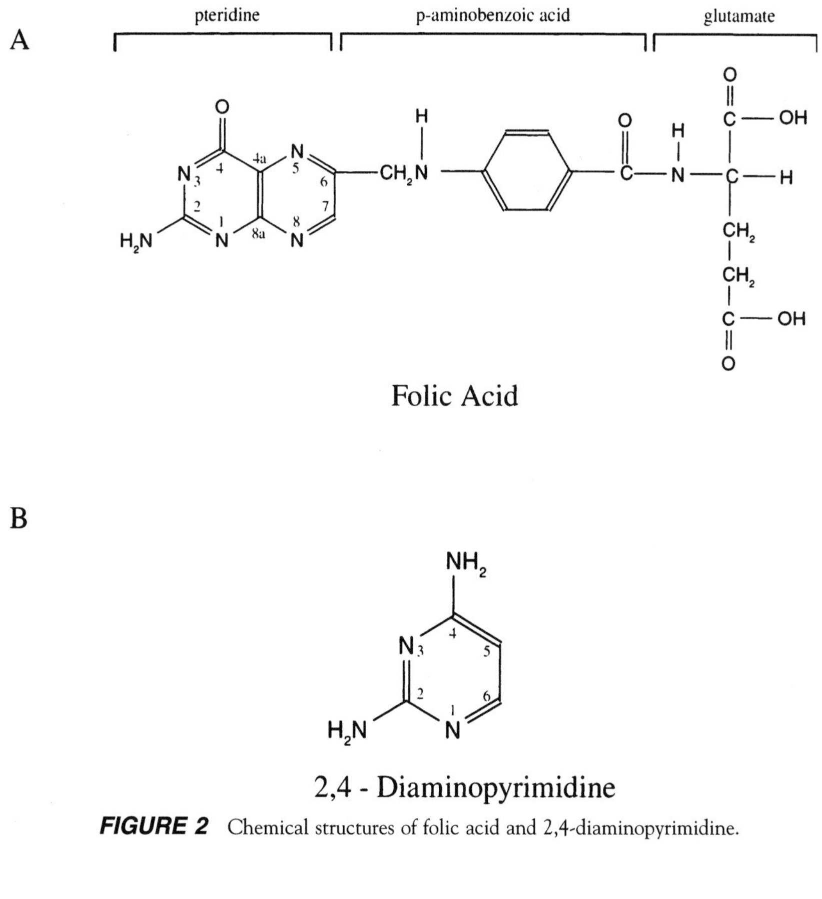

Folic Acid

2,4 - Diaminopyrimidine

FIGURE 2 Chemical structures of folic acid and 2,4-diaminopyrimidine.

TABLE I
Examples of Antifolates That Target DHFR

Drug	Structure	Target enzyme
Classical		
Methotrexate		DHFR
Edatrexate (10-EDAM)		DHFR
MTN (LY231514)		TS DHFR GARFT
PT523		DHFR

continued

TABLE I *Continued*

Nonclassical

Trimetrexate   DHFR

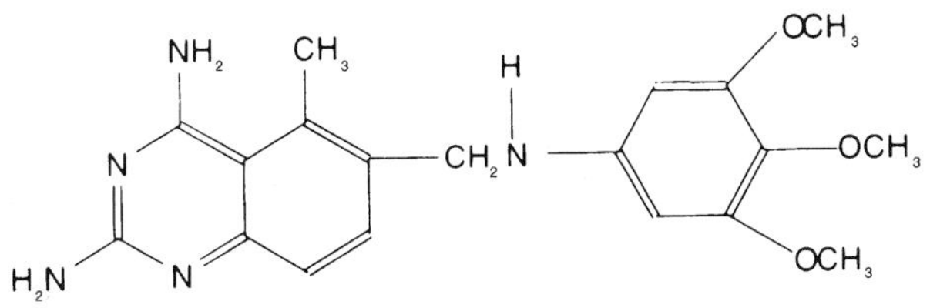

Piritrexim   DHFR

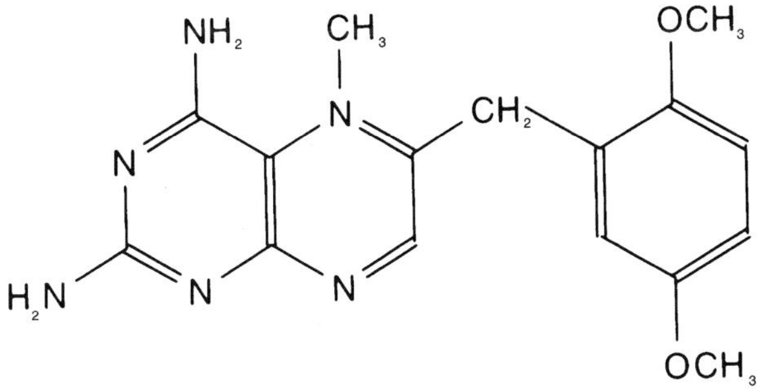

Metoprime   DHFR

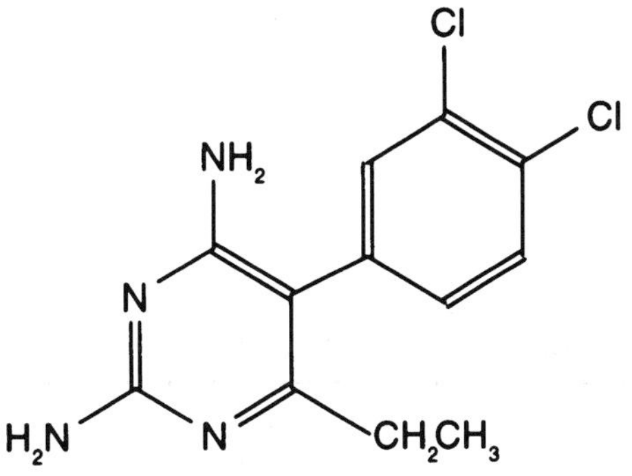

Other antifolates, such as trimetrexate (TMQ), piritrexim (PTX), metoprine, and pyrimethamine, are examples of nonclassical antifolates. In each case the target enzyme is DHFR, but these drugs have been designed as lipophilic compounds and, as a result, enter cells by simple or perhaps facilitated diffusion. They also lack a terminal glutamate residue and, therefore, are not polyglutamylated (Table I). Metoprine, pyrimethamine, and trimethoprim are analogs of 2,4-diaminopyrimidine, not folic acid (Fig. 2B). They were primarily designed as bacterial DHFR inhibitors, and only metoprine approaches MTX in its ability to inhibit the mammalian enzyme.

IV. ACQUIRED DRUG RESISTANCE

Most of the information available concerning mechanisms of resistance to inhibitors of DHFR focuses on

MTX, but in principle pertains directly to all other classical antifolates as well (Table II). Each of these was initially found by the analysis of cell lines selected for resistance and therefore represent acquired phenotypes. In many cases the selection protocol utilized largely determines the phenotype obtained. For example, continuous exposure of cells to MTX during stepwise increases to high doses primarily yields gene amplification-mediated DHFR overexpression mutants accompanied occasionally by altered forms of the enzyme as well, whereas short-term repetitive exposure to moderate- or high-level doses optimizes for the isolation of polyglutamylation mutants. However, single-step selection at low dose primarily yields transport mutants. In terms of clinical relevance, it is the second of these selection strategies that most closely mimics the protocols used for the clinical administration of the drug and which, during selection of MTX-resistant human leukemia cells (CCRF-CEM), led to the identification of a loss in FPGS activity as a mechanism for resistance to classical antifolates. Subsequently, these studies have been extended by attempts to use similar selection strategies *in vivo*. However, when multiple resistant cell lines cloned from the ascites of mice injected with L1210 tumor cells and then treated repetitively with maximum tolerated doses of MTX were analyzed, none displayed lowered FPGS activity. When edatrexate was used in place of MTX, half of the resistant sublines obtained exhibited substantially reduced levels of FPGS activity. These results underscore the fact that resistance phenotypes emerging during drug treatment reflect not only the drug and selection protocol used, but also the cell and the tumor type studied. Indeed, clinical studies show that in relapsed patients with ALL (acute lymphoblastic leukemia) the most prominent form of acquired resistance to MTX is decreased transport, whereas in patients with osteosarcoma, it is the loss of RFC activity and elevated DHFR expression.

Nevertheless, the state of polyglutamylation and the role played by FPGS are important aspects of resistance to classical antifolates. In addition, as evidenced by the loss of the accumulation of polyglutamates, elevation in the activity of GH has been correlated with an increase in cross-resistance to MTX by cells selected for resistance to lometrexol (DDATHF), which is an inhibitor of glycinamide ribonucleotide formyltransferase (GARFT). The extent to which this actually occurs during selection in MTX, however, remains unclear.

Resistance to nonclassical antifolates can also be mediated by a number of mechanisms, some of which are the same as those for classical drugs. These include overexpression of and/or mutation of the target enzyme. Because these drugs are not actively transported and are not polyglutamylated, neither alterations of the reduced folate carrier, or folate receptors for that matter, nor changes in FPGS or GH activity levels

TABLE II

Mechanisms of Resistance to DHFR-Targeted Antifolates

Classical antifolates, i.e., MTX	Nonclassical antifolates, i.e., TMTX
1. Alterations in drug uptake 　a. Changes in RFC expression 　b. Changes in FRα expression 2. Overexpression of DHFR 　a. Gene amplification 　b. Induction of transcription 　c. Increase in translation 3. Mutation of DHFR 4. Inability to form and/or maintain polyglutamates 　a. Lack of normal FPGS activity 　b. Increase in GH activity 5. Use of salvage pathways	1. Overexpression of DHFR 2. Mutation in DHFR 3. Increased efflux 　a. Increase in Pgp1 expression 　b. Increase in MRP 1, 2, or 3 expression 4. Increase in folate pool size 5. Use of salvage pathways

would be expected to confer resistance. Interestingly, however, a phenotype characterized by an inability to accumulate the lipophilic antifolate trimetrexate has been described and found to be associated with an increase in the expression of P-glycoprotein. More recently, a Pgp1-independent mechanism for resistance to both TMQ and another lipophilic antifolate, piritrexim, in cells selected for resistance to the 2,4-diaminopyridine based antifolate, pyrimethamine, has also been reported. In this case, a loss of folic acid exporter activity, coupled with an increase in the activity of the low pH transporter, results in the elevation of folate pools to an extent that provides resistance, presumably by competition with drug for DHFR.

One of the most common forms of resistance to classical antifolates is an alteration in drug transport, caused by changes in the expression of the RFC and, to less extent, FBPs. cDNAs for RFCs cloned from L1210 mouse leukemia cells, CHO cells, and human testis have been shown by transfection to restore MTX accumulation and sensitivity in cells whose resistant is mediated by an RFC defect. RFC genes from mouse, hamster, and human share remarkable conservation in exon/intron structure, attesting to the fundamental nature of the role they play in folate metabolism. Drug resistance is associated with a variety of alterations in RFC gene expression, including point mutations that diminish drug uptake or that increase folic acid uptake to a level that provides resistance by increasing internal folate pools and inhibiting polyglutamylation, possibly through a feedback system evolved to regulate pool sizes. Interestingly, mutations that prevent MTX transport but do not affect the transport of other antifolates also exist, demonstrating the substrate specificity of the carrier and suggesting possible ways to circumvent resistance via novel drug design. Premature termination of the translation of RFC mRNA leading to the formation of a truncated carrier with a rapid turnover rate also leads to impaired transport.

The human RFC gene is located on chromosome 21 (21q 22.2-21q 22.3), and its predominant mRNA transcript is approximately 3.0 kb in length. Different 5'-untranslated regions (UTRs) have been reported, and as many as eight exons, formed by differential splicing, may be involved in their formation. All are attached to exon 2, however, which contains the translational start codon. Hence the same protein is expressed. A similar situation occurs in the mouse, where the different RFC 5' UTRs are tissue specific. Hence differential splicing of the human gene will likely prove to be tissue specific as well. The effect of differential splicing on resistance, however, remains to be determined, as does the reported ability of MTX to induce a transcriptional downregulation of RFC expression. This is particularly interesting because MTX can also induce an upregulation of DHFR expression that alone or in combination with downregulation of the RFC could lead to a transient form of drug resistance.

Resistance to antifolates can also be conferred by FRs. In mouse L1210 cells, adequate expression levels of FRα mediate the transport inward of MTX and folates at rates similar to the RFC. Moreover FR-directed transport of folates and MTX is the prominent route of uptake in human KB cells; in antifolate-resistant clones, it is the reduced level of FR expression that confers MTX resistance. However, in MTX-resistant breast cancer cell lines in which RFC-mediated transport is inactivated, expression of either FRα or β does not appreciably alter resistance to MTX, but does sensitize these cells to other antifolates that have a higher affinity for FRs. Ovarian carcinoma cell lines exposed to the antiepileptic drug carbamazepine display decreased MTX uptake and a concomitant acquired resistance to MTX. These cells downregulate FRα mRNA and protein and exhibit a lowered binding capacity for folic acid. No alterations in RFC, DHFR, TS, or FPGS expression levels occur, indicating that the observed resistance is mediated by downregulation of the receptor.

Although the three isoforms of human FR share approximately 70% amino acid sequence homology, they differ considerably in their affinities for various folates and by 10-fold in the ability of MTX and DDATHF to compete for folic acid binding. Hence, it is likely that differential expression of the receptors could mediate drug transport and resistance. Indeed, studies of the promoters of FRα and FRβ genes, and the multiple transcripts generated from each, confirm that complex transcriptional regulation is a major factor in the control of FR gene expression. Interestingly, this complexity mirrors that of the RFC in that, at least for FRα, the various forms of mRNA differ in their 5′UTRs while maintaining the same protein coding sequence.

In addition to transcriptional regulation, the steady-state level of mRNA for FRα in human KB cells is at least partially regulated by its stability. This has been confirmed in CHL cells, in which the level of receptor expression is regulated by the rate of FRα protein synthesis in response to media folate levels. Naturally occurring mutant forms of FBPs that mediate antifolate resistance have yet to be identified. However, it is clear that a thorough understanding of the manner in which FBPs regulate folate/antifolate uptake will be critical in enhancing the efficacy of antifolate therapy.

Overexpression of target enzymes is another primary mechanism of antifolate resistance and is a very effective means of promoting the survival of cells exposed to high levels of drug and, with less frequency, to low levels as well. Both classical and nonclassical antifolates have been used for the selection of cells that overexpress DHFR by means of somatic cell gene amplification. Depending on the length of exposure and the concentration of drug used, overexpression levels can easily exceed by several hundredfold the wild-type level of DHFR expression found in parental cells. A similar mechanism accounts for TS overexpression in cell lines selected for 5-fluorouracil (5-FU) resistance. DHFR gene amplification is also observed, albeit infrequently, in patients undergoing MTX therapy.

Increased expression of DHFR in the absence of gene amplification also occurs. Transcriptional activation of the DHFR gene promoter takes place in the presence of MTX, 5-flurodeoxy uridine (5-FUdR), or hyroxyurea and leads to transient overexpression *in vitro*. At the protein synthesis level, DHFR can interact with DHFR mRNA to decrease translation *in vitro*. However, the addition of MTX to the reaction destroys the interaction, presumably by binding with DHFR, thus stimulating the translation of DHFR mRNA. Hence a transient increase in DHFR expression ensues. Interestingly, a similar mechanism is involved in the regulation of TS mRNA translation *in vitro*. In this case, dUMP, 5-FudR, or 5,10-methylene-H4PteGlu enhances the translation of TS mRNA by binding to TS, preventing it from associating with TS mRNA. Although neither of these mechanisms has been demonstrated to occur *in vivo*, their presence would help explain reports that DHFR levels acutely

increase during the early stages of drug exposure. This overexpression, albeit at a low level, could provide sufficient survival time for other more substantial forms of resistance to emerge, thus establishing a drug-resistant population.

The occurrence of mutant forms of target enzymes provides still another avenue for acquired antifolate resistance. Mutant forms of DHFR exist in cell lines derived from mouse, hamster, and human cells selected for resistance to MTX or TMQ. Of those reported and representative of independent genetic events, seven involve either Leu_{22} or Phe_{31}, two highly conserved amino acids located within the active site of the enzyme (see Table III and Fig. 3). In all cases, mutations result in enzymes that display lowered affinities for drug, and in all but one, largely preserve enzymatic activity as well. In that one instance, a $Leu_{22} \rightarrow Arg$ mutation in mouse DHFR results in an enzyme that is 210-fold resistant to MTX but maintains only 5% of the wild-type enzymatic activity. Of the remaining six mutants, three are $Leu_{22} \rightarrow Phe$, three are $Phe_{31} \rightarrow Ser$, and one is a $Phe_{31} \rightarrow Trp$ change. Of these, the $Leu_{22} \rightarrow Phe$ mutant from hamster provides a striking contrast to the $Leu_{22} \rightarrow Arg$ mouse mutant in that it is 20-fold resistant to MTX but fully retains the enzymological properties and catalytic activity of the wild-type enzyme.

TABLE III
DHFR Mutations Identified by Independent Selection with Antifolates[a]

Species	Mutation	Selection agent
Human	phe$_{31}$→trp	MTX
Mouse	phe$_{31}$→trp	MTX
	leu$_{22}$→arg[b]	MTX
	gly$_{15}$→trp	MTX
Hamster	leu$_{22}$→phe	MTX
	leu$_{22}$→phe	MQ[c]
	leu$_{22}$→phe	MTX
	phe$_{31}$→Ser	TMQ

[a]In all cases except as noted, selections were carried out by exposing tumor cells in culture to varying drug concentrations.

[b]Selection in this case was carried out *in vivo* by treatment of L1210 leukemia ascites tumors with MTX.

[c]Refers to the quinazoline-based antifolate, methasquin.

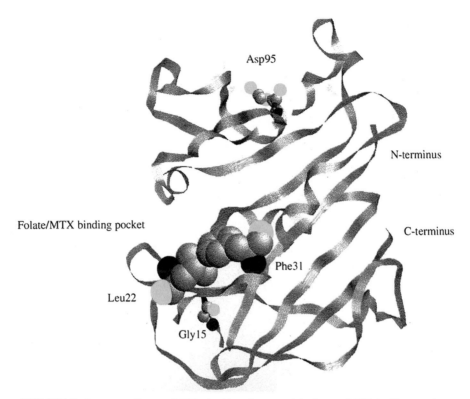

FIGURE 3 Structure of human DHFR. A ribbon diagram of the human DHFR backbone is shown. N- and C-terminal ends are indicated. Amino acids Leu22 and Phe31, both of which are located in the folate-binding pocket, are shown as colored spheres, whereas Gly15 and Asp95, which lie outside of the pocket, are represented by balls and sticks. Dark gray, carbon; light gray, oxygen; black, nitrogen. The structure, 1DRF, was obtained from the Protein Data Bank, and the drawing was prepared using Alchemy 2000 for Windows.

In addition, a Gyl$_{15}$ → Trp mutant obtained from a cell line derived from the ascites of mice injected with L1210 leukemia cells and subsequently treated with MTX has also been described. This mutation results in an enzyme that has an elevated k_m for folate (approximately 20-fold) and a 50% higher catalytic activity resulting in a 12-fold lower catalytic efficiency than the wild type. The k_i of the mutant for MTX is elevated 165-fold, hence as with the other reported DHFR mutants, its sensitivity to MTX has been lowered significantly. Interestingly, amino acid position 15 is not within the active site of the enzyme (Fig. 3) and, therefore, must exert its influence through secondary structure effects that alter the interactions between substrate and/or drug and the active site. The extent to which somatic cell mutation actually plays a role in the acquisition of clinical drug resistance remains obscure.

V. INTRINSIC DRUG RESISTANCE

Other mechanisms of resistance to classical antifolates, such as lowered TS activity and elevation in thymidine and purine salvage pathway enzyme activity, are not generally found by selection but instead represent intrinsic mechanisms that are due to the metabolic differences between cell and tissue types. Moreover, these effects are often exerted indirectly. For example, low TS activity provides resistance to MTX by reducing the need to replenish the H4PteGlu that is normally consumed by the synthesis of TMP. This lowers the requirement for DHFR activity, which in turn reduces sensitivity to MTX. In the case of salvage mechanisms, it is the elevation of nucleoside transporter activity or the inactivation of such transporters by compounds such as dipyridamole that potentiates the activity of antifolates by providing alternate ways of meeting the cells need for nucleotide precursors, obviating *de novo* synthetic routes. Indeed, dipyridamole has been shown to directly sensitize cells to the effects of both MTX and MTA.

Not all forms of intrinsic antifolate resistance exert their efforts indirectly, however. Variation in the level of FPGS activity in acute myelocytic leukemia (AML) and in the extent to which classical antifolates become polyglutamylated in these and other tumor types as well directly mediates resistance by altering the affinity that such structurally modified drugs exhibit for their target enzymes. In soft tissue sarcomas cells, elevated GU activity is correlated with MTX resistance.

The effects of single nucleotide polymorphisms (SNPs) between allelic genes in any of the folate pathway enzymes could also influence intrinsic resistance. As demonstrated in CHL cells, such alleles can encode enzymes with normal catalytic properties that differ in their affinity for a given drug. In this case, due to an Asp → Asn difference at amino acid position 95 (Fig. 3), the two forms of DHFR differ by threefold in their k_d for MTX, and this is sufficient to provide a selective advantage to cells expressing the low-affinity allele (Asp95) during growth in the presence of the drug. By anology, patients containing a similar polymorphism in the human DHFR gene would be intrinsically more resistant to MTX than those carrying an allele that encoded an enzyme with higher affinity. In fact, similar SNPs in any target gene could yield a similar selective advantage. It should be noted, however, that such polymorphic alleles have not been found in human cell lines or patient samples. With the completion of sequencing of the human genome, however, SNPs in DHFR and other folate pathway genes should become more readily discernible.

It may also be argued that the ability of a given cell to amplify a target gene, i.e., DHFR, is an intrinsic property of that cell. The mechanism(s) responsible for gene amplification remains largely speculative, but it is known that the ability to amplify is uncommon in normal cells. Hence transformed cells have acquired a property(s) that destabilizes the genome, a manifestation of which is gene amplification. While it is unclear what that property(s) might be, DNA replication in the presence of clastogenic agents such as MTX in cells in which the wild-type function of the p53 tumor suppressor gene has been eliminated leads to elevated rates of gene amplification, presumably by allowing unrepaired DNA damage, i.e., single and double strand breaks, to be propagated. Such breaks have been associated with the activation of fragile sites and the formation of double minute chromosomes and interstitial HSRs, both of which are known to be cytological manifestations of gene amplification. Thus, transformed cells that have lost p53 function are intrinsically good candidates for the acquisition of antifolate resistance via target enzyme gene amplification.

The expression levels of specific transcription factors such as EF2 that regulate the expression of DHFR can mediate other forms of intrinsic resistance. During the G_2, M, and early G_1 phases of the cell cycle, the unphosphorylated form of the retinoblastoma tumor suppressor protein (Rb) is able to bind and sequester the E2F family of transcriptional activators. These proteins are required for the efficient transcription of several genes involved with DNA synthesis, including DHFR. Phosphorylation of Rb by cyclin/cdk complexes late in G_1 releases these activators, permitting their function. In the absence of Rb, the expression of DHFR is maintained at abnormally high levels throughout the cell cycle, conferring low-level resistance to MTX.

In the final analysis, it is the intrinsic and often subtle differences between cell types and tissues that are critical to the success of chemotherapy. Hence, if the efficacy of antifolate therapy is to be optimized and the promise of new generation drugs realized, it will be necessary to not only understand at the molecular and cellular level the many acquired mechanisms that afford clinical resistance, but also to understand the intrinsic characteristics that define individual tumors and to expolite them for therapeutic gain.

Acknowledgments

This work was supported in part by grants from the NIH and NSF and by Cerbios-Pharma SA. The author thanks the many colleagues and students who have contributed to the overall content of this article.

See Also the Following Articles

FOLATE ANTAGONISTS • PURINE ANTIMETABOLITES • PYRIMIDINE ANTIMETABOLITES • RESISTANCE TO ANTIBODY THERAPY • RESISTANCE TO DNA-DAMAGING AGENTS • RESIS-

Bibliography

Assaraf, Y. G., Babani, S., and Goldman, I. D. (1998). Increased activity of a novel low pH transporter associated with lipophilic antifolate resistance in Chinese hamster ovary cells. *J. Biol. Chem.* **273,** 8106–8111.

Banergee, D., Ercikan-Abali, E., Waltham, M., Schnieders, B., Hochhauser, D., Li, W. W., Fan, J., Gorlick, R., Gorker, E., and Bertino, J. R. (1995). Molecular mechanisms of resistance to antifolates, a review. *Acta Biochim. Pol.* **42,** 457–464.

Calvert, H. (1999). An overview of folate metabolism: Features relevant to the action and toxicities of antifolate anticancer agents. *Semin. Oncol.* **26,** 3–10.

Ercikan-Abali, E. A., Banerjee, D., Waltham, M. C., Skacel, N., Scotto, K. W., and Bertino, J. R. (1997). Dihydrofolate reductase protein inhibits its own translation by binding to dihydrofolate reductase mRNA sequences within the coding region. *Biochemistry* **36,** 12317–12322.

Galivan, J., Ryan, T., Rhee, M., Yao, R., and Chave, K. (1999). Glutamyl hydrolase: Properties and pharmacological impact. *Semin. Oncol.* **26,** 33–37.

Gorlick, R., Cole, P., Banerjee, D., Longo, G., Li, W. W., Hochhauser, D., and Bertino, J. R. (1999). Mechanisms of methotrexate resistance in acute leukemia: Decreased transport and polyglutamylation. *Adv. Exp. Med. Biol.* **457,** 543–550.

Huennekens, F. M. (1994). The methotrexate story: A paradigm for development of cancer chemotherapeutic agents. *Adv. Enzyme Regul.* **34,** 397–419.

Jansen, G., Barr, H., Kathmann. I., Bunni, M. A., Priest, D. G., Noordhuis, P., Peters, G. J., and Assaraf, Y. G. (1999) Multiple mechanisms of resistance to polyglutamatable and lipophilic antifolates in mammalian cells: Role of increased folylpolyglutamylation, expanded folate pools, and intralysosomal drug sequestration. *Mol. Pharm.* **55,** 761–769.

Kinsella, A. R., and Smith, D. (1998). Tumor resistance to antimetabolites. *Gen. Pharm.* **30,** 623–626.

Kool, M., van der Linden, M., de Hass, M., Scheffer, G. L., de Vree, J. M. L., Smith, A. J., Jansen, G., Godefridus, J. P., Ponne, N., Scheper, R. J., Oude Elferink, R. P. J., Baas, F., and Borst, P. (1999). MRP3, an organic anion transporter able to transport anti-cancer drugs. *Proc. Natl. Acad. Sci. USA* **96,** 6914–6919.

Johnson, J. M., Meiering, E. M., Wright, J. E., Pardo, J., Roskowsky, A., and Wagner, G. (1997). NMR solution structure of the antitumor compound PT523 and NADPH in the ternary complex with human dihydrofolate reductase. *Biochemistry* **36,** 4399–4411.

Moscow, J. A. (1997). Methotrexate transport and resistance. *Leukemia Lymphoma* **30,** 215–224.

Moran, R. G. (1999). Roles of folylpoly-gamma-glutamate synthetase in therapeutics with tetrahydrofolate antimetabolites: An overview. *Semin. Oncol.* **26,** 24–32.

Rosowsky, A. (1999). PT523 and other aminopterin analogs with a hemiphthaloyl-L-ornithine side chain: Exceptionally tight-binding inhibitors of Dihydrofolate reductase which are transported by the reduced folate carrier but cannot form polyglutamates. *Curr. Med. Chem.* **6,** 329–352.

Ross, J. F., Chaudhuri, P. K., and Ratnam, M. (1994). Differential regulation of folate receptor isoforms in normal and malignant tissues in vivo and in established cell lines. *Cancer* **73,** 2432–2443.

Shih, C., Habeck, L. L., Mendelson, L., G., Chen, V. J., and Schultz, R. M. (1998). Multiple folate enzyme inhibition: Mechanism of a novel pyrrolopyrimidine-based antifolate LY231514 (MTA). *Adv. Enzyme Regul.* **38,** 135–152.

Sirotnak, F. M., and Tolner, B. (1999). Carrier-mediated membrane transport of folates in mammalian cells. *Annu. Rev. Nutr.* **19,** 91–122.

Smith, P. G., Marshman, E., Newell, D. R., and Curtin, N. J. (2000). Dipyridamole potentiates the in vitro activity of MTA (LY231514) by inhibition of thymidine transport. *Br. J. Cancer* **82,** 924–930.

Yu, M., and Melera, P. W. (1993). Allelic variation in the dihydrofolate reductase gene at amino acid position 95 contributes to antifolate resistance in Chinese hamster cells. *Cancer Res.* **53,** 6031–6035.

Zhu, W.-Y., Alliegro, M. A., and Melera, P. W. (2001). The rate of folate receptor alpha (FRa) synthesis in folate depleted CHL cells is regulated by a translational mechanism sensitive to media folate levels, while stable overexpression of its mRNA is mediated by gene amplification and an increase in transcript half-life. *J. Cell. Biochem.* **81,** 205–219.

Resistance to Topoisomerase-Targeting Agents

John L. Nitiss
Karin C. Nitiss
St. Jude Children's Research Hospital, Memphis, Tennessee

GLOSSARY

camptothecins A class of chemotherapeutic agents that target eukaryotic topoisomerase I. Camptothecins in current clinical use include topotecan, 9-amino camptothecin, and irinotecan.

topoisomerase An enzyme that can change the topological state of DNA through (reversible) breakage and rejoining of DNA strand(s). Topological changes carried out by topoisomerases include changes in DNA supercoiling and catenation and decatenation of DNA molecules.

topoisomerase I A class of DNA topoisomerases that carry out topological changes in DNA by introducing transient single strand breaks in DNA. Type IA topoisomerases generally relax only negatively supercoiled DNA and form a covalent:protein DNA complex in which the enzyme is bound to the 5′ DNA terminus. Type IB enzymes are able to relax both positively and negatively supercoiled DNA.

topoisomerase II A class of DNA topoisomerases that carry out topological changes in DNA by introducing transient double strand breaks in DNA. Because topoisomerase II is the only enzyme that can efficiently decatenate intact double-stranded DNA, it has an essential role in mitosis that cannot be replaced by topoisomerase I. Mammalian cells have two isozymes of topoisomerase II, termed α and β.

topoisomerase poison A drug that targets a topoisomerase and acts by stabilizing the covalent complex intermediate of the enzymes' reactions. Because a topoisomerase poison increases the level of protein:DNA complexes, it converts the enzyme into a form of DNA damage, hence the term "poison."

L ike all anticancer agents, cellular resistance to topoisomerase targeting agents is an important factor that limits the effectiveness of this class of drugs.

Resistance can be intrinsic or acquired by selection in the presence of drugs. In most cases, the mechanisms of intrinsic or acquired resistance are likely to arise from the same molecular mechanisms. The large body of information available concerning the biochemical mechanisms of drug action, and the pathways leading to cell killing by topoisomerase-targeting drugs, has allowed the definition of many mechanisms of drug resistance. This article relates the known mechanisms of cell killing by drugs targeting topoisomerases to pathways of drug resistance. While some pathways of resistance such as changes in drug accumulation or control of apoptosis, are shared (in part) with other classes of anticancer agents, other pathways are very specific for topoisomerase-targeting drugs. Issues relating to general drug resistance pathways are not discussed in detail.

I. INTRODUCTION

DNA topoisomerases are the principal targets for many clinically important antitumor agents. There are two major families of topoisomerases: type I enzymes that introduce transient single strand cuts in DNA and type II enzymes, which in eukaryotes are dimeric enzymes that make double strand cuts in DNA. Both type I and type II enzymes are the targets of important anticancer agents. The principal drugs acting against type I topoisomerases are the camptothecins, including topotecan and irinotecan. A wider range of agents act against eukaryotic topoisomerase II, including the anthracyclines doxorubicin and daunomycin, the epipodophyllotoxins etoposide and teniposide, and other agents, including amsacrine and mitoxantrone. The strong intercalating agent dactinomycin has shown activity against both topoisomerase I and topoisomerase II, as have other experimental agents that have yet to be introduced into the clinic.

DNA topoisomerases participate in a wide variety of cellular functions. The discovery of DNA topoisomerases was motivated by the problem of separating DNA strands following semiconservative DNA replication, and it is clear that topoisomerases play critical roles during this process. Subsequent work has indicated that topoisomerases also play key roles in transcription, chromosome structure, and recombination. The central role of topoisomerases in DNA metabolism, particularly in proliferating cells, might suggest that these enzymes would be potential targets for anticancer agents. While some agents have been identified that act mainly by inhibiting the catalytic activity of topoisomerases, the main action of topoisomerase-targeting drugs in clinical use is to convert the enzyme into a unique form of DNA damage. This unique mechanism of action of topoisomerase-targeting agents dictates many of the potential resistance mechanisms.

II. HOW INTERFERING WITH TOPOISOMERASES CAUSES CELL KILLING

The enzyme reactions of both type I and type II topoisomerases involve transient DNA cleavage. DNA cleavage by topoisomerases is a transesterification reaction, in which a tyrosine residue(s) of the enzymes forms a transient covalent bond with phosphates of the DNA backbone. For eukaryotic topoisomerase I, the tyrosine forms a covalent linkage with the 3′ phosphate of the DNA phosphodiester backbone. Eukaryotic topoisomerase II is a homodimer, and each subunit forms a covalent bond between a tyrosine residue of each subunit and the 5′ phosphate of DNA. Thus, topoisomerase II introduces a transient double strand break in DNA. The break with topoisomerase II has a four base stagger. A third eukaryotic topoisomerase, termed topoisomerase III, is a type I topoisomerase that also forms a phosphotyrosine linkage involving a 5′ phosphate of DNA. No potent inhibitors of topoisomerase III have been described, so this enzyme will not be discussed further. The cleavage reaction of DNA topoisomerases preserves the energy of the broken phosphodiester bond, and the enzymes are able to reseal the DNA breaks by reversing the transesterification reaction, reforming the phosphodiester bond of DNA and allowing the enzyme to dissociate from DNA or initiate a new reaction cycle. This unique mechanism of cleavage allows resealing of the DNA break formed by topoisomerases without a high-energy cofactor. Because the enzyme-mediated break is protein linked, breaks induced by the enzyme are different from DNA breaks arising from DNA damaging agents and do not trigger a DNA damage response that could include induction of recombination events that could lead to deleterious genomic rearrangements.

Inhibitors of DNA topoisomerases in current clinical use as anticancer agents specifically interfere with the breakage–rejoining reactions of the enzymes described earlier. A common mechanism is that drugs targeting a topoisomerase do not interfere with the ability of the enzyme to cleave DNA, but inhibit religation of the DNA strand breaks. These inhibitors therefore lead to an increased level of the transient intermediates where the DNA strands are broken, and the enzyme is covalently bound to DNA. The inhibitors therefore convert the enzyme into a DNA "lesion," which has the potential to interfere with DNA metabolism. Because this type of inhibitor can generate lesions on DNA, they have been referred to as "topoisomerase poisons."

An important property of the covalent complex formed between topoisomerases and DNA in the presence of inhibitors is that the complex can still be reversed. If the drug is removed, the enzymes are capable of rapidly resealing the induced DNA strand breaks. This implies that other processes are required to convert the reversible covalent complex into irreversible DNA damage. The conversion of topoisomerase:DNA covalent complexes into irreversible DNA damage frequently involves DNA replication. Cell killing with camptothecin is schedule dependent. Exposure to even high drug concentrations for brief periods of time causes only limited cell killing, whereas exposure for longer periods of time increases the level of cell killing. Involvement of replication was demonstrated by showing that DNA replication inhibitors such as aphidicolin could completely prevent cell killing by camptothecin. Liu and colleagues proposed that collision of a replication fork with a topoisomerase I covalent complex could lead to DNA double strand breaks. Secondary double strand breaks that arise from collision of a replication fork with a covalent complex would not be reversible by the enzyme. The generation of secondary double strand breaks by fork collision is illustrated in Fig. 1. Hence replication is one factor that can convert topoisomerase I covalent complexes into irreversible DNA

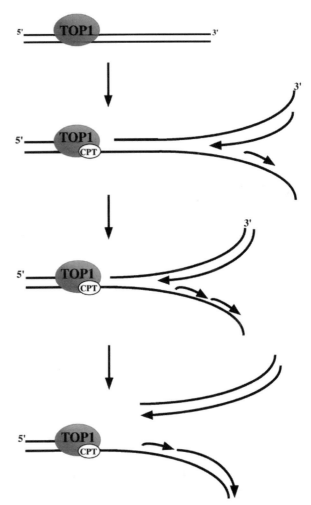

FIGURE 1 Collision of a replication fork with a topoisomerase I covalent complex. During the normal topoisomerase I reaction, the enzyme binds to DNA, carries out its reaction, and then dissociates. In the presence of camptothecin, topoisomerase I is trapped on DNA as a covalent complex that includes a single strand break. A replication fork impinging on the covalent complex can directly lead to a double strand break. A similar mechanism is thought to occur with topoisomerase II (not shown).

damage. It is important to note that the collision of a replication fork with a topoisomerase I covalent complex can lead to a double strand break even though the enzyme makes single strand breaks in DNA.

Similar mechanisms of converting covalent complexes to irreversible DNA damage also apply for topoisomerase II. Schedule dependence is also seen for topoisomerase II-targeting drugs, but it is not as strict as that found with camptothecins. Treatment of cells with replication inhibitors reduces cell killing by topoisomerase II poisons, but does not completely abolish it. These results suggest that collision of a replication fork with a topoisomerase II complex can generate irreversible DNA damage, but that other enzymes that track along DNA can also do this. Because topoisomerase II makes double strand cuts in DNA, collision of a topoisomerase II covalent complex with RNA polymerase or with a DNA helicase could also lead to a double strand break.

Strong evidence for the poison model has been obtained using yeast model systems. A clear example is found with the action of the topoisomerase I specific poison camptothecin. Yeast cells are sensitive to camptothecin, even though topoisomerase I is not essential for the viability of yeast cells. If the gene for topoisomerase I is inactivated, then the yeast cells become completely refractory to camptothecin. These experiments demonstrated that topoisomerase I was the main target for cell killing and that inhibition of enzyme activity per se was not the factor responsible for cell killing. Furthermore, yeast cells that are defective in double strand break repair are hypersensitive to camptothecin, suggesting that in the presence of topoisomerase I, camptothecin exposure leads to double strand breaks. These observations also support the poison model.

A similar set of observations has also demonstrated the importance of poisoning for drugs targeting topoisomerase II. Unlike topoisomerase I, topoisomerase II is essential for viability in yeast. Yeast cells overexpressing topoisomerase II become hypersensitive to topoisomerase II poisons, consistent with the generation of DNA damage in the presence of topoisomerase II targeting drugs. In contrast, yeast cells expressing a topoisomerase II allele with reduced enzyme activity become drug resistant, suggesting that interference with the essential function of topoisomerase II does not play a crucial role in the mechanism of action of this class of drugs. Taken together, results in yeast strongly support a model where the stabilization of covalent complexes leads to DNA damage that can be converted into double strand DNA breaks. Although it is more difficult to manipulate the levels of topoisomerases in mammalian cells, results obtained from cell lines selected for resistance to topoisomerase I or topoisomerase II poisons are also consistent with the poison hypothesis.

III. GENERAL RESISTANCE MECHANISMS

A. Resistance Mechanisms: An Overview

The mechanism of cell killing by topoisomerase poisons indicates that resistance can result from several discrete steps, as illustrated in Fig. 2. First, active drug can be prevented from reaching the nucleus. This can occur either by converting the drug into an inactive form (either extracellularly or intracellularly) or, for prodrugs, by preventing activation of the drug. Reducing drug influx or increasing drug efflux can modify drug accumulation. These mechanisms are not specific for topoisomerase targeting drugs and, as indicated later, general drug resistance mechanisms that have been defined for other classes of anticancer drugs can confer resistance to topoisomerase poisons. A second level of resistance is specific alterations in topoisomerases, either by changing the levels of the proteins or by mutations that render the enzyme drug

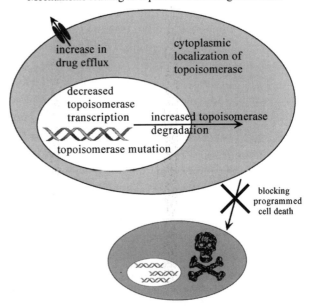

Mechanisms leading to topoisomerase drug resistance

FIGURE 2 Potential mechanisms of resistance to topoisomerase-targeting agents. Several mechanisms have been described that can lead to resistance to topoisomerase-targeting agents. Some mechanisms, such as increased drug efflux or effects on programmed cell death, are important for resistance to many classes of chemotherapeutic agents. Others, affecting topoisomerase levels or mutations in topoisomerases, are specific to topoisomerase-targeting drugs.

insensitive. These changes should primarily affect sensitivity to topoisomerase poisons. Finally, because formation of a trapped covalent topoisomerase:DNA complex by itself is insufficient to cause cell killing, alterations in steps downstream of the generation of the DNA damage can also affect drug sensitivity. The downstream steps, which include cell cycle progression, DNA damage responses, and commitment to cell death, are also not unique to topoisomerase poisons and may therefore affect sensitivity to multiple classes of anticancer agents

B. Changes in Drug Accumulation

It is well established that drug resistance can arise from alterations in drug accumulation. Reduced drug accumulation typically arises from the expression of ATP-dependent transporters, such as the product of the multidrug resistance gene *MDR1* (p-glycoprotein) or the multidrug resistant protein *MRP1*. These two proteins define a superfamily of transmembrane proteins that include transport proteins from bacteria, yeast, and higher eukaryotes. Both p-glycoprotein and *MRP1* have 12 transmembrane domains and two ATP-binding sites. Another related class of transporters has been described that consists of six transmembrane domains and a single ATP-binding site. These proteins have been referred to as a half-transporter because its structure resembles half of p-glycoprotein or *MRP1*. An example of this class of transporter is the BCRP protein. All of these proteins have been demonstrated to be able to transport a variety of cytotoxic drugs, including drugs targeting topoisomerases.

Drug transporters can play important roles in resistance in two major ways. Tumors arising from tissue types that normally express drug transporters can maintain a significant intrinsic drug resistance if they continue to express the transporter. Alternately, selection in the presence of cytotoxic drugs can select for drug resistance that arises from *de novo* expression of transporters or an increase in their expression. In cell lines selected for drug resistance, enhanced expression is frequently accompanied by amplification of the gene encoding a transporter.

Determining the importance of a transporter in conferring resistance can be strongly influenced by details of the experimental system. For example, the ability of topoisomerase I poisons such as topotecan to be transported has been assessed using cell lines expressing very high levels of p-glycoprotein. Such cell lines may show a 200-fold resistance to drugs that are efficiently transported, while showing only 5-fold resistance to agents such as topotecan. Thus, while p-glycoprotein has some potential to confer resistance to topotecan, it is unlikely to play a key role in clinical resistance to this agent.

Table I summarizes the ability of some major transporters to confer drug resistance to drugs targeting topoisomerase poisons. As indicated in Table I, each transporter can efficiently transport some topoisomerase-targeting agents, but not others. BCRP has been the focus of considerable attention, as it is unique among mammalian transporters in its ability to efficiently transport various topoisomerase I poisons of the camptothecin family. Table I does not exhaustively summarize all proteins that play roles in reducing drug accumulation. The ABC superfamily of transporters is quite large, and there are also likely to be other unrelated proteins that can also decrease intracellular concentrations of cytotoxic agents. One example that is still poorly understood is a protein termed lung cancer resistance protein (LRP), which can confer resistance to multiple cytotoxic agents, including topoisomerase poisons. LRP encodes the major protein in a cytoplasmic RNA protein complex that has been termed a "vault." The function of vaults remains to be determined, so it is altogether unclear how overexpression of one protein of this complex can reduce drug accumulation.

C. Roles of p53 and Apoptotic Proteins in Resistance

Exposure of cells to cytotoxic stress, including DNA-damaging agents, triggers a set of complex cellular responses that depend on the cellular environment, the cell type, the amount and type of cellular damage, and a range of other factors. The p53 tumor suppressor gene mediates an important set of cellular responses to DNA damage. In cells carrying a wild-type p53 gene, DNA damage leads to elevated levels of p53 protein. The higher levels of p53 trigger a set of transcriptional responses that include activation of the CDK inhibitor p21, resulting in cell cycle arrest

TABLE I
Drug Transporters That Can Confer Resistance to
Topoisomerase-Targeting Agents[a]

	p-Glycoprotein	MRP1	MRP2	MRP3	BCRP
Topoisomerase I agents					
9-Aminocamptothecin	−	−	?	?	+ +
Topotecan	+	−	+	−	+ +
Irinotecan[b]	−	+ (?)	?	−	+ +
Topoisomerase II agents					
Doxorubicin	+ + +	+ +	?	−	+ +[c]
Etoposide	+ +	+ +	−	+ +	−
Mitoxantrone	+	?	?	?	+ +

[a]−, drug is unable to be efficiently transported by the indicated transporter; +, drug can be transported and expression of the transporter is capable of conferring resistance compared to cells either lacking expression of the transporter or cells that express lower levels of the transporter (additional "+" signs indicate more efficient transport or the ability to confer higher levels of drug resistance); +(?), published reports suggest transport or conferral of resistance, but more direct confirmation is required; ?, currently undetermined whether expression of the transporter can confer resistance.

[b]In general, transport of irinotecan is actually assessed using either SN-38 or irinotecan and a carboxylesterase that is capable of converting irinotecan to SN-38. In most studies, therefore, it is transport of SN-38 that is being assessed.

[c]BCRP can be mutated by a single amino acid change into a form that can transport anthracyclines efficiently. The wild-type allele appears to be unable to efficiently transport doxorubicin or other anthracyclines.

at the G_1/S boundary. As described earlier, DNA replication converts covalent topoisomerase DNA adducts into irreversible DNA damage, suggesting that wild-type p53 might afford cells substantial protection from the cytotoxic effects of these agents. However, p53 can commit cells to undergo apoptosis. p53 therefore has the potential to either protect cells from undergoing DNA replication in the presence of damaged DNA or to cause cells to commit to cell death rather than attempt to repair or tolerate the DNA damage. Because p53 is mutated in a large percentage of human tumors, understanding whether the protective checkpoint function or the apoptotic function of p53 predominates is important in understanding the sensitivity of tumor cells to topoisomerase-targeting agents.

An important reason why the role of p53 in cellular sensitivity to topoisomerase targeting agents (and other chemotherapeutic drugs) remains controversial is that cell death is measured in many in different ways. It is certainly the case that if one exposes $p53^+$ and $p53^-$ cells to topoisomerase II poisons, such as doxorubicin or etoposide, rapid apoptosis is observed in $p53^+$ cells, and considerably less apoptosis is seen on the same time scale in p53-deficient cells. However, cells can die by mechanisms other than apoptosis, and if one measures clonogenic survival as an assay of cell death, differences between p53-proficient and -deficient cells frequently vanish. Advances in the application of transgenic mouse systems have allowed the generation of tumors that differ only in their p53 status and should shed important light on this question; however, the ability to generate isogenic tumors can depend on the use of dominant oncogenes that substantially affect drug sensitivity in their own right.

p53 may play an additional role in both sensitivity both topoisomerase I- and topoisomerase II-targeting agents. Studies have suggested that p53 can regulate topoisomerase II transcription. It has also been suggested that p53 can modulate the activities of both topoisomerase I and topoisomerase II, although these findings have not yet been confirmed. Nonetheless, p53 has the potential to modulate the target of topoisomerase targeting agents, to affect the ability of cells to traverse the cell cycle, thereby converting topoisomerase lesions into irreversible damage, and to determine cell fates in the presence of such damage.

Other events subsequent to the generation of cytotoxic lesions are also potentially important in determining cellular sensitivity to topoisomerase-targeting agents. The pathways of apoptosis include various effectors and antagonists that can sensitize or protect cells from cell death. An important example of an antiapoptotic gene is Bcl-2. In some contexts, overexpression of Bcl-2 prevents the occurrence of apoptosis, which may result in drug resistance. The precise roles of downstream events in resistance to topoisomerase-targeting agents will require an understanding of the entire pathway leading from recognition of DNA damage, activation of signal transduction pathways, and the action of the signaling pathways on effectors or inhibitors of cell death. Kaufmann provides an excellent elaboration of the current controversies relating to the role of cell death pathways in resistance to topoisomerase-targeting agents.

IV. RESISTANCE MECHANISMS SPECIFIC FOR TOPOISOMERASES

Drug resistance arising from changes in drug accumulation or from alterations in apoptotic mechanisms can confer resistance to multiple classes of drugs. It was also observed that cell lines selected for resistance to etoposide or other topoisomerase II-targeting agents could exhibit resistance specific for topoisomerase II-targeting drugs. Beck and colleagues termed this atypical multidrug resistance (atMDR). Subsequent experiments demonstrated that atMDR arose predominantly from alterations in topoisomerase II. Experiments carried out selecting for resistance to topoisomerase I poisons have demonstrated a parallel pattern of resistance, i.e., resistance to drugs targeting topoisomerase I, but normal sensitivity to other cytotoxic agents. As expected, this mode of resistance also arises from alterations in topoisomerase I upon selection for resistance to camptothecins.

The mechanism of cell killing described in Section II predicts that alterations that reduce the level of a drug-sensitive topoisomerase should reduce the sensitivity to topoisomerase poisons. This could occur by various mechanisms, including reducing the level of topoisomerase proteins in the nucleus, which is discussed in Section IV,A, or by a qualitative change in topoisomerase proteins, which is discussed in Section IV,B.

A. Changes in Topoisomerase Levels

A common change in cell lines selected for resistance to either topoisomerase I or topoisomerase II poisons is reduced levels of topoisomerase proteins. For example, cell lines selected for resistance to camptothecin resistance show reduced topoisomerase I levels, whereas cell lines selected for etoposide resistance show reduced levels of topoisomerase II α and/or topoisomerase II β. Frequently, this is due to a reduction in mRNA encoding the protein, suggesting alterations in the transcriptional regulation of the proteins. Transcriptional regulation of the topoisomerases that are the targets of drugs, topoisomerase I, topoisomerase II α and topoisomerase II β, have been characterized in some detail, including a characterization of patterns of expression during the cell cycle and detailed analyses of the respective gene promoters.

Topoisomerase I is expressed at all points in the cell cycle, in both proliferating and quiescent cells, although some studies have suggested stimulation of topoisomerase I transcription when cells are stimulated to proliferate. Promoter analysis of the human topoisomerase I gene has shown that the topoisomerase I promoter, like many housekeeping genes, lacks a TATA box and has binding sites for SP-1, as well as other transcription factors. The functional significance of most of the promoter elements has not been pursued; however, studies have suggested that the transcription factor NF-IL6, a member of the C/EBP family of transcription factors, plays an important role in stimulating topoisomerase I transcription.

The regulation of topoisomerase II α transcription has been studied extensively, partly because expression of this protein is cell cycle and proliferation regulated. Several transcription-binding sites have been identified in the topoisomerase II α promoter, including sites for YB-1, a transcription factor that may regulate the expression of a variety of genes related to proliferation, inverted CAATT boxes, which have also been implicated in the regulation of genes required for cell proliferation, and SP-3, a member of the SP-1 family of transcription factors that can serve as a repressor of transcription. Interestingly, the p53 tumor suppressor has also been shown to affect the transcription of topoisomerase II α. Suttle and colleagues used a temperature-sensitive p53 allele and showed reduced topoisomerase II α gene transcription at the permissive temperature for p53 function. Because a large proportion of human cancers carry p53 mutations, negative regulation of topoisomerase II expression by p53 could improve the therapeutic index of topoisomerase II poisons. However, the role that p53 plays in regulating apoptosis discussed earlier complicates a simple interpretation of how mutations in this central protein affect sensitivity to topoisomerase II poisons.

Topoisomerase II β, like topoisomerase I, is expressed at all points in the cell cycle. Unlike the other two enzymes that are major drug targets, topoisomerase II β is not required for the viability of most cells (although mouse embryos lacking topoisomerase II β are inviable due to a failure to enervate the diaphragm), hence it is possible to completely silence the expression of this enzyme. Studies with mouse fibroblasts derived from transgenic embryos lacking topoisomerase II β are partially resistant to multiple topoisomerase II poisons, indicating that silencing of these genes can lead to drug resistance. Other cell lines selected for resistance to topoisomerase II poisons have also been reported that lack detectable topoisomerase II β, suggesting that silencing of this gene may be a significant factor in acquired drug resistance.

It remains to be established in most cases how topoisomerase gene expression is downregulated in cells that exhibit reduced levels of the enzymes. Two possible mechanisms could be responsible for reduced topoisomerase gene transcription. *cis*-acting changes in topoisomerase promoters can lead to reduced topoisomerase gene transcription and can arise by mutations in key regulatory sites or by epigenetic gene silencing by cytosine methylation. Alternately, *trans*-acting changes in the levels of positive or negatively acting transcription factors could also reduce topoisomerase gene expression leading to resistance. No mutations have been identified in topoisomerase promoters in drug-resistant cell lines, although there have not been many studies examining this question. Similarly, methylation of topoisomerase gene promoters in drug-resistant cells has not been extensively examined. Nor has there been many studies examining changes in transcription factors that regulate topoisomerase expression. In one case, an etoposide-resistant cell line was observed to have reduced topoisomerase

II α transcription and elevated levels of Sp-3, consistent with partial transcriptional silencing of the topoisomerase II α gene promoter. Further studies will be needed to assess whether this represents a general mechanism.

In addition to transcriptional regulation, the posttranslational regulation of DNA topoisomerases has also been observed. Both topoisomerase I and topoisomerase II β are stable proteins. However, topoisomerase II α is considerably less stable, and most of this enzyme is degraded at the time of mitosis. The stability of topoisomerase II α is also regulated by some stress conditions. Glucose starvation leads to the rapid degradation of topoisomerase II α degradation that is mediated by the proteasome. The hypoxic conditions found in many tumors may therefore lead to a destabilization of the enzyme and contribute to intrinsic drug resistance.

Exposure to topoisomerase-targeting drugs themselves may also contribute to destabilization of the topoisomerase enzymes. In some cell lines, exposure to camptothecin results in a substantial decrease in topoisomerase I. Degradation of topoisomerase I may also occur following treatment with other DNA-damaging agents such as ionizing radiation. The degradation of topoisomerase I following DNA damage may be due to the ability of DNA damage to trap topoisomerase I in a manner analogous to topoisomerase I poisons such as camptothecin. Although the reduced levels of topoisomerase I are transient, this regulation may contribute to resistance to regimens that include camptothecins, especially when these drugs are combined with other cytotoxic agents.

Posttranscriptional regulation of topoisomerases can also be accomplished by posttranslational modifications of the enzymes. It is well established that both type I and type II topoisomerases are phosphorylated in eukaryotic cells. Both topoisomerase I and topoisomerase II are also substrates for poly-ADP ribose polymerase, of enzymes that conjugate ubiquitin, or ubiquitin like proteins such as SUMO. It has been hypothesized that some of these posttranslational changes are important for the cell cycle-specific action of DNA topoisomerases. For example, several phosphorylation sites have bee identified in topoisomerase II α and topoisomerase II β that occur specifically in cells progressing from the G_2 to M phase of the cell cycle. Such changes could increase the specific activity of the enzymes at points in the cell cycle that require higher levels of enzyme activity. It would be plausible then that cells resistant to topoisomerase poisons might show alterations in topoisomerase phosphorylation. While changes in topoisomerase phosphorylation have been reported in drug-resistant cell lines, the changes in phosphorylation are also accompanied by changes in protein levels, rates of cell cycle progression, and other variables that make it difficult to definitively ascribe resistance to changes in phosphorylation. Other changes, such as poly-ADP ribosylation or ubiquitination, clearly can affect topoisomerase activity or protein stability, but drug resistance due to alterations in these modifications has not yet been described.

DNA topoisomerases function in the nucleus. Localization of topoisomerases to the nucleus is clearly required for topoisomerase poisons to exert their cytotoxic effects. Topoisomerase I has been further localized to the nucleolus, and recent work suggests strongly that failure to localize topoisomerase I to the nucleolus is sufficient to confer camptothecin resistance. In addition to affecting the stability of topoisomerase I, campotothecin has been reported to cause translocation of nuclear topoisomerase I to the cytoplasm. The mechanistic basis of this observation has not yet been elucidated. Studies have also suggested that topoisomerase I that is trapped on DNA is subject to posttranslational modifications. An intriguing possibility is that the ubiquitin or SUMO modifications target topoisomerase I for degradation or for export from the nucleus. Similar studies have also suggested that topoisomerase II may be targeted for nuclear export when trapped on DNA as a covalent complex. Section IV,B describes mutations in the coding sequence of topoisomerase II α that result in cytoplasmic localization of the enzyme. While it seems plausible that alterations in enzyme targeting could play roles in either intrinsic resistance to topoisomerase-targeting drugs or to acquired resistance following drug exposure, detailed studies directly demonstrating a role in resistance remain to be performed.

B. Mutations in Topoisomerases

The mechanism of cell killing by topoisomerase poisons dictates that mutations in the enzyme that result in drug resistance will have specific characteristics. First, mutations in topoisomerases conferring drug resistance should generally be recessive to the wild-type drug-sensitive allele. The reason for this is that even though a mutation completely eliminates the drug sensitivity of one allele, the remaining wild-type allele(s) can still cause DNA damage and confer drug sensitivity. This is in marked contrast to classical enzyme inhibitors, where a single drug resistant allele providing drug-resistant enzyme activity can confer drug-resistance on a cell. Although data from yeast and cell lines selected for drug resistance are in general agreement with this hypothesis, there is an important additional consideration, particularly for resistance to drugs targeting topoisomerase II. Because topoisomerase II is a dimer, a mutation that renders one allele nonresponsive to a topoisomerase poison will have an unknown effect when the drug-resistant enzyme forms a heterodimer

A second important consideration is that loss of function can give partial drug resistance. As downregulation of the enzymes can confer drug resistance, reduced activity due to mutation of the structural genes should also have the potential for conferring drug resistance. Because topoisomerase I and topoisomerase II α appear to be essential for the viability of all mammalian cells, it should not be possible to generate homozygous mutations in the genes encoding these proteins that result in complete loss of function. Because topoisomerase II β is not required for the viability of all cells, null mutations in the gene encoding this enzyme are possible.

The fact that mutations that reduce enzyme activity can lead to drug resistance also complicates biochemical inferences on why a specific mutation leads to drug resistance. For classical enzyme inhibitors, it would be expected that a mutation conferring drug resistance prevents a drug for inhibiting enzyme activity, e.g., by alteration of a drug-binding site. In contrast, a topoisomerase mutation may confer resistance by reducing enzyme activity, stability, or localization. Because mutations that reduce enzyme function can confer resistance, this also would strongly suggest that there are probably no hot spots for mutations leading to drug resistance in topoisomerase genes. This means that an examination of a topoisomerase gene for potential mutations leading to drug resistance requires an examination of the entire coding sequence.

1. Mutations Leading to Alterations in Enzyme Localization

As discussed in section IV,A, alterations that prevent DNA topoisomerases from being localized to the nucleus can prevent the generation of DNA damage in the presence of topoisomerase poisons. Therefore, a simple loss-of-function mutation that could confer drug resistance would be one that alters the sequences needed for nuclear localization. While this type of mutation remains to be described for mammalian topoisomerase I, several independent alleles of topoisomerase II have been identified from mammalian cell lines selected for resistance to topoisomerase II-targeting drugs that result in the localization of topoisomerase II α to the cytoplasm. These cell lines carry mutations in the gene encoding topoisomerase II α, suggesting that this mislocalization is specific for topoisomerase II α. These cell lines also have relatively normal growth despite the absence of detectable nuclear topoisomerase II, suggesting that a small proportion of topoisomerase II α is able to enter the nucleus, perhaps through other weaker nuclear localization signals located elsewhere in the protein.

2. Mutations in Topoisomerases Leading to Drug Resistance

A series of mutations have been identified in both topoisomerase I and topoisomerase II α that can confer resistance to topoisomerase-targeting drugs. Two major approaches have been applied to identify mutations that can confer resistance to topoisomerase poisons. First, cDNAs encoding topoisomerases from drug resistant cell lines have been sequenced and, in several cases, mutations have been identified in the coding sequence. It is important to note that the presence of a mutation from a drug-resistant cell line is by itself insufficient to prove that the mutation is responsible for drug resistance. Proof that a mutation can confer drug resistance depends on expressing the mutant protein and showing that it encodes an active drug-resistant enzyme. This is most easily accomplished using yeast systems. A second approach has been to directly use yeast systems expressing human topoisomerases and to carry out *in vitro* mutagenesis to identify drug-resistant mutations.

For topoisomerase I, enzymatically active drug-resistant mutations have been found to cluster in two regions. A series of mutations have been identified from amino acids 361–364 and from amino acids 717–729. The region from 717 to 729 includes the tyrosine residue that is involved in the covalent binding of topoisomerase I to DNA. The three-dimensional structure of human topoisomerase I bound to DNA has been reported by Champoux and colleagues, and the region from 361 to 364 is also involved in DNA binding. Although a three-dimensional structure of the drug:protein:DNA ternary complex has not yet been reported, the location of these two clusters of mutations suggests that an important class of mutations conferring resistance alters DNA cleavage, protein:DNA interactions, or drug:protein:DNA interactions. These studies also clearly indicate that it is possible to mutate topoisomerase I by single amino acids changes to generate an enzyme that is insensitive to camptothecins. Again, it is important to stress that the mutations that have been studied extensively are mutations that do not substantially reduce topoisomerase I catalytic activity. Therefore, mutations at other sites in the enzyme can confer resistance to camptothecins, albeit due to reduced enzyme activity. This consideration is especially important in determining whether mutations in topoisomerase I play a role in clinical resistance to camptothecins.

Many mutations conferring resistance to topoisomerase II-targeting agents have also been identified. Mutations leading to resistance to topoisomerase II-targeting agents appear to be spread over a large portion of the breakage/reunion domain of topoisomerase II. A complication in considering the importance of the mutations conferring resistance to topoisomerase II-targeting agents is that the mutations have been selected with several chemically dissimilar agents, such as etoposide, amsacrine, and doxorubicin. Selection of mutants resistant to topoisomerase II agents has clearly demonstrated that it is possible to generate active topoisomerase II enzymes that are insensitive to multiple classes of topoisomerase II-targeting agents, but the biochemical changes in the protein that cause the resistance remain to be fully elucidated. As is the case for topoisomerase I and camptothecin resistance, mutations that reduce topoisomerase II activity will lead to resistance to topoisomerase II-targeting agents. Interestingly, the only mutations in topoisomerase II β that have been reported thus far derived from drug-resistant cell lines are mutations that completely ablate the activity of this enzyme. The significance of this finding remains to be determined.

V. RESISTANCE TO TOPOISOMERASE-TARGETING AGENTS IN THE CLINIC

The previous section defined a set of mechanisms that lead from trapping DNA topoisomerases on DNA to a potentially lethal DNA lesion. An important goal has been to apply the pathways suggested earlier to preclinical models and clinical trials to identify factors that can predict the response of cells to topoisomerase poisons. However, the substantial genetic heterogeneity present in tumor cells has made it difficult to identify single factors predictive of response. An additional complication in many clinical trials has been the inclusion of other agents that act by different mechanisms. Thus clinical resistance is not necessarily due specifically to resistance to topoisomerase-targeting drugs.

One important question that has been addressed extensively has been whether topoisomerase levels are predictive of drug response. From the results described in Section IV,A, one would predict that tumor cells prior to treatment would have higher levels of topoisomerase II α because expression of this protein is increased in proliferating cells. This prediction has been borne out, although substantial heterogeneity in levels of expression are seen. Interestingly, some tumor samples also show elevated expression of topoisomerase I, especially in colon, prostate, ovarian, and lung tumors. In contrast, an elevated expression of topoisomerase II β has not been seen, although it has not been investigated as extensively as topoisomerase I or topoisomerase II α.

In cell lines, the cytotoxicity of topoisomerase poisons frequently correlates with enzyme levels. This holds approximately true whether topoisomerase levels are measured by determining topoisomerase mRNA levels, level of protein by Western blots, or measurement of covalent protein:DNA adducts. However, many exceptions have been described. In clinical samples, the level of topoisomerase has not been predictive of patient response to therapy. This has been the case for levels of topoisomerase I and camptothecin sensitivity, and levels of topoisomerase II, and sensitivity to topoisomerase II-targeting agents.

The inability to correlate topoisomerase levels with sensitivity to topoisomerase-targeting drugs has led to the suggestion that the measurement of topoismerase levels, either indirectly by measuring mRNA levels or directly by measuring protein levels, may not be the most appropriate way to assess resistance at the level of topoisomerases. An alternate approach is to directly measure the levels of topoisomerase:DNA covalent complexes. Unfortunately, there are several difficulties in measuring covalent complexes in patient material. Because topoisomerase:DNA complexes are reversible, time spent in accessing the material and isolating the complexes may cause a substantial reduction in the level of covalent complexes. Current techniques for measuring covalent complexes are relatively insensitive and therefore require substantial amounts of patient material. This type of measurement could conceivably be carried out with leukemia samples, but is unlikely to be applicable to solid tumors. The failure to be able to correlate the levels of topoisomerases with a clinical response also underscores the importance of events downstream of the covalent complex in a clinical response to topoisomerase inhibitors. Appropriate assays for these downstream events that can be applied to patient material are certainly an important priority.

A limited number of studies have searched for putative drug-resistant mutations in tumor samples derived from patients who have relapsed following regimens that include topoisomerase-targeting drugs. No mutations in topoisomerase I have been identified from patients following treatment with camptothecins. The number of samples that have been examined has been limited. Because mutations conferring resistance to topoisomerase I-targeting agents can occur throughout the protein, rigorous examination of a role for mutations will require sequencing of the entire cDNA. This type of study using clinical material has not yet been reported.

Studies examining mutations in topoisomerase II α are subject to the same caveats that apply to mutations in topoisomerase I. In general, few studies have examined the entire cDNA for mutations following drug exposure. Using samples from relapsed AML patients who had been treated with regimens that included etoposide, Kaufmann and colleagues have carried out one major series of studies to look for mutations in topoisomerase II α. This study included samples where the entire topoisomerase II α cDNA was sequenced. No mutations were identified. In contrast, Kubo and colleagues found one sample (from a total of 13 patients) derived from a small cell lung cancer patient treated with etoposide had mutations in topoisomerase II α. The small number of samples examined makes it impossible to determine whether mutations in topoisomerase II α play a significant role in clinical drug resistance. Future studies will be needed in order to answer this question.

VI. OVERCOMING RESISTANCE TO TOPOISOMERASE-TARGETING AGENTS

Whether intrinsic or acquired, the resistance of tumor cells to topoisomerase-targeting agents is an important obstacle to the successful use of this class of anticancer agents. Current studies, especially clinical studies, are trying to discover the optimal ways of combining topoisomerase-targeting agents with other chemotherapeutic agents. While many of the mechanisms of resistance to topoisomerase targeting agents are shared with anticancer agents directed against other targets, some of the mechanisms of resistance that are peculiar to topoisomerases suggest strategies that may minimize the elaboration of drug-resistant tumors.

Because replication plays a key role in the conversion of topoisomerase covalent complexes into irreversible DNA damage, the antitumor effects of both topoisomerase I- and topoisomerase II-targeting agents are strongly schedule dependent. Schedules that include prolonged exposures to the agents are typically more active than schedules that use higher drug concentrations for shorter periods of time, although prolonged exposure can also result in greater toxicity to normal cells. Thus, the development of optimal schedules is particularly critical for drugs targeting either topoisomerase I or topoisomerase II. The use of optimal schedules is an important way in which acquired drug resistance can be minimized.

A second approach to overcoming resistance to topoisomerase poisons has been to try to combine topoisomerase I- and topoisomerase II-targeting agents. As described in Section IV,A, resistance to topoisomerase I targeting agents frequently arises by reduced topoisomerase I levels. Because topoisomerase I plays important roles in cellular processes, cells could compensate for reduced topoisomerase I levels by upregulation of topoisomerase II. Similarly, cells might compensate for downregulation of topoisomerase II by increasing topoisomerase I expression. Although such compensating changes in topoisomerase levels have occasionally been reported, they occur in drug-resistant cell lines only occasionally. Nonetheless, the notion of combining topoisomerase I- and topoisomerase II-targeting agents remains intuitively appealing. Surprisingly, regimens combining topoisomerase I- and topoisomerase II-targeting agents have met with limited success. In many cell lines, the simultaneous administration of a topoisomerase I- and a topoisomerase II-targeting agent results in antagonism rather than synergistic cell killing. The reasons for the antagonism remain obscure. One possibility is that the presence of covalent complexes from both topoisomerase I and topoisomerase II may prevent entry of cells into the S phase or may affect the efficiency with which replication forks convert the complexes into irreversible DNA damage. In other contexts, a combination of topoisomerase I- and topoisomerase II-targeting agents results in regimens with unacceptable toxicity. In these contexts, combining topoisomerase I- and topoisomerase II-targeting agents does cause synergistic cell killing, but the targeting of normal cells results in a loss of therapeutic index.

In order to overcome the antagonism or toxicity of combining topoisomerase I- and topoisomerase II-targeting agents, there has been substantial effort at identifying agents that are able to target both topoisomerase I and topoisomerase II. While several agents have been reported that appear to be able to poison both topoisomerase I and topoisomerase II, it remains to be demonstrated whether these agents kill tumor cells because of their effects on both enzymes. It is also too early to predict whether such agents will have superior antitumor activity.

The third important approach to overcoming resistance to topoisomerase targeting agents will be the identification of new agents that target these enzymes. At present, all topoisomerase I-targeting agents that have been examined extensively in the clinic are camptothecins. While the drugs that target topoisomerase II are more chemically diverse, the topoisomerase II-targeting agents in current use have major undesirable properties that may not be due to their ability to target topoisomerase II. It should also be possible to identify topoisomerase I- or topoisomerase II-targeting agents that are not substrates for drug transporters, although again it is unclear whether such compounds will have a more favorable therapeutic index than compounds in current use.

Acknowledgment

Work in the authors' laboratory was supported by grants from the National Cancer Institute (CA52814 and CA82313), by a core grant from the National Cancer Institute (CA21765), and by the American Lebanese Syrian Associated Charities (ALSAC).

See Also the Following Articles

MULTIDRUG RESISTANCE I: P-GLYCOPROTEIN • MULTIDRUG RESISTANCE II: MRP AND RELATED PROTEINS • RESISTANCE TO DNA-DAMAGING AGENTS • RESISTANCE TO INHIBITOR COMPOUNDS OF THYMIDINE SYNTHASE • RESISTANCE TO INHIBITORS OF DIHYDROFOLDATE REDUCTASE

Bibliography

Arbuck, S. G., and Takimoto, C. H. (1998). An overview of topoisomerase I-targeting agents. *Sem. Hematol.* **35,** 3–12.

Berger, J. M., Gamblin, S. J., Harrison, S. C., and Wang, J. C. (1996). Structure and mechanism of DNA topoisomerase II. *Nature* **379,** 225–232.

Froelich-Ammon, S. J., and Osheroff, N. (1995). Topoisomerase poisons: harnessing the dark side of enzyme mechanism. *J. Biol. Chem.* **270,** 21429–21432.

Kaufmann, S. H. (1998). Cell death induced by topoisomerase-targeted drugs: More questions than answers. *Biochim. Biophys. Acta.* **1400,** 195–211.

Nitiss, J. L. (1998). Investigating the biological functions of DNA topoisomerases in eukaryotic cells. *Biochim. Biophys. Acta.* **1400,** 63–81.

Nitiss, J. L., and Beck, W. T. (1996). Antitopoisomerase drug action and resistance. *Eur. J. Cancer* **32A,** 958–966.

Osheroff, N. (ed.) (1998). DNA topoisomerases. *Biochim. Biophys. Acta* **1400,** 1–354.

Pommier, Y., Pourquier, P., Fan, Y., and Strumberg, D. (1998). Mechanism of action of eukaryotic DNA topoisomerase I and drugs targeted to the enzyme. *Biochim. Biophys. Acta* **1400,** 83–105.

Reid, R. J. D., Benedetti, P., and Bjornsti, M. A. (1998). Yeast as a model organism for studying the actions of DNA topoisomerase-targeted drugs. *Biochim. Biophys. Acta* **1400,** 289–300.

Rubin, E. H., Li, T. K., Duann, P., and Liu, L. F. (1996). Cellular resistance to topoisomerase poisons. *Cancer Treat Res.* **87,** 243–260.

Wang, J. C. (1996). DNA topoisomerases. *Annu. Rev. Biochem.* **65,** 635–692.

Retinoblastoma Tumor Suppressor Gene

Frederick A. Dick
Nicholas J. Dyson
Massachusetts General Hospital Cancer Center

GLOSSARY

cyclin A protein whose expression level is regulated temporally during the cell cycle that dimerizes with kinase catalytic domains for the purpose of regulating activity and directing substrate recognition.

E2F A family of transcription factors capable of regulating cell cycle and adenoviral genes.

G1 The phase of the cell cycle in which commitment to replicate DNA and divide is undertaken.

S phase The phase of the cell cycle in which DNA is replicated.

The retinoblastoma tumor suppressor is functionally inactivated in many tumor cells either by direct mutation of the *RB-1* gene, by viral proteins that bind to pRB, or through changes in a regulatory pathway that controls the activity of pRB. pRB acts during G0 and G1 phases of the cell cycle where it restricts cell cycle progression and facilitates differentiation. pRB interacts with the E2F transcription factor and represses the transcription of genes encoding functions that are needed for cells to enter S phase and functions that are needed for DNA replication.

I. THE RETINOBLASTOMA (RB) TUMOR SUPPRESSOR PROTEIN IS A FREQUENT TARGET FOR INACTIVATION IN CANCER

A. Retinoblastoma Tumor Suppressor Gene Mutations in Cancer

The retinoblastoma tumor susceptibility gene (*RB-1*) was the first tumor suppressor gene to be identified and has served as a prototype for this group of cancer-related genes. The inactivation of both copies of *RB-1* in the developing eye is the critical molecular change underlying the development of retinoblastoma. Although the *RB-1* gene was first identified through its role in a rare pediatric cancer, subsequent tumor studies have shown that this gene is mutated in a wide range of cancers that include osteosarcoma, leukemia, and carcinomas derived from the bladder, prostate, breast, and cervix. These observations suggested that pRB might exert a tumor-suppressor activity in many different tissues. Indeed, the reintroduction of a wild-type pRB gene into a wide variety of RB-deficient tumor cells has been found to suppress their proliferation and/or tumorigenicity. Consistent with the idea that pRB acts in multiple cell types, retinoblastoma patients carrying an inherited *RB-1* mutation, who are successfully treated for retinoblastoma, remain predisposed to other types of cancer later in life.

Microinjection experiments, in which pRB is introduced into $Rb^{-/-}$ tumor cells, have defined a portion of the cell cycle in which pRB blocks cell cycle progression. In these cells the expression of pRB in G0 or G1 is sufficient to prevent S-phase entry, but once cells progress to a point that is close to the initiation of DNA synthesis, they become refractory to the effects of pRB. The time in the cell cycle when cells lose their sensitivity to pRB is roughly coincident with the restriction point, at least within the margin of error of cell synchronization methods. The term "restriction point" refers to a point in the cell cycle where cells are able to complete a cell cycle without further need for mitogen stimulation. $Rb^{-/-}$ cells show a greatly reduced dependence on mitogens and are less responsive to many of the stimuli that arrest wild-type cells in G1. Thus, the inactivation of pRB removes a key negative regulator of cell cycle progression: a protein that normally acts at the critical period when cells integrate positive and negative stimuli and decide whether or not to enter the mitotic cell cycle.

B. The "RB Pathway"

As described later, pRB activity is tightly controlled during the G1 to S transition. In normal cells, pRB is inactivated by multiple inhibitory phosphorylation events each time the cell enters S phase. The analysis of tumor-derived mutations has shown that proteins that regulate the level or timing of pRB phosphorylation are often mutated during carcinogenesis. Thus, pRB is proposed to be a component of a critical regulatory cascade termed the "pRB pathway" that is inactivated in most tumor cells (see Fig. 1).

Evidence for the RB pathway is drawn from three lines of experimentation. First, biochemical studies show that the activities of pRB, cyclin D, cdk4, and p16^{INK4a} are directly linked. The cyclin D1/cdk4 kinase, like most cyclin-dependent kinases, can phosphorylate pRB, and elevated levels of the cyclin D1/cdk4 kinase are sufficient to overcome pRB-induced cell cycle arrest. Cyclin D-associated kinases are likely to be especially significant for pRB regulation because these are the first pRB kinases to become active when quiescent cells are stimulated to proliferate. Hence these kinases are poised to provide some of the initial changes that modulate pRB function. The activity of the cyclin D1/cdk4 kinase is stimulated by mitogenic signals and it, in turn, is also regulated at many levels. One important level of control is provided by the INK4 family of cdk inhibitors that antagonize cyclin D1-associated kinase activity by competing for the kinase subunit. p16^{INK4a}, together with the other members of the INK4 family, provides a buffer or threshold that must be overcome in order to activate the cyclin D1/cdk4 kinase. Thus, biochemical studies show that p16^{INK4a} can inhibit the cyclin D1/cdk4 kinase and that this kinase can inactivate pRB.

A second line of evidence supporting the idea that p16^{INK4a}, cyclin D1, cdk4, and pRB comprise a functional pathway stems from studies of cells lacking pRB. Unlike wild-type cells, pRB-deficient cells are insensitive to the expression of p16^{INK4a} and fail to arrest in G1 in response to elevated levels of this cdk inhibitor. Analogous experiments using antibodies to inhibit the activity of cyclin D1 show that cyclin D-associated kinases are needed for cells to enter S phase.

RB Pathway Components: Mutations in:

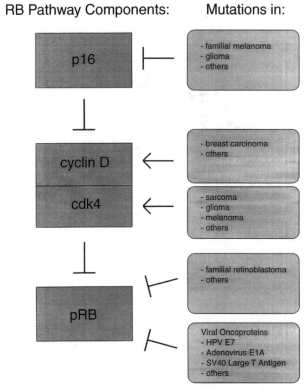

FIGURE 1 The RB pathway. (Left) Components of the RB pathway. Negative regulation of pRB by cyclin D/cdk4 and cyclin D/cdk4 by p16 is depicted. (Right) Tumor types that frequently contain alterations are listed, in addition to pRB inactivation by viral oncoproteins. Tumor mutation data are adapted from Sherr (1996).

However, cyclin D1 is not necessary for S-phase entry if the cells lack a functional pRB. Such experiments clearly show that p16[INK4a]-induced cell cycle arrest requires pRB and that pRB is a critical substrate for cyclin D-associated kinases.

The third line of evidence for the pRB pathway stems from the pattern of mutations of pRB, cyclin D, cdk4, and p16[INK4a] in tumor cells. Loss of function mutations in the INK4a locus, amplification of the cyclin D1 gene, and point mutations in cdk4 that render them insensitive to p16[INK4a] inhibition are all predicted to result in deregulated kinase activity and in reduced pRB activity. Each of these changes has been linked with specific types of cancer. For example, retinoblastomas always have *RB-1* mutations, breast carcinomas typically show cyclin D amplification, and mutations in the INK4a locus and cdk4 have been found in familial melanoma. Other types of tumor, such as glioblastoma, have a more varied spectrum and mutations can be found in several components of this pathway. Re-

markably, mutations in pRB, cyclin D1, cdk4, and p16[INK4a] occur in a manner that is almost always mutually exclusive. This indicates that once one component of this pathway is mutated, there is minimal selective pressure for the mutation of a second component. The importance of the pRB pathway in cancer is underscored by the fact that lesions in this group of genes are found in the majority of cancer cells.

C. The Retinoblastoma Tumor Suppressor Protein Is Targeted by Viral Oncoproteins

An alternative mechanism for pRB inactivation was uncovered by studies of small DNA tumor viruses. Several human adenoviruses, human papilloma viruses (HPVs), and polyomaviruses encode proteins that are normally expressed early during viral infection and that have oncogenic properties. A subset of these proteins (exemplified by SV40 large T antigen, Ad 5 E1A, and HPV type 16 E7) possess a pRB-binding domain that is characterized by a conserved five amino acid motif (LXCXE) at its core. Mutations of single conserved amino acids or deletions within this motif diminish both the pRB-binding activities and the oncogenic properties of these molecules. The correlation between pRB-binding and transforming activity suggests that pRB is a key target for these viral products. The viral proteins are thought to bind to pRB and functionally inactivate it, mimicking the effects of RB-1 mutation in tumor cells (see Fig. 1). Interestingly, each of the viral proteins appears to do more than simply bind to pRB. E1A and SV40 large T antigen contain additional amino-terminal domains that disrupt cellular complexes containing pRB. E7, however, binds to pRB and then uses additional sequences to target pRB for degradation.

pRB is targeted by diverse groups of viruses that are capable of infecting a wide range of hosts in the plant and animal kingdoms. This functional convergence suggests that pRB-related proteins represent a critical target in the battle for the control of an infected cell. Precisely why pRB is such an important target is not certain. As described later, pRB limits the expression of many genes that are needed for efficient DNA synthesis; thus the inactivation of pRB may change the cellular environment to a state that is more conducive for replication of the viral genome.

II. REGULATION OF pRB DURING THE CELL CYCLE

A. pRB Is Inactivated by Phosphorylation

pRB is a stable nuclear protein and is expressed in most cell types. The activity of pRB is controlled by cell cycle-dependent phosphorylation. Biochemical studies have identified three general states of pRB phosphorylation that predominate at different stages of the cell cycle. In truly quiescent cells, such as resting T cells, pRB is almost completely unphosphorylated. When these cells are stimulated to proliferate, pRB can be labeled weakly with ^{32}P-orthophosphate. This "hypophosphorylated" form of pRB associates with E2F (see later) and is tightly bound to the nuclear matrix. pRB becomes heavily phosphorylated as cells approach S phase. This change can be visualized on SDS–polyacrylamide gels by a characteristic mobility shift to a slowly migrating hyperphosphorylated

form. pRB remains heavily phosphorylated throughout the G2 phase and is abruptly dephosphorylated during mitosis. The discovery that SV40 large T antigen specifically targets the hypophosphorylated forms of pRB was the first evidence that the differentially modified forms of pRB might have different activities. Indeed, virtually all of the cellular pRB-binding proteins described to date interact specifically with the un- or hypophosphorylated forms of the protein.

The amino acid sequence of pRB contains at least 16 consensus sites for phosphorylation by cyclin-dependent kinases, including a cluster of sites near the carboxy terminus of the molecule. Phosphopeptide analysis has shown that pRB is phosphorylated *in vivo* on at least 10 distinct sites. Interestingly, phosphopeptide analysis of *in vivo* and *in vitro* phosphorylated pRB results in patterns that are strikingly similar. Mutagenesis studies in which individual phosphorylation sites are altered support the idea that the inactivation of pRB does not depend on the specific modification of a single site but results instead from the accumulation of phosphorylated residues.

Although several different cyclin-dependent kinases can phosphorylate pRB, most attention has focused on complexes containing cyclin D and cdk4 or 6 and on cyclin E/cdk2, as these kinases are activated during the portions of the cell cycle where the phosphorylation of pRB is first apparent. Most cell cycle analyses are carried out on quiescent cells, which have been serum stimulated to reenter the cell cycle. In this type of experiment, D-type cyclins are the first to be expressed as the cells leave quiescence and approach S phase. Interestingly, considerable data suggest that cyclin D/cdk activity alone is not normally sufficient to inactivate pRB and drive S-phase entry. A second round of phosphorylation events by cyclin E/cdk2 appears to be necessary to completely inactivate pRB at the beginning of S phase. *In vitro* kinase assays have demonstrated that cyclin A/cdk2 and cyclin B/cdc2 are also capable of phosphorylating pRB. As these kinases are active in S, G2, and M phases of the cell cycle, their timing precludes them from regulating pRB at the G1 to S-phase transition. However, these kinases are thought to maintain pRB in an inactive state at these later stages of the cell cycle. Evidence that this maintenance role is functionally significant was provided by experiments showing that mutant forms of pRB, which lack multiple cdk phosphorylation sites, can arrest cells in S phase.

B. pRB Integrates the Activity of Multiple Cyclins and Cyclin-Dependent Kinases

Cell cycle progression depends on both the unique functions of the cyclin-dependent kinases and their synergistic effects. Many signaling pathways converge on the cell cycle machinery and these signals need to be integrated into a small number of molecular signals. As the inactivation of pRB is needed for cell cycle progression, and requires the concerted action of multiple cyclin-dependent kinases, pRB appears to be a nodal point in cell cycle regulation. Indeed, a diverse collection of internal and external signals has been found to depend on pRB. For example, $Rb^{-/-}$ cells fail to respond to DNA damage-induced G1 arrest, which is mediated by p53 and p21^{CIP1}, or to TGFβ-induced arrest, which is mediated, in part, by the elevated expression of p15^{INK4b}. Consistent with this, studies of tumor formation in mice have shown that $Rb^{+/-}$ animals develop tumors at an earlier age in a $p27^{-/-}$ background. This type of genetic interaction illustrates that levels of cyclin/cdk activity can influence the rate of tumor formation.

III. A MODEL FOR pRB FUNCTION: pRB REGULATES THE E2F TRANSCRIPTION FACTOR

A. Opposing Roles for pRB and E2F in Cell Cycle Control

The mechanism of pRB action has been the subject of intense investigation for over a decade. In this time more than 130 different cellular proteins have been reported to interact with pRB. Although the relative significance of all of these interactions has yet to be fully resolved, it is clear that the E2F transcription factor is one of the most important pRB partners. This is particularly evident from experiments in which the inactivation of *E2F-1* extends the development of pRB-deficient embryos and reduces the tumor phenotypes associated with $Rb^{+/-}$ mice. Current models for pRB action are drawn largely from studies of the interaction between pRB and E2F.

E2F is a heterodimeric transcription factor that associates with pRB during G0, G1, and early S phase. E2F-binding sites are found in a large number of genes that are normally repressed in quiescent cells. As cells are induced to proliferate, E2F-regulated promoters

are transcribed, pRB becomes phosphorylated, and cell accumulate "free" forms of E2F that are not bound to pRB or pRB-related proteins. When overexpressed, E2F and pRB have antagonistic effects on E2F-dependent transcription (E2F activates transcription, whereas pRB represses transcription) and on S-phase entry (overexpression of E2F genes drives quiescent cells into S phases, whereas pRB blocks S-phase entry). Because pRB binds directly to E2F and masks its transactivation domain, these observations can be combined into a simple model in which pRB prevents S-phase entry by binding to E2F and preventing the transcription of genes needed for this transition. In a normal cell cycle the effects of pRB would be relieved through the phosphorylation of pRB by cyclin-dependent kinases (see Fig. 2).

B. E2F Target Genes

The ability of pRB to regulate E2F activity, as discussed in the preceding section, has established the importance of this regulatory connection in cell cycle control. This has in turn stimulated the search for genes whose transcription is regulated by E2F. In this review the genes known to be regulated by E2F are sorted into four general groups. The first group includes genes whose protein products are necessary for DNA replication. This includes genes encoding ORC and MCM proteins that are needed for the initiation of DNA synthesis, and genes encoding proteins such as dihydrofolate reductase and ribonucleotide reductase that are needed for the enzymatic synthesis of DNA. A second group of genes contains critical cell cycle regulators such as cyclin A, cyclin E, and cdc25c that act to drive cell cycle progression. Because E2F-binding sites are found in the promoters of so many essential genes, it is thought that E2F and pRB exert control of the G1/S transition by coordinately controlling the expression of large programs of transcription rather than by acting on a single essential target.

A third group of E2F-responsive genes is composed of pRB and E2F family members themselves. The ability of E2F to stimulate the transcription of E2F family members provides a mechanism to amplify a proliferative signal. In a similar way, E2F-induced expression of cyclin E and cyclin A genes promotes the synthesis of kinases that inactivate pRB. These positive regulatory feedback loops may be important to ensure that the G1 to S transition is irreversible. From a research point of

Early G1

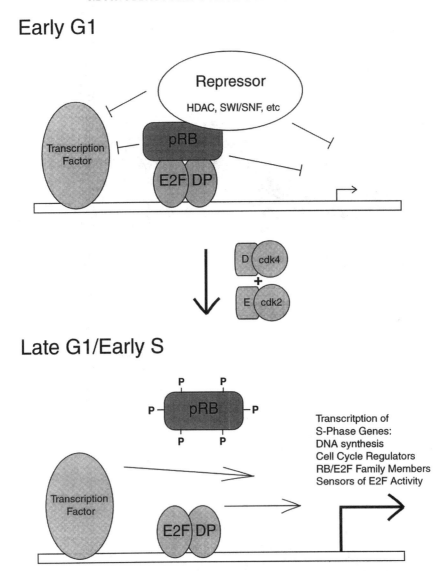

Late G1/Early S

FIGURE 2 RB regulation of G1 to S transition. In early G1, pRB and repressor molecules inhibit transcriptional activation by E2Fs and neighboring transactivators. Following inactivation of pRB by cyclin D/cdk4 and cyclin E/cdk2 phosphorylation, E2F responsive promoters are actively transcribed.

view, these loops blur the view of cdks, pRB, and E2F as components of a linear pathway. For example, in different experimental settings, cyclin E may appear to be upstream or downstream of pRB. Many such feedback loops occur during the G1 to S transition and these may serve to ensure that all the required components are present before DNA synthesis is initiated.

Normal cells that are driven into S phase by elevated E2F activity undergo very high rates of apoptosis, which severely limits the extent of cell prolifera-

tion. In RB-deficient mouse embryos, neurons in the central and peripheral nervous system continue to synthesize DNA and ultimately undergo apoptosis. These inappropriate S phases and apoptosis are suppressed in the central nervous system of mice lacking both pRB and E2F-1, suggesting that the deregulation of E2F-1 activity is key to both of these effects. It is anticipated therefore that a fourth class of E2F target genes must exist to monitor deregulated E2F activity and promote apoptosis. The best-studied example of this type of E2F target is p19ARF. p19ARF activates p53 and can trigger a cell cycle arrest or drive cells toward apoptosis.

C. pRB and E2F Cooperate to Repress Transcription

The ability of pRB to bind to E2F is only part of its role in regulating E2F-dependent transcription. When recruited to a promoter, pRB is an active inhibitor of transcription, i.e., it overrides the activational capacity of other transcription factors that are bound to adjacent sites at the same promoter. The importance of this effect is illustrated by the fact that, in most cases, the mutation of E2F-binding sites results in the derepression of E2F-regulated promoters (G1). Thus the temporal expression of E2F-regulated genes stems in part from E2F-mediated repression of the promoter (in G0/G1) and in part from E2F-mediated activation (in G1/S). Currently, it is unclear whether pRB-mediated, active repression of E2F promoters occurs in every cell cycle or whether this repression is limited to specific situations in which cells are quiescent or exiting the cell cycle. Experiments using decoy E2F-binding sites, or E2F mutants that can bind to DNA but cannot bind to pRB, suggest that active repression is needed for cell cycle arrest induced by TGFβ or p16^{INK4a} or for arrest in response to DNA damage.

The mechanisms of pRB-mediated repression are currently under investigation and several different models have been proposed. pRB has been found to bind directly to histone deacetylase (HDAC) and recruit its associated enzymatic activity to E2F-regulated promoters. HDACs remove acetyl groups from lysine residues at the C termini of histone proteins. This change facilitates a strong interaction between nucleosomes and the DNA that is wrapped around them, allowing chromatin to form a condensed structure that excludes the basal transcriptional machinery and hinders gene expression. Other studies have shown that other transcriptional corepressors, such as RBP1, HBP1, and CtIP, can bind to pRB and might also be involved in the repression of E2F promoters. Another chromatin remodeling protein complex that has been proposed to interact with pRB in repression is the mammalian SWI–SNF complex. This DNA-dependent helicase can transiently alter chromatin to facilitate binding by sequence specific transcription factors. Precisely how this assists pRB in E2F repression is still unknown.

At present it seems likely that multiple mechanisms contribute to the repressor activity of pRB, with the individual modes of repression having variable importance at different promoters. It should also be noted that pRB is also able to repress transcription in ways that are independent of chromatin structure, as it can repress transcription *in vitro* in assay systems that utilize naked DNA templates.

IV. E2FS AND pRB ARE MEMBERS OF MULTIGENE FAMILIES

A. Members of RB and E2F families

Although pRB is often described as if it were a unique molecule in the cell, it is a member of a family of proteins that have a similar structure and perform related functions. Human cells contain two pRB-related proteins, p107 and p130. Like pRB, p107 and p130 proteins contain a "pocket domain" that interacts with E2Fs and is targeted by viral oncoproteins such as E7, E1A, and T antigen. p107 and p130 are also capable of active repression of E2F target genes, and the ectopic expression of either of these proteins is sufficient to arrest $Rb^{-/-}$ tumor cells in G1. p107 and p130 are also substrates for cdks and, much like pRB, they contain clusters of consensus cdk phosphorylation sites. One obvious difference between p107/p130 and pRB is the existence of a cyclin E or A/cdk2-binding site in the spacer region p107 and p130 (see Fig. 3). This site may play a role in targeting cdks to substrates, or potentially in sequestering kinase activity, but its precise role is uncertain.

Another level of complexity has been added by the discovery of multiple E2F family members. The smallest E2F complexes capable of binding to DNA in a sequence-specific manner are heterodimers consisting of an E2F and a DP subunit. Both E2F and DP subunits contact DNA, but the E2F subunit contains transcriptional activation and pRB family-binding domains. The DP family of genes consists of two members: DP1 and DP2. There are no obvious differences in amino acid sequence motifs between these proteins; DP1 is of relatively greater abundance in most cell types. The E2F family consists of six members; E2F1 through 6 contain similar DNA-binding and dimerization domains. E2F1, 2, and 3 contain a cyclin A- or E/cdk2-binding site in

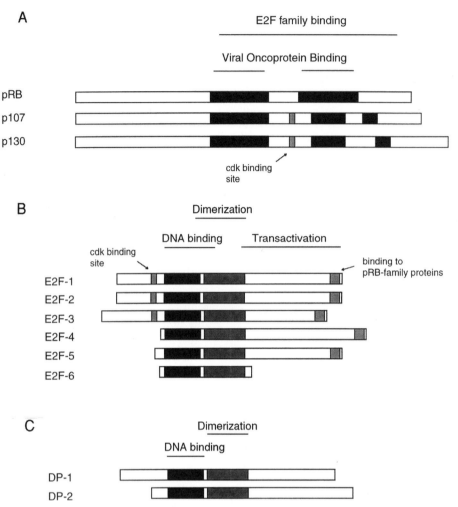

FIGURE 3 RB, E2F, and DP family members are aligned in A, B, and C, respectively. Regions of homology between family members are shaded. Functions of the relevant domains are indicated.

their N terminus that is important for the downregulation of E2F activity in S phase. E2F6 does not appear to bind to pRB family members and lacks the transcription activation domain found in other E2Fs.

pRB family members associate with different subsets of E2F complexes, and these differences may endow the pocket proteins with distinct biological properties. p107 and p130 interact exclusively with E2F4 and E2F5. While pRB can also associate with E2F4, it is the only pocket protein able to regulate E2F1, E2F2, and E2F3. Based on the fact that E2F1, E2F2, and E2F3 are more potent activators of transcription than E2F4 and E2F5 and on the times in the cell cycle when the respective complexes are most apparent, it is generally thought

that p130/E2F4 or 5 and pRB/E2F4 containing complexes are transcriptional repressor complexes that act early in G0/G1, whereas E2F1, E2F2, and E2F3 are important components of the free E2F complexes that actively promote transcription in late G1 or early S phase.

B. Redundancy and Compensation among RB Family Members

Biochemical studies have emphasized the similarities among pRB, p107, and p130, however, the specific mutation of RB in tumor cells indicates that the functions of these family members must be distinct. The clearest evidence for the unique and common functions of the pRB family members has been provided by studies of the loss of function phenotypes of gene targeted knockout mice. Animals deficient for pRB die between embryonic days 13.5 and 15.5. These embryos show defects in cell differentiation, inappropriate proliferation, and a high incidence of apoptosis. In comparison, mice deficient for either p107 or p130 develop normally. However, it is not that the functions carried out by p107 and p130 are unimportant. The absence of both p107 and p130 results in neonatal lethality, and mutant animals show evidence of abnormal cell proliferation in several tissues. Likewise, double mutants lacking pRB and either p107 or p130 die at an earlier developmental stage than the $Rb^{-/-}$ mutants alone. These results clearly demonstrate that p107 and p130 act as negative regulators of the cell cycle and that they have functions that overlap at some level, with each other and with pRB. The interpretation of these results is complicated, however, by evidence that pRB family members may compensate for one another in the knockout cells. Moreover, the phenotypes of p107- and p130-deficient animals have been found to vary greatly between genetic backgrounds.

One of the most surprising results provided by studies of pRB in mice was the finding that mice carrying one mutant RB allele fail to develop retinoblastomas, even though they are predisposed to tumor formation in other tissues. $Rb^{+/-}$ mice typically die between 7 and 9 months of age from pituitary tumors. Examination of these animals usually reveals microscopic tumors in a variety of tissues, but no lesions are found in the retina. This difference between mice and humans may be due, at least in part, to differences in functional overlap between pRB family members. Interestingly, mice that are $Rb^{+/-}$; $p107^{-/-}$ develop retinomas, and retinoblastomas have been found in chimeric embryos containing $Rb^{-/-}$; $p107^{-/-}$ cells. These results indicate that the ability of p107 to compensate for the loss of pRB has an important impact on tumor development and suggest that the degree of compensation varies between cell types. In a similar way, the unique sensitivity of the human developing retina to pRB inactivation may occur, not because pRB has a novel function in these cells, but because these cells are uniquely dependent on pRB.

V. RB AND DIFFERENTIATION

A considerable number of studies have suggested that pRB might normally function to promote cellular differentiation. Rb-mutant embryos show defects in terminal differentiation of neuronal cells and, later in development, pRB appears to be important for some aspects of myogenesis. In tissue culture cells, pRB is able to cooperate with differentiation-specific transcription factors such as C/EBPs and MyoD in transcriptional activation. Additionally, pRB supports the ability of these factors to induce fibroblasts to undergo adipogenesis or myogenesis, respectively. *In vitro*-binding assays suggest that these transcription factors can interact with pRB, and it has even been suggested that the pocket domain of pRB may facilitate DNA binding by these proteins. However, it has not been possible to detect DNA-binding complexes containing pRB and C/EBP or MyoD, and a detailed explanation of the mechanism behind this activational activity of pRB has remained elusive.

Another paradigm of transcriptional activation by pRB is in cooperation with the glucocorticoid receptor. It has been known for some time that activation of transcription by the glucocorticoid receptor occurs through a chromatin remodeling mechanism that involves mammalian homologues of the yeast SWI/SNF complex. More recently, it has been demonstrated that pRB can interact with mammalian SWI/SNF complexes to enhance glucocorticoid receptor activation. These results suggest a mechanism whereby SWI/SNF- and pRB-mediated chromatin remodeling facilitates glucocoritcoid receptor binding to promoters containing its consensus DNA-binding element.

In cell types where the loss of pRB alters the patterns of differentiation, it is uncertain whether this occurs because pRB is directly involved in the expression of differentiation specific genes or whether it occurs because pRB is necessary for differentiating cells to withdraw from the cell cycle. It is striking that primary mouse embryo fibroblasts derived from RB-null embryos can differentiate into myotubes relatively normally despite the absence of RB. However, these myotubes have been found to be incompletely withdrawn from the cell cycle. Myotubes formed from $Rb^{-/-}$ cells differ from wild-type cells in that they can be stimulated to reenter the cell cycle and begin DNA synthesis. Taken together, current data suggest that pRB function is necessary to allow cells to permanently exit the cell cycle and to properly express cell type specific genes. At present it is impossible to determine whether these are completely independent functions of pRB.

VI. FUTURE DIRECTIONS

In recent years, clear models of pRB function have emerged from a combination of biochemical and genetic studies and from the analysis of tumor-derived mutations. This evidence has identified the pRB pathway as an important target during tumorigenesis. The next logical question in the investigation of pRB function is to determine which of the effectors of pRB are most critical for tumor suppression.

Currently, the most obvious candidate is the E2F family of transcription factors. In agreement with this, the inactivation of E2F1 reduces the tumor phenotype and extends the survival of mice that are heterozygous for *Rb*. However, it is unclear that E2F is the only target, or even the most important target, in tumor suppression. Studies of a mutant *RB-1* allele (R661W), which has been associated with only a low predisposition to retinoblastoma, show that this mutation generates a pRB molecule that is unable to bind E2Fs or to regulate cell cycle entry. The partial activity of this mutant suggests that pRB may have additional properties, aside from E2F regulation, that contribute to its tumor suppressor function. Identifying the critical targets that sit downstream of pRB will require the same synergy of biochemical, genetic, and tumor mutation studies that established the upstream regulators of the pRB pathway.

See Also the Following Articles

CELL CYCLE CONTROL • CELLULAR RESPONSES TO DNA DAMAGE • MULTISTAGE CARCINOGENESIS • NEUROBLASTOMA • PEDIATRIC CANCERS, MOLECULAR FEATURES • TP53 TUMOR SUPPRESSOR GENE • TUMOR SUPPRESSOR GENES: SPECIFIC CLASSES

Bibliography

Brehm, A., and Kouzarides, T. (1999). Retinoblastoma protein meets chromatin. *Trends Biochem. Sci.* **24**, 142–145.

Dyson, N. J. (1998). The regulation of E2F by pRB family proteins. *Genes Dev.* **12**, 2245–2262.

He, S., Cook, B. L., Deverman, B. E., Weihe, U., Zhang, F., Prachand, V., Zheng, J., and Weintraub, S. J. (2000). E2F is required to prevent inappropriate S-phase entry of mammalian cells. *Mol. Cell Biol.* **20**, 363–371.

Knudsen, E. S., Buckmaster, C., Chen, T. T., Feramisco, J .R., and Wang, J. Y. (1998). Inhibition of DNA synthesis by RB: Effects on G1/S transition and S-phase progression. *Genes Dev.* **12**, 2278–2292.

Lipinski, M. M., and Jacks, T. (1999). The retinoblastoma gene family in differentiation and development. *Oncogene* **18**, 7873–7882.

Mulligan, G., and Jacks, T. (1998). The retinoblastoma gene family: cousins with overlapping interests. *Trends Genet.* **14**, 223–229.

Park, M. S., Rosai, J., Nguyen, H. T., Capodieci, P., Cordon-Cardo, C., and Koff, A. (1999). p27 and Rb are on overlapping pathways suppressing tumorigenesis in mice. *Proc. Natl. Acad. Sci. USA* **96**, 6382–6387.

Roberts, J. M. (1999). Evolving ideas about cyclins. *Cell* **98**, 129–132.

Ross, J. F., Liu, X., and Dynlacht, B. D. (1999). Mechanism of transcriptional repression of E2F by the retinoblastoma tumor suppressor protein. *Mol. Cell.* **3**, 195–205.

Sherr, C. J. (1996). Cancer cell cycles. *Science* **274**, 1672–1677.

Sherr, C. J., and Roberts, J. M. (1999). CDK inhibitors: positive and negative regulators of G1-phase progression. *Genes Dev.* **13**, 1501–1512.

Vooijs, M., and Berns, A. (1999). Developmental defects and tumor predisposition in Rb mutant mice. *Oncogene* **18**, 5293–5303.

Wang, J. Y. J. (1997). Retinoblastoma protein in growth suppression and death protection. *Curr. Opin. Genet. Dev.* **7**, 39 45.

Weinberg, R. A. (1995). The retinoblastoma protein and cell cycle control. *Cell* **81**, 323–330.

Zhang, H. S., Postigo, A. A., and Dean, D. C. (1999). Active transcriptional repression by the Rb-E2F complex mediates G1 arrest triggered by p16INK4a, TGFbeta, and contact inhibition. *Cell* **97**, 53–61.

Retroviral Vectors

Douglas J. Jolly

Chiron Viagene Inc., San Diego, California

GLOSSARY

env The envelope gene of retroviruses encoding the glyco-protein embedded in the viral lipid envelope from the cell in which the viral particle was made. This protein is also responsible for binding to the cell surface receptor, leading to viral entry into cells. In murine leukemia virus (MLV), the full-length protein is cleaved by a cellular protease to SU (gp70), the external protein, and TM (p15e) which spans the membrane. The two proteins remain joined by uncharacterized interactions.

gag The structural gene of retroviruses in murine retroviruses encoding a polyprotein (Pr 65 in MLV) which makes up most of the viral capsid and is cleaved into four peptides: MA (matrix protein), p12, CA (capsid protein), and NC (nuclear capsid protein) by a viral protease.

gag–pol The gag–pol gene of retroviruses consisting of the gag open reading frame fused to a large, further downstream, in phase, open reading frame with a single stop codon in between. In Moloney MLV, this stop is suppressed about 5% of the time, and read-through creates a polyprotein, Pr 200, which is then processed by the viral protease into the gag proteins, protease, reverse transcriptase, and integrase.

gene therapy The use of gene transfer into a patient's cells, either *ex vivo* or *in vivo*, to treat disease. Originally, this was thought useful for genetic diseases but now it is considered a possibility for all diseases lacking effective therapy.

packaging cell A cell that makes (retro)viral proteins but does not carry a (retro)viral vector, the genome of which would be recognized by these proteins.

packaging signal A segment of the viral or vector RNA genome that is recognized by the viral structural proteins and leads to incorporation of the genome into viral or vector particles.

producer cell A packaging cell into which a vector has been introduced that consequently makes vector particles continuously in culture.

replication-competent virus A term for a wild-type virus that could contaminate nonreplicating vector preparations. Usually this is derived from recombination of the packaging genes and vector to give a complete infectious retroviral structure.

titer The concentration of virus (usually expressed as colony-forming units, cfu/ml). This is normally measured by counting cell colonies resistant to a particular toxic antibiotic after treating a target population of cells with a retroviral vector carrying a gene for resistance to the antibiotic. Because the apparent titer depends on the target cell type, a standardized cell type (mouse 3T3 cells) is normally used.

transduction The process of introducing a gene into a cell using a nonreplicating viral vector.

Retroviral vectors have been used clinically for gene therapy to treat cancer, viral, genetic, and inflammatory diseases. These vectors have generally been made from the murine leukemia virus (MLV) family and have many strengths and some limitations. The vectors are produced in mammalian cells (producer cells) engineered to express the viral structural proteins (packaging proteins) and a vector RNA genome that is recognized and encapsidated by the packaging proteins. Current versions of the system have essentially eliminated the probability that replication-competent retroviruses would contaminate vector preparations. The vectors can have a number of different envelopes, but only one, the amphotropic envelope, has been extensively used. This envelope allows infection of mouse, human, and other mammalian cell types. These vectors have been used as experimental therapies in both *ex vivo* (treatment of cells outside the body) and *in vivo* (direct administration to patients of either vector or producer cell lines) modes, and clinical confidence in the safety of these vectors is building. This system will continue to be used in many clinical trials.

I. INTRODUCTION

The increases in understanding of the molecular and genetic bases of cancer since the mid-1970s have shown that specific differences between cancer cells and normal cells can be defined. This understanding can be potentially exploited in many ways to devise specific therapies, but one method, the transfer of genes to specifically destroy or neutralize cancer cells, has attracted much attention. The basic rationale is that cancer cells have an altered internal environ-

ment and that the transfer of genes into malignant cells is one way to specifically manipulate that altered cellular environment. In general, that manipulation is expected to lead to the death of the cancer cell. However, it will not be possible in the near future to put genes into every or even the majority of cancer cells in a patient. So modalities where the translocation of one cancer cell leads to the death of other tumor cells in addition to the transduced cell are favored. Such modalities include immune manipulation, exploitation of metabolic cooperation between tumor cells, and induction of programmed death (apoptosis). Since the first officially sanctioned gene therapy clinical trial was initiated in 1990, the majority (70%) of clinical gene therapy protocols approved by the U.S. National Institutes of Health Recombinant DNA Advisory Committee are not for genetic diseases as had been expected, but for experimental cancer trials. Most of these cancer protocols used retroviral vectors (derived from the murine leukemia virus family of retroviruses or its relatives) as the gene transfer vehicles. Although other gene transfer vehicles (e.g., lipid vesicles, adenoviral vectors, condensed DNA) are also being tested, retroviral vectors will be a major workhorse for gene transfer in the next few years, at least in clinical settings. It has been suggested that because no cures have been unequivocally demonstrated with gene therapy, it has failed to live up to its promise, and retrenchment is necessary. However, most practitioners in the field recognize that while gene therapy may have been overhyped, in fact it is naive to expect proof of efficacy in small, early stage trials in extremely sick (late stage) patients and that the field is about where one would expect it to be. The proof of general utility will come gradually over the next decades.

II. RETROVIRUSES

Retroviruses are RNA viruses with a positive single-stranded genome; they are generally nonlytic and, in the first step in the replication cycle (Fig. 1) upon infection of a cell, the RNA genome is reverse transcribed into DNA by a reverse transcriptase enzyme present in the viral particle. This DNA is then transported to the nucleus most likely as a nucleus protein

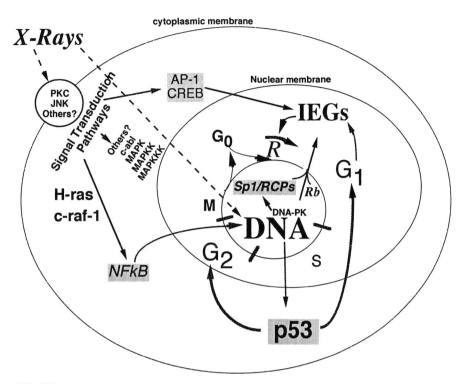

FIGURE 1 Life cycle of a retrovirus. The viral RNA genome is shown at the top. The viral particles carry two copies of this genome which is capped and polyadenylated (A_n) like a conventional messenger RNA. R denotes a repeat sequence at the end of the genome which during reverse transcription is the site of strand switching by the viral reverse transcriptase. U5 and U3 are the 5′- and 3′-terminal portions of the RNA genome that, with R, are converted into long terminal repeats (LTRs) on reverse transcription into DNA. Also shown are the tRNA primer carried in the viral particle and used for the primer in first-strand DNA synthesis and the approximate coding regions of the viral structural gag, gag–pol, and env proteins. The reverse-transcribed DNA is double stranded and is mainly synthesized in the cytoplasm before entering the nucleus and integrating into the host DNA to form the provirus. The provirus is transcribed by the cellular RNA polymerase II to give full-length and spliced transcripts encoding gag-gag/pol and env, respectively. The unspliced transcript also serves as the viral genome in progeny virus and carries Ψ, the packaging signal. The splice donor (SD) and splice acceptor (SA) sites are shown. The cytoplasmic RNA serves as a template for translation into viral proteins which are further modified by processing, glycosylation (CHO) on env, and phosphorylation (P) or myristilation on the gag proteins. The capsid gag and gag–pol proteins recognize the viral genome and enscapsidate it, and this capsid then buds off from the cell with a surrounding lipid envelope carrying the viral envelope gene product, generating new viral particles.

complex and is inserted into the host genome, in an essentially random fashion. This proviral genome is then transcribed by the cellular transcription machinery and gives rise to various transcripts encoding the viral proteins. The full-length transcript also corresponds to the viral genome which is then recognized by certain viral capsid proteins, and the viral capsid particle self-assembles and moves to the membrane of the cell which now carries viral envelope proteins. At the cell membrane the viral capsid particles buds off from the cell, taking with it a piece of the cell membrane as an envelope, and viral envelope proteins are embedded in that membrane. This envelope protein is then capable of interacting with its cognate receptor on a fresh cell to restart the infectious cycle.

Several types of such viruses have been suggested as the bases for vectors: MLV and its relatives such as gibbon ape leukemia virus (GaLV) or feline leukemia virus; the avian viruses, rous sarcoma virus and spleen necrosis virus; human immunodeficiency virus-1 (HIV-1); Mason Pfizer monkey virus (MPMV); primate "foamy" or spuma virus; and mouse mammary tumor virus (MMTV). The archetype, however, is the MLV family. The name is in fact something of a misnomer as many members of this family do not cause leukemia (although some do). Vectors derived from the MLV family are the basis for all the retroviral vectors that have been proposed for clinical trials so far. The basic arrangement of the genomes of all these viruses is shown in Figs. 1 and 3, but some encode more proteins than the gag, gag–pol, and env proteins (HIV-1, e.g., encodes at least nine proteins). These extra proteins usually encode some control functions and, in general, increase the complexity of making vectors. However, some systems such as HIV-1 and MPMV have attracted attention because they apparently have some advantageous properties (i.e., the potential to infect nonreplicating cells and the efficient transduction of blood cells, respectively).

III. RETROVIRAL VECTORS

A. General Description

Retroviral vectors resemble their parent virus except that the genome encodes as a therapeutic gene or gene of interest instead of the viral structural proteins. The capsid proteins, envelope, and envelope protein are essentially identical to a wild-type virus, allowing receptor binding, infection, reverse transcription, transport of the proviral DNA to the nucleus, and integration (Fig. 2). This process is collectively called transduction. After integration, the DNA genome behaves like any cellular gene being transcribed and

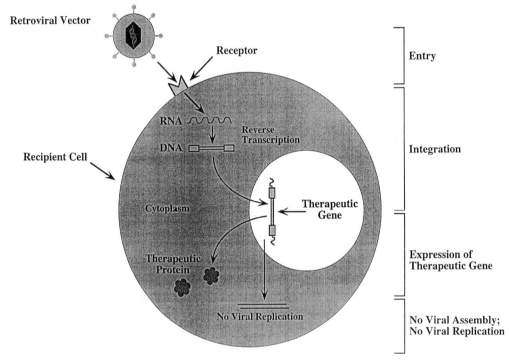

FIGURE 2 Action of a retroviral vector. The vector enters the cell and the RNA genome is reverse transcribed and integrated into the host cell genome by the identical mechanisms as those used by the parent virus (see Fig. 1). However, once integrated, the vector has no capacity to make viral proteins and hence there is no further transmission of the vector or generation of viral or vector particles. Instead, the therapeutic gene carried by the vector is transcribed and expressed by the cellular machinery, usually leading to the presence of the therapeutic protein in the cell for the rest of its life span.

replicating only if the cell replicates. Thus the cell expresses the therapeutic gene and no further viral replication is possible. Vectors are used in preclinical and clinical research in two ways: (1) cells are removed from a patient or animal, treated with a vector, and returned to the animal or patient (*ex vivo* therapy); or (2) vector or vector producer cells are directly administered (*in vivo* therapy) usually physically close to the site where the therapeutic effort is desired.

Although there are other types of gene transfer vectors, retroviral vectors have a number of strengths that make them attractive for clinical use: (1) an expanding clinical record (hundreds of patients have now been treated); (2) long-term expression (made possible by the integration of the incoming gene); (3) relatively well-understood biology; (4) expression of only the desired gene without the production of other irrelevant proteins; and (5) possibility of repeat administration, as normally subimmunogenic amounts of material are administered. The major issue with respect to the use of retroviral vectors has been the possibility of insertional mutagenesis leading to tumorgenesis, but this has been found clinically not to be an acute problem. The long-term effect is unknown, but this information will only become available after many patients have been treated and have survived for decades. Another continuing issue with respect to all gene transfer therapies is the possibility of the undesirable transfer of genes into the germ line. No evidence of this has yet been seen, but it is difficult to know if this is a real issue or not. Other limitations may be the inability of the retroviral vector to transduce nonreplicating cells (although this could be an advantage with cancer treatments), the expectation of relatively modest levels of gene expression per vector copy, and current limitations in the quantity and concentration of the vector that can be produced.

B. Construction and Production of Vectors

The provirus of MLV can be conceptually and physically divided up into (a) the protein-coding region (*trans* acting) and (b) the control sequences (*cis* acting) corresponding to replication, transcription, encapsidation, and integration signals (see Fig. 3). This allows the construction of two types of molecular derivatives: (1) the packaging genomes encoding the viral proteins, but unable to make packagable RNA (Fig. 3A); and (2) the vector genome, including the gene of interest, encoding a packagable RNA genome and nothing else (Fig. 3B). However, many vectors also carry a tissue culture selectable marker (e.g., the gene encoding resistance to the neomycin analog (G418) as a means of finding and titering the vector.

The packaging genomes are used to construct packaging lines which make viral proteins that specifically recognize only their cognate viral RNA genome and not other random RNAs. If a vector genome is now introduced into the packaging cell, it will make viral RNA molecules that are recognized by the viral proteins, and this RNA genome will be packaged into particles and excreted into the external medium. The cell line, derived from the packaging cell, that also encodes the vector is known as a producer cell (although this terminology is not universal in the literature, and packaging, producer, and "helper" lines have been used to mean both types of cell). Thus, vectors are made by mammalian cell culture and the material can be collected from the supernatant.

1. Packaging and Producer Cells

Many different packaging cells have been made over the years, most of them based on mouse 3T3 cells. The two major initial criteria were titer (i.e., how much vector can be made) and lack of replication-competent virus (RCR). As clinical trials have begun, freedom from adventitious agents in general and the ability to scaleup production also have been important.

The original method of making vectors was to superinfect a cell line carrying a vector with a RCR. This yielded a mixture of replication competent virus and vector in the cell supernatant. It soon became apparent that even for research purposes, it would be useful to have preparations of infectious vector particles that were uncontaminated with RCR, and for this purpose several type of defective packaging genomes have been constructed (Fig. 3A).

The first attempts involved construction of packaging genomes that were equivalent to the cloned provirus, but with a single deletion of the packaging sequence located between the 5' long terminal repeat (LTR) and the start of the gag sequence. On introduction into 3T3 cells, this gave cell lines such as ψ2 and PA12 (Table I and Fig. 3A) which were quite efficient but rapidly gave

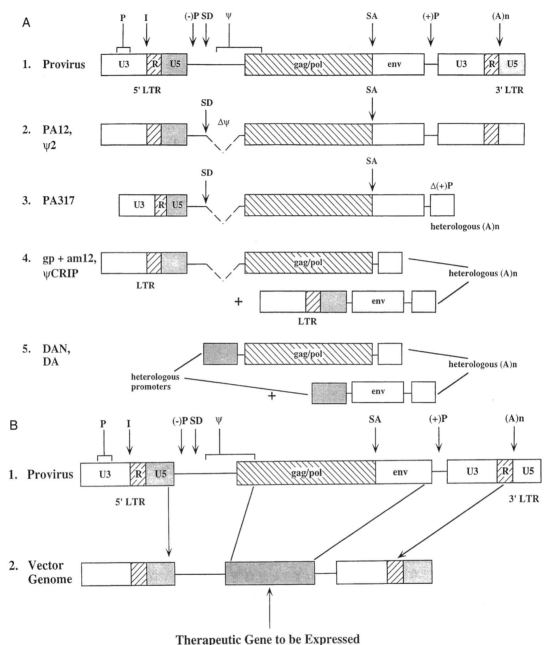

FIGURE 3 Derivation of the molecular components of the retroviral packaging and producer cells from the parent viral genome. (A) Packaging genomes. Various modifications of the provirus (1) are shown, roughly in chronological order and in order of the extent of modification. U3, R, U5, LTR, SD, DA, and A_n are as described in the legend to Fig. 1. P, RNA transcription promoter/enhancer sequences; I, initiation site of RNA transcription; (−) P, start site of first (negative) strand DNA synthesis; (+) P, start site of the second strand (positive) DNA synthesis; and $\Delta\Psi$, deletion of Ψ sequences leading to a nonfunctional packaging signal. The names of various examples of packaging cells corresponding to the packaging structures are shown on the left-hand side in 2–5. (2) Simple packaging signal deletion ($\Delta\Psi$). (3) $\Delta\Psi$, elimination of the 3′ LTR and deletion of some 5′ LTR sequences. (4) $\Delta\Psi$, elimination of 3′ LTR and break up of packaging genomes into two cistrons (gag–pol and env). (5) $\Delta\Psi$, elimination of 5′ *and* 3′ LTRs, two packaging cistrons. (B) Vector genome. The gag–pol and env-coding regions (with the exception of those gag sequences that are part of Ψ) are substituted by heterogolous sequences encoding the therapeutic gene. Often a drug selectable marker (most commonly the neomycin resistance gene which allows selection of transduced mammalian cells with the antibiotic G418) is also included in the heterogenous DNA region, usually with a separate internal promoter such as the SV40 earlier promoter. This allows simple tracking and titering of vector particles, but has no function in most clinical applications.

TABLE I
Properties of Retroviral Vector Packaging Lines

Cell line	Used in clinic	Parent cell	Helper genome	RCR detected	Envelope	Average titer[a] (cfu/ml)
ψ2	No	3T3 (mouse)	One genome	Yes	eco	~10^6 [b]
PA12	No	3T3	One genome	Yes	ampho	~10^6 [b]
PA317	Yes	3T3	One genome, partial LTR deletions	Sometimes	ampho	~10^6
gp + am12	Yes	3T3	Two genomes, includes LTRs	No	ampho	~10^6
ψCRIP	Yes	3T3	Two genomes, includes LTRs	No	ampho	~10^6
PG13	Yes	3T3	Two genomes, includes LTRs	No	GaLV	~10^6
DAN	No	D17 (dog)	Two genomes, LTRs removed	Sometimes	ampho	~10^4
DA	Yes	D17	Two genomes, LTR removed, sequential introduction	No	ampho	~10^6
293/kat	Not known	293 (human)	Two genomes, LTR removed, transient introduction	No	ampho	10^5–10^6 (cocultivation used)

[a]See comments in text about the difficulty in comparing titers.
[b]In general, amphotrophic vectors are more difficult to generate as high-titer preparations, and the rough equivalence shown here represents the greater selection effort involved in generating PA12 as compared to ψ2.

rise to RCR, presumably by the recombination of packaging genomes with the vector when the vector genome was introduced. The next generation of packaging cells, typified by PA317, used packaging genomes that were further deleted but retained the viral 5′ LTR as promoter and the gag–pol–env linear arrangement of the genome. It was thought that these two features might be important in maintaining a correct level of gag and gag–pol messenger RNA compared to the envelope messenger levels and that the extra deletions would require at least two recombination events to give rise to RCR, rendering the appearance of RCR extremely unlikely. In fact, neither of these suppositions turned out to be correct. First, it was demonstrated that the gag–pol and envelope cistrons could be separated and that relative RNA levels did not seem to affect titer. Second, RCR developed after extensive use and scaleup. Despite some RCR problems, the PA317 cell line has been useful for much research and several clinical trials using retroviral vectors. Further measures were taken to essentially eliminate RCR contamination by splitting up the gag–pol and env genes onto different cistrons (gp + am12 and ΨCRIP), stripping the LTR sequences from these (DAN) and sequentially transfecting them into the parent cell (DA). These progressive modifications are summarized in Fig. 3A. Finally, the creation of multilayered banks of producers lines coupled with strict control of the number of replication cycles undergone by a producer line provided physical restraints on the opportunity for rare recombination events. These measures seem to have eliminated the generation of RCR by recombination between the vector and helper as an issue.

At the same time it became useful to vary the parent cell background to the packaging cell line. Mouse cells, such as 3T3, have many homologies to MLV sequences, representing potential recombination targets which could lead to RCR generation. These cells also carry "VL30" sequences which are transcribed, carry LTRs and packaging signals, and can be packaged and transduced into target cells with efficiencies equivalent to vectors. For these reasons, packaging cells with other backgrounds such as dog (D17) or human (HT-I080 or 293 cells) without such homologies or known packagable sequences have been constructed and successfully used. In addition to permanent packaging and producer cell lines, 293 cells can be transiently transfected with packaging and vector genes to yield useful (10^5–10^6 cfu/ml) levels of vector. A list of commonly used packaging cell lines and their properties is shown in Table I.

2. RCR Detection

One of the reasons for the multiple generations of packaging cell lines is that to some extent, the issue of RCR contamination has been of increasing concern. That is, knowledge concerning the sensitivity of testing and the understanding of the limits of testing has gradually built up since the early 1990s (Fig. 4). As the potential for clinical trials appeared, became a reality, and multiple trials began, the issue became of greater importance. RCR represents a safety issue from a general point of view in that it is not de-

sirable to administer a replicating agent that infects human cells to human patients. Furthermore, an RCR infection would seem to increase the likelihood of an insertional mutagenesis event. Direct evidence of the likelihood of this is limited. In one experiment, several monkeys (8) have been infected for over 5 years with a retrovirus that represents a typical RCR gen-

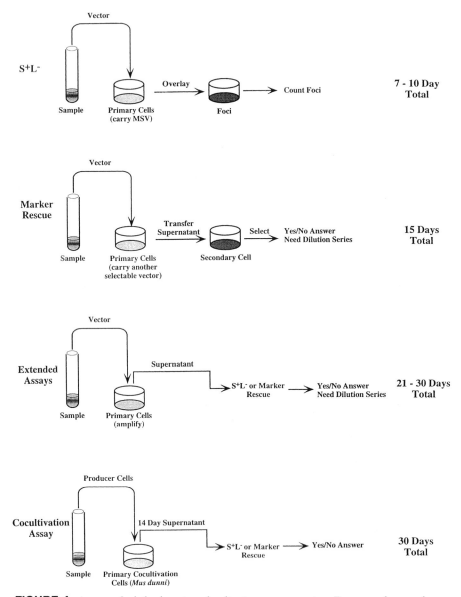

FIGURE 4 Assay methods for detection of replication-competent virus. Four general types of assays are shown and described in the text. The assays are shown in order of increasing sensitivity (from top to bottom). The S⁺L⁻ assay can be used to give RCR titers by counting foci, whereas the other three assays require carrying a dilution series of the initial test sample through the assay, using end point dilution as a readout for quantification.

erated by recombination and no ill effects have been seen. In other experiments, however, 3 out of 10 highly immunosuppressed monkeys given transplants of bone marrow treated with an RCR-contaminated vector gave rise to lymphomas carrying RCR genomes (but no vector genomes). These data suggest that while no evidence of tumorgenesis due to the vector has been observed, RCR may lead to such events. It is thus doubly important to ensure that vector preparations are tested in the best possible way for RCR contamination.

The original RCR assays were (1) the S^+L- assay designed as a titering assay in the seventies for research into murine retroviruses and (2) the marker rescue assay designed in the early days of vector development (see Fig. 4). Both of these assays work off the same principle: a primary cell line carrying a defective virus or vector (murine sarcoma virus for S^+L-, a drug resistance marker for marker rescue) is treated with the test sample of vector and rescue of the defective virus or vector is monitored on a secondary cell line. In the earliest form of the S^+L- test, the primary cell line (such as the mink cell line, $MiCl_1$) is overlaid with the equivalent cell line free of MSV (Mv1Lu, secondary cell line) and transformed foci are identified after 7–10 days. In the marker rescue assay, the test sample is added to a primary cell line carrying the drug resistance marker (e.g., hygromycin resistance) in the form of a vector encoding the resistance gene. The primary cells treated with test sample are grown for 3–7 days, the supernatant is passed onto secondary cells not carrying the marker, and selection is applied to identify those cells that have taken up the vector rescued out of the primary cells by RCR. Variations of these tests have also been used, and the extended format (see Fig. 4), where the test sample is preamplified on a susceptible target cell, appears to increase apparent titers in identically prepared samples by a factor of up to 10-fold for both types of assay. In addition, as the amounts of vector produced increase, it is now clear that interference between the vector and low levels of contaminating RCR can occur at titers of 10^6 cfu/ml and above. Thus it is possible that a negative result in a vector sample may not preclude the subsequent appearance of RCR. The best test available appears to be a cocultivation procedure (Fig. 4) where the primary tester cell line is cocultivated with the producer cell line for up to 14 days, followed by routine testing of the cocultivation supernatant. Using a cell line that amplifies almost all types of MLV (the Mus dunni cell line), this test will detect at least 1 cell making RCR in 10^7 cells. This test seems by far the best, as direct experience shows that vector samples contaminated at a level of 1 RCR in 10^7 vector particles would often pass the vector supernatant test, whereas the cocultivation test of 5×10^5 producer cells gave routine positives. Thus the use of the cocultivation assay gives excellent assurance of absence of RCR. A recent complication with this assay has appeared—namely that Mus dunni cells harbor an endogenous activatable retrovirus that scores in a marker rescue assay. This seems to be induced by halogenated nucleosides, but good controls should allow for the detection of any such artifact during assays.

3. Titers

The ability to make a high-titer vector is important in order to transduce the large numbers of cells necessary in some treatment modalities and to keep costs of vector production down. In addition, for many applications, the concentration of the vector is important.

It is still not clear what the limiting factors are in making vectors. Candidates include the viral proteins, the viral vector RNA genome, tRNA primers, cell membrane, and others. It is likely that most of these can be the limiting factor in different situations. In general terms, titers are measured by making a dilution series of the vector that carries a gene encoding resistance to an antibiotic, then putting the dilutions onto plates of growing target cells (one or more for each dilution), applying selection for the antibiotic resistance marker, and counting the colonies that grow out 10–15 days later by fixing and staining. The titer is then calculated in colony-forming units per milliliter by multiplying back from any one plate with 30–100 colonies on it. Titers can also be performed using a quantitative polymerase chain reaction for vector sequences after transduction of the target cells or by staining for color after transduction of a gene, such as β-galactosidase, that can catalyze a color reaction. A typical titer is 10^6 cfu/ml, but such numbers are difficult to compare from laboratory to laboratory. Depending on the exact protocol used, titers may vary

10-fold or more. In addition, different cell types transduce at vastly different efficiencies for unknown reasons. Thus it is not reliable to compare numbers from different laboratories, and meaningful direct comparisons must be performed with the same vector and in the same laboratory. However, the highest titers from unprocessed vector are around 10^7 to 10^8 cfu/ml. Concentration and/or processing can be this up to approximately 10^{10} cfu/ml. At present, the best clinically available titers are around 10^8 cfu/ml. It is not clear how much further one can go, but MLV is generally only made in tissue culture at 10^7–10^8 biologically active particles or focus forming units (ffu) per milliliter (HIV-1 can be routinely made at 10^9 ffu/ml). A titer of 10^6 cfu/ml generally represents <1 biologically active particle/cell/24 hr, so there would seem to be room for improvement. However, it is likely that, as for wild-type MLV, many defective particles are also made from these packaging cell lines, which may use up valuable cellular resources and limit the production of a high-titer vector.

In terms of increased titers, at least five major steps can be taken. First, in general, maximizing the amount of viral protein made in a packaging cell line seems to help; second, increasing the level of the vector genome also seems useful and introduction of the vector by transduction rather than transfection seems to be one way to do this; third, the actual structure of the vector can have an enormous effect on the titer, although only a few rules are available for general guidance (see *Vector Structure*); fourth, variation and optimization of cell culture conditions can give considerable (up to 100-fold) increases in titer, although this seems more effective at bringing low titers into normal range rather than boosting high titers further; and finally, vector preparations can be processed and concentrated by centrifugation or ultrafiltration to give 10- to 100-fold higher titers than starting material. This may be easier with some types of vector than with others (see Section III.C).

4. Vector Structure

The insert capacity of retroviral vectors is a maximum of 8 kb, although most inserts are smaller than that. The construction of vectors has undergone a comparable evolution to packaging cells but remains to some degree an art, requiring multiple design attempts to achieve a desired goal. The major consistent design features are the requirement for two LTRs, packaging signal, and the first and second strand start synthesis sites (see Fig. 3B). Probably the most generally useful principles, discovered so far are: (1) the packaging signal is not confined to the space between the 5′ LTR and the gag AUG start codon, but extends into the gag coding sequence–vectors using this have 5- to 10-fold increased titers; and (2) the more complex the design of the expression cistrons, the more likely that something will not function as expected (e.g., there will a decrease in titer). Nevertheless, a wide variety of vector structures have been investigated, often with a goal of achieving better control of gene expression. These vectors include simple vectors with the LTR as the promoter and a single gene of interest; vectors that include internal promoters that may be inducible or tissue specific; vectors that include modified locus control regions (LCRs); vectors that express the gene of interest with an internal promoter in the reverse direction (this allows the inclusion of introns that would otherwise be spliced out in the producer cell line); vectors with self-inactivating LTRs so that internal promoters can function free of interference from the LTRs; vectors with pol III expression cassettes; and vectors with the expression cassette inserted in the LTRs (double copy vectors). Generally, the desire for high titers overpowers the urge for the fine control of gene expression and so the recent general trend has been toward simplified vectors. In addition, it has become apparent that the expression of foreign genes as part of gene therapy protocols can lead to immune destruction of the transduced cells in patients. This suggests that even antibiotic resistance genes should be eliminated from vectors for treatments requiring long-term expression.

One issue that now seems to be partially addressed is that of long-term expression in animals and patients. Early experiments suggested that vector expression in animals often shuts down after a few weeks or months. While this is definitely true, empirical varying of vector structures followed by tracking of expression have shown this to be a solvable problem. One example of this is the prolonged expression (up to 6 years) of the introduced adenosine deaminase

(ADA) gene in the T cells of two ADA-deficient patients who participated in the first clinical gene therapy trial.

C. Cell Transduction Efficiencies

Vectors have widely varying abilities to transduce different cell types. One major general limitation (which can also be used as an advantage) is the relative inability to effectively transduce nonreplicating cells (at least 100-fold less than replicating cells). While some of the differences in transduction of different cell types are clearly attributable to LTRs, to gag proteins, and to other unknown factors (e.g., the low efficiency, 0.1–10%, of transduction of human blood cells), a major manipulatable determinant is the envelope protein. For MLV-derived vectors, the original experiments were performed with ecotropic envelopes. This is the natural envelope of Moloney MLV on which many early experiments were performed, and a functional receptor is thought to exist only on mouse cells and some rat cells. Thus these vectors are not useful for human cells or, by extension, genetic therapy. However, at least three other types of envelopes using different receptors from MLV and several other envelopes from related viruses (e.g., GaLV) seem to be interchangeable with the ecotropic envelope in the packaging system. First, the amphotropic envelope allows the infection of mouse and many mammalian species, including humans. This is the type of envelope that has been used for almost all retroviral vector-based clinical gene therapy to date. Second, the xenotropic envelope allows infection of many mammalian cell types, including human but excluding mice. It may have advantages in getting vectors into marrow stem cells or blood cells, but has not been exploited so far and only one or two packaging cell lines have been made. This probably is, in part, due to the fact that everyone's favorite animal model (mice) is not usable with this system. Third, polytropic envelopes allow infection of mouse and rat cells and a small subset of human cells. A couple of packaging cell lines have been made, but no real information is available at present. It is worth noting that these species characterizations for these envelopes are based on a rather narrow information base

with a limited number of cell types in culture. Several cell lines with other envelopes have been made and tested. PG13 is a cell line made with MLV gag and pol and an envelope from GaLV. This cell line has been used to produce vector for clinical trials. Other cell lines based on Friend leukemia virus (an MLV variant) and a hybrid of Friend and MLV protein have been described.

The general rules and mechanism of envelope substitution in vectors and viruses are unclear. Thus, on a wider perspective, although the MLV vectors can be easily pseudotyped (i.e., acquire a modified tropism by means of a substitute envelope protein) with the previously mentioned envelopes, this does not happen with the Sendai virus envelope or even with the HIV-1 envelope (although the reverse, i.e., amphotropic pseudotyping of HIV-1, does work). Nevertheless, it has been possible to pseudotype with the G protein, which is the envelope protein of the unrelated virus, vesticular stomatitis virus (VSV). These pseudotypes seem to have a very broad ability to transduce cells and, furthermore, are somewhat physically more robust and can be easily concentrated 100- to 1000-fold by centrifugation. In addition, VSV G-pseudotyped HIV-1 vectors have been shown to transduce nonreplicating cells *ex vivo* and *in vivo*, leading to new applications for these types of vectors. Unfortunately, the VSV G protein is toxic in almost all cells at levels useful to make packaging cell lines, and so this type of vector is usually made after the transient introduction of the VSV G encoding gene into producer cells. This makes large-scale preparation of such vectors difficult. Permanent cell lines with an inducible expression of VSV G protein have been described, so this may simplify the production of VSVG pseudotypes.

D. Routes of Administration and Targeting

The initial route of administration of retroviral vectors was *ex vivo*, i.e., cells are removed from an animal (or syngenic cells for inbred animals), the gene is introduced, and the cells are returned to the animal. Clearly, such approaches are useful but complex and difficult to use for large numbers of patients. The direct administration of vectors to animals by multiple routes of administration has been shown to lead to biological or therapeutic effects. These include intramuscular injection, intratumor injection, injection into the portal vein of mice to target liver, and endothelial cell transduction. The results have not always been overwhelming, but improved quality and titer of the preparations have shown improved properties. For example, it has been possible to show antitumor effects in rodent models with vectors expressing interferon-γ or herpes thymidine kinase. A further issue that may affect the ability to directly administer vectors is the known susceptibility of conventional ecotropic and amphotropic retroviruses made in mouse cells to inactivation can be avoided by the use of cell lines, mainly human, that confer complement resistance on vectors manufactured from these lines. This is assumed to be due to the presence of complement-suppressing proteins (such as decoy accelerating factor, DAF and CD59) on the surface of these cells and their subsequent transmission to the vector particles. An alternative means of vector delivery (injection of producer cells that make vector) has been used extensively in the clinic after proof-of-principle in animal models. This has been used mainly as an antitumor agent with vectors encoding the herpes thymidine kinase gene. Expression of this gene confers sensitivity to the anti-herpes drug, ganciclovir, on transduced cells, and a poorly understood effect called the "bystander" effect leads to the concomitant death of neighboring nontransduced cells.

Targeting of retroviral vectors (and other gene transfer vehicles) refers to the goal of administering the vectors in some conventional way and arranging that the vectors home to a particular target tissue or cell type (such as a cancer metastasis or a specific hemopoietic cell type), usually by virtue of a specific ligand–receptor interaction. This is the "holy grail" of gene transfer and can conceptually be achieved in at least three ways: (1) alteration of the binding site of the envelope to confer specificity for a target surface receptor (hybrid envelopes); (2) physically attaching new ligands to the vector surface; and (3) incorporating new ligands on the viral lipid envelope by, e.g., expressing them in packaging cells.

So far, targeting has been documented as possible in tissue culture, but with discouragingly low efficiencies of transduction. It has been suggested that the coexpression of wild-type envelopes stabilizes hybrid envelopes and that significantly higher (although still not useful) titers can be achieved (10^3–10^4 cfu/ml). Use of the ecotropic envelope as the stabilizer avoids cell transduction via the wild-type envelope in human applications. Other issues apart from the receptor–ligand bridging are involved in *in vivo* targeting, including the survival of the vector in the body, the availability or accessibility of the target tissue, the transduction efficiency, the expression levels of the therapeutic gene in the target tissue, and whether the effect of the gene product is limited to one cell or to the local area. These issues will have to be addressed before this type of targeting becomes a reality for retroviral vectors, or, for that matter, any gene transfer system.

IV. ANIMAL STUDIES AND THERAPEUTIC USES OF RETROVIRAL VECTORS

There are many modalities that have been proposed to have an effect on disease by gene transfer (e.g., immune stimulation, producing activation by the introduced gene product, ribozymes, dominant negative mutants of viral subunits, etc.). Table II lists some examples of approval clinical trials in the United States using different modalities. In general, theoretical schemes to inhibit disease are not difficult to devise or to show as feasible in tissue culture systems. However, most of the more formidable obstacles seem to be in getting the gene to go where desired. In general, treatments which require a gene for every sick cell are unappealing because of the degree of difficulty involved. An example would be the return of functional tumor suppressor genes to cancer cells in which the endogenous copies of these two tumor suppresser genes are mutated. If the efficiency of the gene transfer system were such as to be able to allow this to have a therapeutic effect (say, putting the gene in 50% of the tumor cells), it is safe to say that the choice of gene to deliver such a therapeutic effect would be quite wide and, for example, the delivery of a toxin or prodrug activating gene (e.g., herpes thymidine kinase for acyclovir) would probably be at least as desirable and effective. Thus, in general, feasible (i.e., current) gene transfer protocols take advantage of situations

TABLE II
Examples of Gene Therapy Protocols Involving Retroviral Vectors with
Complete or Partial Approval in the United States

1. *Ex vivo* administration of retroviral vectors encoding adenosine deaminase to T cells or bone marrow stem cells from adenosine deaminase-deficient children, followed by reinfusion of the transduced cells into the patients
2. Direct injection of producer cells intratumorally into brain cancers, with the vector encoding herpes thymidine kinase, followed by administration of gangciclovir systemically to selectively kill only the cells expressing thymidine kinase
3. Direct intramuscular administration of retroviral vectors encoding HIV-1 env to stimulate anti-HIV-1 cytotoxic T-cell responses in HIV-1-infected individuals
4. *Ex vivo* administration of retroviral vectors encoding a ribozyme or transdominant repressor protein targeted against HIV-1 into T cells followed by reinfusion of these cells into the patient to provide a protected population of T cells
5. *Ex vivo* administration of retroviral vectors encoding cytokines (IL2, IL7, IL12, interferon-γ, GM-CSF) into tumor cells followed by an introduction of the transduced tumor cells into the patient to induce enhanced antitumor immunity capable of clearing unmodified tumor cells
6. *Ex vivo* administration of retroviral vectors encoding an IL1 receptor antagonist into autologous synoviocytes followed by their reintroduction into arthritic joints in rheumatoid arthritis patients

where the effect of the introduced gene is not confined to the cell in which that gene product is made. Examples include (1) the production of ADA in some T cells in ADA$^-$ children to detoxify the blood by removing adenosine; (2) the use of vector to induce active specific cytotoxic T lymphocyte (CTL) responses against tumors or virally infected cells; (3) the modification of a subset of T cell or progenitor cells, making them HIV-1 resistant, then expecting this to give these cells an advantage in HIV-1-positive patients; (4) the delivery of cytokines or other immunomodulation molecules, such as interferon-γ, interleukin (IL)2, IL12, granulocyte–macrophage colony-stimulating factor (GM-CSF), and B7.1 to a small subset of tumor cells to increase their immunogenicity and lead the immune system to clear unmodified cells; (5) the delivery of the genes for ADA and glucocerebrosidase to long-term progenitor marrow cells in patients with genetic deficiency of these enzymes to achieve amplification of these genes through the proliferation of cells from the hemopeotic lineage; and (6) the exploitation of the "bystander" effect (see above) with the HSV TK gene in tumors, where animal models show that transduction of 5–20% of tumor cell results in 100% tumor cell death. The majority of human trials using retroviral vectors have used *ex vivo* approaches, but several involve direct administration protocols and these types of protocols will become more frequent. One involves the injection of retroviral vectors encoding HIV-1 anti-

gens intramuscularly in order to transduce healthy cells *in situ*, leading them to present the HIV antigens in the context of MHC class I and allowing the induction of augmented CTL responses against HIV-1 in HIV-1-infected individuals. This study is now in small-scale efficacy clinical trials (Phase II trial). Another proposal involves the injection of producer cell lines, instead of vector, intracranially into tumor sites in terminal brain cancer (mostly metastatic cancer) patients. The vector encodes the herpes thymidine kinase gene which is expected to be transferred to the only replicating cells available–tumor cells. These can then be killed by administering acyclovir or gangciclovir. Studies in a rat model showed remarkable efficacy and encouraging results have been seen in glioma (primary brain tumor) patients in particular. A large scale efficacy (Phase III) study is currently being planned. In addition, a large number of small studies have been performed using these modalities in multiple tumor types. Other clinical studies involve the direct administration of vectors instead of producer cell lines encoding HSV TK and, in a different study, interferon-γ directly to tumor nodules. No significant clinical data are available from these studies yet.

The net result of these and all the *ex vivo* trials is a renewed confidence in the lack of acute toxicity or tumorgenic potential in humans of retroviral vectors. An example of this is the clinical use of experimental retroviral vector therapy for rheumatoid arthritis. This disease is usually described as non-life-threatening, so this protocol suggests that a much wider use of these vectors may now be acceptable. Thus, the previous use of retroviral vectors gives confidence in their clinical and regulatory acceptability, and therefore their continued utility. It is very likely that therapeutic products based on these vectors will be on the market before the end of the decade.[1]

See Also the Following Articles

ADENO-ASSOCIATED VIRUS: A VECTOR FOR HIGH-EFFICIENCY GENE TRANSDUCTION • GENE THERAPY VECTORS, SAFETY CONSIDERATIONS • RETROVIRUSES • TARGETED VECTORS FOR CANCER GENE THERAPY • TRANSGENIC MICE IN CANCER RESEARCH

---

[1]The FDA "Points to Consider for Somatic Cell and Gene Therapy," "Cell Lines Used to Produce Biologicals," "Biologicals Produced by Recombinant DNA Technology" and "Administration of Activated Leukocytes" can be obtained from the Biologics Information Staff, Office of the Director, Center for Biologics, FDA, Bethesda, MD 20205, USA.

Bibliography

Coffin, J. M. (1990). Retroviridae and their replication. *In* "Virology" (B. N. Fields and D. M. Knipe, eds.), 2nd Ed., pp. 1437–1489. Raven Press, New York.

Friedmann, T. (1992). A brief history of gene therapy. *Nature Genet.* **2,** 93–98.

Human Gene Markers/Therapy Clinical Protocols (1996). *Hum. Gene Ther.* **7,** 567–588.

Jolly, D. (1994). Viral vector systems for gene therapy. *Cancer Gene Ther.* **1,** 51–64.

Leiden, J. M. (1995). Gene Therapy–Promise, Pitfalls, and Prognosis. *N. Engl. J. Med.* **333,** 871–873.

Miller, A. D., Miller, D. G., Garcia, J. V., *et al.* (1993). Use of retroviral vectors for gene transfer and expression. *Methods Enzymol.* **217,** 581–599.

Morgan, R. A., and Anderson, F. (1993). Human gene therapy. *Annu. Rev. Biochem.* **62,** 191–217.

Summers, N. M., and Cooney, C. L. (1994). Gene Therapy: Biotech's n + 1 Technology. *Bio/Technology* **12,** 42–45.

Temin, H. M. (1990). Safety considerations in somatic gene therapy of human disease with retrovirus vectors. *Hum. Gene Ther.* **1,** 111–123.

Verma, I. (1990). Gene therapy. *Sci. Am.* **Nov.,** 68–84.

Retroviruses

Eric O. Freed

National Institute of Allergy and Infectious Diseases
Bethesda, Maryland

GLOSSARY

endogenous retroviruses Sequences integrated into the germline, transmitted vertically from parent to offspring. They often contain defective open reading frames.

envelope glycoproteins Proteins that are embedded in the lipid bilayer of the viral envelope. They are responsible for receptor binding and membrane fusion.

Gag proteins Proteins forming the protein shell that encapsidates the viral RNA genome.

integration The process by which the double-stranded DNA copy of the viral genome splices itself into the host cell chromosome. Catalyzed by integrase.

oncogene A viral or cellular gene capable of inducing neoplastic transformation. Nontransforming cellular forms (also known as protooncogenes) can be converted to oncogenes by mutation or overexpression after transduction by a retrovirus.

protease The viral enzyme that cleaves the Gag and Gag-pol precursors.

provirus The viral genome integrated into the host cell chromosome.

reverse transcription The synthesis of DNA using the retroviral RNA genome as a template. This process is mediated by the enzyme reverse transcriptase.

I. INTRODUCTION

Since the mid 1980s, retroviruses have been the focus of an intensive research effort, due primarily to the causative association between the human immunodeficiency virus (HIV) and the acquired immunodeficiency syndrome (AIDS). Retroviruses are enveloped, contain a diploid RNA genome which is generally between 7 and 11 kb, and possess the ability to convert their RNA genome to double-stranded DNA following infection of the host cell. The process of synthesizing the DNA copy of the RNA genome (known as reverse transcription) is error prone, often leading to a high degree of sequence variation between virus isolates. The double-stranded viral DNA is spliced, or integrated, into the host cell chromosome, thus becoming a permanent part of the host genome. This article provides a brief overview of the classification, structure, and life cycle of retroviruses.

II. CLASSIFICATION

Several years ago, the International Committee on the Taxonomy of Viruses reclassified the retrovirus family into seven genera, based on genome structure and sequence relatedness (Table I). These genera are the spumaviruses, mammalian C-type retroviruses, lentiviruses, D-type retroviruses, B-type retroviruses, bovine leukosis virus (BLV)/human T-cell leukemia virus (HTLV), and avian leukosis virus (ALV) related.

The spumaviruses, or foamy viruses, infect a number of mammalian species, although no definitive link with disease induction has been established. These viruses are characterized by the formation of vacuoles upon infection in tissue culture. This vacuolation (or "foaming") is thought to result from a high level of intracellular assembly and budding, and from syncytium formation induced by envelope glycoprotein expression.

The mammalian C-type genus includes the well-studied endogenous and exogenous murine leukemia viruses. These viruses follow the C-type assembly pathway, i.e., they assemble at and bud from the host cell plasma membrane. Several members of this genus (e.g., Harvey sarcoma virus and Abelson murine leukemia virus) express cellularly derived, transforming genes known as oncogenes. A variety of models for the acquisition of oncogenes by retroviruses have been proposed; the model which currently has the most support postulates the occurrence of nonhomologous recombination between the viral RNA and copackaged cellular RNA during reverse transcription. Sequence and structure/function analysis of the differences between virally encoded oncogenes and their cellular homologs (the protooncogenes) has contributed greatly to modern cancer research. The mammalian C-type viruses, which have acquired cellularly derived oncogene sequences, are noninfectious and thus require the presence of a replication competent "helper" virus. This genus also includes the feline leukemia virus (FeLV), the simian sarcoma

TABLE I
Classification of Retroviruses

Genus[a]	Examples[b]
Spumavirus	Human foamy virus (HFV)
	Feline syncytium-forming virus (FeSFV)
Mammalian C-type	Moloney murine leukemia virus (MoMLV)
	Abelson murine leukemia virus (A-MLV)
	Feline Leukemia virus (FeLV)
	Spleen necrosis virus (SNV)
	Endogenous murine leukemia viruses
Lentivirus	Human immunodeficiency virus type 1 (HIV-1)
	Human immunodeficiency virus type 2 (HIV-2)
	Simian immunodeficiency virus (SIV)
	Feline immunodeficiency virus (FIV)
	Visna/maedi virus
	Equine infectious anemia virus (EIAV)
D-type	Mason-Pfizer monkey virus (M-PMV)
B-type	Mouse mammary tumor virus (MMTV)
	Endogenous viruses
HTLV-BLV	Human T-cell leukemia virus (HTLV)
	Bovine leukosis virus (BLV)
Avian leukosis related	Rous sarcoma virus (RSV)
	Avian myeloblastosis virus (AMV)
	Endogenous viruses

[a] Retroviral genera as classified by the International Committee on the Taxonomy of Viruses.
[b] Partial list of members of the indicated genera, using standard abbreviations.

viruses (SSVs), and the avian retroviruses reticuloendotheliosis virus (REV) and spleen necrosis virus (SNV).

The lentivirus (or "slow" virus) genus includes not only HIV-1 and HIV-2, but also the related simian immunodeficiency viruses (SIVs), which cause an AIDS-like syndrome in several nonhuman primates, the feline and bovine immunodeficiency viruses (FIV and BIV, respectively), and the sheep and horse lentiviruses visna and equine infectious anemia virus (EIAV). The genomes of lentiviruses are more complex than those of other retroviruses, encoding a number of unique regulatory and accessory proteins. The lentiviruses are also distinct in their ability to productively infect nondividing cells. This characteristic is thought to contribute to the pathogenic properties of lentiviruses in that they can infect terminally differentiated cells of the monocyte/macrophage lineage. The viruses in this genus typically follow the C-type assembly pathway, i.e., they assemble at and bud from the plasma membrane.

The prototypic D-type retrovirus is the Mason-Pfizer monkey virus (M-PMV), which was isolated from a simian mammary carcinoma. These viruses assemble in the cytoplasm, forming immature structures known as intracytoplasmic A-type particles. After assembly, these particles are transported to and bud from the plasma membrane. These viruses do not encode oncogenes, but rather induce immune suppression in primates.

Like the D-type retroviruses, members of the B-type genus assemble in the cytoplasm prior to transport to the plasma membrane. B-type viruses include mouse mammary tumor virus (MMTV), which, in addition to Gag, Pol, and Env gene products, encodes a superantigen. This genus also includes a variety of endogenous viruses. Exogenous B-type retroviruses are often transmitted in milk.

The HTLV/BLV genus includes viruses associated with bovine B-cell tumors and human and simian T-cell lymphomas. HTLV is endemic in parts of Japan, the Caribbean, South America, and Africa, and is increasingly common in HIV-infected IV drug users. These viruses encode two regulatory gene products: Tax and Rex.

The prototypic avian leukosis virus is the Rous sarcoma virus (RSV), which was found early in the 20th century to be associated with tumors in chickens. Many avian leukosis viruses encode oncogenes (e.g., *src* in RSV and *myb* in AMV). In the case of RSV, the acquisition of the *src* oncogene did not destroy the ability of the virus to replicate. In other cases, the oncogene-containing virus is replication defective and thus requires the presence of a helper virus. These viruses follow the C-type assembly pathway.

III. GENOME ORGANIZATION

All replication-competent retroviruses encode at least three major open frames: *gag*, *pol*, and *env* (Fig. 1). At the amino terminus of the genome is the gag open reading frame, the primary product of which is the Gag polyprotein precursor. This precursor protein is proteolytically processed by the viral protease (PR) to generate the mature Gag proteins matrix (MA), capsid (CA), and nucleocapsid (NC). The Gag proteins form the proteinacious core within which is packaged the viral RNA genome. Gag expression is necessary and sufficient for particle formation (Table II).

Downstream of *gag* is the *pol* open reading frame. *pol* is initially expressed as a Gag–pol polyprotein precursor, which is processed by PR to generate reverse transcriptase (RT) and integrase (IN). The coding region for PR, which lies between *gag* and *pol*, can be in the *gag* open reading frame (e.g., RSV), the *pol* open reading frame (e.g., HIV and MLV), or in a separate open reading frame (e.g., HTLV). The Gag–pol polyprotein precursor is generated by either a frameshift or by stop codon suppression; as a result, the Pol proteins are synthesized at about 5 to 10% the level of the Gag proteins. RT mediates the conversion of the viral RNA genome to double-stranded DNA, and the IN protein catalyzes the integration of the double-stranded viral DNA into the host cell genome.

At the 3′ end of the viral genome is the *env* open reading frame, which encodes the viral envelope (Env) glycoproteins. Like the Gag and Pol products, Env is synthesized as a polyprotein precursor, which is cleaved by a host cell protease to the mature surface (SU) and the transmembrane (TM) envelope proteins. During transport, the Env precursor oligomerizes into dimers, trimers, or tetramers. SU bears the determinants of receptor binding whereas TM is involved in catalyzing a membrane fusion reaction

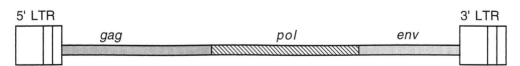

FIGURE 1 Genome organization of simple retroviruses. The three genes common to all replication-competent retroviruses (*gag*, *pol*, and *env*) are indicated. The long terminal repeats (LTRs) are illustrated as boxes at the left- and right-hand ends of the genome.

TABLE II
Retroviral Proteins

Proteins[a]	Primary Function[b]
Gag	
Matrix (MA)	Targeting of Gag to membranes
	Env incorporation into virions
Capsid (CA)	Virus assembly
Nucleocapsid (NC)	RNA binding
Protease (PR)	Cleavage of Gag and Gag-pol precursors
Pol	
Reverse transcriptase (RT)	Reverse transcription of viral genome (RNA → DNA)
Integrase (IN)	Integration of viral DNA into host genome
Env	
Surface (SU)	Receptor binding
Transmembrane (TM)	Membrane fusion

[a]The major proteins common to replication-competent retroviruses. The two-letter standard abbreviations for the mature proteins are indicated.
[b]Partial list of the major functions of the indicated proteins.

between the lipid bilayers of viral envelope and host cell membranes after receptor binding. The SU protein is often heavily glycosylated and is typically the retroviral protein which exhibits the most variation between virus isolates. The SU and TM of some retroviruses (e.g., murine leukemia virus) are linked by disulfide bonds; in other cases (e.g., HIV), SU and TM are held together by noncovalent interactions.

In addition to *gag*, *pol*, and *env*, many retroviruses, in particular the lentiviruses, encode additional open reading frames. These serve a variety of functions in transcriptional activation, regulation of RNA transport, virus assembly and release, and virus infectivity.

At both ends of the retroviral genome are the long terminal repeats (LTRs). The 5′ LTR contains the transcriptional promoter elements; the 3′ LTR provides the polyadenylation signal. The LTRs also play cis-acting roles in reverse transcription and in the integration of the viral DNA into the host cell chromosome.

IV. VIRUS LIFE CYCLE

The infection process is initiated when the SU envelope glycoprotein binds receptor molecules on the plasma membrane of the host cell. The receptors for several retroviruses have been identified; the best-characterized example is the CD4 molecule which serves as the receptor for primate lentiviruses, including HIV. Other retroviral receptors that have been identified include amino acid and phosphate transporters and a molecule that is related to the low-density lipoprotein receptor. Following receptor binding, the envelope glycoproteins catalyze a membrane fusion reaction between the lipid bilayer of the viral envelope and host cell membranes. This fusion reaction can take place, depending on the retrovirus and host cell type, at either the plasma membrane or within low-pH endosomal vesicles following receptor-mediated endocytosis. The membrane fusion reaction delivers the viral nucleocapsid into the host cell cytoplasm.

After the viral nucleocapsid gains entry into the host cell cytoplasm, uncoating occurs, and the single-stranded viral RNA genome is converted to double-stranded DNA by RT. Reverse transcription is primed by a tRNA molecule which is packaged in the virion during assembly. The viral DNA is transported into the nucleus as part of a high molecular weight entity known as the preintegration complex. The preintegration complexes of lentiviruses are able to target and enter the nucleus of the host cell, thereby permitting infection of nondividing cells. Other retroviruses require that the host cell pass through mitosis for a productive infection to become established. In a process known as integration, the viral enzyme IN catalyzes the insertion of the double-stranded viral DNA into the host cell chromosome. Integration ensures that the viral DNA is maintained as a permanent part of the host's genetic material for the lifetime of the infected cell.

The integrated viral DNA, known as the provirus, serves as the template for the synthesis of viral RNAs. These viral RNAs are transported to the cytoplasm, where they are translated into the viral proteins. The Gag and Gag–pol polyproteins, together with full-length viral RNAs (two copies per virion), form the viral nucleocapsid. The nucleocapsids of C-type retroviruses and lentiviruses assemble at the plasma membrane; B-type and D-type retroviruses and spumaviruses assemble in the cytoplasm and are transported to the plasma membrane after assembly. During the budding process, the nucleocapsid is enveloped by a portion of the host cell plasma membrane in which are embedded the viral envelope glycoproteins. During or shortly after budding, the Gag and Gag–pol polyproteins are proteolytically cleaved by the viral PR, leading to core condensation and virion maturation. Cleavage by PR is required for the nascent virions to be infectious.

A schematic representation of mature virion is depicted in Fig. 2; a brief overview of the retrovirus life cycle is shown in Fig. 3.

V. OUTLOOK

Among the major challenges facing biomedical science today is the elucidation of the mechanism by which HIV causes disease in humans, and the effective treatment of patients infected with HIV. The first goal in meeting these challenges is a detailed understanding at the molecular level of the strategies utilized by retroviruses to infect and replicate in the host cell. Several fundamental properties of retroviruses, including the high degree of genetic variation between virus isolates and the ability to integrate into the host cell genome, make the development of vaccines and antiretroviral therapeutics particularly difficult. Understanding the effects of retroviruses on the host immune system, elucidating currently unknown aspects of the virus life cycle, and uncovering the details of the complex interplay between the numerous novel lentiviral gene products may all suggest novel approaches for the treatment of HIV infection. Recent progress in developing drugs which target the viral enzymes RT, NC, and PR

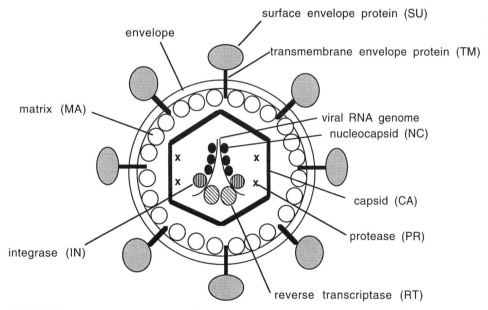

FIGURE 2 A mature retroviral virion. The position of the major proteins is indicated. This diagram is not intended to provide information about the size, abundance, or exact location of the various proteins.

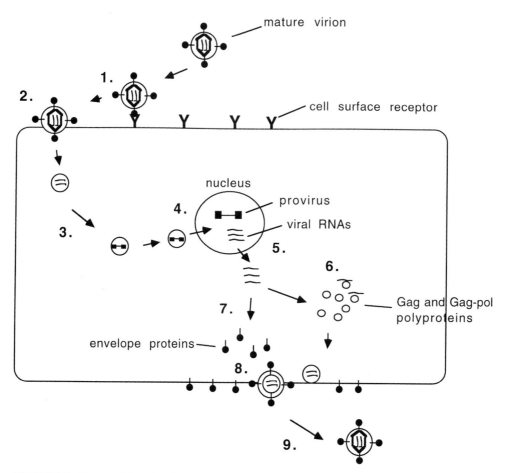

FIGURE 3 The virus life cycle. The virus indicated enters the cell by direct fusion at the plasma membrane and utilizes the C-type assembly pathway (i.e., assembly at the plasma membrane). The steps indicated are (1) receptor binding, (2) membrane fusion and entry, (3) uncoating and reverse transcription, (4) nuclear transport and integration, (5) transcription and RNA transport, (6) translation, Gag and Gag–pol transport, (7) Env transport, (8) virus assembly and budding, and (9) core condensation and virus maturation.

offers some hope for effective anti-HIV therapy in the near future.

See Also the Following Articles

DNA TUMOR VIRUSES: ADENOVIRUS • HEPATITIS B VIRUSES • HIV • HUMAN T-CELL LEUKEMIA/LYMPHOTROPIC VIRUS • IMMUNE DEFICIENCY: OPPORTUNISTIC TUMORS • RETROVIRAL VECTORS • VIRAL AGENTS

Bibliography

Coffin, J. M. (1996). Retroviridae: The viruses and their replication. In "Virology" (B. N. Fields, ed.), pp. 1767–1847. Lippincott-Raven, Philadelphia.

Freed, E. O., and Martin, M. A. (1995). The role of human immunodeficiency virus type 1 envelope glycoproteins in virus infection. *J. Biol. Chem.* **270,** 23883–23886.

Hunter, E. (1994). Macromolecular interactions in the assembly of HIV and other retroviruses. *Semin. Virol.* **5,** 71–83.

Luciw, P. A. (1996). Human immunodeficiency viruses and their replication. In "Virology" (B. N. Fields, eds.), pp. 1881–1952. Lippincott-Raven, Philadelphia.

Martin, M. A. (1993). The molecular and biological properties of the human immunodeficiency virus. In "The Molecular Basis of Blood Diseases" (Stamatoyannopoulos, Neinhuis, Majerus, and Varmus, eds.), pp. 863–908. Saunders, Philadelphia.

Temin, H. M., and Mizutani, S. (1970). RNA-dependent DNA polymerase in virions of Rous sarcoma virus. *Nature* **226,** 1211–1213.

Vaishnav, Y. N., and Wong-Staal, F. (1991). The biochemistry of AIDS. *Annu. Rev. Biochem.* **60,** 577–630.

Rhabdomyosarcoma, Early Onset

R. Beverly Raney
University of Texas M. D. Anderson Cancer Center

Harold M. Maurer
University of Nebraska Medical Center, Omaha

GLOSSARY

alveolar RMS A form of the disease that typically occurs on the extremities and trunk but may be present elsewhere.

botryoid RMS A variety of embryonal RMS that occurs within a hollow space or orifice such as the bladder or nasopharynx.

embryonal RMS A form of the disease that occurs primarily in the head and neck and genitourinary tract, but may arise elsewhere.

rhabdomyosarcoma (RMS) A malignant tumor arising from primitive mesenchyme anywhere in the body (except bone).

R habdomyosarcoma (RMS) is the most common soft tissue sarcoma in the first two decades of life. It is the fifth most common type of solid tumor in children and adolescents, after brain tumors, lymphoma, neuroblastoma, and Wilms' tumor. Seventy percent of the patients are less than 10 years of age at the time of diagnosis, and the male to female ratio is 1.4:1. RMS is a highly heterogeneous tumor that comprises several histologic subtypes and can arise in virtually any tissue of the body other than bone. The major regions affected are the head and neck, extremities, trunk, and genitourinary tract. RMS is highly malignant and can spread directly into surrounding structures, via lymphatics into regional lymph nodes, and/or by venous invasion into the bloodstream. Distant metastases can occur anywhere, but are found most commonly in the lungs, liver, bones, bone marrow, and distant soft tissues and lymph nodes. Because of the multiplicity of primary sites, there are various options for treatment. The most successful approach is multidisciplinary, combining surgery, radiotherapy, chemotherapy, and psychosocial programs for the needs of each individual. Thirty years ago, the likelihood of long-term survival after the diagnosis of RMS was about 20 to 25%, but now this figure is up to 70 to 75%. Much of the success comes from clinical trials conducted by the Intergroup Rhabdomyosarcoma Study Group (IRSG), which was formed in 1972 by pediatric cancer cooperative groups under the guidance of the National Cancer Institute in Bethesda, Maryland.

I. HISTOLOGIC TYPES AND PATHOBIOLOGY

About 60% of patients have the embryonal (E) form of RMS, so designated because of similarity of the tumor cells to those of embryonic muscle cells. Another 5% have the botryoid type of ERMS, so called because the tumor grossly resembles a bunch of grapes; these tumors arise within an orifice or hollow structure of the body such as the vagina, bladder, or nasopharynx. About 20% of patients have alveolar (A) RMS, so designated because the tumor cells are often arranged in a circular formation around what appear to be empty spaces, reminiscent of the architecture of lung tissue. The remaining 15% of the tumors are not readily classified into one of the subtypes because of insufficient tissue or poor preservation of the material.

The relatively unfavorable outlook for patients with ARMS as opposed to ERMS/botryoid RMS was noted in the mid-1970s. The exact basis of the histologic differences is unknown. There are also genetic differences between these types of tumors. The overwhelming majority of ARMS tumors have a translocation involving chromosomes 2 and 13 [t(2;13) (q35;q14)] or 1 and 13 [t(1;13)(p36;q14)]. There are differences in the types of patients affected according to which chromosomal abnormality is present, and eventually there may be a

way to exploit these differences in a therapeutic manner. There is no consistent translocation present in tumors from patients with ERMS. The ability to obtain and store tissue centrally for future research may ultimately provide answers to many questions about etiology and therapy of these different forms of RMS.

II. CLINICAL GROUPING AND STAGING

The initial evaluation of patients requires a detailed physical examination along with complete blood count, chemistries, bone marrow aspirate, and biopsy. Imaging studies of the primary tumor and likely sites of metastases (regional nodes, lungs, and bones, including the liver for those with tumors below the chest cavity) are also needed, as well as a spinal fluid sample from patients with cranial parameningeal tumors. A grouping system was devised by the IRSG in 1972 to categorize patients according to the amount of residual tumor present at the time of diagnosis, prior to initiating chemotherapy. This surgical–pathologic system is shown in Table I. Patients with localized tumors have either no residual disease after surgical removal (group I), microscopic residual and/or removed, tumor-involved regional lymph nodes (group II), or gross residual disease (group III). Patients presenting with metastases are in group IV. The outlook for survival is affected by the initial group, with those in group I having the most favorable prognosis and those with group IV disease the least.

Later it became necessary to devise a complementary system, based on the site and size of the primary

TABLE I
IRSG Surgical–Pathologic Grouping System

Clinical group	Definition
I	Localized tumor, completely removed with pathologically clear margins and no regional lymph node involvement
II	Localized tumor, grossly removed with (a) microscopically involved margins, (b) involved, grossly resected regional lymph nodes, or (c) both
III	Localized tumor, with gross residual disease after grossly incomplete removal, or biopsy only
IV	Distant metastases present at diagnosis

tumor (T) and the presence or absence of regional nodal (N) involvement and of distant metastases (M), called the TNM system. Table II shows the components of this system. Both group and stage are currently used to place patients into different cohorts for treatment purposes, with chemotherapy largely determined by the stage and radiotherapy by the group.

III. SURGICAL CONSIDERATIONS

A. Primary Tumor Removal

It is preferable to remove the tumor completely at the outset with a wide local excision when the result is expected to be acceptable with regard to subsequent function and cosmesis. This procedure is often possible for tumors arising in the extremities or on the trunk, but it may be difficult or inadvisable for tumors arising in the head and neck. In addition, it is important to try to preserve organ function. Thus, in patients with tumors arising in the orbit and bladder, an attempt is made to preserve those structures by using chemotherapy and radiotherapy (XRT) to destroy residual tumor following diagnosis by biopsy. For vaginal tumors, biopsy is followed by chemotherapy because the goal is to avoid XRT in such patients, who are often infants.

Frequently more than one surgical procedure is necessary. The first situation is when the initial procedure was not a wide local excision. IRSG data show that at primary reexcision one can often remove unsuspected residual localized tumor and convert a patient from group II or III into group I, thereby improving prognosis and perhaps avoiding the need for XRT. The other situation occurs in patients with large and/or poorly situated tumors in the intrathoracic/diaphragmatic region or in the retroperitoneum/pelvis. Initiating treatment with chemotherapy, rather than starting with a long and difficult operation, can often produce enough tumor shrinkage that a resection can be more safely and easily performed later.

B. Regional Lymph Node Evaluation

If the regional lymph nodes are large on clinical or radiographic examination, they should be biopsied so as to establish the extent of disease with certainty. XRT is given to the regional lymph nodes if tumor is found within them, but can be withheld if the nodes are merely hyperplastic.

The sentinel lymph node technique is currently the best way to identify a tumor-involved node. This procedure involves injecting both a vital dye (e.g., methylene blue) and a radioactive tracer material (e.g., technetium 99m sulfur colloid) into the region around the primary tumor site. The surgeon then makes an incision over the node-bearing area where the greatest amount of radioemitter is and then removes the node that has been stained by the dye. If that node (including any others that are visibly stained or "hot") is free of tumor on pathologic examination, the patient is considered to have uninvolved regional nodes. This procedure has a high level of accuracy and also obviates the need for lymph node dissection.

TABLE II
IRSG Staging System

Stage	Sites of primary tumor[a]	Tumor width	Regional lymph nodes[b]	Distant metastases[c]
1	Orbit, non-PM head/neck; GU nonbladder/prostate; biliary tract	Any size	N0	M0
2	All other sites	≤ 5 cm	N0	M0
3	All other sites	≤ 5 cm, N1; or > 5 cm, N0 or N1		M0
4	Any site	Any size	N0 or N1	M1

[a]PM, parameningeal; GU, genitourinary.
[b]N0, regional nodes not clinically involved by tumor; N1, regional nodes clinically involved by tumor.
[c]M0, no distant metastases; M1, distant metastases at diagnosis.

A particular subset of patients, those 10 years of age and older with paratesticular RMS, should undergo a modified ipsilateral retroperitoneal lymph node dissection because of an increased risk of disease in those nodes.

IV. RADIATION THERAPY

There are general principles that help to indicate the volume to be treated with XRT. The extent of disease should be imaged carefully at the time of diagnosis, preferably with magnetic resonance scans, so that the margins are clearly defined for subsequent irradiation. Currently, only high-voltage (≥ 4 MV) equipment is used. The tumor volume at the time of diagnosis plus a margin of 2 cm is usually considered the clinical target volume. Exceptions occur when treating an extremity because some of the regional lymphatics should be excluded from the field in order to prevent lymphedema. The volume can also be reduced when treating a pelvic tumor that initially caused bladder obstruction, later relieved by chemotherapy, so as to reduce the amount of radiation to the bladder.

An important new concept is the use of computer-assisted imaging techniques that facilitate planning multiple fields that conform to the often irregular target volume. With this "conformal" approach, the radiation oncologist can design fields that encompass the tumor with acceptable margin but which also minimize the risk of giving a high dose to surrounding normal tissue.

The IRS-IV protocol included a randomized study of twice-daily XRT at 1.1 Gray (Gy) per fraction (total dose, 59.4 Gy) versus conventional, once-daily doses of 1.8 Gy (total dose, 50.4 Gy) for patients with group III (gross residual disease) tumors. The hope was that local control rates would be increased in those receiving the higher dose, twice-daily program. At present, there is no statistically significant difference, and thus conventional fractionation remains the standard.

Members of the International Society of Paediatric Oncology (SIOP) have attempted to avoid giving XRT to patients with orbital tumors to prevent subsequent cataract formation. Their results show that about 40% of children respond to chemotherapy alone and become long-term survivors. The drawback of this approach is that the local recurrence rate is unduly high. Many of

those who relapse will eventually lose the eye, and some will not survive. IRS-III and -IV patients with orbital tumors have a survival rate of nearly 100%, and thus XRT continues to be a part of the treatment plan for nearly all patients with orbital sarcoma in the United States.

V. CHEMOTHERAPY

In four successive randomized clinical trials, the IRSG has attempted to use new agents to improve survival rates for children with gross residual disease and metastases at diagnosis whose outcome is consistently worse than that of children with localized tumors that have been removed prior to beginning chemotherapy. Despite their individual activity against RMS, doxorubicin, cisplatin, etoposide, and ifosfamide have failed to improve survival significantly (i.e., $P > 0.05$) in these studies. The current standard chemotherapeutic approaches are to give vincristine and actinomycin D (VA) to patients with the best prognosis and VAC (VA + cyclophosphamide) to the others.

VI. THE INTERGROUP RHABDOMYOSARCOMA-V STUDY

The IRS-V study combines the group and stage systems to allocate patients to three different therapeutic protocols according to risk of recurrence. Low-risk patients have an estimated 3-year failure-free survival (FFS) rate of 88%, intermediate-risk patients have an estimated 3-year FFS rate of 55 to 76%, and high-risk patients have a 3-year FFS rate of <30%. Multidisciplinary treatment is used, with recommendations specific to the tumors' histologic subtype and primary site, as well as to the patients' extent of disease at diagnosis and response to treatment. The goal is to achieve local control with preservation of as much form and function as possible.

A. Chemotherapy

Low-risk patients have localized ERMS in favorable sites (stage 1) or in unfavorable sites (stages 2 and 3) that have been grossly completely removed, with or without microscopic residual disease and/or resected, tumor-involved regional lymph nodes. Patients with the best prognosis are placed in subgroup A: these have no macroscopic residual disease after surgery (except orbital tumors) and receive VA with or without XRT. The others, placed in subgroup B, receive VAC ± XRT. Intermediate-risk patients have (1) localized ARMS or undifferentiated sarcoma (UDS), stages 1–3; (2) localized ERMS, stages 2 and 3 with gross residual disease; or (3) ERMS with metastases at <10 years of age at diagnosis. They are randomized to receive VAC or VAC alternating with VC plus topotecan, along with XRT. High-risk patients have ARMS or UDS at any age <21 years, or ERMS at <10 years of age, with metastases at diagnosis. They receive a trial of irinotecan plus vincristine over 6 weeks followed by VAC. Irinotecan is continued at intervals for those who responded to it initially, but is omitted for nonresponders. Patients with cranial parameningeal tumors and meningeal impingement at diagnosis receive VAC without irinotecan.

B. Radiation Therapy

Patients with completely excised ERMS (i.e., group I) receive no XRT because giving it provided no statistically significant advantage in FFS. In contrast, patients with completely resected (group I) ARMS and UDS receive XRT to the primary site because the FFS was improved in such patients treated on IRS-I through -III. Other patients receive XRT according to the amount of residual disease. Patients with metastases receive XRT to the primary tumor and to sites of metastases, within the limits of bone marrow tolerance. The total doses are outlined in the respective protocols.

See Also the Following Articles

BONE TUMORS • GERM CELL TUMORS • PAX3–FKHR AND PAX7–FKHR GENE FUSIONS IN ALVEOLAR RHABDOMYOSARCOMA • PEDIATRIC CANCERS, MOLECULAR FEATURES • SARCOMAS OF SOFT TISSUES

Bibliography

Barr, F. G. (1997). Molecular genetics and pathogenesis of rhabdomyosarcoma. *J. Pediatr. Hematol./Oncol.* **19**, 483–491.

Crist, W. M., Anderson, J. R., Meza, J. L., *et al.* (2001). Intergroup rhabdomyosarcoma study-IV: Results for patients with nonmetastatic disease. *J. Clin. Oncol.* **19**, 3091–3102.

Crist, W., Gehan, E. A., Ragab, A. H., *et al.* (1995). The third Intergroup Rhabdomyosarcoma Study. *J. Clin. Oncol.* **13**, 610–630.

Hays, D. M., Lawrence, W., Jr., Wharam, M., *et al.* (1989). Primary reexcision for patients with "microscopic residual" tumor following initial excision of sarcomas of trunk and extremity sites. *J. Pediatr. Surg.* **24**, 5–10.

Kelly, K. M., Womer, R. B., Sorensen, P. H. B., Xiong, Q.-B., and Barr, F. G. (1997). Common and variant gene fusions predict distinct clinical phenotypes in rhabdomyosarcoma. *J. Clin. Oncol.* **15**, 1831–1836.

Lawrence, W., Jr., Anderson, J. R., Gehan, E. A., *et al.* (1997). Pretreatment TNM staging of childhood rhabdomyosarcoma: A report of the Intergroup Rhabdomyosarcoma Study Group. *Cancer* **80**, 1165–1170.

Maurer, H. M., Beltangady, M., Gehan, E. A., *et al.* (1988). The Intergroup Rhabdomyosarcoma Study-I: A final report. *Cancer* **61**, 209–220.

Maurer, H. M., Gehan, E. A., Beltangady, M., *et al.* (1993). The Intergroup Rhabdomyosarcoma Study-II. *Cancer* **71**, 1904–1922.

Michalski, J. M., Sur, R. K., Harms, W. B., *et al.* (1995). Three dimensional conformal radiation therapy in pediatric parameningeal rhabdomyosarcomas. *Int. J. Radiat. Oncol. Biol. Phys.* **33**, 985–991.

Neville, H. L., Andrassy, R. J., Lally, K. P., Corpron, C., and Ross, M. I. (2000). Lymphatic mapping with sentinel node biopsy in pediatric patients. *J. Pediatr. Surg.* **35**, 961–964.

Newton, W. A., Jr., Soule, E. H., Hamoudi, A. B., *et al.* (1988). Histopathology of childhood sarcomas, Intergroup Rhabdomyosarcoma Studies I and II: Clinicopathologic correlations. *J. Clin. Oncol.* **6**, 67–75.

Raney, R. B., Jr., Hays, D. M., Tefft, M., and Triche, T. J. (1993). Rhabdomyosarcoma and the undifferentiated sarcomas. *In* "Principles and Practice of Pediatric Oncology" (P. A. Pizzo and D. G. Poplack, eds.), 2nd Ed., pp. 769–794. Lippincott, Philadelphia.

Rousseau, P., Flamant, F., Quintana, E., *et al.* (1994). Primary chemotherapy in rhabdomyosarcomas and other malignant mesenchymal tumors of the orbit: Results of the International Society of Pediatric Oncology MMT 84 Study. *J. Clin. Oncol.* **12**, 516–521.

Wharam, M. D., Anderson, J. R., Laurie, F., *et al.* (1997). Failure-free survival for orbit rhabdomyosarcoma patients on Intergroup Rhabdomyosarcoma Study IV (IRS-IV) is improved compared to IRS-III. *Proc. Am. Soc. Clin. Oncol.* **16**, 518a. [Abstract 1864]

Wiener, E. S., Anderson, J. R., Ojimba, J. I., *et al.* (2001). Controversies in the management of paratesticular rhabdomyosarcoma: Is staging retroperitoneal lymph node dissection necessary for adolescents with resected paratesticular rhabdomyosarcoma? *Semin. Pediatr. Surg.* **10**, 146–152.

Wolden, S. L., Anderson, J. R., Crist, W. M., *et al.* (1999). Indications for radiotherapy and chemotherapy after complete resection in rhabdomyosarcoma: A report from the Intergroup Rhabdomyosarcoma Studies I to III. *J. Clin. Oncol.* **17**, 3468–3475.

Ribozymes and Their Applications

Helen A. James

University of East Anglia, Norwich

I. Introduction
II. Types of Ribozyme
III. Applications
IV. Future Prospects

GLOSSARY

clinical trial Research study with patients, usually to evaluate a new treatment or drug.

enzymes Catalysts (most commonly proteins) produced by cells that act in specific biochemical reactions, without being destroyed or altered themselves upon completion of the reaction.

gene therapy Treatment of a disease caused by the malfunction of a gene (or a viral gene), by the addition to the cells of a normal gene, or the alteration, elimination, or repair of the abnormal gene.

oncogene A gene that can potentially induce neoplastic transformation (cancer), transforming a normal cell into a cancerous tumor cell.

ribonucleic acid (RNA) A nucleic acid that traditionally plays a role in transferring information from DNA (genes) to proteins of the cell.

ribozyme An RNA with catalytic (enzymatic) capacity, often catalyzing the breakdown of other RNA molecules.

transduction The transfer of a gene to modify the phenotype of a cell.

O ne of the more recent important discoveries in the fields of cell and molecular biology was that of Cech and Altman in the early 1980s. They found that ribonucleic acid (RNA) molecules, once thought to be primarily passive carriers of genetic information, could carry out functions that had been ascribed to proteins. Some RNA molecules are capable of acting as catalysts, acting upon themselves or other RNA molecules. Most naturally occurring ribozymes act upon themselves (intramolecular). However, with the identification of the features that allow ribozymes to bind and cleave their substrates, ribozymes have been designed to cleave novel RNA substrates intermolecularly. These custom-designed RNAs have great potential as therapeutic agents and are becoming a powerful tool for molecular biologists.

I. INTRODUCTION

It has long been recognized that RNA has many roles in the cell. Messenger RNA (mRNA) transfers the information contained within DNA to the protein-forming system of the cell. Transfer RNA (tRNA) is also involved in the information transfer system, in this case by carrying specific amino acids to the ribosome to be added to the growing protein chain. Ribosomal RNA (rRNA) can be considered as having a structural role as part of the permanent structure of the ribosome. It may also have a catalytic role in the formation of peptide bonds during protein synthesis. Small nuclear RNAs (snRNAs) are involved in splicing. This process generates mature mRNA from the original transcript. RNA can also act as a store for genetic information: certain viruses have RNA genomes. More recently, it has been shown that RNA can act as a catalyst, involved in processes such as tRNA maturation and the rolling circle replication of small pathogenic RNAs.

The enzymatic nature of RNA was first identified by Cech and colleagues for the self-splicing group I intron of *Tetrahymena thermophila* and by Altman and colleagues for the RNA moiety of ribonuclease P (RNase P). Since then, catalytic RNA motifs have been found in more examples of group I introns, some group II introns, many small plant pathogenic RNAs and associated RNAs, a satellite RNA from *Neurospora* mitochondria, and in human hepatitis delta virus.

An RNA catalyst, or ribozyme, is an RNA molecule that has the intrinsic ability to break and/or form covalent bonds. Like its protein counterpart, a ribozyme greatly accelerates the rate of a biochemical reaction and shows exquisite specificity with respect to the substrates it acts upon and the products it produces.

Every naturally occurring ribozyme acts upon itself, apart from RNase P. However, the ribozymes can be modified so that they can act on an independent RNA, i.e., act in *trans*. People such as Uhlenbeck, Haseloff and Gerlach, Szostak, and Zaug and Cech pioneered the design of these so-called *trans*-acting ribozymes.

II. TYPES OF RIBOZYME

Ribozymes can cleave either the 3' carbon-phosphate (C-O-P) bond or the 5' C-O-P bond of a phosphodiester linkage in an RNA molecule, resulting in 3' hy-

droxyl (OH) and 5'phosphate or 5'OH and 2'3' cyclic phosphate termini, respectively. The phosphodiester bonds of RNA are normally exceedingly unreactive chemical species. However, it is thought that the folded RNA structure of the ribozyme confers reactivity to selected bonds, making them more prone to nucleophilic attack. Several different catalytic RNA structures, or motifs, have been identified (Table I).

A. Self-splicing RNAs

Within various gene transcripts, several group I and group II introns have been shown to be capable of excising themselves from the exons, subsequently catalyzing the ligation of the exons (self-splicing). This was first demonstrated for the intron of the nuclear 26S ribosomal RNA gene in *Tetrahymena*. The excised intron can be converted into a true enzyme, with the ability to act in *trans* on novel substrates. Some group II introns were also shown to have self-cleaving ability that could be converted to act in *trans*. This has led to the development of *trans*-splicing ribozymes, allowing modification of a target RNA.

B. RNase P

Precursor-transfer RNA (pre-tRNA) molecules are processed by a different type of ribozyme called ribonuclease P. RNase P is a ubiquitous endoribonuclease that consists of both RNA and protein components. It was demonstrated that the RNA moiety had catalytic activity. As such, it is the only true RNA enzyme identified so far to occur naturally. As with catalytic introns, the substrate upon which RNase P acts upon can be changed by desire. This is done by the addition of a short RNA called an external guide sequence (EGS) that is complementary to the target RNA. The EGS–target RNA complex mimics pre-tRNA and acts as a substrate for RNase P cleavage activity.

C. Small Self-cleaving RNAs

A number of small plant pathogenic RNAs (viroids, satellite RNAs, and virusoids), an RNA transcript from satellite II DNA of the newt, a transcript from a *Neurospora* mitochondrial DNA plasmid, and an animal virus, hepatitis delta virus, all undergo a self-cleavage reaction *in vitro* in the absence of protein.

TABLE I

Types of Ribozyme

Ribozyme type	Normal function	Normal products	Cofactors required in vitro[a]	Adaped function	Products
Group I introns e.g., intron in 26S rRNA gene of *Tetrahymena*	Splicing	Spliced exons (3′ hydroxyl, 5′ phosphate intermediates)	GMP, GDP, or GTP Mg^{2+}	*trans* cleavage of novel RNA substrates *trans* splicing	3′ hydroxyl, 5′ phosphate Replaced 3′ part of targeted RNA with new sequence
Group II introns e.g., intron 5γ of the oxi 3 gene	Splicing	Spliced exons	Mg^{2+} spermidine	Cleavage of single–stranded DNA *trans* splicing	3′ hydroxyl, 5′ phosphate Replaced 3′ part of targeted RNA with new sequence
Ribonuclease P e.g., M1 RNA and C5 protein of *E. coli*	Pre-tRNA maturation	tRNA 3′ hydroxyl, 5′ phosphate	Divalent metal ion	Cleavage of novel RNA substrates by means of an external guide sequence	3′ hydroxyl, 5′ phosphate Destruction of target RNA
Self-cleaving RNAs *hammerhead* e.g, +sTRSV[b] *hairpin* e.g., −sTRSV[b]	Rolling circle replication of small pathogenic RNAs	2′,3′ cyclic phosphate 5′ hydroxyl Monomeric RNA transcripts from concatamers	Mg^{2+}	*trans* cleavage of novel substrates	2′,3′ cyclic phosphate, 5′ hydroxyl Destruction of target RNA

[a]GMP, guanosine 5′-monophosphate; GDP, guanosine 5′-diphosphate; GTP, guanosine 5′-triphosphate.
[b]Satellite RNA of tobacco ringspot virus.

The self-cleaving RNAs can be subdivided into groups depending on the sequence and secondary structure formed about the cleavage site. The majority of self-cleaving RNAs share one of two structural motifs, the so-called hammerhead and hairpin motifs.

1. Hammerhead Ribozymes

The hammerhead ribozyme consists of a catalytic core flanked by two arms, the sequence of which can be modified to base pair with the substrate RNA on either side of the cleavage site. Extensive mutagenesis studies have shown that, in theory, any UH sequence (where U is uracil and H is adenine, cytosine, or uracil) in the target RNA can be recognized by the ribozyme and subsequently cleaved. Hence, any RNA can be cleaved by ribozymes. The simplicity of the hammerhead motif has made it a favorite for *trans* cleavage applications.

2. Hairpin Ribozymes

The other favored *trans* catalytic motif is the hairpin ribozyme, which was first identified as the *cis*-cleaving domain of the negative strand of tobacco ringspot satellite RNA. The catalytic motif is slightly more complex than the hammerhead, but the way in which it recognizes its target RNA, by base pairing between complementary sequences either side of the cleavage site, is the same.

III. APPLICATIONS

Through the ability of ribozymes to form base pairs with complementary sequences, they can be designed to interact with any novel RNA. With this, and their ability to subsequently cleave the RNA they are base paired to, ribozymes are ideal specific agents to use against the mRNAs of important genes found to be linked with disease (of both cellular and viral origin).

The identification of specific endogenous or viral gene products as a cause of acute or chronic disease has led to research to develop gene suppression or modification strategies. It is theoretically reasonable to use the gene-suppressing activities of ribozymes for the treatment of such diseases. This gene-suppressing activity can also be used as a tool by molecular and cell biologists to determine the function of an unknown gene. Figure 1 demonstrates the possible approaches for suppressing or modifying gene activity using different types of ribozymes.

A. Delivery of Ribozymes to Cells

There are two general approaches for introducing catalytic RNA molecules into cells: (1) endogenous expression of a ribozyme gene from a transcriptional unit and (2) exogenous delivery of a preformed ribozyme.

Endogenous delivery depends on the efficient transfer of the ribozyme-encoding gene into the cell. This approach, where the ribozyme gene is under the control of an RNA polymerase (pol) II, pol III, or viral promoter, could be described as ribozyme gene therapy. It has been achieved by inserting ribozyme sequences into the untranslated regions of genes transcribed by pol II, such as the actin gene. Pol III promoters such as those from small nuclear RNA or tRNA genes have been successfully used, as have tissue-specific promoters such as the tyrosinase promoter. However, both retroviral-derived and adeno associated virus (AAV)-derived vectors are commonly used to express ribozymes. The advantages with retroviral vectors include high transduction efficiencies and the integration of the ribozyme gene into the host genome. Several studies have compared the expression levels and effectiveness of ribozymes from different promoters. Long terminal repeat (LTR) promoters tend to produce the highest amount of ribozyme transcript, but factors such as ribozyme colocalization with the target mRNA were more important for effectiveness.

Alternatively, ribozymes can be synthesized chemically and delivered to cells already preformed. For this approach, chemical modification of the RNA is required to make the ribozymes stable against ribonucleases. However, stabilization should not compromise catalytic efficiency. Another limitation is the means by which the modified ribozymes cross the cell membrane. Some method for temporarily permeabilizing the cell membrane to facilitate entry (e.g., electroporation) or aiding the ribozyme across the membrane (e.g., liposomes) is required.

B. Ribozymes as a Tool for Molecular and Cell Biologists

Ribozymes can be used to generate loss-of-function phenotypes to elucidate the roles of various genes. This

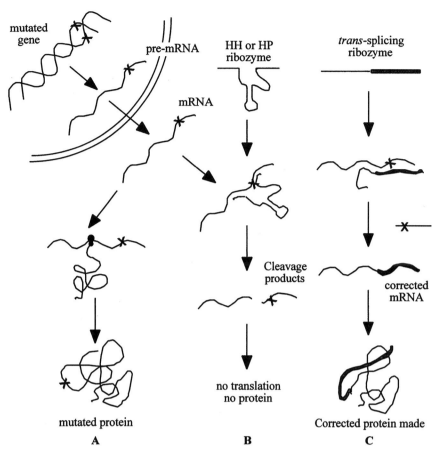

FIGURE 1 Site of action of ribozyme activity. Transcription and translation (A) of a mutated gene (e.g., an oncogene) or a viral gene can be prevented by ribozymes. (B) Binding and subsequent cleavage of the mutated mRNA by a hammerhead (HH) ribozyme [the same would apply for a hairpin (HP) ribozyme]. (C) Correction of the mutated mRNA with a *trans*-splicing group I intron ribozyme. Reprinted with permission from "Therapeutic potential of ribozymes in haematological disorders." *Exp. Opin. Invest. Drugs* **9**(5), 1009–1020 (2000) (Ashley Publications Ltd.).

has been performed for the *fushi targu* (*ftz*) gene in *Drosophila*. The study confirmed the *ftz* gene as a pair-rule gene during development. Ribozymes were also used to attenuate *white* gene expression and suppress eye pigmentation. Gene function analysis has also been carried out with ribozymes in zebrafish. The recessive dominant no-tail gene was effectively inhibited using a transient ribozyme expression system injected into fertilized eggs. A phenotype identical to that of a known defective mutation in the same gene was produced.

Ribozymes have been used to elucidate roles of the c-*fos* protooncogene and the matrix metalloproteinase 2 (gelatinase A) and for demonstrating that p16 (INK4a) has roles in fundamental processes such as homeostatic tissue renewal, protection against onco-genic transformation, and cellular senescence. Several ribozyme transgenic mice have been generated to further examine the roles of various genes *in vivo*. Hammerhead ribozymes have been used in structural studies of ribosomal 5S RNAs.

Through recent advances, it has become possible to tailor the activity of ribozymes to respond allosterically to specific effector compounds. For example, appending a well-characterized RNA motif that specifically binds ATP to the hammerhead ribozyme yields an ATP-sensitive ribozyme whose activity is inhibited 18-fold by ATP binding. Data from such studies suggest that allosteric ribozymes possess significant potential as genetic control elements, biosensor components, or controllable therapeutic agents.

C. Ribozymes as Potential Therapeutic Agents

The therapeutic use of ribozymes in a clinical setting is clearly an attractive goal. Because all genes are expressed via RNA intermediates, the potential applications of ribozymes are only limited by our knowledge of the disease and the genes involved.

1. Cancer

Cancer can be considered a genetic disease that arises from a combination of gain of function of some genes (oncogenes) and loss of function of others (tumor suppressor genes). The mutations that activate oncogenes, be it a point mutation or chromosome translocation, make that sequence unique to the cancer cells. Provided that there is a ribozyme cleavage site adjacent to, or ideally created by, the mutation, ribozymes can be designed to target the oncogenic mRNA and thus cleave and reduce or hopefully eliminate the oncogenic gene expression.

The activating mutation of the oncogene H-*ras* at codon 12, GGU → GUU, creates a cleavage site for the hammerhead ribozyme. The wild-type H-*ras* would not be cleaved by the hammerhead ribozyme, as GGU is not a suitable sequence for cleavage. Such a specific targeting has been demonstrated. The tumorigenicity of H-*ras*-transformed NIHT3 cells in nude mice was abrogated by the expression of an anti-H-*ras* ribozyme. A reduction of mutant H-*ras* expression was concomitant with a partial or complete reversion of the phenotypic characteristics of the cells.

Ribozymes against the nuclear protooncogenes c-*fos* and c-*myc* affected cell proliferation. Targeting of the c-*fos* gene by ribozymes resulted in increased sensitivity to the chemotherapeutic agent cisplatin after expression in resistant cells. Expression of a hammerhead ribozyme against Bcl-2 mRNA induced apoptosis and restored the ability of the cells to respond to secondary apoptotic agents in low and high bcl-2 expressing prostate cancer cell lines, respectively.

Fusion genes created by chromosome translocations are good targets for sequence-specific technologies such as ribozymes. Hybrid genes being targeted by ribozymes include the AML1/MTG8 mRNA that results from the t(8;21) translocation of acute myeloid leukemia (AML) and the bcr-abl mRNA of the

t(9;22) of chronic myeloid leukemia (CML). In the latter case, effects such as a decrease in mRNA and protein levels and a decrease in bcr-abl kinase activity and in cell proliferation due to anti-bcr-abl ribozymes have all been observed. Colony formation suppression and a reduction in tumor formation in SCID mice have been obtained with ribozyme treatment of bcr-abl containing cells. Figure 2 shows an *in vitro* cleavage reaction of bcr-abl RNA by a hammerhead ribozyme.

Reactivation of telomerase is a common event in human tumors. Telomerase is thought to be essential in maintaining the proliferative capacity of tumor cells and therefore represents an attractive target for ribozymes. A hammerhead ribozyme has been shown to inhibit telomerase activity in cell extracts from a human melanoma cell line. This inhibition was also observed when the ribozyme was transfected into the cell line. The transfected cells had a longer doubling time than the control cells, but no telomere shortening was observed.

Metastasis, or the spread and development of secondary tumors, is a huge problem for the treatment of cancer. Ribozymes against MMP-9 (a matrix metallo-

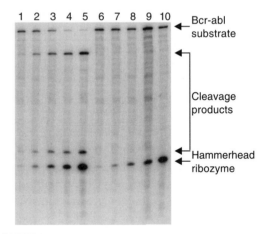

FIGURE 2 *In vitro* hammerhead ribozyme cleavage of a shortened bcr-abl substrate. Substrate RNA was incubated with an active (lanes 1–5) or inactive (lanes 6–10) hammerhead ribozyme at the following ribozyme:substrate molar ratios: 1:5 (lanes 1 and 6), 1:2 (lanes 2 and 7), 1:1 (lanes 3 and 8), 2:1 (lanes 4 and 9), and 5:1 (lanes 5 and 10). Cleavage products can be seen in lanes 1–5 where the ribozyme has cleaved the bcr-abl RNA at the expected position. The reaction was carried out in a buffer of 50 mM Tris–HCl, pH 8.0; 20 mM $MgCl_2$ for 2 h at 50°C. The samples were subjected to electrophoresis in a 4% polyacrylamide/8 M urea/1 × TBE gel.

proteinase involved in metastasis) have been shown to slow down metastasis in a rat sarcoma model system.

The phenomenon of drug resistance of tumor cells to chemotherapeutic drugs is yet another problem to be faced when treating cancers. Many tumors are intrinsically resistant, whereas others acquire resistance. There are a number of causes for the cells' drug resistance, one of which is the increased expression of P-glycoprotein from the multidrug resistance gene *mdr*-1. Hammerhead ribozymes targeted to the *mdr*-1 sequence have been shown to reduce drug resistance in previously resistant cell lines.

The growth of malignant cells from patients with juvenile myelomonocytic leukemia is postulated to be supported by TNF-α autocrine stimulation of granulocyte-macrophage colony-stimulating factor (GM-CSF). A ribozyme against TNF-α was shown to knock out not just TNF-α mRNA but GM-CSF mRNA as well, confirming the hypothesis and potentially opening up a new avenue for treatment.

2. Viral Diseases

Diseases that result from viral infections are suitable targets for ribozyme methodology, as the viral RNA sequences are unique to the infected cell. A number of different viruses are being targeted by both hammerhead and hairpin ribozymes, including the human immunodeficiency virus -1 (HIV-1).

It has been demonstrated several times that anti-HIV-1 hammerhead ribozyme expressing cells are resistant, to varying degrees, to HIV-1 infection and replication. When freshly isolated, noninfected, peripheral blood lymphocytes (PBLs) were transduced with a hammerhead ribozyme gene, they were resistant toward challenge with HIV-1 clones and clinical isolates. Nontransduced cells were fully permissive for HIV infection. Cells from already infected HIV-1 patients have also been examined in this manner. Ribozyme expressing cells can be up to 1000-fold more resistant to HIV-1 replication than unmodified cells. It is not just viral sequences that can be targeted by ribozymes. The receptor CCR5 is crucial for HIV-1 infection of a cell. The CCR5 receptor mRNA is being targeted by ribozymes in order to inhibit infection. All these encouraging preclinical data have led to several clinical trials of ribozymes against HIV-1 (Table II).

Other viruses are also being investigated as potential targets for therapeutic ribozymes. The human T-cell leukemia virus etiologically associated with adult T-cell leukemia has been targeted by ribozymes. Viral mRNA and protein levels were shown to be reduced. Hepatitis B and C viruses, Epstein–Barr virus, and Influenza A virus are also under investigation.

Nonviral infections are another potential application. In one study, a reduction in the viability of the human malaria parasite *Plasmodium falciparum* was achieved after treatment with ribozymes.

3. Hemoglobin Disorders

Sickle cell anemia is the most common heritable hematological disease, yet there is no curative treatment. One proposal is to reduce the overall hemoglobin concentration in the cells to reduce the sickle polymerization potential. One way to do this is to target either the β sickle (β^S) globin or α globin mRNA transcripts with ribozymes. Decreased globin transcript levels have been detected, as has a decrease in β^S globin levels in transgenic mice, but it has yet to be determined whether the ribozymes have an effect on sickling. Recently, a completely different approach has been taken. Instead of using hammerhead ribozymes to cleave a mRNA, a *trans*-splicing group I intron ribozyme has been used. Lan and colleagues have shown that it is possible to replace the region in the β globin mRNA containing the sickle mutation with a fetal γ globin encoding sequence. The *trans*-splicing ribozyme recognizes the β^S mRNA by base pairing between complementary sequences. The β^S mRNA is then cleaved by the ribozyme, and the mutation encoding sequence is released. The ribozyme then joins the replacement γ sequence to the remaining β globin mRNA. This was demonstrated in primary human red blood cell precursors with high fidelity.

4. Coronary Artery Disease

Coronary artery disease remains the most widespread cause of mortality and serious morbidity in developed countries and is increasing in prevalence in the third world. The current treatments consist of medication, coronary bypass, and angioplasty (repair of blood vessel). Stents, tubes to keep the vessel open, are often inserted into the artery during angioplasty. Unfortunately, in-stent restenosis (a stent-induced narrowing

TABLE II

Ribozyme Clinical Trials[a]

Target	Ribozyme type	Company/organization involved	Additional information
HIV	Hammerhead (expressed from ribozyne gene)	Ribozyme Pharmaceuticals, Inc. (RPI)[b] Chiron Corporation[b] City of Hope National Medical Center Children's Hospital, Los Angeles	Phase II trials with CD34[+] cells from AIDS-related lymphoma patients
HIV	Hammerhead (expressed from ribozyne gene)	Gene Shears Pty Ltd., St. Vincent's Hospital, Sydney, Australia Gene Shears Pty Ltd., UCLA School of Medicine, UCLA AIDS Institute, CARE Center Los Angeles	Phase I trial with CD4[+] cells from uninfected twin to give to HIV-infected sibling Phase I trial CD34[+] cells from HIV[+] patients
HIV	Hairpin (expressed from ribozyne gene)	University of California, San Diego (UCSD) San Diego VA Healthcare System UCSD Gene Therapy Production Facility, Magenta Inc. National Gene Therapy Vector Laboratories	Phase I trial
Flt-1 (VEGFr)	Hammerhead (preformed) RPI.4610 or ANGIOZYME	RPI Chiron Corporation	Phase Ia/Ib completed Phase I/II dosing trial started
Hepatitis C virus	Hammerhead (preformed) LY-466700 or HEPTAZYME	RPI Eli Lilly	Phase I trial with normal volunteers completed Phase I trial with chronic hepatitis patients initiated

[a]As of June 2000.
[b]As of April 2000, RPI and Chiron announced that they were discontinuing this trial, City of Hope National Medical Center will continue.

of the artery) often occurs. The use of ribozymes to prevent restenosis is being investigated. Proliferating cell nuclear antigen (PCNA) is an important regulator of cell division, and blocking its expression after angioplasty may limit proliferation of the vascular smooth muscle cells causing restenosis. A hammerhead ribozyme against PCNA inhibited vascular smooth muscle cell growth *in vitro* and reduced restenosis in a porcine coronary model.

Overproduction of apolipoprotein B (ApoB) is positively associated with premature coronary artery diseases. ApoB gene expression has been modulated by hammerhead ribozymes in cell culture. The ribozymes cleaved the ApoB mRNA and a truncated protein was produced, which was subsequently degraded. In a second study, apolipoprotein A was targeted by ribozymes. Selective inhibition of the ApoA gene resulted. These approaches may provide novel therapeutic strategies for high ApoA or ApoB levels.

5. Retinitis Pigmentosa

Approximately 10% of patients with autosomal dominant retinitis pigmentosa (ADRP) carry a substitution at codon 25 in their rhodopsin gene. This causes the synthesis of an abnormal gene product, which results in photoreceptor cell death and, ultimately, blindness. Both hammerhead and hairpin ribozymes have been shown specifically to cleave the mutant rhodopsin mRNA but not the wild-type sequence *in vitro*. More recently, it has been demonstrated that the *in vivo* expression of either ribozyme in a rat model of ADRP considerably slows the rate of photoreceptor degeneration for at least 3 months. Ribozyme-directed cleavage of mutant mRNAs may therefore be an effective therapy for ADRP.

IV. FUTURE PROSPECTS

The examples described earlier by no means represent a comprehensive list of successful ribozyme applications (e.g., ribozymes and plants are not mentioned). They do, however, demonstrate the enormous potential number of applications of ribozymes to treat diseases in particular.

However, transferring ribozymes from the bench to clinical applications faces a number of hurdles to optimize efficacy: stability of the ribozyme, delivery of the ribozyme to the target cell, colocalization of ribozyme and target mRNA, and optimal cleavage. Despite these hurdles, several ribozymes (both hammerhead and hairpin) have been used in preliminary clinical trials (Table II). Four of the six trials have been investigating the potential of either hammerhead or hairpin ribozymes against HIV-1. Phase I trials have been conducted, and in the case of the Ribozyme Pharmaceuticals Inc. and Chiron trial, a more advanced trial is underway to look at the extent to which ribozyme containing cells are engrafted into the bone marrow of patients. In the two Gene Shears' trials, CD4$^+$ or, more recently, CD34$^+$ progenitor cells are being transduced with an anti-HIV-1 ribozyme. The trial at UCSD under the direction of Wong-Staal uses a hairpin ribozyme against HIV-1. Initial results indicate that the procedure is safe and that transduced cells persist for a considerable time.

RPI are also conducting clinical trials to test a hammerhead ribozyme (RPI.4610 or Angiozyme) against Flt-1, the receptor for VEGF (involved in angiogenesis or new blood vessel formation) and a hammerhead ribozyme against hepatitis C (LY-466700 or Heptazyme). A third ribozyme, Herzyme targeting Her-2 is approaching clinical trials. No ribozyme has yet to have a proven therapeutic advantage.

Much research driven by both private companies and publicly funded bodies is currently being undertaken to develop further the potential of the catalytic RNA. The chemical synthesis of RNA has undergone dramatic advances, leading to increasingly stable preformed ribozymes in the inter- and intracellular environments. Advances in vector design (due to the huge interest in gene therapy) have improved the delivery of ribozyme genes to their target cells. Despite these improvements, a clinically useful ribozyme is still some distance off. However, there is considerable enthusiasm and excitement over their potential both as tools to study gene function and as rationally designed therapeutic agents in particular.

Acknowledgments

The author thanks Dr. P. Hawley for her useful comments and suggestions. This work was supported by The Bryan Gunn Leukaemia Appeal, Norwich, UK, and Mrs. Pamela Salter.

See Also the Following Articles

Bibliography.

Amado, R. G., Mitsuyasu, R. T., Symonds, G., Rosenblatt, J. D., Zack, J., Sun, L.-Q., Miller, M., Ely, J., and Gerlach, W. (1999). A phase I trial of autologous CD34+ hematopoietic progenitor cells transduced with an anti-HIV ribozyme. *Hum. Gene Ther.* **10**, 2255–2270.

Cech, T. R., Zaug, A. J., and Grabowski, P. J. (1981). *In vitro* splicing of the ribosomal RNA precursor of Tetrahymena: Involvement of a guanosine nucleotide in the excision of the intervening sequence. *Cell* **27**, 487–496.

Guerrier-Takada, C., Gardiner, K., Marsh, T., Pace, N., and Altman, S. (1983). The RNA moiety of ribonuclease P is the catalytic subunit of the enzyme. *Cell* **35**, 849–857.

Haseloff, J., and Gerlach, W. L. (1988). Simple RNA enzymes with new and highly specific endoribonuclease activities. *Nature* **334**, 585–591.

James, H. A., and Gibson, I. (1998). The therapeutic potential of ribozymes. *Blood* **91**, 371–382.

Kruger, K., Grabowski, P. J., Zaug, A. J., Sands, J., Gottschling, D. E., and Cech, T. R. (1982). Self-splicing RNA: Autoexcision and autocyclization of the ribosomal RNA intervening sequence of Tetrahymena. *Cell* **31**, 147–157.

Lan, N., Howrey, R. P., Lee, S.-W., Smith, C. A., and Sullenger, B. A. (1998). Ribozyme-mediated repair of sickle β-globin mRNAs in erythrocyte precursors. *Science* **280**, 1593–1596.

Sullenger, B. A., and Cech, T. R. (1994). Ribozyme-mediated repair of defective mRNA by targeted *trans*-splicing. *Nature* **371**, 619–622.

Symons, R. H. (1992). Small catalytic RNAs. *Annu. Rev. Bioch.* **61**, 641–70.

Wong-Staal, F., Poeschla, E. M., and Looney, D. J. (1998). A controlled, phase 1 clinical trial to evaluate the safety and effects in HIV-1 infected humans of autologous lymphocytes transduced with a ribozyme that cleaves HIV-1 RNA. *Hum. Gene Ther.* **9**, 2407–2425.

Yuan, Y., and Altman, S. (1994). Selection of guide sequences that direct efficient cleavage of mRNA by human ribonuclease P. *Science* **263**, 1269–1273.

RUNX/CBF Transcription Factors

Dong-Er Zhang

The Scripps Research Institute

RUNX is a family of mammalian DNA-binding transcription factors that contain a highly homologous region to *Drosophila* runt protein, the runt homology domain (RHD) (Fig. 1). There are three members in the RUNX family (RUNX1, RUNX2, and RUNX3). RUNX is also called AML, CBFα, and PEBP2α due to the discovery of these proteins in different systems. The name AML comes from the cloning of its gene from a common form of chromosomal translocation t(8;21) associated with the development of acute myeloid leukemia. CBFα is from the purification of a protein—core binding factor—that interacts with the core site of several virus enhancers. PEBP2α is from the analysis of transcription factors bound to the enhancer of polyomavirus (polyomavirus enhancer-binding protein). RUNX1 = AML1 = CBFα2 = PEBP2αB; RUNX2 = AML3 = CBFα1 = PEBP2αA; and RUNX3 = AML2 = CBFα3 = PEBP2αC. CBFβ is the heterodimer partner of RUNX protein. RUNX and CBFβ are important transcription factors in regulating a variety of genes during cell proliferation and differentiation and have been demonstrated as critical players during animal development and cancer. Studies about their structure, function, and regulation have provided significant information to the fundamental role of transcription factors in gene regulation and animal development.

I. RUNX/CBF: STRUCTURE AND REGULATION OF GENE EXPRESSION

RHDs of three mammalian RUNX proteins are 60–70% homologous to two *Drosophila* runt proteins (runt and lozenge) and are also over 90% homologous to each other. RHD is responsible for the interaction of RUNX with DNA and with its heterodimer partner CBFβ (Fig. 1). Due to the extremely high

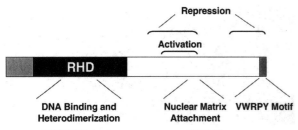

FIGURE 1 Domain structure of RUNX protein.

homology of RHDs of the three RUNX proteins, their binding to DNA is indistinguishable from each other. RUNX binding consensus DNA sequence TGT/$_C$GGT was isolated by polymerase chain reaction-mediated DNA target site selection. RUNX protein has runt homology domain, nuclear matrix attachment domain, transactivation domain, and repression domain (Fig. 1). In addition to binding to DNA and CGFβ, the runt homology domain also interacts with other transcription factors, such as Ets-1, PU.1, Myb, and C/EBP, which have shown a synergistic effect with RUNX in the activation of gene expression. The transactivation domain directly interacts with transcriptional coactivator p300/CBP and plays a critical role in the activation of gene expression by RUNX protein. VWRPY is an extremely conserved region at the end of C terminuses of all three RUNX proteins. VWRPY, with its adjacent region, binds a transcription repressor TLE and is involved in transcription repression. The nuclear matrix attachment domain directly affects the localization of RUNX inside cell nuclei to further regulate its biological function. Furthermore, the mSin3 corepressor binds to RUNX protein in a region probably overlapping with p300/CBP binding and can repress promoter activity. Because mSin3 is involved in condensing chromatin through histone deacetylation and p300/CBP is involved in relaxing chromatin through histone acetylation, such a physical interaction may have a Yin–Yang regulatory effect on RUNX target gene expression. In addition, other proteins, such as Ear2 and YAP, have been identified as cofactors to modify RUNX activity via yeast two hybrid protein–protein interaction analysis. The activity and stability of RUNX proteins are also regulated via protein phosphorylation and ubiquitination.

CBFβ does not directly bind to DNA. However, it significantly enhances the interaction between RUNX

and DNA and facilitates RUNX transactivation. Although there are two *Drosophila* homologues of CBFβ—Brother and Big-brother—only one gene for CBFβ protein has been reported in mammals. A large portion of the CBFβ N-terminal domain (amino acids 1 to 141) is involved in its interaction with RUNX. In addition to binding to RUNX, little is known about whether there are other protein partners of CBFβ.

RUNX regulates the expression of a variety of cellular genes. In general, it is a relatively weak regulator by itself. However, it plays a critical role in cooperating with other transcription factors to control gene expression. Two excellent examples of RUNX involvement in transcription activation are the synergistic effects of RUNX and C/EBP on the regulation of macrophage colony-stimulating factor (M-CSF) receptor promoter activity and of RUNX and Ets on the regulation of T-cell receptor (TCR) enhancer activity. In the absence of RUNX protein, C/EBP barely activates M-CSF receptor promoter; in the absence of C/EBP, RUNX plus CBFβ activates the promoter 5-fold. However, in the presence of RUNX, CBFβ, and C/EBP, over 100-fold activation can be detected in transient transfection assay. DNA-binding domains of RUNX and C/EBP cooperatively bind to their adjacent binding sites. A 50 amino acid fragment at the C-terminal of the runt homology domain directly participates in the synergistic activation. This region may provide a direct surface in association with a domain from the C/EBP protein to stably interact with transcription coactivators. RUNX and Ets-1 bind to the adjacent sites in TCR enhancer. These two proteins directly interact and cooperatively bind to DNA. Using a serial RUNX and Ets-1 deletion constructs in the analysis, it has been proposed that RUNX has an autoinhibitory domain to block its interaction with DNA and/or to mask the function of its transactivation domain. Upon association with Ets-1, the conformation change will expose the DNA-binding domain and the activation domain for its activity.

II. RUNX1 AND CBFβ IN HEMATOPOIESIS AND LEUKEMIA

The RUNX1 gene was originally cloned from human acute myeloid leukemia cells with t(8;21) and was named acute myeloid leukemia 1 (AML1). To easily describe RUNX1 fusion proteins associated with leukemia, AML1 will be used in this section to discuss leukemia-related problems. AML1 and CBFβ are the most frequent targets in human acute leukemia. In chromosomal translocation t(8;21)(q22;q22), the runt homology domain of *AML1* is fused to a protein encoded by a gene termed eight-twenty-one (*ETO*) or myeloid transforming gene 8 (*MTG8*) to form a fusion protein called AML1-ETO. The t(8;21) is found in 12% patients with *de novo* acute myeloid leukemia. Most of these patients are with the FAB-M2 subtype of acute myeloid leukemia. AML1 is also involved in t(3;21)(q26;q22) in the blast transformation of chronic myeloid leukemia and therapy-related acute myeloid leukemia. In this chromosomal translocation, the AML1 runt homology domain is fused to one of three proteins, EAP, MDS1, or EVI1, encoded by genes closely linked on chromosome 3. Another rare type of chromosomal translocation involving AML1 is t(16;21)(q24;q22), which generates an AML1 runt homology domain and MTG16 fusion protein AML1-MTG16. A common form of chromosomal translocation, t(12;21), generates a fusion protein TEL-AML1 with the N-terminal portion of TEL and almost the entire AML1 protein. TEL-AML1 is detected in up to 25% of childhood pre-B-cell acute lymphoblastic leukemia. Furthermore, AML1 is also involved in radiation-related chromosomal translocation in acute myeloid leukemia. CBFβ is involved in chromosomal abnormality inv(16)(p13;q22), which forms a fusion protein with muscle myosin heavy chain (CBFβ-MYH11). This chromosomal inversion is specifically associated with the M4Eo subtype of acute myeloid leukemia. The CBFβ-MYH11 chimeric protein contains the CBFβ N-terminal domain for its dimerization with AML1 and MYH11 C-terminal coiled-coil tail for its multimerization. The frequent appearance of translocations involving AML1/CBFβ in human leukemias indicates that they play a critical function in hematopoiesis.

Aml1 and *Cbf*β knockout mice have been generated. The phenotypes of *Aml1* and *Cbf*β knockout mice are identical. Heterozygous mice are healthy and fertile. Homozygous knockout mice die between 12.5 to 13.5 days postcoitus (dpc) with severe hemorrhage along the central nervous system. The reason for such extensive hemorrhage is still unknown. Furthermore, although these mice have nucleated primitive erythrocytes, they lack definitive hematopoiesis. Cells from embryonic hematopoietic tissues, such as yolk sac and liver, do not show colony-forming units when they are cultured *in vitro*. Chimeric mice made from *Aml1-* or *Cbf*β-deficient embryonic stem (ES) cells and wild-type mouse blastocysts do not show any ES cell contribution to adult hematopoietic cells. Using the reporter gene knockin approach, it has been demonstrated that *Aml1* expression marks the earliest hematopoietic precursor cells. These results indicate that the heterodimer partners *Aml1* and *Cbf*β of the core binding factor complex are equally important for their biological function and they play a fundamental role in the establishment of definitive hematopoietic stem cells.

AML1 haploinsufficiency has been reported in some patients with familial platelet disorder who have a predisposition to develop acute myeloid leukemia (FPD/AML). These patients have nonsense mutations or intragenic deletions in one allele of *AML1*. Mono- or biallelic mutations in AML1 have also been found in sporadic leukemia. The main form of leukemia in these patients is AML FAB-M0. AML1 haploinsufficiency patient bone marrow and periphery blood cells have decreased megakaryocyte, granulocyte–macrophage, and erythrocyte colony formation abilities. However, heterozygous *Aml1* or *Cbf*β knockout mice develop normally and do not get leukemia. Additional studies are necessary to understand the relationship of AML1 heploinsufficiency and leukemia development. From another prospective, overxpression of AML1 causes cell transformation in the mouse fibroblast cell line NIHT3 and is associated with the development of acute myeloid leukemia in mice. Furthermore, amplification of the AML1 gene fragment has been reported in human leukemia. Together, these results indicate that the level of AML1 expression plays a critical role in normal hematopoiesis.

Because chromosomal translocations involving AML1 and CBFβ are commonly associated with leukemia, establishing mouse models of such leukemia will be useful for studying the development and treatment of leukemia. Several approaches have been taken to generate mouse models: bone marrow transplantation of a retrovirus that expresses fusion proteins, knockin fusion protein portions into normal AML1 or CBFβ locus, and transgenic mice. Mice with bone marrow transplantation of cells expressing t(3;21) fusion protein AML1/MDS1/EVI1 have developed acute myeloid leukemia 5 to 13 months after transplantation. t(12;21) fusion TEL/AML1, inv(16) fusion CBFβ-MYH11, and t(8;21) fusion AML1-ETO have been used in bone marrow transplantation in various laboratories. No successful leukemia model has been established yet. However, bone marrow cells with the AML1-ETO retrovirus have shown increased replating efficiency in the *in vitro* colony assay. AML1-ETO and CBFβ-MYH11 knockin mice have been generated. The heterozygous knockin mice died at the embryonic stage with similar phenotypes to AML1 and CBFβ homozygous knockout mice—hemorrhage along the central nervous system and lack of normal definitive hematopoiesis, indicating the dominant-negative effect of AML1-ETO and CBFβ-MYH11 or their wild-type proteins. However, these mice also showed differences from homozygous knockout mice. *In vitro* colony-forming unit assays using cells from the yolk sac and fetal liver of AML1-ETO knockin mice show dysplastic hematopoietic colony formation. Furthermore, CBFβ-MYH11 knockin embryos have an increased number of immature primitive erythroblasts in their circulating blood. Because knockin mice expressing fusion proteins died at the embryonic stage, it is necessary to develop animal models that do not express fusion proteins during early hematopoiesis in the embryo. An animal model with tetracycline-inducible AML1-ETO expression has been generated. These mice give a tight inducible AML1-ETO expression in their bone marrow cells and show an increased replating efficiency of their AML1-ETO expressing bone marrow cells in *in vitro* colony assays. However, throughout the normal life span of 24 months, mice expressing AML1-ETO have not developed leukemia. These results demonstrate that AML1-ETO has a restricted capacity to transform cells. Additional genetic changes are necessary for the development of leukemia in AML1 fusion protein expressing mice. In fact, Castilla and colleagues have clearly demonstrated that an additional mutation(s) is required for the development of leukemia with chimeric mice of CBFβ-MYH11 knockin. Chimeric

mice with cells containing CBFβ-MYH11 knockin cells do not develop leukemia in their first year of life. However, upon injection of a potent DNA alkylating mutagen, N-ethyl-N-nitrosourea (ENU), 84% of chimeric mice developed acute myeloid leukemia. Buchholz and co-workers have reported the generation of mice with the Cre-LoxP conditional AML1 and ETO chromosomal translocation, which make both AML1-ETO and ETO-AML1 fusion proteins to fully mimic t(8;21) in leukemia patients. However, no investigation of hematopoiesis in these mice has been reported.

III. RUNX2 IN BONE DEVELOPMENT AND LEUKEMIA

The critical biological function of RUNX2 is revealed by the analysis of RUNX2 knockout mice and a human autosomal-dominant bone disorder, cleidocranial dysplasia (CCD), which has designated RUNX2 as a master gene for bone development. Runx2$^{-/-}$ mice died shortly after birth due to the inability to breath. These mice do not have normal bone formation. Both membranous bones (bones of the skull and the face derived from bone cells in the connective tissue) and endochondral bones (the rest of the bones of the skeleton generated by the process of endochondral ossification) are absent. Further histochemical analysis demonstrates that Runx2$^{-/-}$ mice lack normal osteoblasts, indicating that RUNX2 plays a critical role in bone development. RUNX2 is strongly expressed in cells related to bone formation. The expression of genes associated with the function of osteoblastic cell function, such as osteocalcin, osteopontin, and alkaline phosphatase, is very low in Runx2$^{-/-}$ mice. The RUNX DNA-binding consensus sequence is present in the promoter of almost all bone-specific expressed genes. Therefore, Runx2 has also been called osteoblast-specific factor 2 (OSF2). It activates the promoters of bone-specific genes in *in vitro* transactivation studies using nonosteoblastic cell lines.

RUNx$^{+/-}$ mice have hypoplasia of the clavicle and have delayed development of membranous bones and delayed ossification of cranial bones, resulting in open anterior and posterior fontanelles, smaller parietal and interparietal cranial bones, and multiple Wormian bones (small bones in the sutures). These are typical features of a human-dominant autosomal disease—CCD syndrome. These same phenotypes also present in the γ irradiation-induced mouse CCD model. The mutation associated with CCD syndrome is located on human chromosome 6p21, which includes the RUNX2 gene. Further studies demonstrate that both human and mouse CCD syndromes are due to mutations in the RUNX2 gene. This finding suggest a critical dosage effect of RUNX2 on bone development.

Northern blot analysis indicates that Runx2 is mainly expressed in the bone and osteoblasts in adult mice. No significant Runx2 expression is detected in the thymus. However, Runx2 has been reported as an oncogene in T-cell lymphoma development. Human CD2 locus control region–human c-myc gene transgenic mice are reported to develop T-cell lymphoma at low frequency. The Moloney murine leukemia virus accelerates this lymphoma development in CD2-myc transgenic mice. Over 30% of the mice with the lymphoma are due to the activation of Runx2 expression with virus integration upstream of the Runx2 promoter. This study demonstrates that Runx2 is a collaborating oncogene of c-myc. A further study using CD2-Runx2 transgenic mice reveals that Runx2 can act in synergy with other oncogenes, such as Pim1, to cause T-cell lymphoma.

IV. RUNX3

Relative to RUNX1 and RUNX2, little is known about RUNX3. It has been cloned due to its high homology to RUNX1 and RUNX2. Among hematopoietic cells, RUNX3 is relatively highly expressed in B-cell and myeloid lineages. No data about RUNX3 expression in normal tissue have been reported. Retinoic acid and TGFβ have been reported as positive regulators for RUNX3 expression. RUNX3 binds to the mouse germline Ig α promoter and activates Ig α transcription. Runx3 knockout mice have been generated. However, no data about their phenotype have been published formally in the literature. It will be very interesting to know the critical function of RUNX3 in normal and disease development.

In summary, RUNX/CBF is a small family of transcription factors. They have important biological functions during animal development and are closely related to human disease, especially in hematopoiesis and bone generation. Studying the molecular mechanism of the regulation of their own expression, their cooperation with other transcription factors, and their target gene expression in cells and animal models has generated and will provide us with further valuable knowledge regarding human health.

See Also the Following Articles

ALL-1 • EWS/ETS Fusion Genes • PAX3–FKHR and PAX7–FKHR Gene Fusions in Alveolar Rhabdomyosarcoma • TLS-CHOP in Myxoid Liposarcoma

Bibliography

Blyth, K., Terry, A., Mackay, N., Vaillant, F., Bell, M., Cameron, E. R., Neil, J. C., and Stewart, M. (2001). Runx2: A novel oncogenic effector revealed by in vivo complementation and retroviral tagging. *Oncogene* **20**, 295–302.

Buchholz, F., Refaeli, Y., Trumpp, A., and Bishop, J. M. (2000). Inducible choromosomal translocation of AML1 and ETO genes through Cre/loxP-mediated recombination in the mouse. *EMBO Rep.* **1**, 133–139.

Castilla, L. H., Garrett, L., Adya, N., Orlic, D., Dutra, A., Anderson, S., Owens, J., Eckhaus, M., Bodine, D., and Liu, P. P. (1999). The fusion gene Cbfb-MYH11 blocks myeloid differentiation and predisposes mice to acute myelomonocytic leukaemia. *Nature Genet.* **23**, 144–146.

Castilla, L. H., Wijmenga, C., Wang, Q., Stacy, T., Speck, N. A., Eckhaus, M., Marin-Padilla, M., Collins, F. S., Wynshaw-Boris, A., and Liu, P. P. (1996). Failure of embryonic hematopoiesis and lethal hemorrhages in mouse embryos heterozygous for a knocked-in leukemia gene CBFB-MYH11. *Cell* **87**, 687–696.

Cuenco, G. M., Nucifora, G., and Ren, R. (2000). Human AML1/MDS1/EVI1 fusion protein induces an acute myelogenous leukemia (AML) in mice: A model for human AML. *Proc. Natl. Acad. Sci. USA* **97**, 1760–1765.

Ducy, P., Zhang, R., Geoffroy, V., Ridall, A. L., and Karsenty, G. (1997). Osf2/Cbfa1: A transcriptional activator of osteoblast differentiation. *Cell* **89**, 747–754.

Gamou, T., Kitamura, E., Hosoda, F., Shimizu, K., Shinohara, K., Hayashi, Y., Nagase, T., Yokoyama, Y., and Ohki, M. (1998). The partner gene of AML1 in t(16;21) myeloid malignancies is a novel member of the MTG8(ETO) family. *Blood* **91**, 4028–4037.

Golub, T. R., Barker, G. F., Bohlander, S. K., Hiebert, S. W., Ward, D. C., Bray-Ward, P., Morgan, E., Raimondi, S. C., Rowley, J. D., and Gilliland, D. G. (1995). Fusion of the TEL gene on 12p13 to the AML1 gene on 21q22 in acute lymphoblastic leukemia. *Proc. Natl. Acad. Sci. USA* **92**, 4917–4921.

Hromoas, R., Shopnick, R., Jumean, H. G., Bowers, C., Varella-Garcia, M., and Richkind, K. (2000). A novel syndrome of radiation-associated acute myeloid leukemia involving AML1 gene translocations. *Blood* **95,** 4011–4013.

Kamachi, Y., Ogawa, E., Asano, M., Ishida, S., Murakami, Y., Satake, M., Ito, Y., and Shigesada, K. (1990). Purification of a mouse nuclear factor that binds to both the A and B cores of the polyomavirus enhancer. *J. Virol.* **64,** 4808–4819.

Kim, W. Y., Sieweke, M., Ogawa, E., Wee, H. J., Englmeier, U., Graf, T., and Ito, Y. (1999). Mutual activation of Ets-1 and AML1 DNA binding by direct interaction of their autoinhibitory domains. *EMBO J.* **18,** 1609–1620.

Komori, T., Yagi, H., Nomura, S., Yamaguchi, A., Sasaki, K., Deguchi, K., Shimizu, Y., Bronson, R. T., Gao, Y. H., Inada, M., Sato, M., Okamoto, R., Kitamura, Y., Yoshiki, S., and Kishimoto, T. (1997). Targeted disruption of Cbfa1 results in a complete lack of bone formation owing to maturational arrest of osteoblasts. *Cell* **89,** 755–764.

Kurokawa, M., Tanaka, T., Tanaka, K., Ogawa, S., Mitani, K., Yazaki, Y., and Hirai, H. (1996). Overexpression of the AML1 proto-oncoprotein in NIH3T3 cells leads to neoplastic transformation depending on the DNA-binding and transactivational potencies. *Oncogene* **12,** 883–892.

Lee, B., Thirunavukkarasu, K., Zhou, L., Pastore, L., Baldini, A., Hecht, J., Geoffroy, V., Ducy, P., and Karsenty, G. (1997). Missense mutations abolishing DNA binding of the osteoblast-specific transcriptional factor OSF2/CBFA1 in cleidocranial dysplasia. *Nature Genet.* **16,** 307–310.

Li, J., Shen, H., Himmel, K. L., Dupuy, A. J., Largaespada, D. A., Nakamura, T., Shaughnessy, J. D., Jenkins, N. A., and Copeland, N. G. (1999). Leukaemia disease genes: Large-scale cloning and pathway predictions. *Nature Genet.* **23,** 348–353.

Liu, P., Tarle, S. A., Hajra, A., Claxton, D. F., Marlton, P., Freedman, M., Siciliano, M. J., and Collins, F. S. (1993). Fusion between transcription factor CBF beta/PEBP2 beta and a myosin heavy chain in acute myeloid leukemia. *Science* **261,** 1041–1044.

Meyers, S., Downing, J. R., and Hiebert, S. W. (1993). Identification of AML-1 and the (8;21) translocation protein (AML-1/ETO) as sequence-specific DNA-binding proteins: The runt homology domain is required for DNA binding and protein-protein interactions. *Mol. Cell Biol.* **13,** 6336–6345.

Miyoshi, H., Shimizu, K., Kozu, T., Maseki, N., Kaneko, Y., and Ohki, M. (1991). t(8;21) breakpoints on chromosome 21 in acute myeloid leukemia are clustered within a limited region of a single gene, AML1. *Proc. Natl. Acad. Sci. USA* **88,** 10431–10434.

Mundlos, S., Otto, F., Mundlos, C., Mulliken, J. B., Aylsworth, A. S., Albright, S., Lindhout, D., Cole, W. G., Henn, W., Knoll, J. H., Owen, M. J., Mertelsmann, R., Zabel, B. U., and Olsen, B. R. (1997). Mutations involving the transcription factor CBFA1 cause cleidocranial dysplasia. *Cell* **89,** 773–779.

Niini, T., Kanerva, J., Vettenranta, K., Saarinen-Pihkala, U. M., and Knuutila, S. (2000). AML1 gene amplification: A novel finding in childhood acute lymphoblastic leukemia. *Haematologica* **85,** 362–366.

Nucifora, G., Birn, D. J., Espinosa, R., Erickson, P., LeBeau, M. M., Roulston, D., McKeithan, T. W., Drabkin, H., and Rowley, J. D. (1993). Involvement of the AML1 gene in the t(3;21) in therapy-related leukemia and in chronic myeloid leukemia in blast crisis. *Blood* **81,** 2728–2734.

Okuda, T., Cai, Z., Yang, S., Lenny, N., Lyu, C., Van Deursen, J., Harada, H., and Downing, J. R. (1998). Expression of a knocked-In AML1-ETO leukemia gene inhibits the establishment of normal definitive hematopoiesis and directly generates dysplastic hematopoietic progenitors. *Blood* **91,** 3134–3143.

Okuda, T., Van Deursen, J., Hiebert, S. W., Grosveld, G., and Downing, J. R. (1996). AML1, the target of multiple chromosomal translocations in human leukemia, is essential for normal fetal liver hematopoiesis. *Cell* **84,** 321–330.

Osato, M., Asou, N, Abdalla, E, Hoshino K., Yamasaki, H., Okubo, T., Suzushima, H., Takatsuki, K., Kanno, T., Shigesada, K., and Ito, Y. (1999). Biallelic and heterozygous point mutations in the runt domain of the AML1/PEBP2αB gene associated with myeloblastic leukemias. *Blood* **93,** 1817–1824.

Otto, F., Thornell, A. P., Crompton, T., Denzel, A., Gilmour, K. C., Rosewell, I. R., Stamp, G. W., Beddington, R. S., Mundlos, S., Olsen, B. R., Selby, P. B., and Owen, M. J. (1997). Cbfa1, a candidate gene for cleidocranial dysplasia syndrome, is essential for osteoblast differentiation and bone development. *Cell* **89,** 765–771.

Petrovick, M. S., Hiebert, S. W., Friedman, A. D., Hetherington, C. J., Tenen, D. G., and Zhang, D. E. (1998). Multiple functional domains of AML1: PU.1 and C/EBPalpha synergize with different regions of AML1. *Mol. Cell Biol.* **18,** 3915–3925.

Rhoades, K. L., Hetherington, C. J., Harakawa, N., Yergeau, D. A., Zhou, L., Liu, L. Q., Little, M. T., Tenen, D. G., and Zhang, D. E. (2000). Analysis of the role of AML1-ETO in leukemogenesis, using an inducible transgenic mouse model. *Blood* **96,** 2108–2115.

Rodan, G. A., and Harada, S. (1997). The missing bone. *Cell* **89,** 677–680.

Shi, M. J., and Stavnezer, J. (1998). CBF alpha3 (AML2) is induced by TGF-beta1 to bind and activate the mouse germline Ig alpha promoter. *J. Immunol.* **161,** 6751–6760.

Song, W. J., Sullivan, M. G., Legare, R. D., Hutchings, S., Tan, X., Kufrin, D., Ratajczak, J., Resende, I. C., Haworth, C., Hock, R., Loh, M., Felix, C., Roy, D. C., Busque, L., Kurnit, D., Willman, C., Gewirtz, A. M., Spec, N. A., Bushweller, J. H., Li, F. P., Gardiner, K., Poncz, M., Maris, J. M., and Gilliland, D. G. (1999). Haploinsufficiency of CBFA2 causes familial thrombocytopenia with propensity to develop acute myelogenous leukaemia. *Nature Genet.* **23,** 166–175.

Stewart, M., Terry, A., Hu, M., O'Hara, M., Blyth, K., Baxter, E., Cameron, E., Onions, D. E., and Neil, J. C. (1997). Proviral insertions induce the expression of bone-specific isoforms of PEBP2alphaA (CBFA1): Evidence for a new myc collaborating oncogene. *Proc. Natl. Acad. Sci. USA* **94,** 8646–8651.

Tracey, W. D., and Speck, N. A. (2000). Potential roles for RUNX1 and its orthologs in determining hematopoietic cell fate. *Semin. Cell Dev. Biol.* **11,** 337–342.

Wang, Q., Stacy, T., Binder, M., Marin-Padilla, M., Sharpe, A. H., and Speck, N. A. (1996). Disruption of the Cbfa2 gene causes necrosis and hemorrhaging in the central nervous system and blocks definitive hematopoiesis. *Proc. Natl. Acad. Sci. USA* **93,** 3444–3449.

Wang, Q., Stacy, T., Miller, J. D., Lewis, A. F., Gu, T. L., Huang, X., Bushweller, J. H., Bories, J. C., Alt, F. W., Ryan, G., Liu, P. P., Wynshaw-Boris, A., Binder, M., Marin-Padilla, M., Sharpe, A. H., and Speck, N. A. (1996b). The CBFbeta subunit is essential for CBFalpha2 (AML1) function in vivo. *Cell* **87,** 697–708.

Wang, S. W., and Speck, N. A. (1992). Purification of core-binding factor, a protein that binds the conserved core site in murine leukemia virus enhancers. *Mol. Cell Biol.* **12,** 89–102.

Yergeau, D., A., Hetherington, C. J., Wang, Q., Zhang, P., Sharpe, A. H., Binder, M., Marin-Padilla, M., Tenen, D. G., Speck, N. A., and Zhang, D. E. (1997). Embryonic lethality and impairment of haematopoiesis in mice heterozygous for an AML1-ETO fusion gene. *Nature Genet.* **15,** 303–306.

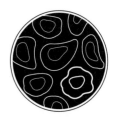

Sarcomas of Soft Tissue

Robert G. Maki

Memorial Sloan-Kettering Cancer Center

GLOSSARY

desmoplastic small round cell tumor Aggressive sarcoma of the Ewing sarcoma family with translocation involving Wilms' tumor gene WT1. It is found exclusively in the abdomen with occasional liver metastasis. It nearly always demonstrates multiple sites of disease within the abdomen at the time of presentation. Only patients who respond well to chemotherapy and who can have their remaining disease completely resected have a chance for long-term survival.

Ewing sarcoma Rare sarcoma of soft tissue or of bone, typically occurring early in the second decade of life. Systemic disease from the outset requires multimodality therapy with chemotherapy, radiation, and usually surgery. Typically CD99+ but this marker is not specific. Ewing sarcoma has the same chromosomal translocation as primitive neuroectodermal tumor and Askin tumor, so believed to represent different aspects of the same tumor.

liposarcoma Soft tissue sarcoma of adipocytes, with highly variable phenotype. The most differentiated forms are called atypical lipomas or low-grade liposarcomas. Dedifferentiated forms show more aggressive behavior. Beyond the normal pattern of metastasis to lung in high-grade lesions, these sarcomas can metastasize to other fatty tissue of the body. Retroperitoneal liposarcomas are nearly impossible to eradicate completely due to their large size and involvement of many nearby organs at the time of presentation.

malignant fibrous histiocytoma Term often used for sarcomas that cannot be otherwise classified. Because therapy is similar for most sarcomas, some pathologists lump together many varieties of sarcomas under this one term. Other pathologists do not use this term, preferring instead to refer to sarcoma (not otherwise specified) with particular histologic features.

rhabdomyosarcoma Typically a pediatric sarcoma that demonstrates skeletal muscle differentiation. It is common in the orbit or genitourinary tract in children, but can occur in any site. A systemic disease that requires chemotherapy in addition to local control.

synovial sarcoma Soft tissue sarcoma with small spindle cells and characteristic t(X;18) translocation. The monophasic type appears monotonous; the biphasic type shows gland formation. It is typically relatively sensitive to chemotherapy (among sarcomas). Ifosfamide is probably the best single drug for this form of sarcoma.

Soft tissue sarcomas (STS) are a very heterogeneous group of tumors that constitute less than 1% of all cancer. STS have widely variable behavior, from localized lesions that grow slowly with no chance of distant recurrence, to aggressive lesions with a high risk of hematogenous spread to lungs and other sites. While many sarcomas show a complex karyotype, some sarcomas show very specific chromosomal rearrangements, which point out key biological features of these tumors. Sarcomas are features of certain genetic cancer syndromes, again pointing out possible genes important in sarcoma development. The new American Joint Committee on Cancer (AJCC) staging system was developed to reflect the biological behavior of these tumors and is based on sarcoma grade, size, location, and spread of disease. Treatment of STS is largely surgical. Radiation can help improve the local control of disease, whereas chemotherapy may help local control as well. Chemotherapy is used for metastatic disease, which develops in half of patients presenting with localized disease only. Debate continues as to the utility of adjuvant chemotherapy to increase survival for patients with sarcomas. Doxorubicin and ifosfamide are the two most active agents in sarcoma, with dacarbazine also showing some activity.

I. INTRODUCTION

Soft tissue sarcomas are a heterogeneous group of cancers developing from connective tissue (i.e., of mesodermal origin). These cancers include tumors of smooth muscle, fat, and other connective tissues, such as fibroblasts, and also include endothelial cells, which give rise to angiosarcomas and support cells of peripheral nerves (Schwann cells). Some 8000 people in the United States will develop sarcomas this year, which gives an incidence of less than 3 cases per 100,000 people. Certain STS are more common in children than adults, such as Ewing sarcoma/primitive neuroectodermal tumor (PNET) and rhabdomyosarcoma; however, overall, sarcomas are much more common in adults than in children.

II. GENETIC SYNDROMES

Some sarcomas occur in association with genetic syndromes (Table I). The best example of a familial sarcoma syndrome is Li–Fraumeni syndrome, which involves mutation in the germline gene encoding p53. As a result, patients with a p53 mutation have a high rate of STS and are also at risk of developing other tumors. A representative list of familial syndromes associated with sarcomas and their associated genes is indicated in Table I.

III. CHROMOSOMAL TRANSLOCATIONS

Interestingly, many hematologic malignancies demonstrate specific chromosomal translocations, and some types of sarcoma demonstrate specific genetic translocations as well. These translocations even occasionally involve some of the same genes seen in translocations noted in leukemias and lymphomas. However, most translocations involve genes unique to connective tissue cells. Many pediatric sarcomas show specific translocations, as do some liposarcomas. However, leiomyosarcomas and tumors designated MFH usually do not have specific translocations. Rarer forms of sarcoma also show specific translocations, as noted in Table II.

IV. HETEROGENEITY

A variety of factors determine the biological behavior of sarcomas. These include histologic type, location of the tumor, histologic grade, size, and evidence of spread of the tumor. Given the heterogeneity of sarcomas (over 50 different types are recognized), there is not uncommonly disagreement on specific grade for specific sarcomas, if not on the subtype of sarcoma recognized. It is suggested that

TABLE I
Genetic Syndromes Featuring Soft Tissue Sarcomas

Syndrome	Gene (chromosome) involved	Clinical syndrome
Li–Fraumeni	*TP53* (17p13)	Soft tissue sarcoma Breast cancer Osteosarcoma Brain tumor Leukemia Adrenocortical carcinoma Germ cell tumors
Neurofibromatosis type I (von Recklinghausen disease)	*NFI* (17q11.2)	Café au lait spots Neuofibromas, including acoustic neuromas Meningiomas Osseous fibrous dysplasia Malignant peripheral nerve sheath tumors
Retinoblastoma	*Rb-1* (13q14)	Retinoblastoma, osteosarcoma Soft tissue sarcomas
Gorlin syndrome (nevoid basal cell carcinoma syndrome)	PTC/NBCCS (9q22.3)	Basal cell carcinomas Pitting of palms and soles Cysts of the jaw Rib and vertebral anomalies Medulloblastoma Rhabdomyosarcoma Fibrosarcoma of the jaw
Werner syndrome (adult progeria)	DNA helicase (8p12)	Premature aging Leg ulcers Scleroderma-like skin changes Soft tissue sarcomas Meningiomas
Gardner syndrome	*FAP* (5q21)	Bowel polyps/carcinoma Desmoid tumors Fibromas, fibrosarcoma Epidermal and sebaceous cysts Lipomas Bony exostoses
Tuberous sclerosis (Bourneville disease)	*TSC1* (9q34) *TSC2* (16q13.3)	Seizures, mental retardation Hamartomas of skin, kidney, heart CNS malignancy Rhabdomyosarcoma

any diagnosis of sarcoma be confirmed by a center familiar with sarcoma pathology. The most common subtypes of sarcoma are sarcomas of fat (liposarcoma) and of smooth muscle (leiomyosarcoma). There is debate as to whether the concept of "malignant fibrosis histiocytoma (MFH)" should be discarded, as many of these lesions can be classified as another type of sarcoma on more careful examination. Some centers refer to an otherwise unclassified sarcoma as MFH, whereas other centers refer to such tumors as sarcomas (not otherwise specified) with spindle cell or epithelioid features,

for example, depending on the microscopic features of the tumor.

V. STAGING AND GUIDELINES FOR CARE

Staging of soft tissue sarcoma is based on a new system developed by the International Union Against Cancer (UICC) and AJCC. The new staging system incorporates some features of two older classification systems from the AJCC and the Surgical Staging

TABLE II

Translocations in Soft Tissue Sarcoma

Tumor histology	Chromosomal alteration	Involved gene(s)	Frequency
Ewing sarcoma family[a]	t(11;22)(q24;q12)	EWS-FLI1	85%
	t(21;22)(q22;q12)	EWS-ERG	5–10%
	t(1;16)(q11-25;q11-24)	Unknown	~10%
	Trisomy 8	Not applicable	~50%
Myxoid/round cell liposarcoma	t(12;16)(q13;p11)	TLS (FUS)-CHOP	>75%
	t(12;22)(q13;q12)	EWS-CHOP	Uncommon
Low-grade liposarcoma	Giant chromosomes, ring chromosomes	Unknown	60%
Alveolar rhabdomyosarcoma	t(2;13)(q35;q14)	PAX3-FKHR	~70%
	t(1;13)(p36;q14)	PAX7-FKHR	~15%
Malignant melanoma of soft tissue (clear cell sarcoma)	t(12;22)(q13;q12)	EWS-ATF1	>75%
Desmoplastic small round cell tumor	t(11;22)(p13;q12)	EWS-WT1	>90%
Synovial sarcoma	t(X;18)(p11;q11)	SYT-SSX1, SYT-SSX2	>90%
Extraskeletal myxoid chondrosarcoma	t(9;22)(q22;q12)	EWS-CHN (TEC)	>75%
Dermatofibrosarcoma protruberans	t(17;22)(q22;q13), ring chromosomes	COL1A1-PDGFB	>50%; ring chromosomes >75%
Congenital fibrosarcoma	t(12;15)(p13;q25)	ETV6 (TEL)-NTRK3 (TRKC)	?
Malignant rhabdoid tumor	del 22 (q11.2)	hSNF5/INI1	~50%
Alveolar soft-part sarcoma	der(17)t(X;17)(p11;q25)	ASPL-TFE3	>90%

[a] Includes Ewing sarcoma, Askin tumor, primitive neuroectodermal tumor (PNET).

System of the Musculoskeletal Tumor Society. The old AJCC system was based largely on tumor grade, whereas the newer staging system takes into account the better biological behavior of specific subsets of sarcomas, being largely based on the work of Brennan and colleagues and their extensive database of several thousand consecutive sarcoma patients. In the new AJCC system, tumors are segregated based on size (≤5 or >5 cm), anatomical location (superficial or deep to investing fascia—most sarcomas are deep lesions), grade (high or low), and nodal and metastatic status. The staging system is shown in Table III.

Guidelines for sarcoma therapy have been proposed by the national Comprehensive Cancer Network (NCCN). These guidelines provide a reasonable consensus as to therapy for STS. Therapy for sarcomas often requires more than one modality of care. Surgery, chemotherapy, and radiation may all be indicated for care of a large sarcoma. The knowledge of the use of multiple modalities of care for STS, combined with the relative rarity of sarcomas, argues that all patients

with sarcomas should be discussed by a team of specialists at a referral center with expertise in sarcoma to achieve an optimal result for the patient.

VI. DIAGNOSIS

Diagnosis of sarcoma is usually achieved by needle biopsy of a suspicious mass. If further tissue is required for diagnosis, an incisional biopsy is generally recommended, as an excisional biopsy can contaminate tissue planes and can result in the need for a far more extensive resection to achieve clear margins. A fine needle aspirate is not sufficient to diagnose a sarcoma due to the very small amount of tissue recovered; however, once diagnosed, a fine needle aspirate can, in many cases, determine if disease is recurrent.

Once diagnosed, complete staging is indicated for higher grade lesions, including complete imaging of the primary tumor (generally by magnetic resonance imaging if feasible) and chest, abdomen, and pelvis

TABLE III
AJCC Sarcoma Staging System

G:Grade			N:Nodes	
GX	Grade cannot be assessed		NX	Nodes cannot be assessed
G1	Well differentiated		N0	No regional lymph node metastases
G2	Moderately differentiated		N1	Regional lymph node metastases
G3	Poorly differentiated			
G4	Undifferentiated		M: Metastases	
			MX	Metastasis cannot be assessed
T: Tumor			M0	No distant metastases
TX	Primary tumor cannot be assessed		M1	Distant metastases present
T0	No evidence of primary tumor			
T1	Tumor ≤5 cm in greatest extent			
	T1a: Superficial			
	T1b: Deep			
T2	Tumor >5 cm in greatest extent			
	T2a: Superficial			
	T2b: Deep			

Stage	Grade	Tumor	Nodes	Metastasis
IA (low grade, small, superficial or deep)	G1-2	T1a-b	N0	M0
IB (low grade, large, superficial)	G1-2	T2a	N0	M0
IIA (low grade, large, deep)	G1-2	T2b	N0	M0
IIB (high grade, small, superficial or deep)	G3-4	T1a-b	N0	M0
IIC (high grade, large, superficial)	G3-4	T2a	N0	M0
III (high grade, large, deep)	G3-4	T2b	N0	M0
IVA (nodal metastasis)	Any G	Any T	N1	M0
IVB (distant metastasis)	Any G	Any T	Any N	M1

Note: SUPERFICIAL lesions lack involvement of the superficial investing fascia in extremity lesions. All retroperitoneal and visceral lesions should be considered DEEP lesions. From Anonymous (1997).

computerized tomography scan. In some instances, where pain is a symptom, bone scans are reasonable modalities for initial staging.

VII. MULTIMODALITY THERAPY FOR SARCOMA

A. Surgery and Radiation (Local Control)

The primary sarcoma is generally treated with surgery and, in many cases, with radiation as adjuvant or neoadjuvant therapy. An important study indicated that morbidity was less and local recurrence no higher when radiation was given after surgery, as opposed to before surgery. However, it should be noted that radiation given before surgery is given to a smaller field than the field used in the postoperative setting, which must include the entire surgical site plus a margin. Radiation is

generally given to patients with intermediate- to high-grade extremity sarcomas to help decrease the risk of local relapse, where it has been proven to be useful. Radiation is of more questionable utility for retroperitoneal sarcomas. The reason for this question of utility is that lower doses of radiation must be given to the abdomen as compared to extremities due to lower radiation tolerance of abdominal viscera. Intraoperative radiation given in addition to external beam radiation is one way to try and increase the local dose of radiation (when viscera can be moved out of the way of the beam of radiation), but this technique remains investigational.

B. Chemotherapy

The use of chemotherapy in the neoadjuvant or adjuvant setting in sarcoma management is still controversial as well. There have been at least 13 published randomized studies of adjuvant chemotherapy for sarcoma that have been published since the 1980s. Only two have shown a benefit for adjuvant chemotherapy, but several studies showed a trend for improved overall survival. A formal meta-analysis of data from these many studies showed improved disease-free survival, local recurrence-free survival, and metastasis-free survival, but not in overall survival. There was a trend of improved overall survival in patients who received chemotherapy, but in this meta-analysis of 1568 patients, the 4% absolute survival benefit for chemotherapy did not reach statistical significance ($P = 0.12$). However, in the subset analysis of 904 extremity patients (58% of cases examined), a significant absolute advantage in overall survival of 7% was seen for patients receiving chemotherapy ($P = 0.03$). It is unclear if this subset analysis is a legitimate way to analyze such data given the different criteria for inclusion for each study, etc. There is a recently published study of adjuvant chemotherapy from Italy showing improved survival for patients receiving chemotherapy in the adjuvant setting; this is in contrast to some older studies examining extremity tumors in which there was no significant improvement in survival in the patients who received chemotherapy, a small study in which there was an improvement in survival in patients who received chemotherapy (but the control group fared worse than expected), and studies in which some control arm patients received preoperative chemotherapy. Thus, it remains controversial if adjuvant chemotherapy is of use for patients with extremity sarcoma.

It should also be noted that patients with uterine sarcomas had no benefit to single agent doxorubicin in the adjuvant setting, and adjuvant chemotherapy is not recommended in this setting. Similarly, there is no evidence that patients with visceral sarcomas benefit in any way from adjuvant chemotherapy. However, pediatric soft tissue sarcomas, such as Ewing sarcoma or rhabdomyosarcoma, are the one type of sarcoma in which adjuvant (and often times neoadjuvant) chemotherapy is warranted, as these diseases are recognized to be systemic in extent at the time of presentation in the overwhelming majority of patients, and pediatric studies indicate that systemic chemotherapy for these sarcomas can improve overall

survival, similar to the situation seen with pediatric osteogenic sarcomas.

VIII. ADVANCED DISEASE

At least half of patients with sarcoma will develop metastatic disease, and the vast majority of these patients will succumb to their disease as a result. In selected instances, surgery can be performed to remove the sole site(s) of metastatic disease. For example, a small fraction of patients with lung metastasis from sarcoma will be alive 3 years after initial resection of metastatic disease. However, in the main, patients with metastatic disease are treated with chemotherapy alone with palliative intent.

Doxorubicin and ifosfamide remain the two best agents for sarcoma in the metastatic setting, with response rates in the 15–25% range as single agents. Dacarbazine (DTIC) is a third agent with modest activity in sarcoma. MAID, the combination of mesna, doxorubicin, ifosfamide, and dacarbazine, has been widely used in metastatic sarcoma, with response rates in the 25–47% range. Doxorubicin plus ifosfamide (with mesna) is the other widely used combination used for patients with metastatic sarcomas, with similar response rates. There is presently no clear evidence that combinations of chemotherapy for metastatic sarcoma are better than single agents in terms of overall survival, despite the higher response rates seen with combinations of agents. It should be noted that patients with gastrointestinal stromal tumor (especially those abdominal sarcomas that mark positively for c-*kit*) do not response to standard agents but 60% do respond to imatinib mesylate. Liposarcomas as a group appear to give a better prognosis overall compared to other subtypes of sarcoma due to their slower rate of growth. Pediatric tumors are a special case and are generally treated with aggressive chemotherapy, surgery, and radiation, with chemotherapy usually being selected from combinations of the following agents: vincristine, doxorubicin, actinomycin D, cyclophosphamide, ifosfamide, and etoposide.

Beyond doxorubicin, ifosfamide, and DTIC, there

are few active agents in sarcoma. There are occasional responses to taxanes or vinorelbine, particularly in some patients with angiosarcoma. Otherwise, patients with refractory sarcoma are candidates for phase I and phase II studies of new agents or new combinations of agents. The recent excitement in antiangiogenic agents seems particularly applicable to sarcomas in light of initial data from the 1970s with tumor necrosis factor in mice, which controls tumor growth through breakdown of the vasculature feeding the tumor.

New chemotherapy agents, antiangiogenic drugs, gene therapy, and immunotherapy will all be considered in the next several years for the treatment of sarcomas. New drugs continue to be tested in phase I and phase II studies and some of these such as ET743 may have relevance to sarcoma therapy. Other studies ongoing today are examining different routes of chemotherapy administration. These studies include chemotherapy given directly through the pulmonary artery for lung metastases, intraperitoneal administration of chemotherapy for recurrent disease within the abdomen, and limb infusion or perfusion for otherwise unresectable extremity sarcoma (already approved in Europe for such a clinical situation), as well as inhalation of chemotherapy for lung metastases.

As for gene therapy, because p53 is frequently mutated or deleted in sarcomas, it is a prime candidate for genetic "correction." It may be quite some time before high percentages of tumor cells can be affected in order to achieve a useful response to such therapy, however. In terms of immunotherapy, vaccine therapy with proteins derived from patient tumors is undergoing study within the next year. It may well turn out that more complex combinations of different forms of therapy will be necessary to try and control this heterogeneous group of tumors.

See Also the Following Articles

Bone Tumors • Ewing's Sarcoma • Li–Fraumeni Syndrome • p53 Gene Therapy • Retinoblastoma Tumor Suppressor Gene • Rhabdomyosarcoma, Early Onset

Bibliography

Anonymous (1997). Soft tissue sarcoma. In "AJCC Cancer Staging Manual" (I. D. Fleming, J. S. Cooper, D. E. Henson, R. V. P. Hutter, B. J. Kennedy, G. P. Murphy, B. O'Sullivan, L. H. Sobin, and J. W. Yarbro, eds.), 5th Ed., pp. 149–153. Lippincott-Raven, Philadelphia.

Brennan, M. F., Alektiar, K., and Maki, R. G. (2000). Soft tissue sarcoma. In "Principles and Practice of Oncology" (V. T. DeVita, Jr., S. Hellman, and S. A. Rosenberg, eds.), 6th Ed. Lippincott-Raven, Philadelphia.

Demetri, G. D., Pollock, R., Baker, L., Balcerzak, S., Casper, E., Conrad, C., Fein, D., Hutchinson, R., Schupak, K., Spiro, I., Wagman, L. (1998). NCCN sarcoma practice guidelines. National Comprehensive Cancer Network. Oncology (Huntingt) **12**, 183–218.

Fletcher, C. D. M. (ed.) (1995). Soft tissue tumors. In "Diagnostic Histopathology of Tumors," pp. 1043–1096. Churchill-Livingstone, Edinburgh.

Frustaci, S., Gherlinzoni, F., De Paoli, A., Bonetti, M., Azzarelli, A., Comandone, A., Olmi, P., Buonadonna, A., Pignatti, G., Barbieri, E., Apice, G., Zmerly, H., Serraino, D., and Picci, P. (2001). Adjuvant chemotherapy for adult soft tissue sarcomas of the extremities and girdles: Results of the Italian randomized cooperative trial. J. Clin. Oncol. **19(5)**, 1235–1237.

Joesuu, H., Roberts, P.J., Sarloma-Rikala, M., Andersson, L.C., Tervahartiala, P., Tuveson, D., Silberman, S., Capdeville, R., Dimitrijevic, S., Druker, B., and Demetri, G. D. (2001). Effect of the tyrosine kinase inhibitor STI571 in a patient with a metastatic gastrointestinal stromal tumor. N. Engl. J. Med. **344(14)**, 1052–1056.

O'Sullivan, B., Davis, A., Bell, R., Catton, C., Turcotte, R., Wunder, J., Chabot, P., Hammond, A., Benk, V., Isler, M., Freeman, C., Goddard, K., Kandel, R., Sadura, A., James, K., and Zee, B. (1999). Phase III randomized trial of preoperative versus postoperative radiotherapy in the curative management of extremity soft tissue sarcoma. Proc. Am. Soc. Clin. Oncol. A2066.

Pisters, P. W. T., and Brennan, M. F. (2000). Sarcomas of soft tissue. In "Clinical Oncology" (M. D. Abeloff, J. O. Armitage, A. S. Lichter, and J. E. Niederhuber, eds.), 2nd Ed., pp. 2273–2313. Churchill-Livingstone, New York.

Sarcoma Meta-analysis Collaboration (1997). Adjuvant chemotherapy for localised resectable soft-tissue sarcoma of adults: meta-analysis of individual data. Lancet **350**, 1647–1654.

Van Glabbeke, M., van Oosterom, A. T., Oosterhuis, J. W., Mouridsen, H., Crowther, D., Somers, R., Verweij, J., Santoro, A., Buesa, J., and Tursz, T. (1999). Prognostic factors for the outcome of chemotherapy in advanced soft tissue sarcoma: An analysis of 2,185 patients treated with anthracycline-containing first-line regimens. J. Clin. Oncol. **17**, 150–157.

Weiss, S. W. (1994). Histological typing of soft tissue tumors. In "WHO International Histological Classification of Tumors." 2nd Ed. Springer-Verlag, Berlin.

Senescence, Cellular

Judith Campisi
Lawrence Berkeley National Laboratory

I. Definitions and Nomenclature
II. History
III. Senescent Phenotypes
IV. Causes of Cellular Senescence
V. Physiological Consequences of Cellular Senescence

GLOSSARY

cellular senescence The process by which cells express the senescent phenotype (irreversible growth arrest and other characteristic features). At least in mammals, cellular senescence may be a fail-safe mechanism that protects normal cells from tumorigenic transformation. Cellular senescence can be induced by telomere shortening, agents that cause DNA damage or alter chromatin, or overexpression of growth stimulatory proteins.

end-replication problem The inevitable loss of 3′ sequences from linear duplex DNA molecules as a consequence of DNA replication. 3′ sequences are lost because DNA replication is bidirectional, and DNA polymerases are unidirectional (5′ to 3′) and require a labile primer for initiation. Mammalian chromosomes lose 50–200 bp of 3′ terminal (telomeric) DNA with each round of DNA replication.

Hayflick limit The replicative life span of a cell population, or number of doublings at which a cell population completely senesces (all cells in the population are senescent).

immortal cells Refers to replicative immortality—cell populations that can divide indefinitely or have an unlimited replicative life span. Immortal cells are also referred to as cell lines.

mortal cells Refers to replicative mortality—cell populations that cannot divide indefinitely or have a limited replicative life span. Mortal cells are also referred to as cell strains.

passage Subcultivation. Cell populations are generally subcultivated or split at a fixed dilution (usually between 1:2 and 1:10) and thus may undergo one or several population doublings at each passage (depending on the split dilution). Cultures that have undergone relatively few passages and are far from the end of their replicative life span are often termed early passage. Cultures near the end of their replicative life span are often termed late passage.

replicative life span The maximum number of doublings that a cell population can complete.

replicative senescence Cellular senescence induced by repeated cell division; senescence that occurs when cells reach the end of their replicative life span.

senescent phenotype The essentially irreversible arrest of cell proliferation and accompanying functional changes that occur upon induction of cellular senescence. For most cell types, functional changes typically include an enlarged cell size, an increase in lysosomes, and expression of a neutral (senescence-associated) β-galactosidase. In addition, cell type specific functional changes occur (e.g., overexpression of metalloproteinases by senescent stromal fibroblasts, or underexpression of cell surface CD28 by senescent T lymphocytes). For some cell types, the senescent phenotype also includes resistance to certain apoptotic stimuli.

telomerase A ribonucleoprotein enzyme that adds telomeric repeats de novo to the 3′ ends of telomeres.

telomere The end of linear eukaryotic chromosomes. Telomeres are composed of a repetitive DNA sequence (TTAGGG in vertebrates) and specialized proteins and are essential for capping chromosome ends and preventing end-to-end fusions.

Cellular senescence is a process that causes mitotically competent cells, i.e., cells that have the potential to divide, to irreversibly lose the ability initiate, much less complete, the mitotic cell cycle. Coupled to this loss of cell division capacity are additional phenotypic changes. Cellular senescence can result from a number of normal and abnormal processes, including repeated cell division, DNA damage, and certain intracellular signaling events. Several lines of evidence suggest that cellular senescence, at least in mammalian species, evolved to suppress the development of cancer.

I. DEFINITIONS AND NOMENCLATURE

The first and most thorough understanding of cellular senescence came from the realization that most eukaryotic cells do not divide indefinitely. The process that limits cell division capacity is termed replicative senescence. Replicative senescence and cellular senescence are often used interchangeably because, to the extent it has been examined so far, cells induced to senesce by different stimuli have similar phenotypes.

Cells that do not divide indefinitely are said to have a finite (or limited) replicative life span. In some cases, they are also called "mortal" cells, and replicative senescence is referred to as cellular aging. The term "mortal" is not strictly accurate in this context

because cellular senescence does not necessarily result in cell death. In fact, some cells become less prone to die after they become senescent. For this reason, the term *replicative* life span is used to denote the number of divisions a cell or cell population can complete and should not be confused with chronological life span or viability. Likewise, although evidence discussed later suggests that cellular senescence may contribute to the aging of organisms, the link between cellular senescence and organismal aging remains tenuous and very likely is indirect. *Cellular* senescence describes a normal cellular response to potentially cancer-causing stimuli. It does not a priori connote the senescence or aging of organisms.

A few cell types do not undergo replicative senescence. Such cells are said to have an infinite or indefinite replicative life span and are often termed "immortal." Again, "immortal" is not strictly accurate because immortal cells may die as readily, or even more readily, than mortal cells. Moreover, DNA damage can induce cellular senescence in some immortal cells.

Three cell types appear to be replicatively immortal. First, the germline (cell lineages that give rise to mature sperm and eggs) has unlimited replicative capacity. Second, certain embryonic stem cells appear to divide indefinitely. Some adult stem cells may also divide indefinitely, but this has not yet been firmly established. Third, most malignant tumors contain cells having an extended or unlimited ability to divide.

II. HISTORY

The finite replicative life span of cells was first formally described by Leonard Hayflick and colleagues in the early to mid-1960s. Since then, replicative senescence has been shown to occur in many cell types from many animal species.

Hayflick and colleagues were culturing human fetal fibroblasts when they noted, and carefully documented, that the cultures progressively and inevitably lost proliferative capacity with each subculture (passage). Thus, cells cultured from tissue explants grew well during initial subcultures (early passages), but proliferation gradually declined. Eventually, the cultures contained only nondividing cells, despite culture conditions that supported the growth of early passage cells. Cultures that have not reached the end of their replicative life span are often termed early (or mid-) passage, whereas replicatively senescent cultures are late passage. The number of doublings at which a cell population senesces is sometimes termed the Hayflick limit.

Replicative senescence is most often studied in culture, where proliferation can be controlled and monitored for the many doublings needed for most or all the cells to senesce. The number of doublings at which complete senescence occurs varies by cell type and species. For example, human fetal fibroblasts senesce after 50–80 doublings, whereas mouse fetal fibroblasts do so after 10–15 doublings, and human adult mammary epithelial cells senesce after 20 or so doublings. Although cell proliferation is not easily controlled or monitored *in vivo*, some cell types have also been shown to have a finite replicative life span in intact organisms.

III. SENESCENT PHENOTYPES

Regardless of the inducer, senescent cells show two, in some cases three, striking phenotypic changes. First, the cells irreversibly stop dividing. Second, in some cases, they become resistant to apoptotic death. Third, senescent cells show selected changes in differentiated function. These changes are linked and define the senescent phenotype.

A. Cell Proliferation

A hallmark of cellular senescence is the irreversible growth arrest. Senescent cells cannot be stimulated to divide by known physiological stimuli. In this regard, they resemble terminally differentiated (postmitotic) cells, such as mature neurons.

Senescent cells arrest growth with a G1 DNA content, similar to quiescent (G0) cells. It is not surprising then that senescent cells fail to express several growth-regulatory or growth-related genes. Examples include cyclins A or B, DNA polymerase α, replication-dependent histones, and phosphorylated retinoblastoma (Rb) protein, among others—proteins normally present only during S phase or G2. The major difference between senescent and G0 cells is the reversibility of the growth arrest. Upon stimulation with mitogens, or conditions that promote proliferation, quiescent cells resume growth. This entails the orderly expression of

genes prior to S phase, e.g., those encoding FOS and MYC, and metabolic enzymes such as ornithine decarboxylase (ODC). Later, genes needed for S phase and completion of the cell cycle are expressed. In contrast, senescent cells do not resume growth upon mitogenic stimulation. Surprisingly, however, many genes remain mitogen inducible. For example, growth factors fully induce c-MYC, c-JUN and ODC in senescent human fibroblasts. However, a few genes whose expression is essential for entry into S phase remain repressed. These include c-FOS, ID1 and ID2 (inhibitors of basic helix–loop–helix transcription factors), and E2F1. The repression of selected growth regulatory genes very likely contributes to the senescence-associated growth arrest, but cannot fully explain it.

Senescent cells also express high levels of certain inhibitors of cyclin-dependent protein kinases (CDKs). CDKs stimulate proliferation by phosphorylating critical cell cycle regulators such as Rb. In contrast, CDK inhibitors (CDKIs) inhibit cell cycle progression. In human fibroblasts, the p21 CDKI increases as cells near replicative senescence. Interestingly, p21 levels slowly decline in senescent cultures, whereas expression of the p16 CDKI, encoded by the INK4a locus, rises. p16 is an affirmed tumor suppressor that is frequently deleted or silenced in mammalian cancers. The INK4a locus encodes a second tumor suppressor and growth inhibitor, p14/ARF, which is not a CDKI. p14/ARF expression also rises during replicative senescence. p21 and the proteins encoded by INK4a are important regulators of senescence. Cells that lack p21 or a functional INK4a locus have an extended replicative life span and an increased probability of immortalization and tumorigenic transformation.

Thus, irreversible senescence growth arrest is maintained by both the suppression of positive growth regulators and the expression of growth inhibitors. The latter very likely explains the dominance of the senescence growth arrest in cell hybrids.

B. Cell Death

Senescent cells remain viable and metabolically active for long periods of time. Thus, cellular senescence is not apoptosis or programmed cell death.

Some cells (e.g., human fibroblasts or T lymphocytes) become resistant to apoptotic death upon senescence. Thus, presenescent fibroblasts or T cells are more likely to die in response to growth factor deprivation or FAS ligand than senescent fibroblasts or T cells. Other cell types (e.g., human endothelial cells or keratinocytes), however, do not appear to resist apoptosis when senescent, although they certainly do not die immediately upon senescence.

C. Cell Function

A striking feature of senescence is the changes in cell function that accompany the growth arrest.

Some of these functional changes occur in most, if not all, senescent cells. These changes include (1) increased cell size and lysosome biogenesis and (2) decreased rates of protein synthesis and degradation. However, some functional changes are cell type dependent. For example, senescent adrenal cortical epithelial cells secrete an altered spectrum of steroid hormones, senescent endothelial cells express high levels of interleukin-1 and the adhesion molecule I-CAM, and senescent fibroblasts secrete high levels of interleukin-1, EGF-like growth factors, and matrix metalloproteinases. Very little is known about how the altered differentiation associated with cell senescence is regulated.

D. Significance

There is strong evidence that cellular senescence is an important mechanism for suppressing tumorigenesis, at least in mammals. Less direct evidence suggests that the accumulation of senescent cells may also contribute to organismal aging.

1. Cancer

The idea that cellular senescence is a tumor suppressive mechanism derives from four major lines of evidence.

First, most naturally occurring or experimentally induced tumors contain cells that have bypassed the limit imposed by replicative senescence. This is not to say that immortality is required for tumorigenesis. Rather, there appears to be a strong selection for cells with an increased proliferative potential in the development of cancer. Immortality, or even extended replicative life span, greatly increases the susceptibility to malignant progression because it permits the extensive cell division that is necessary to acquire successive mutations.

Second, certain oncogenes act, at least in part, by immortalizing or extending the replicative life span of cells. These oncogenes include mutated or deregulated cellular genes (e.g., c-MYC, BMI-1), as well as the oncogenes of certain viruses implicated in some human cancers (e.g., Epstein–Barr or human papilloma viruses). Thus, mutations that lead to tumorigenesis, or the strategies of oncogenic viruses, can and do involve mechanisms that permit cells to escape senescence.

Third, among the genes that are essential for establishing and/or maintaining the senescence growth arrest are those encoding the p53 and Rb tumor suppressor proteins. The activities of these tumor suppressors are together perhaps the most commonly lost functions in human cancer, and both are necessary for cellular senescence.

Fourth, cells from mice with inactivating germline mutations in tumor suppressor genes such as p53 and p16 either do not senesce or have a greatly increased probability of spontaneous immortalization. Needless to say, these animals die prematurely of cancer. Moreover, humans with germline mutations in the tumor suppressors p53, p16, or Rb are cancer prone, and cells from such individuals are prone to spontaneous immortalization. Thus, the cellular phenotype of defective senescence results in a cancer-prone organismal phenotype.

Finally, as discussed later, the events or agents known to induce cellular senescence are potentially oncogenic. This suggests that normal cells are programmed to respond to potentially cancer-causing stimuli by entering a permanent senescence growth arrest.

2. Aging

The link between cellular senescence and aging derives from data that are largely correlative and indirect.

First, cells cultured from old donors tend to senesce after fewer doublings than cells from young donors. With some exceptions, this trend was reported by several independent studies, but, in all cases, there was considerable scatter in the data. This correlation suggests that the replicative life span of cells may become progressively exhausted with chronological age. Second, cells from short-lived species tend to senesce after fewer doublings than cells from long-lived species, suggesting that there may be overlap in genes that control the chronological life span of organisms and replicative life span of cells. Finally, cells from donors with hereditary premature aging syndromes senesce more rapidly than cells from age-matched controls. This has been documented best in cells from donors with Werner syndrome, an adult onset premature aging syndrome caused by defects in a RECQ-like helicase (WRN) that may participate in DNA replication, recombination, and/or repair. This finding supports the idea that the life span of organisms and replicative life span of cells are controlled by common genes.

Replicative senescence is thought to compromise organismal life span because it depletes tissue renewal or repair capacity. This may be the case, but proliferating cells can often be recovered from even very old tissue. Moreover, the proliferative capacities of adjacent tissue biopsies from the same donor can vary considerably. A more recent idea is that cellular senescence may be detrimental because dysfunctional senescent cells accumulate in tissues, where they secrete molecules that can compromise tissue integrity or function.

3. Evolutionary Context

At first glance, the idea that cellular senescence can prevent cancer and yet contribute to aging may seem contradictory. However, the apparent paradox of a trait having both beneficial and detrimental effects is consistent with the evolutionary theory of antagonistic pleiotropy. This theory predicts that, because the force of natural selection declines with age, traits that are selected to improve fitness in young organisms (e.g., forestalling cancer) can have unselected deleterious effects late in life. In this context, the senescence growth arrest may be the selected trait that suppresses tumorigenesis, whereas the altered function of senescent cells may be an unselected deleterious feature of the senescent phenotype.

IV. CAUSES OF CELLULAR SENESCENCE

Repeated cell division is not the only cause of cellular senescence. A senescent phenotype can also be induced by certain types of DNA damage and intracel-lular signals. In all cases, there is an irreversible arrest of cell division and changes in cell function. Close examination of the senescent phenotypes induced by different stimuli will undoubtedly uncover differences, as indeed early microarray analyses indicate, but, in general, the senescent phenotypes induced by diverse stimuli are similar.

A. Telomere Shortening

Telomeres are nucleoprotein structures at the ends of linear eukaryotic chromosomes, consisting of a repetitive DNA sequence and specialized proteins. Telomeres are essential for preventing chromosome end-to-end fusions and genomic instability. Due to the biochemistry of DNA replication, each S phase leaves unreplicated 50–200 bp of 3′ telomeric DNA. This inevitable loss of DNA is termed the end-replication problem. The enzyme telomerase solves the end-replication problem by adding telomeric repeats directly to the 3′ telomeric end. However, most somatic cells do not express this enzyme. Thus, for most cells, telomeres shorten with each cell cycle.

It is now clear that telomere shortening is a critical determinant of replicative senescence, at least in human cells. Human telomeres are 15–20 kb in the germline and somewhat shorter in neonatal and adult cells. Human cells senesce when the telomeres reach 5–7 kb. Both telomere shortening and replicative senescence can be prevented by ectopic expression of telomerase. Thus, telomere shortening limits the number of divisions that human cells can complete, and senescence ensues before the telomeres shorten enough to cause genomic instability. The telomeres of laboratory mice are much longer than human telomeres. However, for reasons that are not understood, mouse cells senesce after fewer doublings than human cells. One possibility is that mouse cells contain only one or very few short telomeres, which limit their replicative life span.

Telomerase is expressed in the germline, early embryonic cells, some stem cells, and most cancer cells. Thus, telomerase is the major means by which immortal cells solve the end-replication problem to divide indefinitely. However, telomerase is not necessarily sufficient for replicative immortality. Some somatic cells, such as T lymphocytes, express telomerase. In such cells, telomere loss is retarded, but not prevented, and the cells senesce. Moreover, telomerase did not immortalize some human epithelial cells unless p16 was silenced. Data suggest that telomere-associated proteins can regulate whether and to what extent telomerase accesses the 3′ telomeric end. Conversely, telomerase is not absolutely essential for preventing telomere loss. A minority of immortal cancer cells do not express telomerase. Such cells have long heterogeneous telomeres that are very likely maintained by recombination.

Short telomeres may resemble DNA double strand breaks, which can also induce senescence (discussed later). Telomere shortening may also alter heterochromatin, which could explain why inhibitors of DNA methylation or histone deacetylase inhibitors can induce senescence within a few doublings. Finally, telomere shortening may cause the redistribution of telomere binding proteins that can alter gene expression when present at nontelomeric sites.

B. DNA Damage

Normal cells respond to certain types of DNA damage by arresting growth with a senescent phenotype. Human fibroblasts, for example, irreversibly arrest growth with senescent-like characteristics within a few doublings after exposure to agents that cause oxidative DNA damage, or single or double strand DNA breaks. In addition, some human tumor cells underwent a senescent-like arrest after exposure to DNA-damaging chemotherapeutic agents. The senescence response to DNA damage may explain why mouse cells senesce more rapidly than human cells. Mouse cells may be more sensitive to the oxidizing environment of cell culture, and senesce due to DNA damage.

Some types of DNA damage may induce cellular senescence by accelerating telomere shortening. Human fibroblasts senesce after a few doublings when under oxidative stress. Under these conditions, cells acquired genome-wide single strand breaks, and the damaged telomeres shortened at a much-accelerated rate.

C. Intracellular Pathways

Normal cells have been shown to respond to potentially oncogenic signals by adopting a senescent phenotype. This response was first shown for activated RAS, and subsequently for other components in RAS-mediated signaling (RAF and MEK) and for the E2F1 transcription factor. All these proteins are potent stimulators of cell cycle progression and induce tumorigenic transformation or apoptosis when overexpressed in immortal cells. Normal human cells, however, responded to overexpression of these proteins by undergoing senescence within a few doublings. This senescence response was mediated by pathways controlled by p53 and pRb. Thus, RAS, MEK, or E2F1 had little effect, or stimulated growth, when cells were deficient in p53, pRb, or INK4a proteins. These findings support the idea that the senescence response is a fail-safe mechanism that protects normal cells from oncogenic transformation.

V. PHYSIOLOGICAL CONSEQUENCES OF CELLULAR SENESCENCE

Many mammalian cell types have been shown to senesce in culture. These include many epithelial cells, endothelial cells, smooth muscle cells, and lymphocytes. Because there are few markers that distinguish senescent from quiescent or terminally differentiated cells, there are only a few reports of cells with senescence characteristics *in vivo*. A senescence-associated β-galactosidase distinguishes senescent fibroblasts and keratinocytes from their quiescent or differentiated counterparts in culture. Cells expressing this marker were found in human skin and increased with donor age. Similarly, T lymphocytes with surface characteristics of senescent T cells (lacking CD28) were found in human blood, and their prevalence increased with donor age. Thus, senescent cells probably exist *in vivo* and accumulate with age.

Senescent cells secrete molecules that can have deleterious effects and act at a distance within tissues. These molecules include proteases that degrade stromal and basement membrane components, inflammatory cytokines, and even growth factors that can disrupt proliferative homeostasis. This feature of senescent cells may be responsible for their role in aging.

Carrying this idea a step further, cancer incidence is thought to rise exponentially with age because several mutations are required for malignant transformation. There is little doubt that mutations are a necessary and critical feature of cancer. However, it is now clear that tumors harbor a plethora of mutations and that the tissue microenvironment can control cell growth and differentiation, even in the face of potentially oncogenic mutations. Cells harboring such mutations may not express a malignant phenotype until they are released from the constraints of the microenvironment. Because senescent cells can destroy the organization, and hence constraints, of the microenvironment, neoplastic growth may be initiated, or at least favored, by the presence of senescent cells. Indeed, senescent fibroblasts have been shown to stimulate the ability of premalignant and malignant epithelial cells to proliferate and form tumors in mice. It has been proposed that the age-dependent accumulation of senescent cells may synergize with the accumulation of mutations to explain the exponential rise in cancer incidence. Hence, cellular senescence, despite its ability to suppress tumorigenesis early in life, may contribute to tumorigenesis later in life.

See Also the Following Articles

CELL CYCLE CHECKPOINTS • CELL CYCLE CONTROL • CELLULAR RESPONSES TO DNA DAMAGE • P16 AND ARF • TELOMERES AND TELOMERASE • TP53 TUMOR SUPPRESSOR GENE

Bibliography

Bacchetti, S., and Wynford-Thomas, D. (ed.) (1997). Telomeres and telomerase in cancer. *Eur. J. Cancer* **33**, 703–800.

Campisi, J. (1997). Aging and cancer: The double-edged sword of replicative senescence. *J. Am. Geriatr. Soc.* **45**, 482–488.

Campisi, J., Dimri, G. P., and Hara, E. (1996) Control of replicative senescence. *In* "Handbook of the Biology of Aging" (E. Schneider and J. Rowe, eds.), 4th Ed., pp. 121–149. Academic Press, New York.

Dimri, G., Lee, X., Basile, G., Acosta, M., Scott, G., Roskelley, C., Medrano, E.E., Linskens, M., Rubelj, I., Pereira-Smith, O., Peacocke, M., and Campisi, J. (1995) A novel biomarker identifies senescent human cells in culture and aging skin *in vivo. Proc. Nat. Acad. Sci. USA* **92**, 9363–9367.

Dimri, G. P., Itahana, K., Acosta, M., and Campisi, J. (2000). Regulation of a senescence checkpoint response by the E2F1 transcription factor and p14(ARF) tumor suppressor. *Mol. Cell. Biol.* **20**, 273–285.

Hayflick, L. (1965) The limited *in vitro* lifetime of human diploid cell strains. *Exp. Cell Res.* **37**, 614–636.

Krtolica, A., Parrinello, S., Lockett, S., Desprez, P., and Campisi, J. (2001). Senescent fibroblasts promote epithelial cell growth and tumorigenesis: A link between cancer and aging. *Proc. Natl. Acad. Sci. USA* **98**, 12072–12077.

Lin, A.W., Barradas, M., Stone, J.C., van Aelst, L., Serrano, M., and Lowe, S.W. (1998) Premature senescence involving p53 and p16 is activated in response to constitutive MEK/MAPK mitogenic signaling. *Genes Dev.* **12**, 3008–3019.

Pawelec, G., Effros, R. B., Caruso, C., Remarque, E., Barnett, Y., and Solana, R. (1999). *Front. Biosci.* **4**, 216–269.

Sager, R. (1991). Senescence as a mode of tumor suppression. *Environ. Health Perspect.* **93**, 59–62.

Serrano, M. (2000). The INK4a/ARF locus in murine tumorigenesis. *Carcinogenesis* **21**, 865–869.

Shelton, D. N., Chang, E., Whittier, P. S., Choi, D., and Funk, W. D. (1999). Microarray analysis of replicative senescence. *Curr. Biol.* **9**, 939–945.

Stanulis-Praeger, B. (1987). Cellular senescence revisited: A review. *Mech. Ageing Dev.* **38**, 1–48.

Stein, G. H., Drullinger, L. F., Soulard, A., and Dulic, V. (1999). Differential roles for cyclin-dependent kinase inhibitors p21 and p16 in the mechanisms of senescence and differentiation in human fibroblasts. *Mol. Cell. Biol.* **19**, 2109–2117.

von Zglinicki, T., Pilger, P., and Sitte, N. (2000). Accumulation of single-strand breaks is the major cause of telomere shortening in human fibroblasts. *Free Radic. Biol. Med.* **28**, 64–74.

Yeager, T. R., DeVries, S., Jarrard, D. F., Kao, C., Nakada, S. Y., Moon, T. D., Bruskewitz, R., Stadler, W. M., Meisner, L. F., Gilchrist, K. W., Newton, M. A., Waldman, F. M., and Reznikoff, C. A. (1998). Overcoming cellular senescence in human cancer pathogenesis. *Genes Dev.* **12**, 163–174.

Signal Transduction Mechanisms Initiated by Receptor Tyrosine Kinases

Peter Blume-Jensen

Serono Reproductive Biology Institute

Tony Hunter

The Salk Institute

GLOSSARY

anchoring protein Protein that simultaneously binds to subcellular structures and to a complement of protein kinase(s) and protein phosphatase(s), thereby bringing the latter close to their substrate(s).

cross talk Mechanisms whereby activated signaling molecules in a primary signal transduction pathway can regulate signaling molecules in another primary signal transduction pathway.

feedback regulation Mechanisms by which activated signaling molecules can regulate upstream components within the same signal transduction pathway.

growth factor A molecule, in most cases a polypeptide, which binds specifically to a cell membrane receptor, thereby regulating cell growth and differentiation.

kinase An enzyme that catalyzes phosphorylation of a protein, a lipid, or a carbohydrate. A majority of protein kinases are specific for either tyrosine residues or serine/threonine residues.

oncogene A gene whose protein product can lead to malignant transformation.

phosphatase An enzyme that catalyzes dephosphorylation of a protein, a lipid, or a carbohydrate. A majority of protein phosphatases are specific for either phosphotyrosine residues or phosphoserine/phosphothreonine residues.

protein module A conserved three-dimensional structure, often with a conserved primary amino acid sequence, found in several otherwise unrelated proteins. Its function is independent of the surrounding amino acid sequence.

protooncogene The normal cellular counterpart of an oncogene. Protooncogenes can become oncogenes upon structural alterations.

receptor protein tyrosine kinase A subgroup of tyrosine-specific protein kinases that are transmembrane receptors for growth factors and have intrinsic, ligand-stimulatable tyrosine kinase activity in their cytoplasmic parts.

scaffold protein A protein that simultaneously associates with several enzymes, often protein kinases, of a signaling pathway in a modular fashion, permitting sequential activation of each enzyme.

signal transduction Molecular events that take place in response to extracellular biological stimuli to elicit specific cellular responses.

Intercellular communication is of paramount importance in multicellular organisms. Signals transmitted between cells stimulate cell surface receptors to activate intracellular signaling pathways that are precisely regulated, controlled, and organized. Perturbation of the normal regulation of intracellular signaling underlies most, if not all, diseases, including cancer. One large subfamily of transmembrane cell surface receptors is endowed with intrinsic protein tyrosine kinase activity and is of particular importance for the regulation of intracellular signaling pathways. These receptor protein tyrosine kinases (RPTKs) catalyze transfer of the γ phosphate from ATP to hydroxyl groups on specific tyrosine residues of intracellular target proteins. In particular, RPTKs phosphorylate specific phosphotyrosine residues in their own intracellular regions, and this autophosphorylation serves to create specific phosphotyrosine-binding sites for cytoplasmic substrates. The specificity in RPTK-initiated signaling is achieved by several means. First, there is specificity in the upstream activating event, where a ligand binds its cognate RPTK. Second, catalytic specificity of the activated RPTK and downstream kinases and phosphatases provides the basis for site-specific phosphorylation and dephosphorylation of proteins within the cell. Specific tyrosine and serine/threonine phosphorylation sites and their surrounding sequences are involved in transient and stable protein–protein interactions with conserved protein modules found in most cytoplasmic signaling molecules. Moreover, anchoring and scaffold proteins are involved in organization of the intracellular signaling pathways into multiprotein complexes by selective binding to pro-

tein serine/threonine kinases and phosphatases. Both the selectivity in binding and the affinity of all these protein–protein interactions control the signaling paths. Third, there is compartmentalization of signaling molecules, and the correct subcellular localization is a prerequisite for specific interactions to occur. Modular binding domains as well as posttranslational modifications of signaling molecules dictate their localization within the cell. Moreover, the duration, amplitude, and kinetics of signals are critical for the cellular response. Protein phosphorylation is a key regulator because it can sustain or attenuate signals via amplification, feedback, and cross talk. Finally, but not least, there is cell type specificity in signaling. Based on the constellation and expression of signaling proteins in a particular cell type, specific molecules can be ascribed different roles in cellular responses. With a focus on mammalian proteins, this article serves to illustrate the main principles of RPTK-initiated signal transduction and the different mechanisms whereby specificity and coordination of signaling are achieved.

I. INTRODUCTION

The proper regulation of cell growth, differentiation, migration, survival, and apoptosis in multicellular organisms is crucial for normal embryonic development and in adult life. The mediators of intercellular communication are the molecules involved in cell–cell and cell–matrix interactions, as well as extracellular signaling molecules. The specific binding of the extracellular molecules to either cell adhesion molecules or transmembrane receptors on the cell surface initiates a cascade of intracellular biochemical events. These culminate in a cellular response, which, depending on the particular signaling pathways activated, may involve cell cycle progression and changes in cellular gene expression, cell survival, cell differentiation, protein trafficking, migration, cytoskeletal architecture, adhesion, and metabolism. Even cell death is programmed in numerous tissues (so-called apoptosis) and can be activated by specific signaling pathways, both during development and in adults. Signal transduction (of Latin: *trans*, over or through; *ductus*, tube, line, something that leads) is this whole scenario of molecular events that takes place to convey information from the exterior of the cell to its cytoplasm or nucleus, eliciting a cellular response.

Conservative estimates based on the approaching completion of the human genome project suggest that as much as 20% of human genes encode proteins involved in signal transduction. These include transmembrane receptors, G protein subunits, and signal-generating enzymes. The latter group includes more than 700 protein kinases and 180 protein phosphatases. Intracellular signal transduction pathways are made up of phosphorylation cascades that are reversibly and tightly controlled by these enzymes. Protein kinases and phosphatases exist as transmembrane as well as intracellular molecules, and a majority of both categories of enzymes can be subdivided into tyrosine or serine/threonine specific based on their preferred catalytic activity. However, some possess dual specificity for both tyrosine and serine/threonine residues, and a few members of the phosphoinositide (PI) kinase family, lipid kinases that phosphorylate the inositol ring of phosphatidylinositol (PtdIns) or specific PIs, exhibit protein serine/threonine kinase activity as well.

Tyrosine phosphorylation is rare in cells; it probably constitutes less than 0.05% of the total amount of protein phosphorylation, the majority of which occurs on serine and threonine residues. However, the importance of protein tyrosine kinases (PTKs) in normal cell growth regulation is evident from the fact that many of them are encoded by cellular protooncogenes. Protooncogenes are the normal cellular counterparts of oncogenes (*oncos*, Greek for "mass"), cancer-causing genes originally identified in RNA viruses. While numerous retroviruses carrying oncogenes cause cancer and other malignancies in avian and rodent cells, so far only the RNA virus human T-cell lymphotropic virus (HTLV-1) has been directly implicated in oncogenesis in humans, in the form of T-cell lymphomas. Rather, human protooncogenes become altered and activated by irradiation (e.g., UV exposure), chemical carcinogens (e.g., in cigarette smoke), unrepaired replication errors, or aging, resulting in the development of cancer.

Today more than 150 oncogenes are known, most of which encode components of the signal transduction chain from the cell exterior to the nucleus. Examples include homologues of growth factors, growth factor receptors of the RPTK type, cytoplasmic PTKs and serine/threonine (S/T) kinases, small GTP-binding proteins of the Ras superfamily, nuclear proteins (mostly transcription factors), and cell cycle regulators. In addition, loss-of-function mutations in so-called tumor suppressor proteins can lead to malignant transformation. These molecules are not oncogenes, but rather their normal function is important to prevent oncogenesis by counteracting some of the oncogenic insults or stimuli mentioned earlier. Interestingly, PTKs comprise a major group of oncoproteins, and many RPTKs have been isolated as retroviral oncogene intermediates, such as v-*ErbB* (EGF receptor), v-*fms* (CSF-1 receptor), or v-*kit* (Kit/SCF receptor).

The mechanisms for oncogenic activation of signaling molecules are varied, but in all cases they involve constitutive or deregulated protein activity. The normal intracellular regulation is thereby perturbed, resulting in malignant transformation. Activation or deregulation of protooncogenes in humans can occur by three mechanisms: mutations, as mentioned earlier; chromosomal rearrangements, which cause altered expression or activity of any oncogene involved in the rearrangement; or amplification, which results in protooncogene overexpression. It is believed that cancer arises via a multistep process, usually over many years, and that cooperation between oncogenes and simultaneous inactivation of tumor suppressors is necessary for malignant transformation. More recently, this concept has been slightly challenged by findings in inducible transgenic tumor mouse models, indicating that constitutive activation of a single oncogene is sufficient for at least morphological signs of malignant transformation of specific tissues without other detectable genomic alterations. Interestingly, the lesions in these mice remain dependent on expression of the oncogenic transgene and regress when expression is switched off. However, those findings need to be substantiated significantly, in particular it needs to be demonstrated that true metastases are formed, a hallmark of malignant tumors, and that the tumors in these mice are not mere examples of monoclonal hyperproliferative disorders. A few well-established examples of oncogenic conversion of signaling molecules are provided under the individual sections that follow.

II. RECEPTOR PROTEIN TYROSINE KINASES (RPTKs)

PTKs are found in all multicellular eukaryotic organisms examined, but not in yeast, possibly reflecting their key role for the evolution of multicellular organisms where they function in intercellular communication. There are two classes of PTKs: cytoplasmic PTKs and transmembrane receptor PTKs (RPTKs). The latter are endowed with ligand-stimulatable intrinsic protein tyrosine kinase activity in their cytoplasmic domains and are all activated by polypeptide ligands called growth factors. Accordingly, RPTKs are sometimes referred to as growth factor receptors, but it is now clear that not all stimulate growth per se. Most known ligands for RPTKs are secreted, soluble proteins, but transmembrane, membrane-bound, and extracellular matrix-bound forms also activate RPTKs. In addition to classical, single transmembrane-spanning RPTKs, there are also binary receptors with ligand-inducible PTK activity. These multicomponent receptors are composed of a transmembrane ligand-binding molecule devoid of PTK activity, with an associated cytoplasmic PTK. Many cytokine receptors are binary receptors, and a typical example is the interferon (IFN) receptor, which interacts with *Janus* kinase (JAK), a cytoplasmic PTK, via its intracellular domain. In response to ligand stimulation, JAK becomes activated, resulting in tyrosine autophosphorylation and tyrosine phosphorylation of the receptor subunit, and the receptor phosphotyrosine residues, in turn, bind to so-called signal transducers and activators of transcription (STATs) that mediate signaling to the nucleus. The following sections mainly discuss signaling mechanisms from classical RPTKs, but the same main principles govern binary receptor signaling.

The classification of RPTKs is based largely on their structural organization. There are at present a total of almost 60 RPTKs identified, which can be divided into 20 distinct subfamilies (Fig. 1). For 8 or 9 of these, the so-called orphan receptors, the ligand is still not identified. All RPTKs are type I transmembrane proteins with a single membrane-spanning region and have several characteristic features in common. The extracellular ligand-binding domain is the most distinctive feature in RPTKs. It is several hundred amino acids in length and is composed of different patterns of cysteine residues and various structural sequence motifs, e.g., immunoglobulin (Ig)-like domains, fibronectin type III-like domains, and leucine-rich sequences, among others. Most RPTKs are modified by N- and sometimes O-linked glycosylations. Following the hydrophobic stretch of amino acids traversing the membrane are a few basic amino acids. The cytoplasmic part of the receptors is composed of a juxtamembrane region of 50 to 100 amino acids, which precedes the catalytic domain. In some RPTKs the kinase domain is split by a hydrophilic insert sequence up to 150 amino acids long. Finally, there is a region C-terminal to the catalytic domain, which is from a few up to 200 amino acid residues in length (Fig. 1). Most of the tyrosine autophosphorylation occurs in the regions outside the catalytic domain proper, including the kinase insert region, and these phosphotyrosine residues serve as substrate-binding sites. However, a major tyrosine autophosphorylation site(s) is located within the catalytic domain proper and its phosphorylation is in most cases essential for kinase activation.

The conserved catalytic domain is composed of approximately 250 amino acid residues. It is shared by all protein kinases in the protein serine/tyrosine kinase superfamily and has been delineated by sequence similarities. Within the RPTK catalytic domains, the sequence similarities range from 32 to 95%, and 13 amino acid residues are totally conserved and crucial for kinase activity. Accordingly, RPTKs such as ErbB3 and of the RYK (related to tyrosine kinases) family, such as H-Ryk and its Drosophila orthologue Derailed, each of which has a substitution(s) of one or more of these conserved residues, are kinase inactive. The crystal structures of the catalytic domains for several S/T kinases and PTKs, including those of cAMP-dependent protein kinase (PKA), cyclin-dependent kinase 2, extracellular-regulated kinase 2 (ERK2), the insulin receptor, the type I FGF receptor, and c-Src, among others, have been solved. They show a similar overall structure. The kinase domain is composed of two lobes with a cleft in between where Mg^{2+}/ATP and the substrate are brought together. The distance of the substrate peptide backbone from the active site residues and the γ phosphate within the cleft in which the phos-

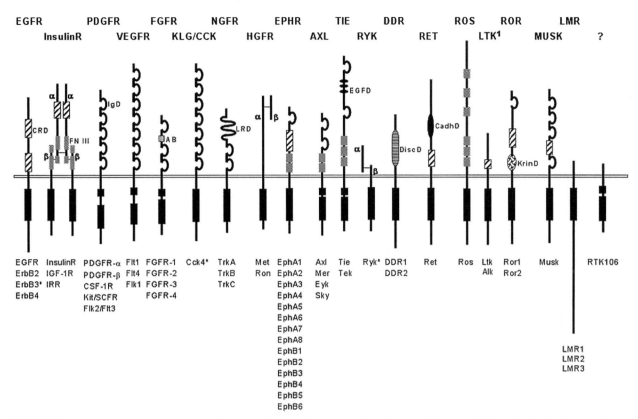

FIGURE 1 Human receptor protein tyrosine kinase families. Based on structural similarities, 59 human RPTKs can be divided into 20 distinct subfamilies. The prototypic receptor for each family is indicated above the receptor, and the known members below. AB, acidic box; CadhD, cadherin-like domain; CRD, cysteine-rich domain; DiscD, discoidin-like domain; EGFD, epidermal growth factor-like domain; FNIII, fibronectin type III-like domain; IgD, immunoglobulin-like domain; KrinD, kringle-like domain; LRD, leucine-rich domain. α and β denote distinct RPTK subunits. Notes: [1] RPTKs Ltk and Alk were originally classified as InsR family members, but they have distinct structural characteristics and form a separate RPTK subfamily. * These RPTKs are devoid of intrinsic kinase activity due to mutation of one or several highly conserved amino acid residues in the core catalytic domain. KLG/CCK indicates that colon carcinoma kinase-4 (CCK-4) is homologous, or possibly orthologous, to chick KLG. ? indicates that RTK106 is still uncharacterized. Figure not drawn to scale.

photransfer reaction occurs determines the substrate preference for either tyrosine or serine/threonine.

III. RPTK-INITIATED SIGNAL TRANSDUCTION

In outline, signaling by RPTKs involves ligand-induced receptor oligomerization, which results in tyrosine autophosphorylation of the receptor subunits. Tyrosine phosphorylation acts as a molecular switch for the RPTKs in two ways: it activates their catalytic activity and simultaneously the tyrosine autophosphorylation sites mediate the specific binding of

cytoplasmic-signaling molecules. In this way, signaling molecules are translocated to the membrane. Several of these act as substrates and become phosphorylated and, in some cases, activated by the RPTK as well. These translocated and phosphorylated targets and substrates can, in turn, create specific binding sites for other signaling molecules, and in this way networks of interacting signaling molecules are stimulated.

A. Ligand Binding and Ligand-Induced Receptor Oligomerization

The polypeptide ligands reach their target cells and cognate receptors via the bloodstream by diffusion between neighboring cells or by basement membrane or extracellular matrix deposition. They may also be presented in cell-bound forms from neighboring cells. Ligand binding to the extracellular part of the receptors is reversible, specific, and occurs with high affinity, often in the nanomolar range. The specificity in binding is conferred by specific regions of the growth factors interacting with specific regions of the extracellular domains of the receptors, and, conversely, only part of the extracellular domain of RPTKs is required for ligand binding. It is now well established that ligand binding induces a specific oligomeric conformation and that this is tightly linked to RPTK kinase activation. Most of our initial knowledge regarding ligand-induced receptor-oligomerization has come from studies on members of the platelet-derived growth factor (PDGF) and epidermal growth factor (EGF) receptor subfamilies of RPTKs (see Fig. 1).

Ligands in the PDGF receptor subfamily are all dimeric in nature, existing as disulfide-bonded homo- and heterodimers of an A and a B chain. Biochemical and cell biological studies revealed that the A chain of PDGF binds only PDGF α receptors, whereas the B chain of PDGF binds both α and β receptors. Based on the isoform-specific properties of the ligands and their receptors, PDGF-AA stimulates the formation of αα receptor homodimers, PDGF-AB induces both αα receptor homodimers and αβ receptor heterodimers, whereas PDGF-BB induces all three possible combinations of receptor dimers. Importantly, the different dimeric PDGF receptor complexes transduce specific biological signals. The structurally related receptors for colony-stimulating factor-1 (CSF-1) and stem cell factor (SCF), for which both of the ligands are noncovalent dimers under physiological conditions, dimerize by a similar mechanism: one ligand dimer binds to two receptors by each ligand subunit contacting one receptor, causing a 2:2 ligand subunit:receptor complex. Other growth factors, such as vascular endothelial growth factor (VEGF), are also physiological dimers, and both biochemical and structural data show that they induce receptor dimerization by a similar mechanism. In all these cases the dimerization process is driven by each ligand subunit binding independently to each of the receptors in the dimer, thereby bringing them together initially. However, homophilic receptor–receptor interactions of

extracellular, and sometimes intracellular, juxtamembrane regions are involved in the stabilization of receptor dimers, resulting in a tight, specific conformation of receptor subunits, compatible with receptor kinase activation. This was initially shown by Yarden and co-workers in a series of elegantly conducted studies on the Kit/SCF receptor and was later supported by structural evidence from other ligand–receptor systems. This has led to a sequential dimerization model involving an initial step of monovalent ligand binding with unstable dimer formation. The subsequent stabilization of the dimers involves conformational receptor changes, allowing for homophilic receptor–receptor interactions via the fourth Ig-like domain in the extracellular part. This conformational change is transferred to the intracellular domains, enabling juxtaposition of the kinase domains and transphosphorylation. Only correct orientation of the receptor subunits and juxtaposition of the kinase domains within dimers allow for kinase activation (see Fig. 2 and later).

More recent mutational studies of the ErbB2 receptor, together with structural predictions, support such a model of induced protein proximity for RPTK activation. Hence, productive ErbB2 dimerization requires a precise rotational coupling of the receptor monomers within a dimer, again enabling juxtaposition and transphosphorylation of the kinase domains. In the EGF/ErbB subfamily of receptors (Fig. 1) the ligands are monomeric, but they might bind in a bivalent fashion. The ligands, including EGF and NDF/heregulin, induce both homo- and heterodimers of their receptors. In this case, different domains of the ligands can participate in receptor binding. For instance, EGF induces homodimers of ErbB1, as well as heterodimers between ErbB1 and ErbB2 or ErbB3. NDF/heregulin, a ligand for ErbB3 and ErbB4, induces heterodimers between each of these and the orphan receptor Neu/ErbB2. The presence of either ErbB3 or ErbB4 is necessary for NDF/heregulin-induced tyrosine phophorylation and activation of ErbB2.

Ligand-induced dimerization by certain monomeric ligands involves ligand aggregation or clustering. Thus, heparin and heparan sulfate proteoglycan, present in the extracellular matrix, make numerous contacts with monomeric FGFs and with FGFR. Crystal structure studies have shown that receptor–receptor

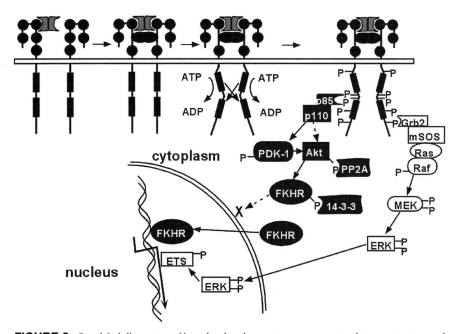

FIGURE 2 Simplified illustration of ligand-induced receptor protein tyrosine kinase activation and signal transduction. The dimeric ligand binds to its receptor, resulting in unstable dimer formation. Conformational changes in the receptors ensue, allowing for homophilic receptor–receptor interactions, which stabilize the receptor dimers. This leads to receptor autophosphorylation and subsequent binding of SH2-containing signaling molecules that act in different signaling pathways, including the PI 3′-kinase and Ras-Raf-ERK pathways illustrated here. p85, the adaptor subunit of PI 3′-kinase, binds through its SH2 domain to the activated RPTK, causing activation of the catalytic p110 subunit. Stimulated p110, in turn, causes activation of the protein serine/threonine kinases PDK-1 and Akt, and activated Akt subsequently phosphorylates the apoptosis-promoting transcription factor FKHR, resulting in binding to 14-3-3 and cytoplasmic sequestration. This prevents nuclear translocation of FKHR and transcriptional activity (illustrated with a dashed arrow and an "X"). Activated Akt also translocates to the nucleus where it could possibly phosphorylate nuclear FKHR as well. For simplicity, this possibility has been omitted. PP2A has been shown to associate with and dephosphorylate T308 in activated Akt. The adaptor protein Grb2 is also recruited to activated RPTKs through its SH2 domain, in association with the Ras exchange factor mSOS, bound to the SH3 domains of Grb2. The Grb2/mSOS complex subsequently stimulates the classical Ras-Raf-ERK cascade. Activated ERK translocates to the nucleus where it phosphorylates the ETS family of transcription factors through direct phosphorylation. For simplicity, arrows indicate an activating event. However, note that most of the illustrated proteins form large, multimeric complexes. For instance, the kinase suppressor of Ras (KSR) binds simultaneously Ras, Raf, MEK, and ERK in complexes with 14-3-3 and Hsp90. Basic events known for the PDGF receptor subfamily of receptors are illustrated. For further details, see text.

and receptor–heparin interactions facilitate the dimer formation induced by the heparin-bound FGF, resulting in a 2:2 FGF:FGFR complex. Clustering of the membrane-attached ligands for the Eph class of RP-TKs facilitates receptor oligomerization, aided by homophilic receptor–receptor interactions through intracellular SAM domains, a specific type of protein interaction domain (see later). Oligomerization of proteins by induced protein proximity is a general phenomenon in signaling, being also observed for cy-

tokine receptors, antigen receptors, serine/threonine kinase receptors, and cytoplasmic signaling molecules and transcription factors.

B. Receptor Protein Tyrosine Kinase Activation

While it is well established that ligand-induced receptor oligomerization leads to receptor tyrosine kinase activation, it is also clear that receptor oligomerization per se is not always sufficient for RPTK activation. For instance, a majority of unstimulated RPTKs exist as monomers in the cell membrane in equilibrium with a few transient and unstable receptor dimers, and most of these dimers are inactive. However, experimental evidence based on RPTK tyrosine phosphorylation induced by protein tyrosine phosphatase inhibitors and receptor overexpression would indicate that, at least under these circumstances, a few active receptor dimers exist, despite an absence of ligand. The current consensus is that only receptor oligomers with stabilized unique configurations of the extracellular and cytoplasmic domains are kinase active and that the main function of ligand binding is to aid in stabilizing a kinase-active conformation of receptor dimers. Ligand-induced receptor dimerization leads to juxtaposition of the receptor cytoplasmic domains, resulting in tyrosine autophosphorylation by an intermolecular mechanism. Based on the crystal structures of the catalytic domains of the insulin receptor and the FGFR tyrosine kinases, a *cis* inhibition and *trans* activation model for receptor activation has been proposed. The initial phosphorylation event occurs on one or more conserved tyrosine residues in the activation loop in the C-terminal lobe of the kinases. These tyrosine residues represent the major autophosphorylation site(s) in protein tyrosine kinases. In the case of the insulin receptor, one of these residues is buried in *cis*, i.e., that is within the same receptor subunit, in the active site, preventing access of Mg^{2+}/ATP. This conformation serves as an autoinhibition mechanism, in principle similar to the intramolecular pseudosubstrate inhibition commonly found in S/T kinases, like protein kinase C, although mediated by another region in this case. The conformational changes induced by receptor binding and dimerization favor tyrosine disengagement, upon which Mg^{2+}/ATP can bind in the cleft and *trans* phosphorylation of the major tyrosine residue in the other receptor in the complex can occur. Such a conformational change-based mechanism for RPTK activation also explains receptor activation in certain cases of receptor heterodimer formation between ligand-bound and -unbound RPTKs. For instance, no ligand has been identified for the EGF receptor member ErbB2, but upon EGF or neuregulin stimulation, ErbB2 is recruited into heterodimers with either

EGFR or with ErbB3 or ErbB4, respectively. It has suggested that two ErbB2 molecules are recruited into a tetrameric complex with the ligand-bound receptor dimer. Within this complex, the ErbB2 receptor dimers are stabilized in an active conformation through extensive contacts with the ligand-bound RPTK dimer partner in the complex, allowing ErbB2 kinase activation and tyrosine autophosphorylation in *trans*. Again, stabilization of conformational changes in the receptor subunits is key to tyrosine kinase activation.

For most RPTKs the initial autophosphorylation event is involved in activation of the kinase. In the case of EGFR it has been reported that phosphorylation of Y845 in the activation loop is mediated by the cytosplasmic tyrosine kinase Src, and this phosphorylation results in enhanced EGFR signaling. Subsequently, phosphorylation of additional tyrosine residues in the RPTKs, mostly located outside the catalytic domain, occurs. These tyrosine autophosphorylation sites serve as molecular switches to specifically recruit and bind cytoplasmic-signaling molecules, containing Src homology 2 (SH2) and protein tyrosine-binding (PTB) domains. In many cases, the SH2 and PTB proteins become phosphorylated on tyrosine residues by the receptors, which modulate their activity. Docking proteins such as insulin receptor-stimulated-1 (IRS-1) and fibroblast growth factor receptor substrate-2 (FRS-2) serve as platforms for binding of yet other SH2 and PTB domain-containing proteins through their phosphotyrosine residues. Finally, in some cases, the recruited molecules serve as adaptor molecules by bringing preassociated molecules close to the membrane. These RPTK-regulated substrates and binding molecules thereby initiate specific cytoplasmic signaling cascades leading to cellular responses (Fig. 2).

It is obvious that receptor activation by the mechanisms just described allows for a high degree of specificity coupled with diversity in signaling. First, not only is there specificity in the ligand binding to its receptor, but receptor heterooligomerization increases the number of possible ligand–receptor combinations, thereby allowing for an increased diversity in signaling pathways stimulated by one ligand. The actual ligand–receptor complexes formed in a particular target tissue in the body will obviously depend on the receptor combinations expressed in it. Furthermore, the individual tyrosine autophosphorylation sites and their immediate surrounding sequence constitute specific binding sites for individual SH2- and PTB-containing signaling molecules, thereby initiating different signaling pathways. Based on this insight, much of our current knowledge about RPTK-initiated signaling pathways has come from studies using cell lines expressing receptor point mutants, where individual tyrosine phosphorylation sites have been identified and mutated to nonphosphorylatable amino acids. This specifically interrupts the association with specific signaling molecules and the pathways in which they act. Technological advances have made it possible to introduce single amino acid changes in the germline of mice, enabling a similar analysis to be undertaken for the first time *in vivo* in mammals.

As an illustration of how specificity and diversity is achieved by some of the mechanisms just described, the ErbB family of receptors serves again as an excellent example. NDF/heregulin-induced tyrosine phosphorylation of ErbB2 is dependent on heterodimerization of ErbB2 with either ErbB3 or ErbB4. The individual tyrosine residues phosphorylated in ErbB2 differ, depending on whether the dimeric receptor partner is ErbB3 or ErbB4. Furthermore, the tyrosine phosphorylation of ErbB3, which is itself devoid of intrinsic kinase activity, is mediated in *trans* by ErbB2 or EGF receptors in the receptor complexes. This provides docking sites for SH2 proteins such as phosphoinositide 3'- (PI 3'-) kinase, which does not directly bind either the EGF receptor or ErbB2.

C. Dimerization and Oncogenic Activation of Receptor Protein Tyrosine Kinases

Oncogenic activation of RPTKs, whether it be due to mutations, DNA rearrangements, or amplification, has been associated with ligand-independent dimerization and constitutive kinase activation. Some examples of such gain-of-function (GOF) mutations follow.

Overexpression, due to gene amplification, of the ErbB1/EGF receptor or ErbB2 has been associated with mammary and ovarian cancer in humans. No recurrent mutations have been identified. However, based on *in vitro* systems, the overexpression per se is likely to result in the formation of receptor dimers even in the absence of ligand. A chemically induced Val664Glu mutation in the transmembrane region of the Neu/ErbB2 receptor has been shown to give rise to tumors in rodents. The corresponding mutation introduced *in vitro* leads to constitutive dimerization and activation of Neu/ErbB2.

In patients with myelodysplastic syndromes, recurrent activating point mutations have been identified in the receptor for CSF-1 involving codon 301 in the extracellular part of the receptor and, in particular, codon 969 at the C terminus. The codon 301 mutation causes constitutive dimer formation and kinase activation, while the codon 969 mutation might specifically abolish binding of c-Cbl, which is a negative regulator of RPTK signaling. Thus, it has been demonstrated that c-Cbl has ubiquitin ligase activity and associates with activated RPTKs through its SH2 domain, causing their degradation via the proteasome pathway (see Section V,A). When transfected into cells, these mutated receptors exhibited ligand-independent kinase activation, focus formation in soft agar, and tumorigenesis in nude mice.

More than 30 GOF mutations, either single amino acid changes or deletions of a few amino acids, have been identified in the Kit/SCF receptor, and they are associated with several highly malignant tumors in humans. Mutations clustered in the juxtamembrane region are associated with gastrointestinal stromal tumors, certain acute myeloid leukemias, and myelodysplastic syndromes, whereas a recurrent D816V or D816H mutation in the kinase domain of Kit is associated with mast cell leukemia or seminoma/dysgerminoma, respectively. The expression of the mutant form of Kit in these cases is associated with more aggressive forms of these malignancies. In most cases examined, the tumor tissue is heterozygous for the mutant form of c-*kit*. This indicates a dominant-positive phenotype, consistent with the formation of heterodimers between constitutively active mutant Kit with wild-type Kit receptors. All the Kit GOF mutations have been demonstrated to cause constitutive, ligand-independent kinase active dimers.

In the case of TrkA, the receptor for NGF, and Met/HGFR, most cases seem to involve fusions of the cytoplasmic domain of TrkA or Met/HGFR with either tropomyosin or translocated promotor region (Tpr), a component of the nuclear pore. The N-terminal fusion partners mediate dimerization and constitutive kinase activation. These oncogene rearrangeements have been implicated in papillary thyroid carcimomas (Tpr/Met, Tpr/TrkA and tropomyosin/TrkA), and gastric carcinomas (Tpr/Met).

Another illustrative example of oncogenic activation of RPTKs is provided by the Ret oncogene product. Ret ("rearranged during transfection") is part of a multicomponent receptor for glial-derived neurotrophic factor (GDNF). In response to GDNF stimulation, Ret becomes activated by heterodimer formation with GDNF receptor-α, a glycosylphosphatidylinositol-linked cell surface receptor, which binds GDNF directly. Somatic rearrangements of Ret lead to three common N-terminal truncations and subsequent GDNF-independent receptor activation caused by constitutive dimerization of the three resulting proteins, RetPTC1, RetPTC2, and RetPTC3. RetPTCs are involved in a high proportion of papillary tumors, the most common form of thyroid tumor. The prevalence of this tumor form is rising at an alarming rate in rather young people exposed to radiation fallout following the 1986 Chernobyl accident. More than 60% of these patients have the RetPTC-activated oncogenes.

In addition to sporadic tumors, germline mutations in Ret are involved in three familial tumor syndromes: multiple endocrine neoplasia 2A (MEN2A), MEN2B, and familial medullary thyroid carcinoma (FMTC). MEN2A is characterized by medullary thyroid carcinoma, parathyroid hyperplasia, and pheocromocytoma. MEN2B is similar to MEN2A, but is distinguished by the absence of parathyroid hyperplasia and the presence of mucosal ganglioneuromas of the digestive tract. Strikingly, almost 100% of patients with MEN2A and FMTC have mutations in one of the five conserved cysteine residues in the extracellular domain of Ret. This leads to the formation of intermolecular disulfide bonds between adjacent Ret molecules and constitutive receptor dimerization and activation.

In contrast, the MEN2B syndrome constitutes an exception to all these examples of oncogenic activation by receptor dimerization. MEN2B is due to a Met918Thr mutation. Met918 corresponds to a highly conserved Met in the substrate binding pocket of RP-TKs, whereas a Thr at this position is typical for cytoplasmic tyrosine kinases. It has been shown that this replacement increases the activity of Ret without constitutive dimer formation. In this case the oncogenic mechanism can be ascribed to an altered substrate specifity of the Ret/MEN2B receptor toward optimal peptide substrates of Src and Abl, two cytoplasmic tyrosine kinases. This altered specificity leads to autophosphorylation of Ret on novel tyrosine residues and tyrosine phosphorylation of in particular Crk and Nck-associated substrates, such as paxillin, substrates not phosphorylated by the activated wild-type Ret receptor. In addition, there is increased activation of PI 3'-kinase, an important mediator of mitogenic and survival signaling.

Finally, numerous naturally occurring activating point mutations in FGF receptor genes cause at least 15 genetic disorders, including skeletal dysplasias such as Apert syndrome and achondroplasia. These are not malignancies, but can be considered hyperproliferative or dysplastic bone disorders. All these examples illustrate how even minimal structural changes of RP-TKs can cause grossly altered quantitative and qualitative signaling, resulting in perturbed growth regulation and often malignant cell transformation.

IV. PROTEIN–PROTEIN INTERACTION MODULES AND COMPARTMENTALIZATION

One of the most significant discoveries in signal transduction research has been the realization that diverse families of protein modules direct the specific molecular interactions in signal transduction pathways. These conserved sequences, including Src homology 2 (SH2), protein tyrosine binding (PTB), Src homology 3 (SH3), WW, pleckstrin homology (PH), FYVE, PDZ, EVH1, and sterile α motif (SAM) domains, among others, range in size from ~50 to 140 amino acids. For an updated database overview of the rapidly growing family of modular protein domains found in intracellular signaling proteins, see http://smart.embl-heidelberg.de/. The crystal structures have been obtained for several of these interaction domains in their bound form. Each of them folds into a compact globular and functional module independently of surrounding sequences. They generally bind short primary amino acid sequence motifs, in some cases in a phosphorylation-dependent manner. Various combinations of domains are frequently found in a single protein (Fig. 3), enabling the formation of networks of signaling complexes downstream of RPTKs. Detailed knowledge about domain-binding consensus motifs has enabled investigators to specifically block signaling pathways at discrete points. The protein modules are also involved in locating proteins to the proper subcellular localization during signal transduction. Other ways to achieve intracellular organization of signaling molecules include binding to anchoring and scaffolding proteins, as well as posttranslational modifications. Compartmentalization of signaling

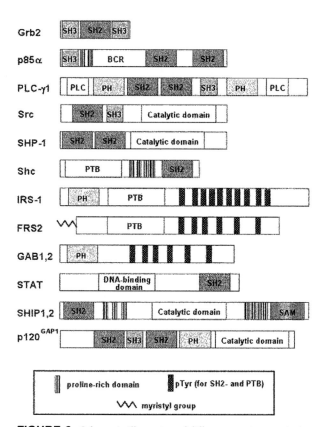

FIGURE 3 Schematic illustration of different protein–protein interaction domains in cytoplasmic signaling molecules discussed in the text. Note that different types of domains often reside within the same signaling molecule, allowing for multiple interactions at once. Proline-rich domains are often involved in binding SH3 and WW domains. The pTyr motif indicates phosphotyrosine residues involved in binding SH2 and/or PTB domains. Myristyl groups mediate binding to the inner leaflet of the plasma membrane. Figure not drawn to scale.

molecules is a very important aspect in the regulation of intracellular signaling pathways.

A. Src Homology 2 and Protein Tyrosine-Binding Domains

SH2 and PTB domains recognize short phosphotyrosine-containing motifs and their binding is inducible by the tyrosine phosphorylation of target proteins. Consequently, SH2- and PTB-containing proteins are directly involved in tyrosine kinase-regulated signaling pathways. SH2 domains are the most well characterized of these and are found in numerous signaling molecules involved in phospholipid metabolism, tyrosine phosphorylation and dephosphorylation, activation of Ras-like GTPases, gene expression, protein trafficking, and cytoskeletal architecture (see Fig. 3). SH2 domains have been identified in ~150 mammalian signaling proteins deposited in the databases to date. SH2 domains are conserved regions of about 100 amino acids that were first identified as regions of homology between v-Src and v-Fps, which lie outside the catalytic domain and are not required for catalytic activity. They bind specifically to phosphotyrosine and the immediate carboxy-terminal 3–6 amino acids in a sequence-specific fashion. Accordingly, autophosphorylated tyrosine residues in RPTKs bind specifically to one or more SH2 proteins. The binding is of high affinity, with K_d being in the high nano- to submicromolar range. Binding specificities of SH2 domains have been determined by the incubation of different SH2 domains with degenerate phosphotyrosine-containing peptide libraries and subsequent sequencing of the bound peptides. By this means, a binding code has emerged for the different SH2 domains, which is generally pY-X-A-X or pY-A-X-A, where pY is phosphotyrosine, A is a specific amino acid, and X is any amino acid. Resolution of the three-dimensional structures of several SH2 domain has revealed that the SH2 domain exists as a folded, globular structure protruding from the rest of the protein, with the N- and C-terminals closely together. The phosphopeptide binding site is a bipartite pocket on the surface of the SH2 domain. One part of the pocket is lined by conserved basic amino acid residues and binds the phosphotyrosine. The second binding surface is more variable and allows the specific recognition of the amino acids immediately C-terminal to the phosphotyrosine. SH2 domains can be divided into three major groups with similar recognition motifs based on this second binding surface. PLC-γ-like SH2 domains bind phosphopeptides with neutral amino acids followed by carboxy-terminal residues fitting into a hydrophobic cleft, Src-like SH2 domains selects for charged residues at the +1 and +2 position, and a hydrophobic amino acid at position +3, and finally, Grb2-like SH2 domains recognize preferentially peptides with a +2 Asn. Interestingly, the catalytic specificity of SH2-containing PTKs fits with the preferred binding consensus for their own SH2 domains.

The PTB and the closely related PTB–IRS-like (PTBI) domains are conserved domains of approximately 110 and 135 amino acids, respectively. A PTB domain is found in molecules such as the adaptor molecule Shc and the scaffolding protein JNK-interacting protein (JIP) and PTBI in docking molecules such as insulin receptor-stimulated-1 (IRS-1) and fibroblast growth factor receptor substrate 2 (FRS2; see Fig. 3 for examples). Based on *in vitro* binding of tyrosine-phosphorylated peptides and receptor-binding studies, a recognition consensus motif has been identified for PTB. In contrast to SH2 domains, PTB domains bind phosphotyrosine in the context of 3-5 N-terminal, rather than C-terminal, amino acid residues. In addition, some PTB domains bind to unphosphorylated tyrosine residues, or to both unphosphorylated and phosphorylated tyrosine residues. The minimal binding motif is B-X-N-P-X-pY or B-X-N-P-X-Y, respectively, single letter code for amino acids, where B represents a large hydrophobic residue, X is any amino acid, and pY is phosphotyrosine. Accordingly, the PTB domain of Disabled1 (Dab1) has been suggested to bind to the internalization signals of transmembrane glycoproteins (GYXNPXY), whereas the PTB domain in FRS2 binds both phosphorylated and unphosphorylated motifs. The binding affinity of PTB domains is ~100-fold lower than that of SH2 domains, i.e., in the midmicromolor range. Interestingly, the overall topology of PTB domains is very similar to that of PH domains, which bind PtdIns(3,4,5)P$_3$ and EVH1 domains, which bind proline-rich motifs, indicating functional overlap. In accordance with this, PTB domains have been shown to also bind acidic phospholipids *in vitro*, as do PH domains.

The SH2 and PTB domain-containing proteins can be subdivided into four categories on a functional basis (see Fig. 3): proteins possessing a catalytic domain, pure adaptor or docking molecules, structural proteins, and translocated transcription factors. The enzymatic activities of the catalytic domain-containing SH2 proteins are diverse and include protein-tyrosine kinase activity, phospholipase activity, GTPase-enhancing activity, guanine nucleotide exchange activity, and protein-tyrosine phosphatase (PTPase) activity.

Four main mechanisms prevail for the activation of signaling pathways by SH2 proteins: (1) activation of catalytic activity by tyrosine phosphorylation by the activated RPTKs (e.g., phospholipase C-γ), (2) activation by conformational changes induced upon binding (e.g., the heterodimeric PI 3′-kinase), (3) activation by recruitment to the membrane where many substrates are located (e.g., Grb2, Shc, and most others), and (4) activation by translocation to the nucleus leading to DNA binding and gene transcription (e.g., STATs).

B. Src Homology 3 and WW Domains

Both of these modules bind to short, proline-rich sequences. The SH3 family of proteins is large; almost 300 mammalian proteins with SH3 domains have been deposited in the databanks thus far. SH3 domains are found in many proteins with SH2 and other protein–protein interaction domains, cytoskeletal components, formin-binding proteins, and subunits of the neutrophil oxidase (see Fig. 3). They are conserved domains of approximately 60 amino acid residues, originally identified in v-Crk, phospholipase C-γ (PLC-γ), and Src. SH3 domain binding to targets is normally constitutive, although it is regulated in some instances by phosphorylation of the SH3 domain. SH3-binding sites consist of proline-rich peptides of approximately 10 amino acids. They bind to SH3 domains with a K_d in the micromolar range. The core ligand is a seven residue peptide containing the minimal consensus P-p-X-P (single letter code for amino acids; X tends to be aliphatic and p tends to be proline). The crystal structure of SH3 domains has shown them to contain elongated binding clefts, where hydrophobic pockets contact the polyproline type II helix of peptides. Type I and II SH3 ligands differ mainly in the position of an Arg in the polyproline helix, which determines their relative binding orientation; each ligand binds in only one orientation relative to the SH3 domain, i.e., from the N toward the C terminus or from the C toward the N terminus. The ligand orientation will determine the spatial organization of the resulting complex, which may be critical for signaling. SH3 domains are involved in the binding of cytoskeletal components, guanine nucleotide exchange factors, regulation of cytoplasmic tyrosine kinases, and recruitment of specific substrates.

WW domains are ~35 amino acids long, conserved sequences involved in the binding of proline-rich sequences similar and sometimes identical to those bound by SH3 domains, but the preferred binding consensus sequence is P-P-X-Y or P-P-L-P. The name WW refers to two highly conserved tryptophan residues, one close to each end of the consensus motif. WW ligands can bind in either the N- to the C-terminal direction or the C- to the N-terminal direction, such as SH3 ligands. The WW domain is a small, monomeric, triple-stranded antiparallel β-sheet protein domain that is stable in the absence of disulfide bonds, despite its small size. This motif has been found in a variety of proteins, including formin-binding proteins, Yes-kinase-associated protein, dystrophin, and the peptidyl-prolyl isomerase Pin-1. A subset of WW domain-containing proteins, including Pin-1 and the ubiquitin ligase Nedd4, also recognizes phosphorylated Ser or Thr residues followed by a Pro. WW and SH3 domains can compete with each other *in vitro* for binding to proline-rich sequences. The cellular functions of WW domain-containing molecules are varied and include targeting of proteins for degradation, modulation of SH3 domain function, and modulation of the function of proteins containing a phosphorylated S-P or T-P motif.

C. Pleckstrin Homology Domains

The PH domain is about 100 amino acid residues long, of limited primary sequence conservation, and found in a large family of signaling molecules, including protein tyrosine kinases, protein serine/threonine kinases, phospholipase C isoforms, guanine nucleotide exchange factors of the Dbl family, the GTPase dynamin, and cytoskeletal proteins. The

structures of several PH domains have been solved and, interestingly, contain an overall fold very similar to that of PTB domains. All PH domains consist of a seven-stranded β sandwich with a positively charged lobe at the open end, in some cases involved in binding anionic ligands. Generally, PH domains bind with specificity to diverse lipid second messengers. Of particular interest to RPTK signaling is their binding to phospholipids, including mainly phosphatidylinositol-3,4,5-trisphosphate [PtdIns(3,4,5)P$_3$], but also PtdIns(3)P, PtdIns(3,4)P$_2$, and PtdIns(4,5)P$_2$. Protein binding is more of an exception, but it is well documented that a separate region from the lipid-binding surface of some PH domains binds to $\beta\gamma$ subunits of heterotrimeric GTP-binding (G) proteins. For instance, an extended C-terminal region of the PH domain of the β-adrenergic receptor kinase (β-ARK) binds $\beta\gamma$ subunits with high affinity, and the PH domains of PLC-β1 and 2, which bind neutral membrane lipids independent of PtdIns(4,5)P$_2$, associate with $\beta\gamma$ subunits of G proteins while bound to phosphatidylcholine membranes *in vitro*. Upon binding to PtdIns(3,4,5)P$_3$, PH domains are also able to homodimerize, an important mechanism for the activation of many PH domain-containing kinases, which often rely on dimerization for full activation. Thus, in many instances, PH domains mediate both recruitment of signaling molecules to the inner leaflet of membranes and aid in the activation of their host molecules. For instance, the serine/threonine kinases phosphoinositide-dependent kinase-1 (PDK-1) and Akt both contain a PH domain. They are important mediators of RPTK-initiated PI 3'-kinase signaling. Activation of PI 3'-kinase leads to the phosphorylation of PtdIns lipids at the D-3 position of the inositol ring, producing mainly PtdIns(3,4,5)P$_3$ and subsequently PtdIns(3,4)P$_2$, with the latter produced mainly by the action of a D5-specific phosphoinositide phosphatase, SHIP. PtdIns(3,4,5)P$_3$ binds with high affinity to the PH domain of PDK-1, leading to a conformational change of the protein and subsequent PDK-1 kinase activation through relief of an autoinhibitory constraint and concomitant dimerization. Akt is also recruited to the cell membrane by binding of PtdIns(3,4,5)P$_3$ to its PH domain, and activated PDK-1, in turn, phosphorylates the lipid-bound Akt on Thr308 in the kinase activation loop, causing partial activation of Akt. PDK-1 and Akt form homo- and heterodimers through their PH domains, which is probably important for their full activation. Deletion of the PH domains in either PDK-1 and Akt prevents their proper membrane localization and prevents their normal regulation. PDK-1 and Akt are major targets of PI 3′-kinase signaling mediating control of cell proliferation, growth, survival, and differentiation, as well as protein and glycogen metabolism.

PH domains in other proteins are also targets of PI 3′-kinase signaling. For instance, the PH domain-containing docking proteins GAB1 and 2 are also recruited to the cell membrane by binding to PtdIns(3,4,5)P$_3$ upon RPTK-induced PI 3′-kinase activation. Here they serve as direct substrates for several RPTKs, and phosphorylated tyrosine residues within GAB1 and 2, in turn, can bind PI 3′-kinase and other signaling molecules through their SH2 and PTB domains. Another example is the binding of PtdIns(3,4,5)P$_3$ to the PH domain of PLC-γ, which stimulates its phospholipase activity. Although PI 3′-kinase lipid products are not substrates for PI-specific PLCs, they use PtdIns(4,5)P$_2$ as a substrate, which links RPTK-induced PI 3′-kinase and PLC-γ activation. Finally, binding of PtdIns(3,4,5)P$_3$ to the PH domain in Bruton's tyrosine kinase (Btk) is required for its normal activation and provides yet another example. Lipid binding to the PH domain stabilizes Btk in a dimeric state, enabling efficient transphosphorylation. Mutations in the PH domain of Btk have been linked to X-linked agammaglobulinemia and other B-cell immunodeficiencies in humans. Most of these proteins that bind PtdIns(3,4,5)P$_3$ also bind PtdIns(3,4)P$_2$, albeit with lower affinity. Distinct PH domains found in proteins such as the Ras guanine nucleotide exchange factor Sos-1, β-spectrin, and PLC-δ$_1$ isoforms bind exclusively PtdIns(4,5)P$_2$, the substrate for PLCs. These few examples clearly illustrate how PH domain-containing proteins are central points of convergence for lipid-mediated signaling pathways.

D. PDZ, FYVE, EVH1, and Sterile α Motif (SAM) Domains

The PDZ domain is found in a variety of signaling proteins implicated in ion channel and receptor clustering and the linking of RPTKs to their effector substrates, including cytoplasmic protein phosphatases, GTPase-activating proteins, and tight junction structural proteins. It is at least as common as the SH2 domain. PDZ domains (also known as DHR domains or GLGF repeats) are approximately 90 residue protein recognition modules. They bind to diverse motifs, including the tripeptide motif S/T-X-V$_{COOH}$, a short hydrophobic peptide motif found at the extreme carboxyl termini of transmembrane proteins, including RPTKs. PDZ domains also undergo homophilic interactions to form homotypic dimers. A typical PDZ domain, composed of an antiparallel β barrel flanked by α helices, has a groove over the surface that ends in a conserved hydrophobic pocket, which creates the binding site for the C-terminal peptide. PDZ domains are involved in organizing synaptic signaling pathways. Several PDZ domain-containing molecules bind to RPTKs, including Kit/SCF receptor, PDGFR, Eph family receptors, and ErbB4 in a regulated, often tyrosine kinase-dependent, fashion. Their binding to RPTKs serves at least two functions: regulation of RPTK activity through a conformational change and localization of RPTKs (and/or the PDZ molecule) to specific subcellular sites. For instance, binding of the multiple PDZ domain-containing protein MUPP to the C terminus of Kit is inversely correlated with Kit kinase activity, and binding of the ErbB2-interacting protein, ERBIN, through its PDZ domain to ErbB2 localizes the receptor to the basolateral membrane of intestinal epithelial cells. Interestingly, a PDZ domain-binding site is also found in the intracellular carboxyl terminus of the transmembrane class of ephrins, the Eph receptor ligands, where it has been shown to bind several intracellular signaling molecules. This might suggest a novel "receptor-induced ligand activation" mechanism, where receptor binding induces conformational changes in the cytoplasmic part of ephrin, causing altered substrate specificity and subsequent activation of signaling.

The FYVE domain has been identified in a rather limited number of proteins. FYVE domains were named after the founding four protein members of this family: Fab1p, YGLO23, Vps27, and EEA1. All these proteins are involved in vesicle and endosomal trafficking, from the Golgi apparatus to the vacuole. The FYVE domain is ~60 amino acids and contains two Zn^{2+}-binding clusters with structural similarities to regions in RING finger domains. However, FYVE members have unique characteristics, including the very basic sequence motif R/K-R/K-H-H-C-R, which is conserved in more than 30 proteins from yeast to mammals. FYVE domains specifically bind to vesicles containing PtdIns(3)P, but not to vesicles containing other PtdIns species. The basic motif region in the FYVE domain forms a highly charged basic pocket on the surface of the domain that is required for the lipid binding. Hence, FYVE domains are essential for the role of PtdIns(3)P in vesicle trafficking and possibly other signaling events. For instance, SARA is a FYVE domain-containing protein involved in recruiting SMAD domain proteins to the TGFβ receptor. It seems likely that PH domains and FYVE domains through binding to PtdIns(3,4,5)P$_3$ and PtdIns(3)P, respectively, provide an important means for both regulated recruitment to membranes and activation of their host proteins.

The Enabled/VASP homology 1 (EVH1; also called WH1) domain is an interaction module found in several proteins implicated in actin-based cell motility. The overall structure is very similar to that of PH, PTB, and Ran-binding domains. EVH1 domains specifically bind the consensus proline-rich motif FPPPP found in the mammalian zyxin and vinculin proteins and are required for targeting the actin assembly machinery to sites of cytoskeletal remodeling. Membrane association may play an auxiliary role in EVH1 targeting. Hence, the EVH1 family of proteins acts as molecular adaptors linking the cytoskeletal system to signal transduction pathways and is important in the regulation of neuronal development.

The SAM domain is found in more than 70 diverse eukaryotic proteins that reside in the cytoplasm and/or nucleus and are involved in signal transduction or transcriptional repression. It is a ~70 amino acid compact structure, consisting of five helices without any binding pockets or exposed conserved aromatic residues, but with two major homotypic interaction interfaces. SAM domains are able to homo- and heterodimerize and possibly tetramerize, and also to mediate other specific protein–protein interactions. It was originally described as a homotypic interaction domain in the Ets family transcription factor TEL (TEL-SAM). In many human leukemias, chromoso-

mal translocations render the TEL-SAM domain fused to tyrosine kinase domains of Abelson leukemia virus kinase, the PDGFR-β kinase and Janus kinase (JAK) 2, and AML, a transcription factor. The self-oligomerization of TEL-SAM causes constitutive activation of the fusion partners, resulting in malignant cell transformation. A conserved subclass of SAM domains are found at the extreme, intracellular C terminus of all 14 Eph receptors, the largest subfamily of RPTKs. These receptors are important for axonal pathfinding and establishment of normal tissue boundaries. Each of the Eph-contained SAM domains has a highly conserved tyrosine autophosphorylation site. Upon ligand-induced phosphorylation, this phosphotyrosine residue and its surrounding sequence can bind specifically to cytoplasmic signaling molecules, such as Grb2, Grb10, and Nck through their SH2 domains. The same phosphorylated tyrosine residue, Y929 in EphB1, also binds and recruits low molecular weight protein tyrosine phosphatase (LMW-PTP). Binding of LMW-PTP, in contrast to SH2 domain-containing proteins, is strengthened upon ephrin-induced Eph receptor oligomerization and provides a mechanism of oligomerization- and tyrosine phosphorylation-dependent recruitment of a protein tyrosine phosphatase. A cytoplasmic inositol polyphosphate 5′-phosphatase, SH2 domain-containing inositol 5′-phosphatase-2 (SHIP-2), contains a carboxy-terminal SAM domain. It binds to several tyrosine-phosphorylated cytoplasmic proteins through its SH2 domain. The SAM domain might be involved in the regulation of SHIP-2 phosphatase activity.

E. Binding Proteins, Intracellular Organization, and Compartmentalization

SH2- and SH3-binding proteins, including the IRS-1, FRS2, and Shc docking proteins, serve as platforms for the assembly of multimolecular signaling complexes of PTKs and PTPases and target them to subcellular localizations as well. However, organization into molecular complexes and targeting is just as important for other classes of signaling molecules activated downstream of RPTKs, including serine/threonine kinases, small GTP-binding proteins, and other molecules that are not directly involved in phosphotyrosine-directed interactions.

Several phosphoserine/phosphothreonine interaction motifs have been identified, and they operate in a manner very similar to that described for SH2 and PTB domains in binding phosphotyrosine motifs. The dimeric 14-3-3 proteins bind to phosphoserine in a specific basic sequence context (see later) in a variety of proteins, including transcription factors, proapoptotic molecules, and protein serine/threonine kinases, among others. The WW domain of the isomerase Pin1 and the ubiquitin ligase Nedd4 specifically bind to phosphorylated Ser or Thr residues followed by a Pro (see earlier discussion). Finally, Forkhead-associated (FHA) domains, originally found in members of the Forkhead-type transcription factor family, bind specifically to phosphoserine, phosphothreonine, and possibly phosphotyrosine. The FHA domain is a ~120–140 amino acids long conserved interaction domain found in a variety of protein kinases, protein phosphatases, and transcription factors. FHA domains bind to proteins involved in DNA repair, cell cycle arrest, or pre-mRNA processing. The exact binding motif for FHA is not clearly defined yet, but peptide-binding studies with the DNA damage repair protein Rad53 and others suggest that amino acid residues from the −2 to the +3 position relative to the phosphorylated Ser or Thr are important for binding specificity. In particular, the +3 position determines specificity for different FHA domains, reminiscent of what is seen for SH2 domain:phosphotyrosine peptide interactions. In addition to these three families of binding domains, there are other examples of phosphoserine-dependent interaction motifs, but they do not always require phosphorylated residues for binding. For instance, the coactivator CREB-binding protein (CBP) contains a phosphoserine-binding domain, called KIX, which interacts with the protein kinase A-phosphorylated form of the cyclic AMP-responsive factor CREB. However, the KIX domain can also bind to unphosphorylated sequences in proteins, e.g., a sequence in c-Myb.

In addition to these phosphorylation site interaction motifs mediating simple protein–protein interactions, serine/threonine kinases and phosphatases are also organized into larger complexes via binding to two classes of adaptor molecules: scaffold and anchoring proteins. In some cases, binding is mediated in part by the phosphoserine/phosphothreonine motifs within these complexes. Scaffold proteins simultaneousy bind several protein kinases in a pathway, forming an organized module allowing for sequential action of each enzyme, whereas anchoring proteins bind to subcellular structures via a targeting locus bringing their bound enzymes to the site of action.

The 14-3-3 family of ubiquitously expressed proteins is involved in binding Raf-1, a serine/threonine kinase, as well as numerous other proteins, including PI 3′-kinase, Bcr, PKC isoforms, PLC isoforms, transmembrane receptors, protein phosphatases, and the proapoptotic molecules Bad and the Forkhead transcription factor FKHRL1. The 14-3-3 proteins bind to Raf-1, Bad, and FKHRL1 via phosphoserine or phosphothreonine within the minimal consensus recognition motif R-s-X-pS/pT-X-P (single letter code for amino acids), where s tends to be serine, X is any amino acid, pS is phosphoserine, and pT is phosphothreonine. Interestingly, this is part of the phosphorylation consensus motif for the protein serine/threonine kinase Akt, R-x-R-x-x-pS/pT, and, accordingly, Akt has been shown to phosphorylate Raf-1, Bad, and FKHRL1, inducing their subsequent binding to 14-3-3 through the Akt phosphorylation sites. However, 14-3-3 proteins are also bound constitutively to Raf-1, and this binding is necessary, but not sufficient, for Raf-1 activation. 14-3-3 proteins are dimeric and can therefore, in principle, bind two phosphorylated proteins. 14-3-3 proteins have been shown to simultaneously mediate binding in ternary complexes of Raf-1 with PKC-α, Ras, or Bcr. Ternary complexes indicate a major role for 14-3-3 as a scaffold in mammalian ERK/MAP kinase signaling pathways, bringing together molecules into signaling complexes in a phosphoserine-regulated manner. However, in the case of Bad and FKHRL1, the binding of 14-3-3 leads to sequestration of these molecules in the cytosol. Binding of 14-3-3 to Bad inhibits its death function through preventing it from binding to and neutralizing the survival function of Bcl-XL, and binding of 14-3-3 to FKHRL1 masks its nuclear localization signal and prevents its nuclear entry and transcription of target genes. One of the best characterized scaffold proteins is the yeast Ste5p protein, which binds enzymes in the MAP kinase pathway involved in the pheromone mating response. The yeast homologues of MEKK, MEK, and MAPK are organized in a complex together with two upstream molecules. Each enzyme binds to a distinct region of Ste5p, which is itself a dimer, and they are organized in a modular fashion. This allows for tight regulation of the pathway, one protein kinase activating the next in the chain. Several mammalian MAPK scaffolds are known, including MAPK kinase (MEK) partner 1 (MP1), c-Jun N-terminal kinase (JNK) interacting proteins (JIP1/2), JNK/SAPK (stress-activated protein kinase) activating protein (JIP3/JSAP), kinase suppressor of Ras (KSR), and others. KSR binds simultaneously Ras, Raf, MEK, and ERK, forming a high molecular aggregate, including 14-3-3 and hsp90. JIP1, JIP2, and JIP3/JSAP bind JNK, MKK7, and other kinases in the JNK and p38 MAPK pathways. It is postulated that scaffolds such as KSR, JIP, and JSAP exert inhibition or enhancement of signaling, depending on their local cellular concentration relative to the bound components. In all cases, scaffolds help organize the interacting components of a signaling cascade.

Examples of anchoring proteins include the "A-kinase anchoring protein" (AKAP) and the family of "receptors for activated C kinase" (RACKs). AKAPs associate with cAMP-dependent protein kinase (PKA) by binding to the regulatory subunit (RII) in PKA. However, AKAPs are multivalent and simultaneously anchor other protein kinases and phosphatases. For instance, in neurons, an AKAP isoform, AKAP79, binds not only PKA, but also Ca^{2+}–calmodulin-dependent protein phosphatase 2B (calcineurin) as well as PKC-α and PKC-β. AKAP79 targets these enzymes to substrates, e.g., ion channels, in the postsynaptic membrane. Stimuli leading to increased levels of the second messenger cAMP, e.g., G protein-coupled receptor activation, will then result in PKA activation through binding of cAMP to the two PKA catalytic subunits, which are released to phosphorylate the substrate(s) bound to the AKAP protein complex. Organization of the AKAP79 signaling complex is modular, suggesting a model for reversible phosphorylation by opposing effects of the kinases and phosphatase. Yotiao is an adaptor protein that maintains PKA and protein phosphatase-1 (PP1) in complex with the NR1A subunit of the N-methyl-D-aspartate (NMDA) receptor subtype of glutamate receptors. When bound to Yotiao, PP1 is active, keeping the NMDA ion channel closed. When PKA is activated through generation of cAMP, the released cAMP-bound catalytic subunits phosphorylate, and hence activate the NMDA channel. In this case, Yotiao serves to keep the protein kinase, phosphatase, and their common substrate in close proximity. Similarly, the RACKs seem to target PKC to subcellular localizations. In this case, only activated PKC binds, and there is no evidence for other molecules bound in the complex. While RACK is not a substrate for PKC, all of the PKC substrates identified are themselves anchoring proteins. Each of them, including vinculin, talin, myristoylated alanine-rich C kinase substrate (MARCKS), annexins, and adducins, bind PKC in a phosphatidylserine-dependent manner. They are involved in linking membranes with cytoskeletal structures, where PKC is targeted into complexes with its substrates.

Targeting of calcium–calmodulin-dependent kinases is also anchoring protein-mediated, and many other enzymes than PKC become targeted indirectly by interaction with their substrates. A different means, finally, for proper targeting of molecules is via post-translational modifications of proteins or via the biochemical properties of the molecule itself. Examples include myristylation and isoprenylation of Src and Ras, respectively, glycosylations and phosphorylations, nuclear targeting signals, and so on. Research into the role of subcellular targeting and compartmentalization is still in its infancy, but is fundamental for understanding the regulation and organization of signaling pathways. Clearly, signaling is organized into complexes of interacting proteins rather than into linear one-component paths.

V. NEGATIVE REGULATION AND TERMINATION OF RPTK SIGNALING

Mechanisms that precisely regulate and coordinate the quenching of RPTK-initiated signaling are just as important as the fine-tuned activation mechanisms. Termination and attenuation of RPTK signaling are achieved by several means, including receptor internalization and degradation of the signaling complex, receptor tyrosine dephosphorylation, negative feedback loop regulation, and other inhibitory mechanisms. Finally, under certain pathological conditions, signaling from wild-type RPTKs is attenuated by dominant-negative mechanisms through hetero-dimerization with the corresponding loss-of-function receptor mutants.

A. Ligand-Induced Receptor Endocytosis

An immediate and fast-acting mechanism for RPTK downregulation is ligand-induced endocytosis. Growth factor binding to its cognate RPTK leads to receptor aggregation (clustering) in clathrin-coated pits, and subsequently the ligand–receptor complex is internalized by endocytosis and contained within cytoplasmic vesicles. These vesicles develop into so-called multivesicular bodies, which eventually fuse with lysosomes, within which the ligand and receptor are degraded by the action of lysosomal proteases and other enzymes. The process of ligand-induced endocytosis occurs within minutes and immediately leads to attenuated signaling due to a decreased number of cell surface receptors. There is also a low level of constitutive, unstimulated RPTK internalization and endocytosis. The typical half-life for cell surface expression of RPTKs is in the order of 4–6 h at 37°C for unstimulated receptors and in the order of 20–40 min for ligand-stimulated receptors. For several RPTKs it has been shown that degradation is dependent on RPTK activity and that kinase-negative receptors recycle to the cell surface for reutilization. For instance, EGF or neuregulin stimulates heterodimer formation between kinase-active receptors (EGFR, ErbB2, or ErbB4) and kinase-inactive ErbB3 receptors. While the kinase active receptor in the dimer is degraded through the proteasome, ErbB3 is recycled to the cell surface. Likewise, certain naturally occurring kinase-inactive mutants of the Kit/SCF receptor are recycled to the cell surface, often leading to higher expression levels of mutant than of wild-type receptor in cells heterozygous for the mutation. This causes further signal attenuation, via simple out-titration of signaling active Kit dimers by an excess mutant receptor. One possible mechanism for the degradation of kinase-active RPTKs involves the protooncogene product c-Cbl. c-Cbl binds to activated PDGF and EGF receptors through its SH2 domain, thereby causing receptor ubiquitination by its RING finger domain, which exhibits ubiquitin ligase activity. Ubiquitinated proteins are subsequently degraded by the proteasome

or are otherwise targeted to the lysosomal degradation pathway. Accordingly, the CSF1-R has a longer half-life in CSF-1-treated c-Cbl-/- macrophages. However, additional mechanisms are at play for RPTK ubiquitination and not all RPTKs require ubiquitination for degradation. Future studies using c-Cbl knockout cells, SH2 deletion mutants of c-Cbl, and mutation of the amino acid residues in RPTKs ubiquitinated by c-Cbl should clarify the role of c-Cbl for RPTK degradation in general and whether its negative effect on RPTK signaling also occurs by other mechanisms. Based on the number of ubiquitin ligase family members and the different lysosomal degradation mechanisms identified to date, one can foresee the identification of several other important ubiquitin ligases, as well as other degradation mechanisms for RPTKs in the near future.

B. Protein Phosphatases in RPTK Signaling

Tyrosine dephosphorylation is another fast-acting mechanism for the inhibition or termination of signaling from RPTKs. Protein phosphorylation in signal transduction is reversible, and PTKs act in concert with PTPases in determining the initiation, extent, and termination of tyrosine phosphorylation. Downregulation of RPTK signaling occurs not only through direct phosphotyrosine dephosphorylation of the RPTK itself (i.e., the RPTK is a substrate for the PTPase), but also through dephosphorylation of a crucial downstream target of the RPTK. Because tyrosine-phosphorylated proteins, serine and threonine-phosphorylated proteins, and even phospholipids are mediators of RPTK signaling, there are examples of protein serine/threonine-specific phosphatases and phosphoinositide-specific lipid phosphatases that mediate the downregulation of RPTK-intiated signaling as well. Some examples follow, as well as a short, general description of protein phosphatases.

All identified PTPases contain a conserved, ~280 amino acid long PTPase domain. Their specific catalytic activity is approximately 1000-fold higher and much less specific than that of PTKs. As is the case for PTKs, PTPases can be divided into transmembrane and cytoplasmic PTPases. Transmembrane PTPases contain extracellular regions with motifs such as fibronectin type III-like repeats, cadherin-like repeats, and immunoglobulin-like domains. They have a single transmembrane-spanning region usually followed by two PTPase domains, only one of which seems to contribute catalytic activity. As their extracellular region would indicate, certain transmembrane PTPases, such as PTPκ and PTPμ, are involved in homophilic cell–cell adhesion, and PTPμ may stabilize cell–cell contacts by dephosphorylating catenins and cadherins. These and other transmembrane PTPases have not been implicated in the direct dephosphorylation of RPTKs, in contrast to the cytoplasmic PTPases, of which several are capable of directly dephosphorylating RPTKs.

The hematopoietically expressed, cytoplasmic protein tyrosine phosphatase SHP-1 is one of only two SH2 domain-containing PTPases identified. SHP-1 binds to activated RPTKs, like CSF-1 and Kit/SCF receptor, through either of its two SH2 domains. The SH2 binding of SHP-1, and of the structurally related SHP-2 (see later), relieves an autoinhibitory constraint on the PTPase domain. Accordingly, it has been shown that both the CSF-1 and the Kit/SCF receptors are direct substrates for SHP-1 and that SHP-1 is important for the normal downregulation of Kit and CSF-1 receptor signaling. This has also physiological relevance. Hence, mice with the motheaten (*me*) phenotype, which is due to naturally occurring loss-of-function (LOF) mutations in SHP-1, have numerous hematopoietic abnormalities due to the hyperproliferation of myeloid/monocytic and mast cells. The deregulated CSF-1 and Kit receptor signaling is thought to cause these defects, which is supported by studies showing that the phenotype of dominant white-spotting (W) mutant mice, which have naturally occurring LOF mutations in Kit, is alleviated by crossing with the *me* mutant mice, and vice versa. These and more recent data showing alternative transcripts causing either truncations of SHP-1 or frameshift mutations resulting in the loss of SHP-1 in primary Kit-expressing tumor cell lines established from leukemic patients, indicate that SHP-1 is a tumor suppressor.

The protein tyrosine phosphatase PTP1B is another cytosolic phosphatase, which is involved in the direct downregulation of RPTK signaling. PTP1B binds to the activated insulin and IGF-1 receptors through its N-terminal catalytic domain through an unknown mechanism. Upon binding, PTP1B directly dephosphorylates the insulin receptor itself and its major associated docking protein, insulin receptor substrate-1 (IRS-1). Accordingly, the targeted deletion of PTP1B in mice causes hyperphosphorylation of insulin receptor and IRS-1 and sensitization of insulin signaling. PTP1B also dephosphorylates STAT5a and STAT5b, thereby preventing their nuclear translocation and transcriptional activity. STAT5a and STAT5b are phosphorylated by JAKs activated by cytokine receptors, but are also phosphorylated directly by several RPTKs.

However, PTP1B, as well as the receptor-like PTPα, and SHP-2, another SH2 domain-containing phosphatase, have also been implicated in the enhancement of signaling downstream of RPTKs. PTP1B is overexpressed in breast cancer cell lines where it causes dephosphorylation of Tyr527 at the C terminus of c-Src. This leads to enhanced Src kinase activity, as phosphorylation of this site is inhibitory for Src activity through an allosteric, autoinhibitory mechanism. The transmembrane RPTPα is tyrosine phosphorylated *in vivo* at Tyr789, which creates a binding site for c-Src, enabling RPTPα to dephosphorylate Tyr527 in Src *in vitro*. Interestingly, both binding and dephosphorylation of Src are dependent on phosphorylation at Tyr789, and a phosphotyrosine displacement mechanism has been proposed for the activation of Src by RPTPα. Accordingly, kinase-defective or Tyr789Phe mutants of RPTPα abrogate neoplastic transformation by overexpressed RPTPα, and targeted disruption of RPTPα causes a decreased activity of Src family members in cells from the mutant mice, which correlates with increased phosphorylation levels of Tyr527. SHP-2, which is ubiquitously expressed, associates *in vivo* via its SH2 domains with numerous RPTKs and PTK substrates, including the receptors for PDGF, EGF, insulin-like growth factor-1 (IGF-1), and SCF, as well as the docking protein IRS-1. SHP-2 becomes tyrosine phosphorylated in response to stimulation with several growth factors, and tyrosine-phosphorylated SHP-2 binds to the receptors for either PDGF or SCF, as well as the adaptor molecule Grb2. The bound SHP-2, in turn, has been shown to selectively dephosphorylate tyrosine residues in the PDGFR-β important for binding of PI 3'-kinase and the GAP for Ras. Moreover, microinjection of blocking antibodies to SHP-2 or expression of SHP-2 SH2 domains or of catalytically inactive SHP-2 inhibits mitogenesis stimulated by EGF, insulin, and IGF-1. These findings suggest that SHP-2 is an upstream activator of Ras signaling and other Grb2-regulated signaling pathways and is possibly a modulator of RPTK-induced PI 3′-kinase signaling. Similar to SHP-1, binding of SHP-2 might activate its catalytic function. SHP-2 is also claimed to dephosphorylate Tyr527 in the C terminus of Src, which provides additional positive regulation of signaling.

Several protein serine/threonine kinases and substrates thereof are dephosphorylated by the major serine/threonine-specific phosphatase PP2A. This is a cytoplasmic and nuclear heterotrimeric phosphatase, consisting of a structural A subunit, a regulatory B subunit, and a catalytic C subunit. PP2A is bound to numerous scaffold proteins through its regulatory subunit, and its activity is tightly regulated in the context of assembled scaffolds. One of the important substrates in RPTK signaling is the PI 3′-kinase target Akt, a protein serine/threonine kinase mediating cell survival in part through phosphorylation of the Bcl-2 family member Bad. PP2A dephosphorylates the activating phosphorylation site T308 in Akt, crucial for kinase activity. In addition, PP2A might dephosphorylate the antiapoptotic molecule Bcl-2, abrogating its survival function. Numerous other substrates for PP2A have been identified, many of which are important downstream targets of RPTKs.

Two phosphoinositide-specific phosphatases, PTEN and SHIP1/2, respectively, specifically dephosphorylate the D-3 and the D-5 position of the inositol ring in PtdIns(3,4,5)P_3, one of the main effectors of PI 3′-kinase signaling. This counteracts RPTK-initiated PI 3′-kinase signaling, and, accordingly, PTEN has been shown to be a frequently mutated human tumor suppressor gene. Inactivating mutations in PTEN are instrumental in certain neuronal, breast, and germ cell tumors in humans, which is associated with increased activity of Akt.

C. Inhibition of RPTK Signaling by Negative Feedback Loop Regulation

Several RPTKs are negatively regulated by feedback loop inhibition through the action of downstream-activated or -induced proteins. For instance, the receptors for EGF, HGF, and SCF insulin and IGF-1 are all regulated by negative feedback loops.

The EGF receptor is phosphorylated at Thr654 located in the intracellular juxtamembrane region by activated PKC, resulting in intracellular sequestration of the receptor. Other protein serine/threonine kinases, such as ERK/MAPK and calcium/calmodulin-dependent kinase II (CAMKII), phosphorylate additional intracellular sites, including Ser1046/1047 and Thr669, respectively. This phosphorylation results in decreased ligand-binding affinity and inhibition of kinase activity of the EGFR. This provides a means for transmodulation of EGFR activity by G protein-coupled receptors, PDGF receptors, phorbol esters, and other activators of PKC. The EGF receptor itself is only a weak activator of PKC. In the case of the Kit/SCF receptor, SCF-induced Kit activation results in PKC activation, which is in part dependent on PI 3′-kinase. Activated PKCα, in turn, directly phosphorylates Ser741 and Ser746 in the kinase insert region, causing inhibition of Kit kinase activity and SCF-induced mitogenesis. PKC has also been implicated in negative feedback loop phosphorylation of the Met/HGF receptor and the insulin and IGF-1 receptors. However, in these cases, the evidence is mainly obtained from *in vitro* studies.

A family of proteins induced in response to cytokines is involved in negative feedback loop regulation of cytokine signaling. These suppressors of cytokine signaling (SOCS) proteins, which are transcriptionally induced within minutes of stimulation, bind to the protein tyrosine kinase JAK through their SH2 domains, thereby inhibiting JAK activity. SOCS proteins are also induced by RPTKs, and SOCS-1 binds to the activated Kit/SCF receptor, whereas SOCS-3 binds to the insulin and IGF-1 receptors. SOCS-1 inhibits SCF-induced mitogenesis, possibly through binding to Grb-2 and the Rho-GEF Vav, whereas SOCS-3 inhibits insulin-induced STAT5b activation, possibly through competition to a common binding site on the insulin and IGF-1 receptors. In addition, a so-called SOCS box motif mediates degradation of the bound proteins by the proteasome pathway. Finally, a family of signal regulatory proteins (SIRPs) have been identified. They can be divided into two subtypes distinguished by the presence or absence of a SHP-2-binding domain. SIRPα1 is a transmembrane polypeptide and a substrate of activated RPTKs and JAKs. It contains four cytoplasmic tyrosine phosphorylation sites. SHP-2 and, to a lesser extent, SHP-1 and Grb2 bind to the C terminus of SIRP1α through their SH2 domains in a phosphorylation-dependent manner; interestingly, SIRP1α serves as a substrate for the bound SHP-2. SIRPs in general have a tyrosine phosphorylation-dependent negative regulatory role on RPTK and JAK signaling, and the ability of SIRPα1 tyrosine mutants to negatively regulate RPTK signaling correlates with their ability to bind SHP-2.

D. Inhibition of RPTK Signaling through Heterodimerization

RPTK signaling can also be inhibited through a dominant-negative effect by heterodimerization with receptor variants or mutants with decreased or abolished kinase activity. A wealth of experimental data, where kinase-deleted or ATP-binding site mutant, kinase-inactive RPTKs have been coexpressed in cells at similar levels together with their wild-type partners, shows a dominant-negative effect of the mutant RPTK on signaling. This is most likely due to the formation of signaling-defective heterodimers. Thus, assuming equal expression levels of mutant and wild-type protein, a 1:2:1 ratio of wild-type (wt)/wt homodimers: wt/mutant heterodimers:mutant/mutant homodimers should form in response to ligand, meaning that only 25% of the dimers are signaling active. This mechanism for a dominant-negative function has been causally implicated in the phenotype induced by several heterozygous RPTK mutations in mice and humans. Thus, many tissues express truncated, kinase-inactive RPTK variants that might serve to inhibit signaling through heterodimer formation with the wild-type RPTK. Mammals with inactivating point mutations in the kinase domain of Kit/SCF receptor provide the best characterized example of negative dominance due to mutant RPTKs. Thus, mice and humans heterozygous for such naturally occurring loss-of-function mutations in Kit exhibit severe anemia, depigmentation, sterility, and constipation with variable tissue penetrance of different mutations. This phenotype is more severe than would be expected from a true dosage effect. More recently, it has been reported that several human diseases are caused by heterozygous LOF mutations in other

RPTKs. For instance, missense LOF mutations in the vascular endothelial growth factor receptor-3 (VEGFR-3) cause a dominant form of primary human lymphoedema. Likewise, humans heterozygous for LOF mutations in the orphan RPTKs ROR2 and Mer, the latter an Axl family member, suffer from the Robinow syndrome, a form of short-limbed dwarfism and retinitis pigmentosa, respectively. In all cases, this is probably due to heterodimer formation and a dominant-negative effect of the mutant receptors. However, heterodimerization with kinase-inactive RPTKs does not always inhibit signaling, but in some cases it might provide more diversity in signaling through recruitment of a different spectrum of substrates. For instance, in the EGF receptor family of RPTKs, the kinase-inactive ErbB3 is transphosphorylated on tyrosine residues by its kinase-active heterodimeric partner. Some of these mediate recruitment and activation of PI 3′-kinase, which does not bind directly to any of the kinase-active ErbB partners (see earlier discussion).

VI. CONCLUDING REMARKS

The identification of modular domains in signaling proteins involved in protein–protein interactions has revolutionized the field of signal transduction. Together with highly advanced protein chemical and molecular biological techniques, this knowledge has made it possible to identify numerous novel signaling molecules and to specifically interfere with and manipulate the function of signaling molecules in intact cells. By this means, the molecular details of several entire signal transduction pathways have been elucidated. To analyze the physiological role of individual RPTK-initiated signaling pathways, novel technologies have been developed enabling the introduction of single amino acid changes into RPTK phosphorylation sites in the mouse genome, causing disruption of specific ligand-induced signaling pathways. It is likely that specific interruption of the function of deregulated signaling molecules involved in malignant cell transformation can prevent tumorigenesis. Examples of such molecular signal transduction therapy include the use of the small molecule Bcr-Abl inhibitor STI571 for the therapy of chronic myeloid leukemia. It is also in phase trials for glioblastoma and gastrointestinal stromal tumors based on its ability to inhibit the Kit/SCF receptor. Several "specific" RPTK inhibitors are currently in clinical trials to prevent tumor angiogenesis and leukemic cell growth in patients.

Acknowledgments

P.B.-J. is a Special Fellow of the Leukemia and Lymphoma Society of America and T.H. is a Frank and Else Schilling American Cancer Society Professor.

See Also the Following Articles

Bibliography

Burack, W. R., and Shaw, A. S. (2000). Signal transduction: Hanging on a scaffold. *Curr. Opin. Cell Biol.* **12,** 211–216.

Edwards, A. S., and Scott, J. D. (2000). A-kinase-anchoring proteins: Protein kinase A and beyond. *Curr. Opin. Cell Biol.* **12,** 217–221.

Forman-Kay, J. D., and Pawson, T. (1999). Diversity in protein recognition by PTB domains. *Curr. Opin. Struct. Biol.* **9,** 690–695.

Fruman, D. A., Rameh, L. E., and Cantley, L. C. (1999). Phosphoinositide binding domains: Embracing 3-phosphate. *Cell* **97,** 817–820.

Heldin, C.-H. (1995). Dimerization of cell surface receptors in signal transduction. *Cell* **80,** 213–223.

Hunter, T. (2000). Signaling—2000 and beyond. *Cell* **100,** 113–127.

Jordan, J. D., Landau, E. M., and Iyengar, R. (2000). Signaling networks: The origins of cellular multitasking. *Cell* **103,** 193–200.

Pawson, T., and Nash, P. (2000). Protein–protein interactions define specificity in signal transduction. *Genes Dev.* **14,** 1027–1047.

Pawson, T., and Saxton, T. M. (1999). Signaling networks—do all roads lead to the same genes? *Cell* **97,** 675–678.

Plowman, G. D., Sudarsanam, S., Bingham, J., Whyte, D., and Hunter, T. (1999). The protein kinases of *Caenorhabditis elegans*: A model for signal transduction in multicellular organisms. *Proc. Natl. Acad. Sci. USA* **96,** 13603–13610.

Schlessinger, J. (2000). Cell signaling by receptor tyrosine kinases. *Cell* **103,** 211–225.

Skin Cancer, Non-Melanoma

Leslie Robinson-Bostom
Charles J. McDonald
Brown Medical School and Rhode Island Hospital

GLOSSARY

basal cell carcinoma A slow-growing, invasive but usually nonmetastasizing neoplasm recapitulating normal basal cell of the epidermis or hair follicles, most commonly rising in sun-damaged skin of the elderly and fair skinned.

carcinoma Any of the various types of malignant neoplasm derived from epidermal tissue.

immunosuppression Prevention or interference with the development of immunologic response; may reflect natural immunological unresponsiveness (tolerance) may be artificially induced by chemical, biological, or physical agents, or may be caused by disease.

squamous cell carcinoma A malignant neoplasm derived from stratified squamous epithelium; variable amounts of keratin are formed in relation to the degree of differentiation.

ultraviolet Denoting electromagnetic rays at higher frequency than the violet end of the visible spectrum at 210–400 nm.

Nonmelanoma skin cancers are the most common malignancies in the United States, with a projected incidence of up to 1,300,000 cases for 2001 alone. Basal cell carcinomas (BCC) account for approximately 80%, whereas squamous cell carcinomas (SCC) account for 20%. A sharp rise in the incidence of nonmelanoma skin cancer has been documented with basal cell carcinoma increasing by 153% since the late 1980s.

I. NEOPLASMS OF THE SKIN

Ultraviolet (UV) light is the single most important etiologic agent in the development of nonmelanoma skin cancer. Sunburn and carcinogenesis are induced by UV, B and C (250 to 320 nm). Ultraviolet light A (320 to 440 nm) can also produce sunburn and augment the sunburn effects of UVB, but it is approximately 1000 to 10,000 times less mutagenic than either UVB or UVC. Absorption of UV light by DNA induces the formation of pyrimidine dimers. Ineffective excisional repair leads to partial defect repair, mutation and carcinogenesis, altered metabolism, or cell death. Ultraviolet light also causes mutations in the p53 tumor suppressor gene, which is found in squamous cell carcinomas. This protein acts as a tumor suppressor by promoting apoptosis of cells with DNA damage. UVB, as well as UVA, also appears to promote tumor formation by selective immunosuppression. Ultraviolet light C (wavelengths less than 290 nm) is filtered by the ozone layer in the stratospheric atmosphere and effectively does not reach the surface of the earth. It has been estimated that a 1% decrease in stratospheric ozone may increase the prevalence of nonmelanoma and melanoma skin cancers by 2.3%. X-ray exposure, burns, scars, and chronic ulcers (Marjolin's ulcer) also play a significant role in the pathogenesis of SCC.

Numerous potential chemical carcinogens have been extensively studied as risk factors and include polycyclic and aromatic hydrocarbons and, to a lesser extent, tar, pitch, soot, creosol, asphalt, and diesel oils among others. The actual incidence of carcinomas attributable to these substances is unknown. Cutaneous malignancies, particularly squamous cell carcinoma, have long been associated with arsenic exposure through medicines as well as pesticides. This has been especially problematic in Asian countries where arsenic was used in proprietary medications and may be an underrecognized factor in this country. Arsenic exposure is also associated with internal malignancies, especially of the lung and bladder that classically present after the skin cancers are apparent.

Skin color is the most important host factor in the development of nonmelanoma skin cancer. Melanin gives skin its color and is our principal cutaneous sun protector. An increased risk of basal cell carcinoma is strongly associated with fair skin color, inability to tan, birth or early age of arrival in Australia, northern European ancestry, presence of multiple nevi, and presence of solar elastosis (cutaneous sun damage). Immunosuppression also increases the risk for nonmelanoma skin cancer. This has been especially well studied among renal transplant patients. The overall risk of developing nonmelanoma skin cancer is 40% at 20 years status postrenal transplant. Renal transplant recipients have a 250 times increased risk of developing cutaneous squamous cell carcinoma. The risk is 43.8% at 7 years after heart transplant. Risk is further increased in both cases in light skin types and with a history of prolonged UV exposure. Although the incidence of BCC is also increased in this population, the normal ratio of BCC vs SCC is maintained. An increased risk of nonmelanoma skin cancer has also been associated with chronic corticosteroid treatment and altered immune states, such as that caused by lymphomas and leukemia.

Human papillomavirus infection has been associated with nonmelanoma skin cancer, especially in immunosuppressed individuals. Human papilloma virus is frequently found in precancerous lesions and squamous cell carcinomas in renal transplant patients. Human papillomavirus type 16 has been associated with Bowen's disease and squamous cell carcinoma of the fingers, whereas virus types 16 and 18 have been associated with squamous cell carcinoma of the genital tract. Other cutaneous disorders that predispose to an increased risk of nonmelanoma skin cancer include epidermodysplasia verruciformis, xeroderma pigmentosum, basal cell nevus syndrome, and albinism.

II. ACTINIC KERATOSES

Actinic keratoses are the most common epithelial precancerous lesions, developing almost exclusively in Caucasians. Actinic keratoses are almost always located on sun exposed skin with the vast majority occurring on the head and neck followed by the extensor upper extremities, trunk, and lower extremities.

Actinic cheilitis is a lesion of the lip that is analogous to actinic keratosis. As with actinic keratoses, it is widely accepted that this lesion is due to excessive sun exposure. Lesions occur almost exclusively on the lower lip, predominantly at the vermillion border, thus reinforcing its direct relationship with the sun. Chronic skin irritation (i.e., from tobacco, poor hygiene, ill fitting dentures) has also been associated with an increased risk of actinic cheilitis. As with actinic keratoses, actinic cheilitis has been associated with malignant transformation into squamous cell carcinoma. The relative risk is estimated at 2.5.

A. Clinical Manifestations

Actinic keratoses present initially as ill-defined pink to red macules or papules with adherent scale that is difficult to remove (Fig. 1). Left untreated, the scale becomes hypertrophic. A cutaneous horn may eventually develop. Actinic cheilitis may also present early on as persistent lip erythema. Dry and scaling skin subsequently develop and may involve the entire lower lip. Some areas may develop thickened white plaques known as leukoplakia. An ill-defined vermillion border, atrophy, ulceration, and nodularity are warning signs for malignant transformation, although apparently insignificant surface change may represent carcinoma.

B. Treatment

Multiple modalities are available for the treatment of actinic keratoses. Cryosurgery with liquid nitrogen is a highly effective method. In thicker hyperkerotic lesions, curettage with or without desiccation may be more effective. In widespread lesions, topical 5-fluorouracil (5-FU) available as 1–5% cream and solutions applied for 3–4 weeks will result in a significant reduction of precancerous lesion. In exceptional refractory and extensive cases, medium depth chemical peeling, dermabrasion, and laser resurfacing can be utilized. As an adjunctive therapy, daily sunscreen alone appears to modulate squamous cell cancer development. Topical retinoids are reported to decrease the number of actinic keratosis. Photodynamic therapy with 5-aminolevulinic acid is also effective. Systemic retinoids can be selectively used in severe and extensive cases.

III. BOWEN'S DISEASE

Bowen's disease, or squamous cell carcinoma *in situ*, is a premalignant neoplasm that occurs on both sun-exposed and nonsun-exposed areas of the body. Bowen's disease is typically a disease of elderly Caucasians, but may present as early as the third decade. Bowen's disease also has been reported in black patients and may be underdiagnosed because it is asymptomatic and mimics other dermatoses. Bowen's tumors are known to be associated with chronic trivalent arsenic exposure from medicinal and environmental sources.

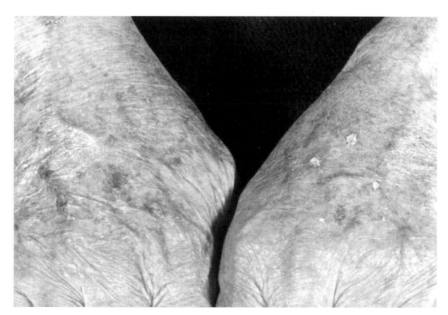

FIGURE 1 Actinic keratoses: Ill-defined papules with adherent scale on the dorsal hands.

A. Clinical Manifestations

Clinically the lesions appear as sharply demarcated red to brown plaques with a very fine scale or crust. When the lesions occur on the fingers they may mimic an eczematous reaction.

B. Treatment

Treatment with topical 5-FU, simple destruction with cryosurgery, electrodestruction, or CO_2 laser vaporization are all effective. However, microinvasion or spread down hair follicles results in a variable response. Excision may be the treatment of choice in larger lesions because of the high risk of focal invasion. Mohs surgery can be selectively employed in recurrent, poorly defined tumors or if wide resection is not desired, such as on a digit. Interferon has been used successfully in Bowen's disease. Photodynamic therapy can also be used. A combination of isotretinoin and interferon has been reported useful in extensive or multiple lesions.

IV. KERATOACANTHOMA

Keratoacanthoma (KA) is a relatively common, rapidly growing tumor of the elderly with a clinical and histologic pattern similar to squamous cell carcinoma. These tumors rarely progress to squamous cell carcinomas and often resolve spontaneously. They are grouped into solitary and multiple types.

Ultraviolet light probably plays a role in the genesis of these lesions as the majority occur on sun-exposed skin. The face, extensor surface of the hands, and the forearms are the most common sites. Tumors of the lower leg are found almost exclusively in women. Tumors of the hands are more common in men.

An increased risk of keratocanthomas has been associated with Muir–Torre syndrome, xeroderma pigmentation. Immunosuppressed patients are at increased risk of developing keratocanthomas as well as other cutaneous malignancies.

A. Clinical Manifestations

Solitary keratocanthoma presents initially as a small domed papule with a central keratotic umbilication that grows rapidly over a period of 6 to 8 weeks. Most keratocanthomas measure 1.0 to 2.5 cm. Mature nodules exhibit a smooth pink to red surface. The majority of lesions spontaneously resolve over a period of 3 to 6 months, leaving an atrophic scar.

B. Treatment

Treatment of keratoacanthoma is the same as SCC. In an early lesion, cryosurgery and electrodessication and curettage can be used with reported success. Although a KA will follow a self-limited course and regress spontaneously, the behavior cannot be predicted and many act as a squamous cell carcinoma, showing rapid growth regional spread and metastasis. Excision is generally the treatment of choice. Mohs surgery is reported with a very low recurrence rate of 2.4%.

The tumors are very sensitive to radiation and its use may avoid local deformity. Interferon interlesionally has great appeal but larger studies need to be performed. Intralesion responses to numerous agents have been reported, including fluorouracil, methotrexate, and bleomycin. Systemic retinoids have been reported as helpful in patients with multiple lesions.

V. SQUAMOUS CELL CANCER (EPIDERMOID CARCINOMA)

Squamous cell cancer is the second most common skin neoplasm in Caucasians and accounts for 20% of skin cancers. The incidence among Australians is 201 per 100,000. In nonwhite races, squamous cell carcinoma is the most common skin cancer. Squamous cell carcinoma is generally a disease of the middle aged and elderly. Most squamous cell cancers that occur in Caucasians arise on sun-exposed areas, principally the head, neck, and extremities. In general, squamous cell carcinomas in African-Americans occur on sun-protected areas and areas exposed to frequent external trauma.

A. Modes of Spread

Squamous cell carcinoma is locally invasive and destructive. In transit metastasis can occur. Local invasion can occur by lymphatic, perineural, and rarely intravascular means. All are associated with a significantly worse prognosis.

Several factors affect the prognosis of squamous cell carcinoma, including presence of a precancerous lesion, anatomic location, depth of invasion, and histologic grade. Tumors associated with actinically damaged skin tend to be slow growing and rarely metastasize. Estimates for rates of metastases in these lesions range from less than 0.1% of cases to less than 2.6%. Tumors that arise from apparently normal skin or from precancerous lesions other than actinic keratoses act more malignant and frequently metastasize. They are more invasive and frequently involve surrounding tissues producing large, firm nodules. The rate of metastases also depends on the location of the tumor. The overall rate of metastases for squamous cell carcinoma by meta-analysis is 5.2%; the rate for ear and lip lesions is 11 and 13.7%, respectively. Lesions occurring on the head and neck area tend to invade locally and extend along peripheral nerves. Perineural tumor may be associated with symptoms, such as pain, but usually is initially asymptomatic. Recurrences are very common and a high mortality is associated with perineural SCC. Poorly differentiated tumors and deeply invasive tumors also have a worse prognosis (greater than 4 mm in thickness).

B. Clinical Manifestations

The clinical presentation of squamous cell carcinomas depends on the site of origin and type of precursor lesion. Cutaneous squamous cell cancers are usually asymptomatic. Tumors that evolve from actinic keratoses appear as red, slightly elevated, scaling plaques. They are differentiated from actinic keratoses by the presence of induration (Fig. 2). As these tumors enlarge they become firm and occasionally smooth with subsequent ulceration. Early squamous cell carcinomas are freely mobile. As they invade surrounding tissues they become more indurated and fixed.

Squamous cell carcinoma of the lip is frequently subtle. Palpable induration is not a prominent feature of this tumor and is not as helpful in assessing for malignancy as it is in squamous cell carcinoma of other sites. If induration is present, it is a sign of long-standing disease. These tumors often present early as an innocuous white patch with a small fissure or ulceration.

Tumors arising in burn scars tend to occur on the periphery of the scars in hyperkeratotic areas. Multiple squamous cell carcinomas can occur in former radiation ports and in individuals exposed to chemical carcinogens. Tumors arising in chronic ulcers and along sinus tracts can be diagnostic dilemmas.

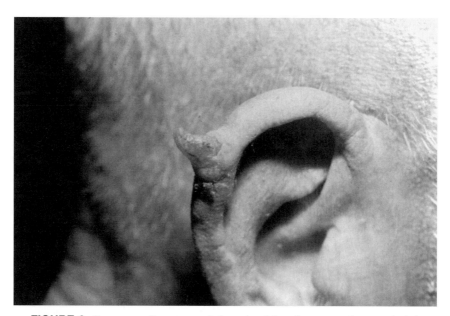

FIGURE 2 Squamous cell carcinoma: Indurated nodule with cutaneous horn on the helix.

Certain tumors are at risk of local recurrence. Recurrent tumors, tumors in the mid facial/embryonic fold, large tumors greater than 2 cm, tumors greater than 4 mm in depth, poorly differentiated or spindle cell variants, and neurotrophic tumors are all at higher risk of recurrence.

C. Treatment

The treatment of squamous cell carcinoma is primarily surgical. Small, thin actinically derived tumors in low risk sites are amenable to a destructive approach, but excision is the standard treatment. With standard excisions, minimal margins are in the 4- to 5-mm range and should be increased according to the clinical risk of the situation. Wide margins are needed in more aggressive tumors because skipping of tumor "in transit metastasis."

Mohs micrographic surgery may be helpful to define the tumor and offers a cure of primary tumors of approximately 95%. Tissue conservation is noted in early lesions of the ear and lip with cures of 100 and 95%, respectively. However, in aggressive extensive cases, an additional margin after Mohs resections is recommended.

Perineural invasion occurs in 14–36% of squamous cell carcinoma. The risks of both metastasis and recurrence are increased. Mohs surgery may be helpful to define perineural tumor having up to a 12% local recurrence. However, adjunctive radiation is a good option in this situation.

In the aggressive tumor, clinically and radiographic screening (CT scanning, MRI) should be performed to evaluate nodal spread. Clinical staging of local nodes is a very important predictor of outcome. In head and neck lesions, suspicious nodes can be addressed with needle biopsy or surgical node evaluation. Neck dissection is indicated in cases with evidence of local spread. Radiation may offer additional control as an adjunct to neck dissection, either prior to or after surgery, and chemosensitization can be utilized as an adjunctive method. In the absence of nodal spread but with a high-risk tumor, nodal dissection or adjunctive radiation may be prudent, such as deep tumors, especially on the extremities, lip, and ear.

Interlesional interferon has been used with complete responses and low recurrence reported. Ikuc reported only 2/31 squamous cell carcinoma reoccurred after being treated intralesionally. Interferon has been used subcutaneously with 13 cis-retinoic acid for refractory inoperative tumors with a 93% response. In distally spread tumors, a partial regional response and one complete response was reported.

Refractory or metastatic disease has been treated with retinoids, traditional chemotherapy radiation, and interferon. Systemic retinoids have been reported to have a modulating effect on both refractory and metastatic disease, often causing temporary regression of the tumor. Chemotherapy, predominately cisplatinum based, with the addition of 5-FU, bleomycin, or doxirubincin, has been utilized and offers a palliative response. Radiation can be used as a sole agent or as an adjuvant to aggressive tumor.

VI. BASAL CELL CARCINOMA

Basal cell cancer is the most common neoplasm of Caucasians and the incidence is increasing. It is uncommon among African-Americans. The head and neck areas are by far the most frequent sites of basal cell carcinoma in both men and women, with 80% of lesions occurring here. Basal cell carcinomas have been reported to occur in nonsun-exposed areas.

Basal cell carcinomas do occur in nonwhite races, but are less common than squamous cell carcinoma. In a comprehensive study of skin cancer in African-Americans conducted in 1988 at Howard University, 89% of basal cell carcinomas were found to be on sun-exposed areas. Most lesions occur at or after age 50.

Basal cell carcinomas originate in the epidermis and tend to grow slowly and remain confined to this area. Basal cell carcinomas are often referred to as basal cell epitheliomas because of their indolent nature. These tumors do have the potential over decades to become deeply invasive into soft tissue and erode into blood vessels, bone, cartilage, and sinuses. Recurrent tumors tend to be more aggressive than primary tumors. They display a worse histologic subtype and grow in irregular patterns. Large tumors (greater than 2 cm) and tumors arising in a midfacial location are at a higher risk of recurrence. Infiltrating basal cell carcinomas (morpheaform/sclerotic, micronodular, adenocytic, metatypical/basosquamous, and superficial "multifocal" types) are associated with a higher risk of recurrence. A perineural spread of basal cell cancer often occurs and is a prominent risk factor for recurrence, but is not associated with the mortality of perineural squamous cell carcinoma.

Metastatic basal cell carcinoma is rare but reported. Sites of metastases include the bloodstream, regional lymph nodes, bone, lung, liver, and other viscera. Metastases occur at an incidence of 0.1%.

A. Clinical Manifestations

Basal cell carcinomas are categorized in subtypes that have characteristic clinical presentations. These categories include nodular, morpheaform, superficial, and pigmented.

Nodular basal cell carcinomas present as translucent pearly papules of various sizes that are traversed by tortuous telangiectatic blood vessels (Fig. 3). As the lesion ages, the center becomes flat and potentially crusted and the peripheral borders are raised and pearly. The center may eventually ulcerate, producing a rodent ulcer. Nodulocystic tumors may have the appearance of pustules or epidermal cysts. Morpheaform basal cell carcinomas present as ill defined, white, waxy, and sclerotic plaques (Fig. 4). They are usually

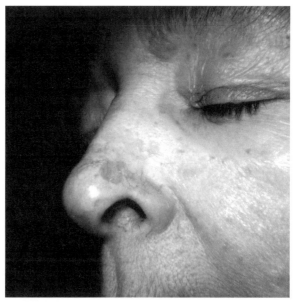

FIGURE 4 Morpheaform basal cell carcinoma: Subtle sclerotic plaque on the lower nasal bridge.

devoid of telangiectasias and may be only slightly raised above the surrounding normal skin. The lesions tend to be firm, depressed, and smooth. They often resemble scars or localized patches of scleroderma.

Horizontal spread, rather than vertical, occurs in superficial basal cell carcinoma. These lesions present as ill-defined, erythematous, scaling plaques without telangiectasias. These tumors are potentially confused with Bowen's disease or localized eczema.

Pigmented basal cell carcinomas are clinically dentical to nodular basal cell carcinomas, but are sprinkled with pigment or may be entirely pigmented. They occur more frequently in people with dark skin types and are easily confused with malignant melanoma.

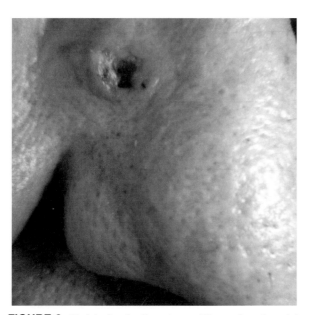

FIGURE 3 Nodular basal cell carcinoma: Ulcerated pearly nodule on the nose.

B. Treatment

All the previously described techniques of skin cancer treatment have been reported effective. Algorithms for selection of modalities based on location, histology, size, tumor history, and other factors have been described. Destructive techniques such as cryosurgery and electrodessication and curettage are useful in many of the uncomplicated tumors, having an effectiveness of cure approximating 93%. Excisional surgery is the standard to which all modalities need to be compared. All of the techniques just described offer 5-year cure rates around 90%. In tumors at risk for recurrence, as defined previously, intraoperative fresh frozen or Mohs micrographic surgery offers an improved cure rate. The efficacy of Mohs surgery is well documented with exceptional cure rates of 97–99% in all types of basal cell cancer. This high cure rate is sustained in recurrent tumors and tumors at risk of recurrence; therefore, Mohs surgery is the treatment of choice for problematic tumors.

Topical 5-FU is limited by the depth of skin penetration and has a high failure rate in all but the most superficial lesions. Radiation is effective in primary and recurrent tumors and offers a nonsurgical, nonmutilating method, and thus some believe it should be the treatment of choice. However, long-term problems may occur after radiation therapy, thus limiting its use. Among these are radiation scar, scar contraction, radiation dermatitis, and occasional secondary radiation-induced tumors.

A subtotally respected tumor is a common occurrence in clinical practice. Selection of proper margins based on location, histology types, and other considerations is essential. The significance of residual tumor is debated, but it is clear that histologic types such as infiltrating or multicentric types are at a higher risk of recurrence, as are tumors of the midfacial area and the ears. Observation can be practiced in a low-risk location and situation, but reexcision or Mohs surgery should be utilized in tumors with high risk factors for recurrence. Adjunctive radiation has also been used in this situation.

Intralesional interferon has been reported in several small series with high clinical response rates of 67–96%. In more aggressive tumors, the response rate is low, 27% with complete response and 33% showing reduction of tumor. Cosmetic outcomes are excellent and a nonsurgical approach is appealing. However, cost, side effects, lower cure rates, and less documented experience than traditional approaches limit the use of interferon in the treatment of basal cell carcinoma.

Systemic retinoids (isotretinate and etretinate) modulate the growth and differentiation of basal cell carcinoma treatment of patients with multiple lesions, resulting in regression of tumors. Used prophylactically in high-risk patients, such as those having basal cell nevus syndrome or xeroderma pigmentosa, significant long-term improvement can be expected.

Photodynamic therapy is undergoing evaluation and offers some promise in extensive disease. Early reports have been promising with up to 88% complete response. Topical leuvulonic acid is effective. Indications, limitations, and parameters are not yet fully developed. At this time, patients with numerous superficial tumors may prove to be the best candidate for this therapy.

See Also the Following Articles

INTERFERONS: CELLULAR AND MOLECULAR BIOLOGY OF THEIR ACTIONS • MELANOMA: EPIDEMIOLOGY • PAPILLOMAVIRUSES • PHOTODYNAMIC THERAPY: BASIC PRINCIPLES AND APPLICATIONS TO SKIN CANCER • TP53 TUMOR SUPPRESSOR GENE: STRUCTURE AND FUNCTION

Bibliography

Alam, M., and Ratner, D. (2001). Primary care: Cutaneous squamous-cell carcinoma. *N. Engl. J. Med.* **344**(13), 975–983.

Albright, S. D. (1982). Treatment of skin cancer using multiple modalities. *J. Am. Acad. Dermatol.* **7**(2), 143–171.

Cohen, P. R., Kohn, S. R., Davis, D. A., and Duzrock, R. (1995). Muir-Torre syndrome. *Dermatol. Clin.* **13**(1), 79–89.

Dufresne, R. G., and Curlin, M. U. (1997). Actinic chelitis. A treatment review. *Dermatol. Surg.* **23**, 15–21.

Elder, E., Elenitas, R., Jaworsky, C., and Johnson, B. (1997). Tumors and cysts of the epidermis. *In* "Lever's Histopathology of the Skin" (D. Elder, R. Elenitas, C. Jaworsky, and B. Johson, Jr., eds.), 8th Ed., p. 730. Lippincott-Raven, Philadelphia.

España A., Redondo, P., *et al.* (1995). Skin cancer in heart transplant recipients. *J. Am. Acad. Dermatol.* **32**, 458–465.

Halder, R. M., and Bang, K. M. (1988). Skin cancer in blacks in the United States. *Dermatol. Clin.* **6**(3), 397–405.

Hartevelt, M. M., Bavinck, J. N., Kootte, A. M., Vermeer, B. J., and Vandenbroucke, J. P. (1990). Incidence of skin cancer after renal transplantation in the Netherlands. *Transplantation* **49**(3), 506–509.

Kawashima, M., Favre, M., *et al.* (1990). Premalignant lesions and cancers of the skin in the general population: Evaluation of the role of human papillomaviruses. *J. Invest. Dermatol.* **95**, 537–542.

Ko, C. B., Walton, S., Keszkes, K., Bury, H. P. R., and Nicholson, C. (1994). The emerging epidemic of skin cancer. *Br. J. Dermatol.* **130**, 269–272.

Kossard, S., and Rosen, R. (1992). Cutaneous Bowen's disease: An analysis of 1001 cases according to age, sex, and site. *J. Am. Acad. Dermatol.* **27**, 406–410.

Kraemer, K. H., Di Giovanna, J. J., Moshel, A. N., Tarone, R. E., and Peck, G. L. (1988). Prevention of skin cancer in xeroderma pigmentosum with the use of oral isotretinoin. *N. Engl. J. Med.* **318**(25), 1633–1637.

Kricker, A., Armstrong, B. K., and Parkin, D. M. (1993). Measurement of skin cancer incidence. *Health Rep.* **5**(1), 63–66.

Kricker, A., Armstrong, B. K., English, D. R., and Heenan, P. (1991). Pigmmentary and cutaneous risk factors for nonmelanocytic skin cancer: A case control study. *Int. J. Cancer* **48**, 650–662.

Kwa, R. E., Campana, K., and Moy, R. L. (1992). Biology of cutaneous squamous cell carcinoma. *J. Am. Acad. Dermatol.* **26**, 1–26.

Lund, H. Z. (1965). How often does squamous cell carcinoma of the skin metastasize? *Arch. Dermatol.* **92**, 635.

Marks, R., Rennie, G., and Selwood, T. S. (1988). Malignant transformation of solar keratoses to squamous cell carcinoma. *Lancet* **1**(8589), 795–797.

Marks, R. (1995). An overview of skin cancers. *Cancer* **75**, 607–612.

Moan, J., and Dahlback, A. (1992). The relationship between skin cancers, solar radiation and ozone depletion. *Br. J. Cancer* **65**, 916–921.

Rank, B. K., and Dixon, P. L. (1979). Another look at keratoacanthoma. *Aust. New Zeal. J. Surg.* **49**, 654–658.

Rowe, D. E., Carrol, R. J., and Day, C. L., Jr. (1992). Prognostic factors from local recurrence, metastasis, and survival rates in squamous cell carcinoma of the skin, ear, and lip: Implications for treatment modality selection. *J. Am. Acad. Dermatol.* **26**(6), 976–990.

Swanson, N. A. (1983). Mohs surgery: Technique, indications, applications, and the future. *Arch. Dermatol.* **119**(9), 761–773.

STAT Proteins in Growth Control

Jacqueline F. Bromberg
Memorial Sloan-Kettering Cancer Center

James E. Darnell, Jr.
Rockefeller University

GLOSSARY

—COOH Regions implicated in transcription activation.
DNA Deoxyribonucleic acid, the substance that constitutes the genetic material of cellular organisms.
SRC Sarcoma virus gene, a family of protooncogenes (*c-src, v-cer, erb*).

S TAT (signal transducers and activators of transcription) proteins are a group of transcription factors that transmit signals from the extracellular surface of cells to the nucleus directing gene-specific transcription. Quite often, human malignancies have lost control of these signaling systems. This article discusses the importance of dysregulated STAT signaling in the pathogenesis of cancer.

I. INTRODUCTION

Growth control and survival of the normal cells in a developing or an adult mammal is exquisitely balanced. Many of the signals that influence this balance are delivered by circulating polypeptides, the binding of which to cognate cell surface receptors govern gene-specific transcription. Very often, human cancer cells can be shown to have lost normal control of these signaling systems. For example, the first oncogene described, v-src, is a mutant tyrosine kinase that is persistently activated, while its cellular wild-type counterpart, c-src, is only transiently activated in response to specific mitogens or growth factors.

Alternatively, and in addition to persistent unregulated mitogenic signaling, the lack of suppressive signals (tumor suppressors) is also critical in the development of cancers. The loss of suppressors occurs either by mutation or complete deletion of the tumor suppressor gene. While there is no argument that deleterious mutations of either protooncogenes or tumor suppressor genes seem to be universally involved in human cancer, there are very likely key cellular regulators that remain intact which are required for the unleashed cancer cell phenotype to be expressed. This chapter will discuss the importance of dysregulated STAT (Signal Transducers and Activators of Transcription) signaling is involved in the pathogenesis of cancer. We believe it likely that these proteins, particularly Stat3, may act as required targets of oncogenes without themselves being mutant. We first briefly describe the mechanisms by which STAT proteins become activated and regulated and describe the molecular anatomy of the STAT proteins which allows precision in the aim of many functional studies of the STATs.

II. STAT DOMAINS: STRUCTURE AND FUNCTION

STAT proteins were originally discovered as DNA binding proteins that mediate interferon (IFN) signaling, but they also play a central role in cytokine, growth factor, and oncogeneic tyrosine kinase signaling. There are seven known mammalian STAT family members that are latent in the cytoplasm of cells, become activated by phosphorylation on a single tyrosine residue (~700), and dimerize by virtue of a reciprocal −SH2 phosphotyrosine interaction. The dimeric STAT protein accumulates in the nucleus and binds DNA to drive transcription. (Fig.1). The STAT proteins are subsequently inactivated by tyrosine dephosphorylation and return to the cytoplasm.

The three-dimensional structures of the core of Stats 1 and 3 (from residues ~130 to 712; lacking an N-terminal and C-terminal domain) bound to DNA revealed four domains. From residues ~130 to 320 there are four long helical coils, which interact with each other and provide large surfaces to interact with other proteins; residues ~320 to 490 comprise the

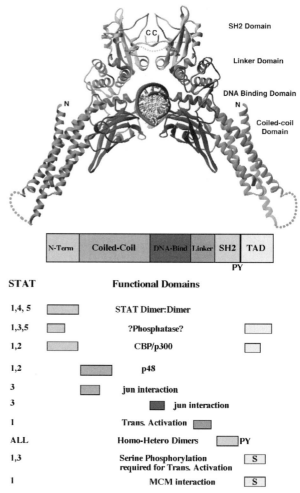

FIGURE 1 Three-dimensional structure of the core of Stat 1 (from residues 130 to 712; lacking an N-terminal and C-terminal domain) bound to DNA. The structure of truncated Stat 3 is virtually superimposable with that of Stat 1. Locations for the functional domains of each STAT protein (depicted from N terminus to C terminus) are shown in the lower half of the figure.

DNA-binding domain, a region of β-sheet structures connected by unstructured loops; and a linker domain from 490 to 575 that contains several α helices followed by a classical −SH2 domain. Reciprocal phosphotyrosine−SH2 interactions hold the dimer together so that DNA contacts on the dyad symmetrical-binding site can occur. Regions implicated in transcription activation are the −COOH-terminal 38 amino acids of Stat 1 and the terminal ~75 amino acids of Stat 3. Included in the COOH-terminal region of Stats 1 and 3 is a critical serine (S727 in both proteins) and a critical leucine residue

(L724 in Stat1). Interaction of this −COOH terminal region from both Stat1 and Stat 2 with histone transacetylases has been established. In addition, the Stat1 −COOH terminus interacts with MCM proteins in a serine phosphorylation-dependent fashion. MCM proteins are known to be important in initiating DNA replication origins, most likely as a dimer of two hexamers, which act as a helicase, but their role in RNA synthesis is unknown. While all STAT molecules depend on this -COOH terminal segment for transcriptional activation, other regions of the STAT molecule can contribute to transcriptional activation. The NH_2 terminus is required in transcription as judged by defective stimulation in transfection experiments of NH_2-terminal deletions. Also, there is a known interaction with histone transacetylases (CBP/p300 proteins) by the −NH_2-terminal end of Stat 1, which may contribute to transcription activation. Furthermore, mutations in the linker domain of Stat1 (connecting the DNA-binding domain with the −SH2 domain) result in a protein that can be phosphorylated on tyrosine, dimerize, accumulate in the nucleus, and bind DNA but fail to activate transcription. In addition, many natural Stat-binding sites (and in fact the most frequently used transfection target) contain closely spaced tandem Stat-binding sites. When two such sites are occupied there is Stat dimer–dimer interaction (tetramer) mediated by the N terminus that is necessary for maximal transcriptional stimulation (Fig. 1). The dimer–dimer interaction was demonstrated for a natural DNA element most clearly for the Stat 5 sites in the gene encoding the α chain of the IL-2 receptor.

III. STATS AS TRANSCRIPTIONAL REGULATORS

In addition to these studies, which suggest how STATs engage transcriptional machinery, there is considerable evidence of STAT interactions with other transcription factors bound to neighboring sites in the promoter segments of various genes. For example, Stat 1 and Sp1 interact on the ICAM promoter; Stat 5 and the glucocorticoid receptor (GR) interact on the β-casein promoter; and Stat 3, c-Jun, and GR interact on the α_2-macroglobulin promoter. A number of other genes

have been found to have closely spaced required DNA-binding sites for a Stat protein and some other transcription factors. These interactions in the STAT family of proteins undoubtedly comprise enhanceosomes and promise to be of great importance as they are known to be in IFN-β promoter and in the promoter for the α chain of the T-cell receptor.

IV. MECHANISMS OF STAT ACTIVATION AND REGULATION

STAT proteins become tyrosine phosphorylated or activated by over 40 different ligands via tyrosine kinases such as JAKs (Janus kinases) associated with cytokine receptors and G-protein receptors; by receptor tyrosine kinases such as the epidermal growth factor receptor and platelet-derived growth factor receptor; and through nonreceptor tyrosine kinases (i.e., Src and Abl) either directly or via other associated tyrosine kinases (Fig.2). STATs form homodimers (most commonly) as well as heterodimers (e.g., Stats 1:2, in response to IFNα). Other heterodimers can form (i.e., Stats 1:3); however, their exact function as transcriptional activators is not known.

In normal cells and in animals, ligand-dependent activation of STATs is a transient process, lasting for several minutes to several hours. In contrast, in many cancerous cell lines and tumors, where growth factor dysregulation is frequently at the heart of cellular transformation, STAT proteins (in particular Stats 1, 3, and 5) are persistently tyrosine phosphorylated, i.e., activated. It is therefore not surprising that a number of regulators that normally serve to decrease STAT activity have been described (Fig. 3). For example, the tyrosine phosphatases SHP-1 and SHP-2 can interact with the intracytoplasmic portion of cytokine receptors and inhibit Jak kinase activity. Such phosphatases could be required to combat unregulated growth. For example, a number of HTLV-1-infected T-cell leukemia cell lines, which have become IL-2 independent, have undetectable levels of SHP-1.

A group of cytokine-inducible proteins have been discovered and determined to negatively regulate STAT phosphorylation. These proteins are known as the CIS/SOCS/JAB/SSI family of negative regulators [CIS1 (cytokine inducible src homology 2 domain

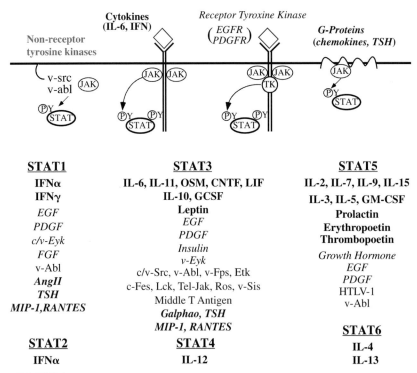

FIGURE 2 STAT proteins become tyrosine phosphorylated by at least four different mechanisms, including (1) nonreceptor tyrosine kinases (2) cytokine-mediated activation of Jaks (in bold), (3) receptor tyrosine kinases (in italics), and (4) G-protein-mediated activation of the Jaks (in bold italics). Listed beneath each mammalian STAT are the cytokines, growth factors, kinases, and ligands (typeface according to mechanism) that lead to their activation.

containing protein), SOCS-1, SOCS-2, SOCS-3 (suppressor of cytokine signaling-1, -2, and -3), JAB (Jak-binding protein), or SSI-1 (STAT-induced STAT inhibitor-1)]. Some of these proteins are transcriptionally regulated by STATs, suggesting that activated STATs negatively regulate their own phosphorylation state. The mechanism(s) by which these proteins inhibit STAT activation is not precisely known. For example, CIS1 can bind to phosphorylated cytokine receptors and either inhibit Jak activity or block STATs from binding to the receptor. However, SOCS-1 and SOCS-3 block Jak activity by binding to the kinase activation loop. Mice deficient for SOCS-1 die perinatally with stunted growth, degeneration and necrosis of the liver, diminished cellularity of the thymus, and a marked loss of maturing B lymphocytes. These phenotypic abnormalities were reversible when SOCS-1 mice were crossed to IFNγ-deficient animals (which were normal in appearance), arguing that the failure of Stat 1 negative regulation in the SOCS-1 knockout caused the phenotypic changes noted ear-

lier. SOCS-3-deficient animals die during embryogenesis with marked fetal erythrocytosis, thus suggesting that SOCS-3, which inhibits Stat 3 and Stat 5 activation, is important in regulating erythropoietin signaling. As with STAT and JAK knockout animals, SOC-deficient animals have very defined phenotypes, which is surprising given the number of cytokines that lead to their upregulation.

In addition to SHPs and SOCs, another group of proteins known as protein inhibitors of activated stats (PIAS) have been found to inhibit *in vitro* the ability of dimerized phosphorylated STATs (Stat 1 and Stat 3) to bind DNA. Furthermore, cultured cells overexpressing PIAS 1 or 3 proteins inhibit transcription mediated by activated Stats 1 or 3, respectively. Animals deficient in PIAS proteins have not yet been described. Finally, an as yet undefined nuclear tyrosine phosphatase(s) will undoubtedly play a critical role in decreasing active STAT. This conclusion rests on the persistent nuclear location of tyrosine-phosphorylated Stat1 when all phosphatase action is

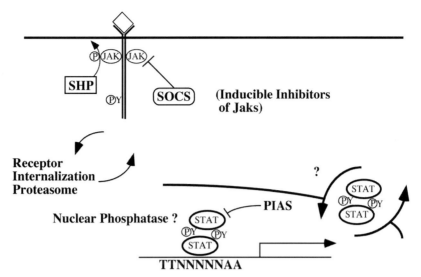

FIGURE 3 Some of the known and presumed negative regulators of STAT activation. The SH2 protein tyrosine phosphatases (SHP) dephosphorylate Jaks. SOCS inhibit Jak activity. Growth factor receptors are internalized via the ubiquitin proteosome pathway. Nuclear import and export of dimeric STATs are undoubtedly regulated. Protein inhibitors of activated STATs (PIAS) inhibit dimeric STATs from binding DNA. A nuclear tyrosine phosphatase has yet to be identified.

inhibited by vanadate. A deletion on chromosome 16p, which contains SOCS-1(JAB1), has been found in 46% of primary hepatocellular carcinomas. We speculate that these negative regulators of STATs, e.g., SHP, SOCS, and PIAS, will play important roles in the control of tumor incidence and/or progression.

V. STATS AS REGULATORS OF GROWTH, DIFFERENTIATION, AND APOPTOSIS

That STATs play an important role in controlling cell cycle progression and apoptosis comes from three sources: (1) cell culture experiments, (2) animal experiments, and (3) clinical observations on human cancer cells. From such studies it can be concluded that Stat 1 is important for growth restraint and can be considered the mediator of a tumor suppressor pathway, whereas Stat 3 and possibly Stat 5 promote tumor cell development and/or growth.

A. Stat 1 in Growth Restraint

Shortly after the discovery of the antiviral activity of IFN, the effect of interferon on the growth of culture

cells was noted. This growth restraint depends on fully transcriptionally activated Stat 1. Strong support for a growth-restraining role of Stat 1 in the whole animal has come from studies on Stat $1^{-/-}$ animals ("knockout" animals). First, Stat $1^{-/-}$ animals develop tumors in response to lower doses of methylcholanthrene than normal mice. Furthermore, when the Stat $1^{-/-}$ genotype is coupled with removal of the tumor suppressor gene, p53 spontaneous mouse tumor formation is greatly increased. The growth-restraining properties of Stat 1 are not limited to mouse cells. A number of human tumor cells show a defective response in the activation of Stat 1 by IFN-γ and also fail to slow growth in culture. Schreiber and colleagues therefore concluded that an IFN-γ-mediated, Stat 1-dependent, tumor surveillance system is important in preventing tumors. Furthermore, established tumors can escape suppression by avoiding the growth restraint imposed by IFN-γ.

Further results implying growth restraint due to Stat 1 have been described. In mutant chondroblasts, where the FGF receptor is constitutively activated, persistent activation of Stat 1 is observed, and profound growth arrest is associated with the activation of the Cdk inhibitor, p21. Furthermore, in A431 cells, growth inhibition by EGF correlates with Stat 1 but not Stat 3 activation. Thus, there is mounting evidence that Stat 1 activation frequently provides an antiproliferative effect and may partially explain why the lack of this molecule *in vivo* leads to increased tumor formation.

Tumor formation may of course require a constant growth stimulus, but cells that are accumulating mutations, as is typical of cancer cells, must also escape apoptosis. Stat 1 in a number of cell types of this kind promotes apoptosis and its removal could also promote tumor cell survival and establishment of tumors.

B. Possible Roles of Stats 3 and 5 in Human Oncogenesis

For a number of years, reports have accumulated showing that clinical tumor samples contain activated Stat 3 and 5 proteins. These include lymphomas, leukemias, mycoses, fungoides, multiple myeloma, brain, prostate, breast, lung, and head and neck cancers (Fig. 4). Two of the best-studied cases of persistently activated STAT proteins in primary tumor samples involve persistent Stat 3 activation in squamous cell head and neck cancer and in multiple myeloma. In the case of squamous cell carcinomas, constitutive Stat 3 activation is due to aberrant EGF/EGFR signaling, whereas in multiple myeloma, IL-6 signaling is abnormally regulated. In both of these tumor types, introduction of the dominant-negative Stat 3 protein leads to apoptosis of the tissue or cells. However, in most of the other clinically reported cases of persistent activation of Stat 3 the cause is not known.

In cell culture, Stat 3 was shown to be persistently activated (tyrosine phosphorylated and capable of binding DNA) in all *src*-transformed cell lines. This finding set the stage for determining whether Stat 3 activation was a necessary part of transformation in culture or merely an accompaniment. Using dominant-negative Stat 3 molecules, it was found that *in vitro* transformation by *src* required Stat 3 activation.

The potency of Stat 3 as a sole transforming agent was tested by engineering a constitutively active Stat 3 molecule (Stat 3-C; constitutive dimerization was achieved through cysteines inserted in the −SH2 region). This molecule spontaneously dimerizes and accumulates in the nucleus where it can bind DNA and

Solid Tumors — Activated STAT

Tumor	Activated STAT
Prostate Cancer	Stat3
Lung Cancer	Stat1/Stat3
Breast Cancer	Stat1/Stat3/Stat5
Head and Neck Cancer (EGF/EGFR)	Stat1/Stat3
CNS Tumors	Stat3

Liquid Tumors

Lymphomas	Stat1/Stat3/Stat5
AML	Stat1/Stat3/Stat5
Multiple Myeloma (IL-6/IL-6R)	Stat1/Stat3
CLL	Stat1/Stat3/Stat5
CML (bcr-abl)	Stat1/Stat3/Stat5
Mycosis fungoides	Stat3
Burkitts Lymphoma	Stat1/Stat3

Oncogenes

Oncogene	Activated STAT
Middle T Ag	Stat3
v-erbB	Stat1/Stat3/Stat5
v-sis	Stat3
c-Fes	Stat3/Stat5
v-Fps	Stat3
v/c-src	Stat3
Etk	Stat3
Lck	Stat3
c-fms	Stat1/Stat3/Stat5
c-kit	Stat1/Stat5
Tel-Jak	Stat1/Stat3/Stat5
bcr-abl	Stat1/Stat3/Stat5
HTLV-1	Stat3/Stat5
Galphao	Stat3

Potential STAT Target Genes

Target Gene	STAT
p21 (CIP1)	Stat1
Caspase 1	Stat1
CyclinD1	Stat3/Stat5
Bcl-xL	Stat3/Stat5
Bcl-2	Stat3
myc	Stat3

FIGURE 4 STAT proteins are persistently activated in human tumors and by oncogenes. If Associations between activated STATs and tumors are indicated by dashed lines, whereas solid lines indicate a known mechanism of STAT activation. A number of potential STAT target genes are listed on the bottom.

drive transcription. As a result, immortalized mouse and rat cells in culture can be transformed, and the resulting transformed cells are capable of forming tumors in nude mice. Thus by uniting mounting clinical evidence with cell culture evidence it appears highly likely that Stat 3 regularly participates in human tumors. In general, Stat 3 activation has been associated with proliferation, protection against apoptosis, and cellular transformation. However, there are a number of examples where activated Stat 3 appears to play a role in differentiation and promoting apoptosis. These observations, although confusing, are not necessarily surprising given the evidence that proteins (e.g., *myc*) controlling cell proliferation are tightly linked to those that drive cell death.

The transcriptional specificity of STATs is undoubtedly determined in part by their interaction with other transcription factors. An interesting possible connection between Stat 3 and tumorigenesis is its association with c-Jun, the first discovered nuclear protooncogene. c-Jun does not interact with Stat 1. Furthermore, there are a number of enhancer elements that contain c-Jun and Stat 3 sites but no reported cases of genes driven by Stat 1 and c-Jun.

Stat 5, like Stat 3, also appears on the basis of cell culture, animal, and clinical results to be involved in tumorigenesis, apoptosis, and cell proliferation. For example, a number of oncogenes, such as BCR/ABL tyrosine kinase and HTLV-1 responsible for chronic myelogenous leukemia and T-cell leukemias, respectively, lead to persistent tyrosine phosphorylation of Stat 5. Furthermore, a dominant negative Stat 5 protein in murine bone marrow cultures can abrogate cellular transformation by BCR/ABL. Activated Stat 5 can promote cell cycle progression in T cells and protects certain cell types from apoptosis, possibly through upregulation of Bcl-xL.

VI. CONCLUSIONS

The control of growth involves, in part, the recognition of external signals and transmitting these appropriately, and STATs are critical mediators of these cellular processes. Abnormal growth, including the development of cancer, is frequently a consequence of persistent abnormal signaling. Many external factors lead to STAT activation, and therefore, not surprisingly, persistent STAT activation is very commonly found in association with cancers and is partly responsible for transformation in a few tested cases either by preventing apoptosis and possibly by altering cell cycle progression. We suggest that targeting therapeutics to disrupting Stat 3 and Stat 5 activation will likely prove to be useful by blocking tumor growth and enhancing apoptosis of cancer cells and tissue.

See Also the Following Articles

DNA DAMAGE, DNA REPAIR, AND MUTAGENESIS • *FOS* ONCOGENE • INSULIN-LIKE GROWTH FACTORS • JAK/STAT PATHWAY

Bibliography

Becker, S., Corthals, G. L., Aebersold, R., Groner, B., and Muller, C. W. (1998). Expression of a tyrosine phosphorylated, DNA binding Stat3beta dimer in bacteria. *FEBS Lett.* **441**, 141–147.

Bromberg, J., and Darnell, J. E., Jr. (1999). Potential roles of STAT1 and STAT3 in cellular transformation. *In* "Cold Spring Harbor Symposium on Quantitative Biology," Cold Spring Harbor Laboratory Press, Cold Spring Harbor, NY, pp. 425–428.

Bromberg, J., and Darnell, J. E., Jr. (2000). The role of STATs in transcriptional control and their impact on cellular function. *Oncogene* **19**.

Catlett-Falcone, R., Dalton, W. S., and Jove, R. (1999). STAT proteins as novel targets for cancer therapy. Signal transducer an activator of transcription. *Curr. Opin. Oncol.* **11**, 490–496.

Chen, X., Vinkemeier, U., Zhao, Y., Jeruzalmi, D., Darnell, J. E., Jr., and Kuriyan, J. (1998). Crystal structure of a tyrosine phosphorylated STAT-1 dimer bound to DNA. *Cell* **93**, 827–839.

Darnell, J. E., Jr. (1997). STATs and gene regulation. *Science* **277**, 1630–1635.

Decker, T., and Kovarik, P. (1999). Transcription factor activity of STAT proteins: Structural requirements and regulation by phosphorylation and interacting proteins *Cell Mol. Life Sci.* **55**, 1535–1546.

Evan, G., and Littlewood, T. (1998). A matter of life and cell death. *Science* **281**, 1317–1322.

Fu, X. Y. (1999). From PTK-STAT signaling to caspase expression and apoptosis induction. *Cell Death Differ.* **6**, 1201–1208.

Garcia, R., and Jove, R. (1998). Activation of STAT transcription factors in oncogenic tyrosine kinase signaling. *J. Biomed. Sci.* **5**, 79–85.

Hilton, D. J. (1999). Negative regulators of cytokine signal transduction. *Cell Mol. Life Sci.* **55**, 1568–1577.

Hoey, T., and Schindler, U. (1998). STAT structure and function in signaling. *Curr. Opin. Genet. Dev.* **8**, 582–587.

Hueber, A. O., and Evan, G. I. (1998). Traps to catch unwary oncogenes. *Trends Genet.* **14**, 364–367.

Ihle, J. N., Thierfelder, W., Teglund, S., Stravapodis, D., Wang, D., Feng, J., and Parganas, E. (1998). Signaling by the cytokine receptor superfamily. *Ann. N. Y. Acad. Sci.* **865**, 1–9.

Kaplan, D. H., Shankaran, V., Dighe, A. S., Stockert, E., Aguet, M., Old, L. J., and Schreiber, R. D. (1998). Demonstration of an interferon gamma-dependent tumor surveillance system in immunocompetent mice. *Proc. Natl. Acad. Sci. USA* **95**, 7556–7561.

Maniatis, T., Falvo, J. V., Kim, T. H., Kim, T. K., Lin, C. H., Parekh, B. S., and Wathelet, M. G. (1998). Structure and function of the interferon-beta enhanceosome. *Cold Spring Harb. Symp. Quant. Biol.* **63,** 609–620.

Shuai, K. (1999). The STAT family of proteins in cytokine signaling. *Prog. Biophys. Mol. Biol.* **71,** 405–422.

Starr, R., and Hilton, D. J. (1999). Negative regulation of the JAK/STAT pathway. *Bioessays* **21,** 47–52.

Zhang, J. J., Zhao, Y., Chait, B. T., Lathem, W. W., Ritzi, M., Knippers, R., and Darnell, J. E., Jr. (1998). Ser727-dependent recruitment of MCM5 by Stat1alpha in IFN-gamma-induced transcriptional activation. *EMBO J.* **17,** 6963–6971.

Stem Cell Transplantation

Keren Osman
Raymond L. Comenzo
Memorial Sloan-Kettering Cancer Center

GLOSSARY

allogeneic stem cell transplantation A method for delivering high-dose chemothreapy followed by bone marrow or stem cells from a donor. These stem cells are expected to reconstitute the marrow as well as aid in preventing relapse of the disease.

autologous stem cell transplantation (SCT) A supportive measure that allows delivery of high-dose chemotherapy. Autologous stem cell transplant involves collection of the patient's own stem cells for later use after high-dose chemotherapy in order to decrease the time of potentially life-threatening cytopenias.

donor lymphocyte infusions In patients with chronic myeloid leukemia or multiple myeloma who relapse after allogeneic SCT, infusions of lymphocytes from their SCT donors can result in durable remissions.

graft-versus-disease effect A potentially beneficial effect of transplant in which donor lymphocytes recognize the disease of the recipient as foreign and aid in the reduction of tumor burden as well as prolongation of remissions.

graft-versus-host disease A potentially fatal complication of allogeneic transplantation in which immune cells of the donor graft mount an immune response against tissues of the recipient.

hematopoetic stem cells (HSC) Pluripotent progenitor cells capable of both self-renewal and differentiation, and usually $CD34^+$. HSC may be found in the bone marrow, peripheral blood and umbilical cord blood.

stem cell mobilization The process of increasing the availability or peripheralization of $CD34^+$ cells in the blood, allowing repeated leukapheresis procedures to be performed, if needed, for the collection of $CD34^+$ stem cells.

I. OVERVIEW

A. Hematopoietic Stem Cells (HSC)

HSC are $CD34^+$ pluripotent cells found in the blood and bone marrow that have the capacity to self-renew as well as differentiate. The outcomes of stem cell cycling and division are regulated by adhesion molecules and cytokines in poorly understood ways. With hematopoietic stem cell support in either allogeneic or autologous stem cell transplantation (SCT), high doses of chemotherapy and radiation can be administered to patients meeting standard criteria for SCT without incurring prolonged life-threatening periods of pancytopenia. Standard criteria for allogeneic or autologous transplantation usually include an age threshold (less than 55 for allogeneic and 70 for autologous), adequate cardiac, pulmonary, hepatic, and renal function, no significant comorbid disease, and the capacity to understand and consent to the treatment. Allogeneic stem cell transplantation is useful in the treatment of chronic myeloid leukemia (CML), acute myeloid and lymphoid leukemia (AML, ALL), aplastic anemia (AA), myelodysplasia, multiple myeloma (MM), severe combined immunodeficiency disorder (SCID), and congenital anemias. Allogeneic grafts contain T lymphocytes that may respond to recipient or host antigens. The success of allogeneic transplant is therefore limited by potentially lethal graft-versus-host disease (GVHD). However, the alloreactive potential of the graft may facilitate a graft-versus-disease effect. This effect has been developed further in the form of donor lymphocyte infusions (DLI) given months posttransplant in order to treat relapse in CML and MM. Autologous stem cell transplantation has been successful in non-Hodgkin's lymphoma and Hodgkin's disease (NHL, HD), multiple myeloma, primary systemic amyloidosis (AL), and some solid tumors.

B. Stem Cell Components

Cytotherapeutic components used in SCT include bone marrow, blood mononuclear cells collected after mobilization (peripheral blood stem cells, PBSC), and umbilical cord blood stem cells (Table I). Until the early 1990s, the most commonly used component was bone marrow. After harvesting bone marrow from the donor, the marrow was either immediately infused (allogeneic) or cryopreserved for later use (autologous). Over the past decade it has become routine to use stem cells mobilized and collected from the peripheral blood for autologous transplantation. Moreover, it is likely that mobilized peripheral blood stem

TABLE I
Donors, Sources, and Characteristics of Hematopoietic Stem Cell Components

Donors	Sources	Characteristics
Normal individuals	Bone marrow	Requires general anesthesia and transfusion-transmissible disease testing (TTDT) and is usually used fresh. Component collected in a single procedure. Dosing based on total nucleated cells/kg. Contains potentially alloreactive T cells. Neutrophil recovery in 2 to 3 weeks
	Peripheral blood	Requires cytokine stimulation usually with G-CSF, leukapheresis with the possible need for a central venous catheter, TTDT, is usually used fresh and may be used after cryopreservation. Component may be collected in multiple procedures. Dosing is based on CD34 cell counts/kg recipient weight, and usual target is >5 × 10^6 CD34 cells/kg. Contains large numbers of T cells possibly made less alloreactive by indirect G-CSF effect. Neutrophil recovery in 10 to 12 days
	Umbilical cord blood	Collected at delivery and requires predelivery planning and consent, TTDT, may be contaminated with maternal lymphocytes, and useful primarily in small recipients because of low cell numbers per component. Dosing guidelines therefore are less well defined. Neutrophil recovery in 3 to 6 weeks. Long-term cryopreservation needed
Patients	Bone marrow	Requires general anesthesia. Component collected in a single procedure. Dosing based on total nucleated cells/kg. May contain tumor cell contamination. Neutrophil recovery in 2 to 4 weeks. Cryopreservation usually needed
	Peripheral blood	Requires mobilization that usually can piggyback onto salvage chemotherapy, and leukapheresis with central venous catheter placement. Component may be collected in multiple procedures. Dosing is based on CD34 cell counts with a minimum dose of 2 to 2.5 × 10^6 CD34 cells/kg needed to assure trilineage recovery. Extent of prior therapy may impair mobilization capacity. Cryopreservation needed

cells will also replace bone marrow for allogeneic transplantation. Autologous stem cell mobilization and collection are often associated with the recovery phase following myelosuppressive salvage therapy. After chemotherapy, patients receive hematopoietic growth factors such as granulocyte colony-stimulating factor (G-CSF) or GM-CSF to enhance rebound hematopoiesis. Stem cell mobilization can also be performed with growth factors alone in either cancer patients or, on an investigational basis, in prescreened healthy donors for allogeneic transplant. Another source of stem cells is umbilical cord blood. To date there have been over 600 transplants performed using umbilical cord blood and the preliminary reports are encouraging. However, technical and ethical aspects of umbilical cord blood collection, storage, and use are not yet comprehensively delineated.

Limitations of autologous SCT include the potential for relapse secondary to contamination of stem cell components by clonal tumor cells and the lack of an alloreactive graft-versus-disease effect. Although purging or the selection of CD34$^+$ HSC may reduce tumor cells in autologous grafts, a clear-cut benefit for such manipulations has not been defined prospectively in randomized trials (Fig. 1). In addition, another area of active investigation remains the manipulation of the immune system after autologous SCT by means of immune modulators such as interleukin-2 or with cancer vaccines.

II. ALLOGENEIC STEM CELL TRANSPLANTATION

A. Chronic Myeloid Leukemia

CML is characterized by a translocation between chromosomes 9 and 22 known as the Philadelphia chromosome [t(9;22)]. This cytogenetic abnormality is important in diagnosis, following response to therapy, and in detecting relapse posttherapy. Left untreated, the median survival from time of diagnosis is approximately 2 to 4 years. Standard therapies include palliative cytoreduction with hydroxyurea, interferon, and allogeneic SCT. Numerous centers have reported the results of allogeneic SCT for CML with HLA identical sibling donors. The overall probabilities of long-term disease-free survival and relapse are about

60 and 20%, respectively. Thus allogeneic SCT is currently recommended for patients under 55 in chronic phase with an HLA identical donor. In the case of patients in the accelerated phase or blast phase, age plays a larger role. The survival of patients transplanted in the accelerated phase is worse than that of chronic phase patients. Patients in blast phase have very poor post transplant survival and a high probability of relapse. In patients who relapse after allogeneic SCT for CML, lymphocyte infusions from their SCT donor (DLI) can be effective treatment.

B. Acute Myeloid and Lymphoid Leukemia

Unlike CML where SCT works during the chronic phase, the role of transplantation in AML remains controversial. Sixty-five to 80% of patients with AML achieve complete remission (CR) with anthracycline-based induction regimens. However, just under half of these patients will remain in durable remissions with standard consolidation therapy. Following SCT in first CR the disease-free survival is 46 to 62%. In one study of 95 patients who received allogeneic SCT in first CR, the 5-year disease-free survival was 52% and the relapse rate was 18%. The advantage of SCT in first CR was that these patients had only limited exposure to chemotherapy before transplant. Therefore, they tolerated the preparatory regimen better and had fewer infectious complications than more heavily pretreated patients.

The issue of timing continues to be debated. In current practice the most significant prognostic factor is cytogenetics. t(8;21), t(15;17), and inv16 are associated with a favorable prognosis. Eighty-four percent of these patients achieve a CR following high-dose cytarabine treatment. 46(XY), 46 (XX), and deletions of chromosome Y are associated with an intermediate prognosis, and all other cytogenetic abnormalities with a poor prognosis. It is reasonable, then, to perform allo SCT in first CR for patients with intermediate or poor prognosis and in first relapse or second CR for those with favorable prognosis.

The use of allogeneic SCT for pediatric patients with ALL usually has involved patients in second CR, as the majority of children with ALL experience long-term disease-free survivals with intensive chemotherapy. Allogeneic SCT may be appropriately considered, however, in those patients who have at

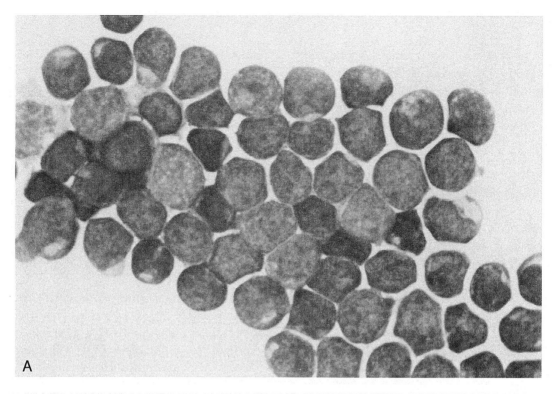

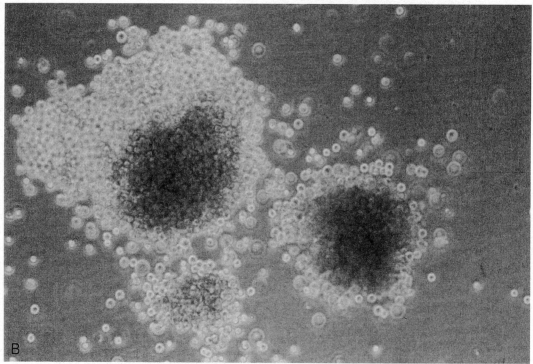

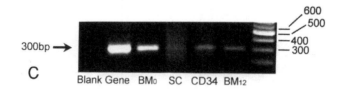

diagnosis a white blood cell count $> 20,000/\mu l$ or poor prognosis cytogenetics such as t(4;11), t(8;14), or t(9;22). The presence of extramedullary disease or failure to respond to initial chemotherapy may also provide a basis for consideration of allogeneic SCT. The use of allogeneic SCT in adults with ALL has been complicated by high rates of GVHD and relapse and by the lack of randomized trials in which patients receive allogeneic SCT in first CR or at relapse.

C. Aplastic Anemia and Paroxysmal Nocturnal Hemoglobinuria (PNH)

AA is a relatively rare disease with an annual incidence of three cases per million persons in the United States and Europe. Despite best supportive care, 50% of patients die within 6 months of diagnosis. The only effective therapies are either immunosuppression with antithymocyte globulin or allogeneic hematopoietic cell transplantation. PNH is also a rare disease, and approximately 25% of PNH patients develop AA. Allogeneic SCT is potentially curative for AA and PNH patients. The largest experience with transplant for AA and PNH has been with HLA-matched sibling donors. The 20-year survival for these patients now exceeds 85%. Survival has improved because of recognition that graft rejection decreases proportionately to the number of transfusions prior to transplant and because of improvements in conditioning regimens and GVHD prophylaxis with cyclosporine and methotrexate.

D. Myelodysplasia

Myelodysplastic syndromes (MDS) encompass a series of clonal stem cell disorders characterized by the impaired maturation of hematopoietic cells, periph-

eral cytopenias, and a tendency to progress to AML. The pathogenesis of MDS is not completely understood. MDS are associated with certain cytogenetic abnormalities and usually occur during the sixth and seventh decade. The percentage of blasts in the marrow and cytogenetics, where available, remain the most useful prognostic indicators at this time. Many therapies have been used to treat MDS, including hormones, differentiation agents, growth factors, and combination chemotherapy. Chemotherapy has been toxic in older patients with MDS. Experience with SCT for MDS began in the 1980s and, as of 1996, 251 patients had been transplanted at Fred Hutchinson Cancer Center (FHCC) in Seattle, Washington. The 3-year cumulative nonrelapse mortality was 42%, the disease-free survival was 41%, and the incidence of relapse was 17%. Predictors of nonrelapse mortality were increased patient age and disease duration, whereas predictors of relapse were advanced disease and poor risk cytogenetics (>3 abnormalities, −7). Good prognostic indicators associated with increased disease-free survival were youth, good risk cytogenetics (normal, deletion Y, isolated abnormalities of 5 or 20), and less advanced disease morphology. Currently, it is recommended that allogeneic SCT be considered for patients under 55 years of age who have life-threatening cytopenias, increased blasts, poor risk cytogenetics, and an appropriate HLA-matched related donor.

E. Non-Hodgkin's Lymphoma

Data on allogeneic SCT in patients with NHL are difficult to evaluate because there have been few controlled trials. There has been one study comparing allogeneic and autologous SCT in NHL. Results demonstrated a decreased relapse rate in the allogeneic group,

FIGURE 1 (A) CD34$^+$ selected HSC from a patient with multiple myeloma are shown. CD34$^+$ cells are heterogeneous with respect to proliferative capacity and lineage commitment. Totipotent stem cells comprise about 5% of the total and have the appearance of small lymphocytes. CD34$^+$ cells that are committed to become myeloid or erythroid progenitors appear blastic. (B) A myeloid colony is shown, a colony-forming unit granulocyte–macrophage (CFU-GM) having grown in semisolid medium innoculated with mobilized blood CD34$^+$ cells. CFU-GM represents the progeny of a single CD34$^+$ cell committed to the myeloid lineage. (C) Polymerase chain reaction results using patient-specific primers for the clonal myeloma light chain gene show that contamination is present even after CD34 selection (Gene, plasmid containing patient sequence; BM$_0$, bone marrow at diagnosis; BM$_{12}$, bone marrow at 1 year). A randomized prospective phase III trial in myeloma failed to demonstrate that CD34 selection to purge contaminating tumor cells increased the response rate or provided a survival benefit, although tumor cell contamination of stem cell components was reduced by several logs. See color insert in Volume 1.

albeit with a higher treatment-related mortality in that group as well. Furthermore, there was no survival advantage for the allogeneic SCT group. Preliminary studies have been conducted with minimally myeloablative regimens supported with allogeneic PBSC. Twenty-one patients with recurrent or primary refractory DLCL were treated and 42% survived disease free beyond 1 year. Further study of so-called mini-allo transplants using allogeneic PBSC are clearly warranted in this population. Allogeneic SCT has been employed in select NHL patients who have relapsed after autologous SCT.

F. Multiple Myeloma

Standard allogeneic SCT has also been performed in MM patients, usually under the age of 55. Thirty-five to 60% of all patients receiving HLA-matched allografts achieved CR. The peritransplant mortality in historical cohorts, however, is 40 to 60%, with female gender, stage I disease, one course of prior treatment, and CR prior to SCT being favorable prognostic factors for allogeneic SCT. The long-term survival is about one-third. Encouraging results have been obtained employing allogeneic SCT with less aggressive conditioning regimens, often including Fludarabine and Melphalan instead of cyclophosphamide and total body irradiation, and allogeneic PBSC instead of marrow. Reduced regimen-related toxicities and mortality have been observed in several small studies.

G. Severe Combined Immunodeficiency

In 1968, allogeneic bone marrow transplantation was shown to be life-saving treatment in infants with SCID. It appears that T-cell function becomes normal in the majority of patients receiving related HLA identical or HLA haploidentical T-cell depleted marrow grafts. B-cell function, however, remains abnormal in many recipients of haploidentical marrow, leaving a long-term requirement for intravenous immunoglobulin.

H. Congenital Anemias

Thalessemia major, sickle cell anemia, and Fanconi's anemia are among the congenital anemias that have been successfully treated with allogeneic SCT. The is-

sues of timing and patient selection, however, remain controversial, particularly since transfusion therapy alone can provide significant benefits for decades. The development of improved forms of iron chelation therapy, as well as the promise of gene therapy, may influence the decision to seek early allogeneic SCT. At the same time, however, the availability of SCT with umbilical cord blood stem cells provides enhanced opportunities for successful allogeneic SCT at an early age in many cases.

III. AUTOLOGOUS STEM CELL TRANSPLANTATION

A. Non-Hodgkin's Lymphoma

NHL is the sixth most common cancer in the United States. A subset of patients will be cured with standard chemotherapy but most are not. The rationale for high-dose cytotoxic therapy in NHL began with experimental evidence using mouse models. The survival of murine lymphoma cells was shown to be inversely proportional to the dose of alkylating agents. These data suggested that chemotherapy resistance may be a relative rather than an absolute property, one that could be overcome by high-dose therapy. The rationale, therefore, for autologous transplant was to escalate the doses of chemotherapy and radiation beyond the limits of marrow toxicity in order to overcome resistance to standard-dose therapy.

The autologous SCT experience in diffuse large cell lymphoma (DLCL) began in 1995 when a multinational trial in relapsed DLCL compared chemotherapy alone to chemotherapy followed by high-dose therapy with SCT. The EFS at 5 years was found to be 46% for SCT patients and 12% for those who received chemotherapy alone. The criteria for entry into this study were very strict and thus this study suffered from selection bias. Such studies, therefore, have generated debate in the field regarding the timing of transplant for relapsed DLCL. Currently, data support high-dose therapy with SCT for patients with chemosensitive DLCL for whom primary treatment has failed. Phase III trials are in progress now comparing high-dose therapy with conventional therapy in selected high-risk patients with previously untreated DLCL.

In the case of follicular lymphoma, the results of phase II studies indicate that remission duration may be prolonged in relapsed follicular lymphoma after HCT as compared with those patients who received standard chemotherapy. However, no survival advantage has been demonstrated. Because median survival is longer for patients with follicular lymphoma than for patients with other NHL, the long-term effect of transplant, such as secondary AML or MDS, should be considered. Consideration therefore should be given to delaying SCT until relapse.

The major cause of treatment failure in NHL is relapse of disease. In the future, approaches to SCT for NHL may remedy this problem by providing better cytoreductive regimens, by performing SCT earlier in the disease process, and finally by consolidating therapy with either radiation or immunotherapy prior to or after SCT.

B. Hodgkin's Disease

HD is one of the success stories of modern oncology. With conventional chemotherapy, approximately 50% of patients can be cured. However, 25% of patients with HD never achieve CR and a similar percentage of patients who achieve CR will relapse. The poor results in some relapsed patients with salvage chemotherapy led to an interest in high-dose chemotherapy followed by autologous SCT based on the theory that increased dose intensity would increase cell kill. Despite intercenter variability in patient selection, numerous phase II studies reported CR rates greater than 40% after SCT, some reporting rates as high as 70%, with disease-free survival rates as high as 50% at 5 years. Overall, based on these robust phase II results, high-dose chemotherapy with SCT has become an accepted modality of treatment for relapsed or primary refractory HD. Randomized studies have not been performed, but the responses are clearly better than those achieved with conventional salvage chemotherapy. Moreover, the transplant-related mortality is under 5%, making SCT an approach whose safety may be superior to salvage chemotherapy. It is hoped that more effective preparative regimens will be found in the future to improve the survival curve and decrease the rate of relapse.

C. Multiple Myeloma and Primary Systemic Amyloidosis

MM accounts for 1% of all, and 10% of hematologic, malignancies; it also accounts for 20% of the deaths due to hematologoic malignancies annually in the United States. MM is the second most common hematologic malignancy after chronic lymphocytic leukemia. In the year 2000, 13,700 new cases of MM were diagnosed in the United States. The median age at diagnosis is 63 but is getting younger. MM is a clonal B-cell tumor of plasma cells often sensitive to steroids, radiation, and alkylating agents. However, cure has not been achieved with conventional chemotherapy and the median survival remains only 3 to 4 years. The experience with autologous SCT began in the 1980s after it was observed that significant cytoreductive responses could be achieved in refractory MM patients with increasing doses of intravenous melphalan. The role of autologous SCT for MM has now been firmly established based on the landmark phase III trial conducted by the French Myeloma Study Group published in 1996. Two hundred previously untreated MM patients less than 65 years of age were randomized at diagnosis to receive conventional chemotherapy or high dose therapy with SCT. The response rate (57% vs 81%), the event-free survival at 5 years (10% vs 28%), and the overall survival (12% vs 52%) were significantly superior in the high-dose therapy group. Interestingly, in a population-based setting, the Nordic Myeloma Study Group has reproduced these findings. With the use of mobilized blood stem cells, double or tandem transplants have been performed but have not yet been formally assessed in a trial comparing single to double SCT. In addition, the question of the optimal timing of SCT, i.e., early, following induction therapy versus as later as salvage after relapse, has yet to be elucidated. At this time, purging clontypic myeloma contamination from stem cell components with CD34 selection does not increase the complete response rate or provide a survival benefit.

Primary systemic or AL amyloidosis is a clonal plasma cell and protein conformation disorder in which monoclonal immunoglobulin light chains are deposited as amyloid in critical organs leading to organ dysfunction and early death. By eliminating the cells responsible for producing these light chains, investigators hypothesized that one could halt the deposition process. In patients eligible for autologous SCT, this hypothesis was confirmed using G-CSF for stem cell mobilization and intravenous melphalan for high-dose therapy. CR was achieved in over half of the patients and improvements in all types of amyloid-related organ dysfunction were documented. However, the initial experience at multiple centers was complicated by a 100-day mortality rate that averaged 25%. It became obvious that because of visceral reserve limited by deposition disease, AL patients have greater toxicity in SCT than patients with MM receiving the same high-dose therapy. This has led to improvements in patient selection. One current recommendation is that SCT should not be offered to AL patients with symptomatic cardiac amyloid and recurrent pleural effusions or syncope, or to patients over the age of 50 with more than two major systems compromised by AL (of heart, liver, kidneys, and peripheral nerves). Therefore, autologous SCT for select patients with AL is a new and often effective therapy for an otherwise uniformly fatal disease. Future directions include the development of clinical trials of SCT following heart or liver allografts.

D. Chronic and Acute Myeloid Leukemia

There has also been interest in autologous SCT for CML and AML. Autologous SCT may be a reasonable second line therapy in patients with CML who are not eligible for allogeneic transplant and do not respond to interferon. Randomized studies comparing the two have not been performed, but clinical experience demonstrates that although autologous SCT does not cure CML, it may be associated with longer survival compared with conventional treatment.

In 1989, a randomized trial in AML patients compared allogeneic and autologous SCT to consolidation chemotherapy. There was no survival advantage or lower relapse rate for chemotherapy or autologous transplant. Further studies were done comparing allogeneic with autologous SCT and salvage chemotherapy. In all studies, patients received allogeneic SCT if they had an HLA-matched sibling and were under 50 years of age. In a major European study at 4 years, allogeneic SCT patients had a disease-free survival of 55%, autologous 48%, and chemotherapy 30%, with a statistically significant improvement in survival for allogeneic and autologous SCT as compared with chemotherapy. However, the North America study group conducted a similar study and found that the 4-year DFS for chemotherapy, autologous HCT, and allogeneic HCT was 35, 37, and 42%, respectively. The most important pretransplant prognostic factor was cytogenetics. Patients with poor risk cytogenetics did better with allogeneic transplant. Overall studies indicate that for patients with AML who lack an HLA-matched sibling donor and who are older than 50, autologous SCT may be a viable option in those with either standard risk or poor risk cytogenetics. In patients with good risk cytogenetics, however, SCT likely represents a form of first-line salvage therapy if a chemotherapy regimen containing high-dose cytarabine fails.

E. Solid Tumors

Given its success in other diseases, high-dose therapy with autologous SCT has also been attempted in germ cell tumors, neuroblastoma, and breast cancer. Beginning at Indiana University in 1986, a small percentage of patients with germ cell tumors who had multiple relapses were shown to respond to high-dose therapy with SCT. These results were confirmed in multiple other studies, and, more recently, high-dose therapy with SCT has been studied as primary therapy for patients with poor risk primary mediastinal germ cell tumors.

Neuroblastoma is a tumor of the peripheral nervous system that affects children under the age of 15. Forty percent of patients have low or intermediate risk tumors and can be treated with conventional therapy to achieve substantial long-term survival. The other 60%, however, cannot achieve long-term survivals with conventional therapy. High-dose therapy and autologous SCT have improved the long-term survival of some high-risk patients. Studies to enhance long-term survival for a larger percentage of patients are ongoing. These involve improved induction regimens, the use of biological agents such as monoclonal antibodies as adjuncts, and modulation of drug resistance.

The use of SCT in patients with metastatic (and high-risk) breast cancer is one of the most revealing medical stories of the recent past. Mobilized blood stem cells made SCT less morbid at a time when American hospitals sought to expand services and income, transplant physicians to develop SCT programs, and biotech companies to find new markets. Concurrently, breast cancer medicine became a major political affair and breast cancer patients and their families struggled as part of a growing community with decisions about what the best treatments might be. The initial justification for high-dose therapy with SCT was that there was no other therapy that achieved complete responses in metastatic disease. Unfortunately, the appropriate phase III trials, designed to determine whether a survival benefit attached to SCT, were difficult to perform for many reasons. Finally, upon their completion (a credit to oncology as a clinical science), overall survival in metastatic breast cancer was not shown to be improved with SCT. Whether the use of autologous SCT for high risk breast cancer will be revisited with new drugs such as bone chelating radiopharmaceuticals is unclear at this time.

IV. TOXICITIES

A. Graft-versus-Host Disease

Tissue compatibility between human recipients and donor grafts is controlled by the genes of the major histocompatibility complex on chromosome 6. Proteins encoded by these genes are called human leukocyte antigens (HLA), and the HLA system is vastly complex and polymorphic, meaning that related individuals who are HLA identical share haplotypes that have the same genes in them, whereas unrelated individuals who are HLA identical likely have different versions of the same genes (polymorphisms). Scientific interest in graft-versus-host reactions began in the 1950s when the recovery of animals after splenic cell transplants was found to be complicated by a "runting" syndrome soon to be observed in humans after allogeneic bone marrow transplantation. The development of GVHD is influenced by the immunocompetence of the recipient, the degree of HLA similarity between donor and recipient, and the number of functional lymphocytes infused.

As a rule, GVHD in the setting of allogeneic SCT increases in frequency with the degree of HLA disparity between donor and recipient. GVHD can occur early in SCT and be immediately life-threatening (acute GVHD), involving the skin, gastrointestinal tract, and liver, or it can occur months after SCT (chronic GVHD) as a deleterious and often debilitating syndrome similar to severe scleroderma, requiring chronic steroid treatment. Selective CD8$^+$ T-cell depletion or improved prophylactic regimens, including the use of intravenous cyclosporine and new immunosuppressive agents, such as mycophenolate, may help decrease the incidence of acute GVHD in the HLA identical setting. Moreover, the use of T-cell-depleted grafts in the setting of related HLA haploidentical SCT can decrease the incidence of GVHD. Of note, the use of unmanipulated allogeneic PBSC appears to be associated with no increase in acute GVHD but possibly with an increased incidence of chronic GVHD.

B. Regimen-Related Toxicities

The toxicities of both allogeneic and autologous SCT are primarily related to the treatment regimens and include acute bacterial, fungal, or viral infections. Furthermore, the convalescent phase is often marked by gastrointestinal incapacities, marked fatigue, and cognitive difficulties. As cytotherapies emerge as a major force in the treatment of cancer, these side effects will become targets for novel drugs and trials, particularly involving the use of agents promising to protect the gastrointestinal tract, such as keratinocyte growth factor.

C. Long-Term Risks and Outcomes

Some of the long-term side effects include a small risk of secondary malignancies and myelodysplasia; late-onset pulmonary problems such as interstitial pneumonitis or bronchiolitis obliterans; disruption of normal growth and development in children; and endocrine, psychosexual, and adjustment disorders. In young patients, the impact of transplantation on fertility may be profound, and cryopreservation of sperm or ova may be a useful option where appropriate. In addition, patients who successfully undergo stem cell transplantation do not necessarily have normal life spans compared to controls with no history of malignancy.

The future of SCT, then, will involve research to help decrease the risks and improve the long-term outcomes so that patients who are free from disease may go on to lead full and normal lives.

V. CONCLUSIONS

Stem cell transplantation has been established as a useful therapy for hematologic malignancies and some solid tumors. Some patients, however, still die in allogeneic SCT because T lymphocytes cause fatal GVHD and many are not cured in autologous SCT because disease recurs post-SCT. Disease may recur because the tumor was not completely eliminated or because the stem cell component was contaminated with tumor cells that home to sites of prior disease. For these reasons, manipulated or engineered stem cell grafts continue to attract interest. Approaches to graft engineering include methods of T-cell depletion designed to minimize GVHD without compromising the potential for graft-versus-disease effect, as well as purging with monoclonal antibodies or selection of CD34$^+$ stem cells in order to eliminate contaminating tumor cells. However, to date, no form of engineered graft has shown itself to be superior to unmanipulated components with respect to survival in phase III trials in autologous SCT or allogeneic HLA identical SCT. In allogeneic-related HLA haploidentical SCT, it is generally agreed that T-cell depletion is required to reduce the risk of acute GVHD. With the apparent superiority of mobilized allogeneic peripheral blood stem cells over bone marrow in a recent large trial, and the promise of minimally myeloablative allogeneic SCT using PBSC, continued success with unmanipulated components is likely to continue. Nevertheless, should the CR rates for autologous SCT in NHL, HD, and MM increase due to advances in treatment, such as the use of new agents or of post-SCT tumor vaccines, the role of tumor cell contamination of stem cell components in disease recurrence post-SCT will likely increase as well.

The applications of cytotherapies will evolve and expand over the coming decades. Hematopoietic stem cell transplants may provide methods for inducing lifelong tolerance to xenografts or allow novel treatment of autoimmune diseases, whereas the discovery and use of nonhematopoietic stem cells may help minimize the toxicities of cancer therapy or cure nonmalignant disorders. For example, the infusion of fetal islet cell progenitors may provide a treatment for severe diabetes. The future of stem cell transplantation and cytotherapies in general will require advances in our understanding of stem cell biology and transplantation immunology and will continue to depend on patients courageous enough to participate in well-designed clinical trials.

See Also the Following Articles

ACUTE LYMPHOBLASTIC LEUKEMIA IN ADULTS • ACUTE MYELOCYTIC LEUKEMIA • CHRONIC LYMPHOCYTIC LEUKEMIA • CHRONIC MYELOGENOUS LEUKEMIA • GRAFT VERSUS LEUKEMIA AND GRAFT VERSUS TUMOR ACTIVITY • MULTIPLE MYELOMA • NEUROBLASTOMA • TRANSFER OF DRUG RESISTANCE GENES TO HEMATOPOIETIC PRECURSORS • TRANSGENIC MICE IN CANCER RESEARCH

Bibliography

Anderson, J. E., and Thomas, E. D. (1997). The Seattle experience with bone marrow transplantation for myelodysplasia. *Leukemia Res.* **21S1**, 51a.

Appelbaum, F. R. (1997). Allogeneic hematopoietic stem cell transplantation for acute leukemia. *Semin. Oncol.* **24**, 114–123.

Apperley, J. F. (1998). Hematopoietic stem cell transplantation in chronic myeloid leukemia. *Curr. Opin. Hematol.* **5**, 445–453.

Attal, M., *et al.* (1996). A prospective, randomized trial of autologous bone marrow transplantation and chemotherapy in multiple myeloma. *N. Engl. J. Med.* **335**, 91–97.

Aversa, F., *et al.* (1998). Treatment of high-risk acute leukemia with T-cell-depleted stem cells from related donors with one fully mismatched HLA haplotype. *N. Engl. J. Med.* **339**, 1186–1193.

Bensinger, W., *et al.* (1999). A prospective, randomised trial of peripheral blood stem cells (PBSC) or marrow (BM) for patients undergoing allogeneic transplantation for hematologic malignancies. *Blood* **94**, 368a.

Buckley, R., *et al.* (1999). Hematopoietic stem-cell transplantation for the treatment of severe combined immunodeficiency. *N. Engl. J. Med.* **340**, 508–516.

Cassileth, P., *et al.* (1998). Chemotherapy compared with autologous or allogeneic bone marrow transplantation in the management of acute myeloid leukemia in first remission. *N. Engl. J. Med.* **339**, 149–156.

Comenzo, R. L. (2000). Hematopoietic cell transplantation for primary systemic amyloidosis: What have we learned. *Leukemia Lymphoma* **37**, 245–258.

Comenzo, R., *et al.* (1998). Dose intensive melphalan with blood stem cell support for the treatment of AL amyloidosis: Survival and responses in 25 patients. *Blood* **91,** 3662–3670.

Dazzi, F., Szydlo, R., and Goldman, J. (1999). Donor lymphocyte infusions for relapse of chronic myeloid leukemia after a stem cell transplant: Where we now stand. *Exp. Hematol.* **27,** 1477–1486.

Gluckman, E., *et al.* (1997). Outcome of cord-blood transplantation form related and unrelated donors. *N. Engl. J. Med.* **337,** 378–381.

Good, R. A. (1987). Bone marrow transplantation for immunodeficiency diseases. *J. Med. Sci.* **294,** 68–71.

Kyle, R. A. (1999). High-dose therapy in multiple myeloma and primary amyloidosis: An overview. *Semin. Oncol.* **26,** 74–83.

Moore, M. A. (1999). Turning brain into blood: Clinical applications of stem-cell research in neurobiology and hematology. *N. Engl. J. Med.* **341,** 605.

Moskowitz, C., *et al.* (1999). The International Prognostic Index predicts for outcome following autologous stem cell transplantation in patients with relapsed and primary refractory intermediate-grade lymphoma. *Bone Marrow Transplant* **23,** 561–567.

Nimer, S., *et al.* (1994). Selective depletion of CD8$^+$ cells for prevention of graft-versus-host disease after bone marrow transplantation: A randomized controlled trial. *Transplantation* **57,** 82–87.

Shpall, E. J. (1999). The utilization of cytokines in stem cell mobilization strategies. *Bone Marrow Transplant* **23S2,** 13–19.

Stadtmauer, E., *et al.* (2000). Conventional-dose chemotherapy compared with high dose chemotherapy plus autologous hematopoietic stem cell transplantation for metastatic breast cancer. *N. Engl. J. Med.* **342,** 1069–1077.

Thomas, E. D. (1999). Does bone marrow transplantation confer a normal life span)? *N. Engl. J. Med.* **341,** 50.

Thomas, E. D., Blume, K., and Forman, S. (1999). "Hematopoietic Cell Transplantation," 2nd Ed. Blackwell, Oxford.

Vescio, R., *et al.* (1999). Multicenter phase III trial to evaluate CD34$^+$ selected versus unselected autologous peripheral blood progenitor cell transplantation in multiple myeloma. *Blood* **15,** 1858–1868.

Weissman, I. (2000). Translating stem and progenitor cell biology to the clinic: Barriers and opportunities. *Science* **281,** 1442–1446.

Stereotactic Radiosurgery of Intracranial Neoplasms

Yoshiya Yamada

Memorial Sloan-Kettering Cancer Center

I. Introduction
II. Management and Outcomes of Specific Lesions
III. Complications Associated with Stereotactic Radiosurgery
IV. Conclusion

GLOSSARY

ateriovenous malformations Potentially fatal congenital vascular space-occupying intracranial lesions that can be treated with surgery, embolization, external beam radiotherapy or stereotactic radiosurgery

fraction Dose of radiation. Radiation therapy is often divided up into fractions.

isocenter Common point through which all radiation beams intersect.

radiotherapy The use of ionizing radiation as a treatment for cancer and other diseases.

stereotactic Derived from the term *stereotaxis*, the Greek roots, "stereo," which comes from the Greek *stereos*, meaning solid or a solid state; and *taxis*, an orderly state. The philosopher and mathematician Rene Descartes described the concept of localizing any point in space as the intersection of three perpendicular planes in the 17th century, laying the theoretical groundwork for stereotactic radiosurgery

stereotactic radiosurgery Single large fractions of radiotherapy delivered via stereotactic localization techniques.

S tereotactic radiosurgery refers to single large fractions of radiation delivered via stereotactic localization techniques. Stereotactic radiotherapy refers to fractioned radiotherapy delivered with stereotactic methods.

I. INTRODUCTION

The term *stereotaxis* is derived from two Greek roots, "stereo," which comes from the Greek *stereos*, meaning solid or a solid state; and *taxis*, an orderly state. The philosopher and mathematician Rene Descartes described the concept of localizing any point in space as the intersection of three perpendicular planes in the 17th century, laying the theoretical groundwork for stereotactic radiosurgery. Sir Victor Horsley devised a stereotactic system based on Cartesian coordinates to reliably place electrodes into dentate nucleus of a monkey in 1908. Through the 1950s, other investigators devised stereotactic systems designed originally to provide accurate localization of probes for electrical ablation of critical pathways for the treatment of pain, movement disorders, emotional or behavioral problems, and convulsive diseases. Proton beams were applied to patients in the 1950s at Boston and Berkeley using sterotactic techniques. Lars Leskell, a Swedish neurosurgeon, performed animal experiments with radiotherapy using stereotactic techniques and first coined the phrase "radiosurgery." The first operational "gamma knife" utilizing 179 cobalt-60 sources for radiation therapy became operational in Stockholm in 1968. In these machines, every cobalt source emits a beam of radiation, which converges at a common point. Megavoltage linear accelerators have been modified for stereotactic radiosurgery, in which the machine rotates and emits radiation at a common set point in space (the isocenter), and have dramatically increased the availability of stereotactic therapy in North America and around the world. Charged particle radiation therapy is also given stereotactically in select centers.

Stereotactic radiosurgery refers to single large fractions of radiotherapy delivered via stereotactic localization techniques. Stereotactic radiotherapy refers to fractionated (multiple dose) radiotherapy delivered with stereotactic methods.

Large single doses of radiotherapy are more apt to induce more significant effects in slowly proliferating "late response" tissues. Conversely, breaking up the dose into smaller fractions will lessen the impact of radiation upon such tissues. Thus acoustic neuromas, meningiomas, arterial venous malformations, pituitary adenomas, and craniopharyngiomas are slowly proliferating tissues and therefore are more likely to show radiation effects if large single fractions are given. However, structures such as the brain parenchyma, optic chiasm, and brain stem also respond as late responding tissues. These structures are able to tolerate higher radiation doses when administered in smaller "fractions." The effects on normal tissue are also dependent on the volume of tissue that is irradiated. When half brain single fraction irradiation was administered to a dog, 15 Gy resulted in no blood–brain barrier disruption, 30 Gy caused blood–brain barrier disruption in 10 months, and 60 Gy caused blood–brain barrier disruption in 10 weeks. When a small volume of brain was irradiated using an 8-mm collimator, 20 Gy to a monkey brain caused no MRI changes, 50 Gy produced MRI changes within 6 months, and 150 Gy resulted in MRI changes within 6 months. Thus large doses can be administered when the volume of radiation is small. A recently reported dose escalation study completed by the Radiation Therapy Oncology Group (RTOG) also found a dose–response relationship predicated upon volume. In terms of toxicity, no upper dose limit was found for small lesions (less than 2 cm in diameter). The maximum tolerated dose for lesions measuring 2.1–3.0 and 3.1–4.0 cm was found to be 18 and 15 Gy, respectively. The dose that can be safely delivered is dependent in part on the volume of the target.

Stereotactic radiosurgery delivers a highly conformal radiation dose to the target lesion by using multiple beams of radiation that intersect through the center of the lesion. Typically, these beams are noncoplanar. Care is taken to choose beam angles that do not pass through or exit out of radiosensitive structures such as the optic apparatus. These beams may be fixed, as in the case of gamma knife treatment machines, or rotate around a fixed isocenter, as in the case of linac (linear accelerator)-based stereotactic setups. An isocenter is the center of axis of rotation of a liner accelerator. In these cases, the beams may be delivered as arcs through an isocenter or as multiple beams that intersect through a given isocenter. Whether a gamma knife or linear accelerator unit is utilized, the lesion must be placed at the point of intersection of all the radiation beams. The end result is a tight concentration of radiation dose to the tumor with relative sparing of surrounding normal tissue. Stereotactic techniques are able to produce very steep dose gradients. Thus a high dose of radiation can be given to a lesion with a significantly less radiation dose to the adjacent normal structures. For example, a lesion 5 mm away from the optic chiasm can be comfortably treated to full dose while sparing the chiasm of significant radiation dose. Given the very conformal and exact nature, as well as the high doses typically associated with stereotactic radiosurgery, any error in lesion localization, patient setup, or dose calculation could result in maladministration of therapy. Thus, stereotactic radiosurgery can only be successfully performed when the following criteria are met.

1. The target lesion must be locatable in three-dimensional space
2. The target lesion must be immobilized or target motion must be accurately tracked and corrected.
3. The lesion must be accurately placed at the isocenter.
4. Radiation doses must be accurately and predictably delivered.

Lesions are identified using at least computed tomography (CT) imaging. CT data sets identify the lesion in X, Y, and Z coordinates in reference to fiducial markers. These fiducial markers have been a series of carbon fiber posts set in parallel and oblique angles (see Figs. 1 and 2). The distances between these posts in relation to each other define any plane in three-dimensional space. Thus any point can be defined in relation to any plane defined within this series of posts.

The posts are attached to a ring (Fig. 3), which is attached to the patient's skull in four points. This ring serves to immobilize the skull in a reproducible and reliable manner, and as a base for attachment of the fiducial "bird cage" for target localization.

Intracranial lesions are ideally suited for stereotactic radiosurgery. If the skull can be fixed securely, there is very little target motion. Stereotactic treatment of liver metastasis, however, is problematic because a liver metastasis may move several centimeters in the caudal/cranial direction with respirations alone.

Noninvasive relocatable stereotactic frames have been developed that accurately fix the skull with 1–3 mm accuracy. Although these frames have greater setup error and less reliable position reproducibility, they are more easily tolerated by patients who require multiple fractions, which would otherwise require multiple fixation. Others have been developed systems based on real-time imaging to correct for changes in patient position.

When appropriate, intravenous contrast dye is used at the time of CT to help identify the target lesion. Magnetic resonance imaging (MRI) scans are often helpful in localizing the lesion(s) as well as structures such as the optic chiasm. MRI scans can be digitally

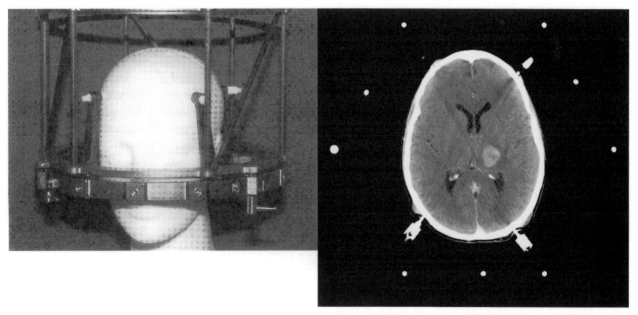

FIGURE 1 CT localization with a Brown Robertson Wells (BRW) frame has nine imaging rods: six vertical and three diagonal rods, which define a unique set of intersections through rods for any image plane and a unique transformation from a two-dimensional image to a three-dimensional BRW coordinate space.

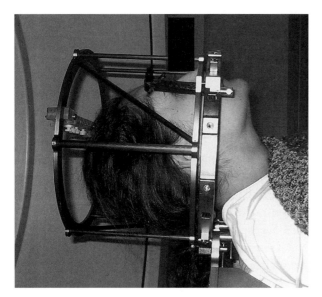

FIGURE 2   Patient with a localizing "bird cage" and frame.

fused with CT scans. These images are reconstructed in three dimensions in a computerized treatment planning system. The treating physician works closely with medical physicists to develop a treatment plan that respects normal tissue tolerances while given a very high dose of radiation in a conformal manner to the target lesion. The size of the treatment portals can be manipulated by utilizing different size collimators. Circular collimators can shape stereotactic beams into spheres of radiation dose. When complex shapes are targets, a number of different size spheres may be used additively to encompass the target by utilizing several different isocenters. Alternatively, linac-based systems may further refine treatment conformality by using micromultileaf collimators, which are able to shape individual beams to the outline of the target when the target presents as a nonspherical shape. Micromultileaf collimators are narrow (3 mm) fingers of tungsten shielding, which are attached to individual computer-controlled motors. Intensity-modulated radiotherapy (IMRT) is also possible with micromultileaf collimation, making it easier to safely treat lesions around sensitive areas and targets with complex three-dimensional shapes.

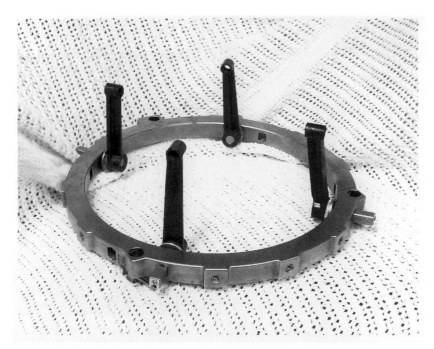

FIGURE 3   A BRW stereotactic frame with carbon fiber posts.

II. MANAGEMENT AND OUTCOMES OF SPECIFIC LESIONS

A. Ateriovenous Malformations

Ateriovenous malformations (AVM) are potentially fatal congenital vascular lesions. Radiosurgery results in lumenal obliteration. Thrombosis and gliosis have also been noted. These changes occur over a length of time of at least 1–2 years. Complete angiographic obliteration has been reported in 40 and 80% of patients at 1 and 2 years after stereotactic radiosurgery, respectively. The likelihood of complete response is smaller in larger lesions.

B. Meningioma

Meningiomas are managed with either surgical resection and/or radiation therapy. Surgical resection of the meningioma and its dural base is the preferred treatment approach in many centers, but over one-third of meningiomas are in areas not amenable to complete resection because of a close association with critical vascular, cranial nerve, or normal brain parenchyma. In these cases, stereotactic radiosurgery or fractionated external beam irradiation should be considered.

After complete resection, there is a 9% recurrence rate, but a 19% recurrence after tumor removal and the dural base was only coagulated. The University of Pittsburgh has reported their experience in 99 patients with 5–10 years of follow-up. The median prescribed dose was 15 Gy. Ninety-seven patients had serial imaging available, and 63% of the tumors were smaller, 32% were unchanged, and 5% increased in size. Neurological deficits attributable to radiosurgery were noted in 5% of patients. In most cases, neurological changes are transient. Hakin and colleagues reported a 5-year actuarial control rate of 89% for those with benign histologies using stereotactic radiosurgery as primary therapy. If the lesion was atypical or malignant, the overall 4-year survival was only 22%. These rates of local control compare favorably with incompletely resected lesions treated with fractionated external beam radiotherapy. There is little published data on the use of fractionated stereotactic radiotherapy for the management of meningiomas. However, the use of standard fraction sizes should reduce the risk of serious morbidity to critical structures.

The long natural history of meningiomas, as well as late radiation reactions, mandates data with long term follow-up (10–15 years) to adequately evaluate single fraction vs multifraction stereotactic radiation therapy. Optimal dose fractionation schedules have yet to be elucidated.

C. Vestibular Schwannoma

Vestibular schwannoma (acoustic neuroma) less than 3 cm in size are often suitable for stereotactic radiosurgery or surgical resection. CT imaging alone does not always adequately demonstrate the intracanalicular portion of these lesions, therefore, MRI imaging should be incorporated into the treatment planning. A comprehensive prospective evaluation of 162 patients with at least 5 years of follow-up has been reported. Nine patients experienced tumor enlargement, but 5 of these patients were found to have tumor necrosis. Those patients with 5–10 years of follow-up demonstrated tumor regression in 72%. The University of Florida has reported tumor regression in 55%, stable disease in 39%, and enlargement in only 7%.

The expected rate of long-term facial or trigeminal nerve deficits with careful treatment planning and dose selection in the modern era is 0–8% for intracanalicular and extracanalicular lesions. Most post-treatment morbidity occurs within the first 3 years of treatment. Surgical series report approximately 50% hearing preservation for small lesions. Modern radiosurgical series using MRI treatment planning report hearing preservation in 68% of patients.

D. Pituitary Adenoma

Neurosurgical advances in transphenoidal approaches and microsurgical techniques have made surgery the most common modality of treatment for most pituitary adenomas. However, radiation therapy often has an important role in the management of these patients. Conventional radiotherapy utilizing a dose of 45 Gy will provide long-term local control in over 80% of cases. Although hormonal levels may normalize, it may take many years to realize the benefits of conventional radiotherapy. It is uncommon to reverse visual deficits or other neurological disturbances. Kjellburg and co-workers have reported 28% normalization of growth hormone levels within 2 years, 75% in 5 years, and 93% within 20 years after proton beam stereotactic radiosurgery, demonstrating the slow response to acromegalic lesions to radiotherapy. The cure rate for Cushing's disease has been reported to be 55, 80, and 90% at 5, 10, and 20 years, respectively. Rhan and colleagues reported an 82% overall cure rate with radiosurgery, and the University of Pittsburgh has reported 62% were either cured or improved after radiosurgery. The largest series of prolactinomas included 23 patients, with a 95% cure/improvement rate.

Potential toxicities related to pituitary radiosurgery include hypopituitarism, visual loss, and hypothalamic dysfunction. Rates of hypopituitarism have ranged from 0 to 55%. The actual incidence of hypopituitarism in the modern age with MRI imaging and modern treatment planning and dosimetry is likely very low, but remains an unknown entity.

Most series have reported very low rates of visual changes secondary to therapy. Levy and co-workers and Kjellburg and Abbe have reported a 1% increase in visual disturbances. Rocher and colleagues, however, have reported visual toxicity in 39% of cases (6% were blinded). In the modern era, where the optic chiasm can be clearly visualized and contoured with MRI assistance, careful treatment planning and meticulous dosimetry should keep the risk of this devastating complication very low.

The University of Pittsburgh group has reported on death attributed to hypothalamic injury. Voges and colleagues have also reported on cases of severe hypothalamic syndrome. These complications are rare in the setting of pituitary radiosurgery.

E. Solid Tumor Metastatic Lesions

Almost 200,000 patients will be afflicted with brain metastasis annually in the United States. Brain metastases are particularly well suited for stereotactic radiosurgery. These lesions are not typically infiltrative and are quite stationary. Therefore, a tight margin around the lesion itself will not risk marginal recurrences. It is a highly effective noninvasive therapy with a low probability of significant toxicity.

If not controlled, brain metastases will cause significant morbidity. In two randomized trials, Patchell and colleagues demonstrated that surgery and whole brain radiotherapy were superior to whole brain radiotherapy alone or surgical resection alone for a single metastasis. These studies also demonstrated that radiotherapy increased the time of remaining functionally independent and delayed the time to neurologic death, underscoring the importance of local control of disease in the brain.

In medically operable patients, surgical resection of solitary metastases has been the standard of care. Although no randomized trial comparing the efficacy of complete resection and stereotactic radiosurgery has been performed, available data suggest that radiosurgery and resection should give equivalent rates of local control and survival. Randomized trials of whole brain radiotherapy and surgical resection for solitary metastasis have found local control rates between 80 and 90%, with overall survival rates between 40 and 48 weeks. Similarly, randomized trials for patients with greater than one metastases, in which whole brain radiotherapy and stereotactic radiosurgery have one of the treatment arms, have found local control rates between 79 and 92%. Overall survival rates were found to be 9–11 months. The median survival of well-selected patients with single brain metastases treated with whole brain radiotherapy and resection or radiosurgery was found to be comparable in a multi-institutional outcome and prognostic factor analysis. Furthermore, retrospective data for stereotactic radiosurgery alone consistently demonstrate rates of local control greater than 80%.

F. High-Grade Gliomas

High-grade gliomas are aggressive primary brain malignancies that are difficult to eradicate with surgery, radiotherapy, and chemotherapy. These cells tend to infiltrate into surrounding brain parenchyma, making total resection very difficult. They also demonstrate significant radiation resistance. Typically, these patients are offered fractionated radiotherapy after subtotal surgical resection in an attempt to improve local rates and improve survival. Radiation dose escalation has resulted in a higher likelihood of toxicity without a significant improvement in outcomes. Single institution series have found improved outcomes with the use of a stereotactic radiosurgery boost after conventional fractionated radiotherapy. These reports have found a mean survival of 20 months with the use of stereotactic boosts, significantly better than those traditionally reported with standard external beam radiotherapy alone. However, 35% of cases experienced radionecrosis, which required reoperation. Also, patients offered radiosurgery boosts in these series may be a more favorable population, thus reflecting selection bias. Randomized trials testing boost strategies using brachytherapy techniques have failed to show a survival benefit, but show similar toxicity profiles to stereotactic boosts. These results draw into question the actual benefit of localized radiation boosts. Therefore, stereotactic boosts can be considered in selected cases only.

III. COMPLICATIONS ASSOCIATED WITH STEREOTACTIC RADIOSURGERY

There are few anticancer therapies in which the likelihood of benefit is as high and the probability of toxicity is as low as those expected with stereotactic radiosurgery. Acute complications, which may occur within the first week of stereotactic radiosurgery, are uncommon. Joseph and co-workers reported a 2.3% incidence of seizures within 12 h of stereotactic radiosurgery, and all three patients were found to have subtherapeutic levels of anticonvulsants. Breneman and colleagues reported that 3/84 patients suffered grand mal seizures within 72 h of stereotactic radiosurgery. All three patients had lesions in the motor cortex and had subtherapeutic levels of anticonvulsants. In another single institutional series, 12 out of 196 patients (6.7%) had seizures within 24 h postradiosurgery. Ten of these patients had a history of prior seizure disorder and had subtherapeutic levels of anticonvulsants. Other acute effects include transient worsening of preexisting neurologic symptoms or nausea, and occur less than 6% of the time. These symptoms often respond to steroid therapy. It would seem prudent to carefully monitor the anticonvulsant levels of patients with a history of seizures and use prophylactic steroids for patients demonstrating perilesional edema. It has also been suggested to premedicate patients with lesions in the posterior fossa with antiemetics to minimize the likelihood of nausea.

Subacute complications, which occur within the first 6 months of treatment, are also relatively rare. Alopecia was noted in 5% of patients who received at least 4.4 Gy to the scalp. A prolonged use of steroids was noted in less than 3% of patients.

Chronic complications include radiation necrosis, cranial nerve palsies, and chronic steroid dependency. Radiation necrosis has been reported in approximately 4–8% of patients who undergo stereotactic radiosurgery. Chemotherapy such as methotrexate may increase the likelihood of radiation necrosis. In such cases, surgical resection is often required. Cranial nerve injury usually presents 7–8 months after radiosurgery is performed. It was noted in 1% of cases reported by Loeffler and Alexander. Persistent edema requiring steroid use longer than 6 months has been reported in 7–8% of patients. In most cases, vasogenic edema improves as lesions respond favorably to stereotactic radiosurgery.

IV. CONCLUSION

Stereotactic radiosurgery should be considered in the management of most intracranial neoplasms. Stereotactic therapy is able to deliver high doses of radiation to small volumes safely. In most cases, the expectation of success is high, while the likelihood of significant toxicity is relatively low. Precision in target localization, patient setup, and quality assurance are important factors in stereotactic therapy. Careful attention to detail is imperative, as a few millimeters can be the margin of error between success and failure, both in tumor control and in avoidance of toxicity. Patients must be carefully selected to ensure safe treatment with a reasonable expectation of benefit.

See Also the Following Articles

Brain and Central Nervous System Cancers • Brain Cancer and Magnetic Resonance Spectroscopy • Dosimetry and Treatment Planning for Three-Dimensional Radiation Therapy • Proton Beam Radiation Therapy • Radiobiology, Principles of

Bibliography

Adler, J. R., Murphy, M. J., Chang, S. D., and Hancock, S. L. (1999). Image guided robotic radiosurgery. *Neurosurgery* **44**(6), 1299–1306.

Alexander, E., Moriarty, T. M., Davis, R. B., *et al.* (1995). Stereotactic radiosurgery for the definitive, noninvasive treatment of brain metastases. *J. Natl. Cancer Inst.* **87**, 34–40.

Auchter, R. M., Lamond, J. P., Alexander, E., *et al.* (1996). A multiinstitutional outcome and prognostic factor analysis of radiosurgery for resectable single brain metastasis. *Int. J. Radiat. Oncol. Biol. Phys.* **35**, 27–35.

Breneman, J. C., Warnick, R. E., Albright, R. E., *et al.* (1996). Stereotactic radiosurgery for the treatment of brain metastases: Results of a single institution series. *Cancer* **79**, 551–557.

Buiatti, J. M., Friedman, W. A., Bova, F. J., *et al.* (1995). Treatment selection factors for stereotactic radiosurgery treatment of intracranial metastatses. *Int. J. Radiat. Oncol. Biol. Phys.* **32**, 1161–1166.

Chougule, P. B., Burton-Williams, M., Saris, S., *et al.* (2000). Randomized treatment of brain metastasis with gamma knife radiosurgery, whole brain radiotherapy or both. *Int. J. Radiat. Oncol. Biol. Phys.* **48**(S), 114.

Colombo, F., Benedetti, A., Pozza, F., *et al.* (1989). Linear accelerator radiosurgery of cerebral arteriovenous malformations. *Neurosurgery* **24**, 833–840.

Degerblad, M., Rahn, T., Bergstrand, G., *et al.* (1986). Long-term results of stereotactic radiosurgery to the pituitary gland in Cushing's disease. *Acta Endocrinol.* **112**, 310–314.

Flickinger, J. C., Kondziolka, D., Lunsford, L. D., *et al.* (1994). A multi-institutional experience with stereotactic radiosurgery for solitary metastasis. *Int. J. Radiat. Oncol. Biol. Phys.* **28**, 797–802.

Foote, K. D., Friedman, W. A., Buatti, J. M., *et al.* (1999). Linear accelerator radiosurgery in brain tumor management. *Neurosurg. Clin. North Am.* **10**, 203–242.

Foote, R. L., Coffey, R. J., Swanson, J., *et al.* (1995). Stereotactic radiosurgery using the gamma knife for acoustic neuromas. *Int. J. Radiat. Oncol. Biol. Phys.* **32**, 1153–1160.

Hakim, R., Alexander, E., III, Loeffler, J. S., *et al.* (1998). Results of linear accelerator-based radiosurgery for intracranial meningiomas. *Neurosurgery* **42**, 446–454.

Joseph, J., Adler, J. R., Cox, R., *et al.* (1996). Linear accelerator-based stereotactic radiosurgery for brain metastases: The influence of number of lesions on survival. *J. Clin. Oncol.* **14**, 1085–1092.

Kjellburg, R. N., and Abbe, M. (1988). Stereotactic Bragg peak proton beam therapy. *In* "Modern Stereotactic Neurosurgery" (L. D. Lunsford, ed.), pp. 463–470. Martius Nijhoff, Boston.

Kjellburg, R. N., Hanamura, T., Davis, K. R., *et al.* (1983). Bragg peak proton beam therapy for arteriovenous malformations of the brain. *N. Engl. J. Med.* **309**, 269–274.

Kondziolka, D., Flickenger, J. C., Bissonette, D. J., *et al.* (1997). The survival benefit of stereotactic radiosurgery for patients with malignant glial neoplasms. *Neurosurgery* **41**, 776–785.

Kondziolka, D., Levy, E., Niranjan, A., *et al.* (1999). Stereotactic radiosurgery for meningiomas. *Neurosurg. Clin. North Am.* **10**, 317–325.

Kondziolka, D., Lunsford, L. D., McLaughlin, M., *et al.* (1998). Long term outcomes after acoustic tumor radiosurgery. *N. Engl. J. Med.* **339**, 1426–1433.

Kondziolka, D., Patel, A., Lunsford, L. D., *et al.* (1999). Stereotactic radiosurgery plus whole brain radiotherapy versus radiotherapy alone for patients with multiple brain metastases. *Int. J. Radiat. Biol. Phys.* **45**, 427–434.

Laperriere, N. J., Leung, P. M., McKenzie, S., Milosevic, M., Wong, S., Glen, J., Pintilie, M., and Bernstein, M. (1998). Randomized study of brachytherapy in the initial management of patients with malignant astrocytoma. *Int. J. Radiat. Oncol. Biol. Phys.* **41**(5), 1005–1011.

Larson, D. A., Flickenger, J. C., and Loeffler, J. S. (1993). The radiobiology of radiosurgery. *Int. J. Radiat. Oncol. Biol. Phys.* **25**, 557–561.

Levy, R. P., Fabrikant, J. I., Frankel, K. A., *et al.* (1991). Heavy charged particle radiosurgery of the pituitary gland: Clinical results of 840 patients. *J. Stereotact. Funct. Neurosurg.* **57**, 22–35.

Loeffler, J. S., and Alexander, E. (1993). Radiosurgery for the treatment of intracranial metastases. *In* "Stereotactic Radiosurgery" (E. Alexander, J. S. Loeffler, and D. Lunsford, eds.), pp. 139–141. McGraw Hill, New York.

Loeffler, J. S., Alexander, E., Siddon, R. L., *et al.* (1989). Stereotactic radiosurgery for intracranial arteriovenous malformations using a standard linear accelerator. *Int. J. Radiat. Oncol. Biol. Phys.* **17**, 673–677.

Lunsford, L. D., Aschuler, E. M., and Flickinger, J. C. (1999). *In vivo* biological effects of stereotactic radiosurgery: A primate model. *Neurosurgery* **27**, 373–382.

Lunsford, L. D., and Linskey, M. E. (1992). Stereotactic radiosurgery in the treatment of patients with acoustic tumors. *Otolaryngol. Clin. North Am.* **25**, 471.

Lunsford, L. D., Witt, T. C., Kondziolka, D., *et al.* (1995). Stereotactic radiosurgery of of anterior skull base tumors. *Clin. Neurosurg.* **42**, 99–118.

McCord, M. W., Buatti, J. M., Fennell, E. M., *et al.* Radiotherapy for pituitary adenomas: Long-term outcome and sequelae. *Int. J. Radiat. Oncol. Biol. Phys.* **39**, 437–444.

McCoullogh, W. M., Marcus, R. B., Rhoton, A. L., *et al.* (1991). Long term follow-up of radiotherapy for pituitary adenoma: The absence of late recurrence after greater than or equal to 4500 centigray. *Int. J. Radiat. Oncol. Biol. Phys.* **21**, 607–614.

Patchell, R. A., Tibbs, P. A., Regine, W. F., *et al.* (1998). Postoperative radiotherapy in the treatment of single metastases to the brain. *JAMA* **280**, 1485–1489.

Patchell, R. A., Tibbs, P. A., Walsh, J. W., *et al.* (1990). A randomized trial of surgery in the treatment of single metastases to the brain. *N. Engl. J. Med.* **322**, 494–500.

Rahn, T., Thoren, M., Hall, K., *et al.* (1980). Stereotactic radiosurgery in Cushing's syndrome: acute radiation effects. *Surg. Neurol.* **14,** 85–92.

Rocher, F. P., Sentenac, I., Berger, C., *et al.* (1995). Stereotactic radiosurgery: The Lyon experience. *Acta Neurochir. Suppl. (Wein)* **63,** 109–114.

Samii, M., and Mathies, C. (1997). Management of 1000 vestibular schwannomas (acoustic neuromas) function in 1000 tumor resections. *Neurosurgery* **40,** 248–260.

Shaw, E., Scott, C., Souhami, L., Dinapoli, R., Kline, R., Loeffler, J., and Farnan, N. (2000). Single dose radiosurgical treatment of recurrent previously irradiated primary brain tumors and brain metastases: final report of RTOG protocol 90-05. *Int. J. Radiat. Oncol. Biol. Phys.* **47**(2), 291–298.

Souhami, L., Olivier, A., Podgorsak, E. B., *et al.* (1990). Radiosurgery of cerebral arteriovenous malformations with the dymaic stereotactic irradiation. *Int. J. Radiat. Oncol. Biol. Phys.* **19,** 775–782.

Sperduto, P. W., Scott, C., Schell, M., *et al.* (2000). Preliminary report of RTOG 9508: A phase III trial comparing whole brain irradiation alone versus whole brain irradiation plus stereotactic radiosurgery for patients with two or three unresected brain metastases. *Int. J. Radiat. Oncol. Biol. Phys.* **48**(S), 113.

Thoren, M., Rahn, T., Guo, W. Y., *et al.* (1991). Stereotactic radiosurgery with the Colbalt-60 gamma unit in the treatment of growth hormone-producing pituitary tumors. *Neurosurgery* **29,** 663–668.

Voges, J., Sturm, V., Deub, U., *et al.* (1996). LINAC radiosurgery in pituitary adenomas: Preliminary results. *Acta Neurochir. Suppl. (Wein)* **65,** 41–43.

Steroid Hormones and Hormone Receptors

Thomas S. McCormick
Clark W. Distelhorst
Case Western Reserve University, Cleveland, Ohio

GLOSSARY

autoregulatory control A process in which steroid hormone receptors may cause their own upregulation or downregulation.

DNA regulatory element A site on DNA molecule where steroid receptors bind and affect downstream transcriptional events.

endonuclease An enzyme that functions in apoptotic cells to degrade chromosomal DNA.

neoplastic cell A cell in which growth is uncontrolled, i.e., a cancer cell.

oncogene Any gene that regulates a product that can transform a normal cell to a tumor cell.

Steroid hormones are hydrophobic molecules derived from cholesterol that diffuse through the plasma membrane and bind reversibly to specific receptors in the cytoplasm or nucleus. On binding ligand, the hormone–receptor complex associates tightly with the nucleus, where it interacts with specific regulatory DNA sequences. The binding of receptor complexes to DNA increases or decreases the transcription rates of nearby genes. The products of these regulated genes may in turn lead to further transcriptional regulation, or they may directly effect cellular processes such as growth and differentiation. Defects in steroid receptors contribute to the pathogenesis of malignancies such as prostate cancer and breast cancer. Likewise, hormones such as estrogen can promote the growth of breast cancer cells mediated by the estrogen receptor. Therefore, steroid hormones and their receptors may have important oncogenic potential.

I. INTRODUCTION

Steroid hormones promote the growth of certain malignancies, most notably prostate carcinoma and breast carcinoma. Likewise, endocrine manipulations such as orchiectomy for prostate cancer and ovariectomy or hypophysectomy for breast cancer were among the earliest successful approaches to treating cancer. Similarly, recognition that glucocorticosteroid hormones induce atrophy of normal lymphoid tissues led to the first successful use of these hormones in the treatment of lymphoid malignancies. Until relatively recently, the mechanisms that allowed the success of these early treatments were unknown. However, the molecular events associated with the regulation of tumor cell growth by steroid hormones have begun to yield to the search for answers. The first description of the estradiol receptor by Jensen and colleagues in 1960 opened the door for increased understanding of the fundamental mechanisms by which steroid hormones interact with cells. Cloning of the genes for various steroid hormones receptors revealed that steroid hormone receptors are members of a large superfamily of ligand-regulated transcriptional regulatory molecules and led to new insight into the potential oncogenic role of steroid hormones and their receptors.

II. STEROID HORMONE ACTION AT A MOLECULAR LEVEL

A steroid hormone acts in conjunction with its specific receptor, binding to DNA and regulating transcription. Steroid hormone receptors are ligand-regulated transcriptional regulatory molecules that either induce or repress the transcription of target genes. In the absence of hormone, the receptor molecules are inactive; on binding their hormonal ligand, the receptors undergo a conformational change (receptor activation) that allows them to interact with specific transcriptional regulatory elements on DNA. Each class of steroid receptors possess a distinct regulatory element, and the regulatory elements for most of the major steroid hormones have been described. These include the glucocorticoid response element (GRE), the estrogen response element (ERE), and the thyroid response element (TRE). Through interaction with these sequences, receptor molecules regulate the rate of transcription initiation from nearby promoters, causing either an increase or decrease in the transcription of specific genes.

The first receptor to be well characterized was the glucocorticoid receptor. Interaction of this receptor with DNA was studied using the DNA of the mouse mammary tumor virus (MMTV). This virus increases its transcription rate in the presence of glucocorticoids. The direct binding of the glucocorticoid receptor complex to the MMTV DNA was demonstrated using both DNA binding assays and electron microscopic studies. Purification of the glucocorticoid receptor and subsequent production of a cDNA encoding the receptor allowed for intense study of the mechanism by which this receptor operates. Subsequent cloning of the receptors for other members of the steroid receptor superfamily has provided additional information relevant to all steroid receptors.

Comparison of the amino acid sequence corresponding to the cloned receptors revealed that the hormone receptors are part of a large superfamily of genes that encode ligand-responsive transcription factors. Each of the members of this family share a high degree of homology (ranging from 42 to 94%) in a central core sequence that is rich in cysteine, lysine, and arginine residues. The region appears to form a zinc finger structural motif in which multiple cysteine- and histidine-rich repeating units fold into a fingered structure coordinated by a zinc ion. This zinc finger region interacts with DNA and constitutes the DNA-binding domain.

The presence of a highly conserved sequence element corresponding to the DNA-binding domain initiated searches for cryptic receptor genes by low-stringency hybridization; through this technique, a number of ligand-dependent transcription factors have been identified, including the gene that encodes the retinoic acid receptor and a gene that encodes a receptor closely related to the retinoic acid receptor that has been implicated in the etiology of hepatocellular carcinoma (HAP).

The other major structural feature shared by all members of the steroid receptor family is a C-terminally located ligand-binding domain. The ligand-binding domain has at least two important functions. First, this domain confers specificity on the receptor molecule by defining which class of ligands it will bind. Thus, for example, the estrogen receptor binds estrogens but not glucocorticoids. Second, this domain has a protein inactivation activity that represses other receptor activities. For example, in the absence of hormonal ligand, the glucocorticoid receptor is held in the cytoplasm in an inactive, non-DNA-binding form. The repressive effect of the ligand-binding domain is relieved on hormone binding, inducing nuclear localization and DNA binding. The repressive effect of the ligand-binding domain has been elegantly demonstrated by experiments in which mutant forms of the glucocorticoid receptor were expressed in cells; these studies revealed that deletion of the ligand-binding domain produces a constitutively active receptor that binds DNA and regulates gene transcription, even in the absence of hormone.

The mechanism of the protein inactivation displayed by the ligand-binding domain has not been fully elucidated. However, studies suggest that it may be mediated through an interaction of the ligand-binding domain with nonreceptor proteins known as molecular chaperones. This group of proteins, which includes the 90-kDa heat-shock protein (HSP-90), aids in the folding and assembly of proteins. In addition to HSP-90, the glucocorticoid receptor has also been shown to associate as an inactive complex with both the p59 and p23 proteins. HSP-70 has also been thought to associate with this complex, although this interaction has not been defined. It appears that this interaction not only represses receptor activity by preventing DNA binding, but is also responsible for maintaining the receptor in a conformation that is able to bind ligand. In contrast to the glucocorticoid receptor, most of the steroid receptors, including the estrogen receptor, the progesterone receptor, and the androgen receptors, are resident proteins in the nucleus. Indeed, the exact location of the glucocorticoid receptor in the absence of hormone is still the topic of some controversy.

III. REGULATION OF STEROID HORMONE RECEPTOR LEVELS

The effect of any steroid hormone on its target cell is ultimately determined by the ability of the target cell to bind the steroid hormone. This is accomplished on the basis of the intracellular concentration of the specific steroid receptor expressed in the target cell. The extent of a structural alteration in the chromatin at a characterized glucocorticoid response element, as well as the magnitude of several transcriptional responses elicited by the receptor, is roughly proportional to the number of receptor molecules per cell. Thus, factors that regulate the intracellular level of steroid hormone receptors in tumor cells may be important determinants of hormonal responsiveness *in vivo*.

There is considerable evidence that different classes of steroid hormone receptors in tumor cells are under autoregulatory control; thus, the dominant factor regulating steroid hormone receptor levels in tumor cells appears to be the cognate hormonal ligand itself. This type of autoregulatory control has been extensively investigated for the estrogen and progesterone receptors.

In breast cancer cells estrogen receptors are not upregulated by growth factors but rather are regulated by the steroid hormonal ligand itself. The response of the receptors to ligand binding, either upregulation or downregulation, is dependent on the individual cell line tested. Thus, in one particular cell line, the T47D breast cancer line, the estrogen hormone estradiol induces a significant increase in the level of estrogen receptors; in the MCF-7 breast cancer line, however, estradiol induces a decrease in the level of estrogen receptors. The regulation of the receptor levels is also dependent on the nature of the hormonal ligand. For example, in the T47D breast cancer cell line, estradiol induces a 2.5-fold increase in estrogen receptor mRNA levels; in contrast, the progestin hormone R5020 induces a marked decrease in estrogen receptor mRNA levels. The mechanisms of differential autoregulatory control in different cell lines by different ligands are not understood at present. In the MCF-7 cell line, the mechanism of estrogen receptor downregulation by estradiol is complex and appears to involve inhibition of estrogen receptor gene transcription at early times and at later times a posttranslational effect on receptor mRNA.

Progesterone receptors, like estrogen receptors, are also under autoregulatory control. In breast cancer cell lines, progesterone receptors are downregulated by progestins and upregulated by estrogens. Receptor autoregulation is not a phenomenon unique to breast cancer cell lines, as progesterone has been found to downregulate its own receptor in rat prostate carcinoma cells as well. The mechanism of downregulation by progestins involves both a decrease in the rate of receptor synthesis and a decrease in receptor half-life. The mechanism of upregulation by estrogens involves an increase in the rate of receptor synthesis, rather than modulation of the rate of receptor degradation.

Glucocorticoid hormones are an additional class of hormonal steroids that appear to downregulate the level of their own receptor in cells. A variety of mechanisms appear to be involved in glucocorticoid receptor autoregulation, including decreased rate of receptor gene transcription and decreased receptor mRNA half-life. Intriguingly, the glucocorticoid receptor gene appears to contain several internal glucocorticoid receptor-binding regions that may mediate receptor autoregulation. In addition, in certain cell lines, but not others, glucocorticoids appear to induce a reduction in receptor half-life. Finally, it should be noted that regulation of the glucocorticoid receptor by its cognate ligand may be tissue specific; in certain cell lines, glucocorticoids upregulate rather than downregulate the level of their own receptor.

IV. HORMONAL REGULATION OF TUMOR CELL GROWTH

The possibility that certain steroid hormones, mainly estrogens, play a role in both carcinogenesis and tumor progression has intrigued investigators for many years. On the basis of both epidemiological and experimental studies, the length of exposure of the mammary glands to estrogen appears to be proportional to breast cancer risk. Thus, an increased incidence of breast cancer has been linked to diethylstilbestrol exposure during pregnancy and estrogen treatment for postmenopausal symptoms. Also, the risk of both localized and widespread endometrial cancer has been linked to both the long-term use of conjugated estrogens and tamoxifen. Cell culture experiments have demonstrated that estradiol stimulates the proliferation and invasiveness of the MCF-7 human breast cancer cell line. Endometrial cell cultures also respond to estrogens with increased proliferation. This situation has been likened to the process thought to occur *in vivo* during long-term estrogen therapy.

The mechanisms responsible for promotion of tumor cell growth and invasion by estrogens appears to be complex. Estrogens have a direct mitogenic effect on breast cancer cells, causing them to divide more rapidly by shortening their cell cycle. Also, estrogens induce a large number of enzymes and other proteins involved in nucleic acid synthesis in isolated breast cancer cell lines. The induced proteins include DNA polymerase, the c-*myc* protooncogene, thymidine and uridine kinases, thymidylate synthetase, carbamoyl-phosphate synthase, aspartate transcarbamylase, dihydroorotase, glucose-6-phosphate dehydrogenase, and dihydrofolate reductase. Also, a role for polyamines in estrogen-regulated breast cancer cell growth has been suggested by the observation that inhibition of polyamine synthesis in the MCF-7 breast cancer cell line inhibits estradiol-induced cell proliferation. Each of these estrogen-induced effects could potentially contribute to direct stimulation of tumor cell growth.

Estrogenic stimulation plays a critical role in the developing normal mammary epithelium; thus, it is not surprising that neoplastic mammary epithelium should also respond to estrogenic stimulation, possibly through many of the same mechanisms. One of the mechanisms used to control breast tumor growth by estrogens is induction of pituitary synthesis and secretion of prolactin. Estrogens may also permit breast cancer cells to overcome growth inhibiting agents in their environment. Another way that estrogens can control breast tumor growth is by inducing the synthesis and release from breast cancer cells of polypeptide growth factors that mediate growth of breast cancer cells in either an autocrine or paracrine fashion.

Several prominent growth factors have been implicated in regulating breast cancer growth in response to estrogens, including transforming growth factor alpha (TGF-α), epidermal growth factor (EGF), insulin-like growth factors (IGF-I and IGF-II), transforming growth factor beta (TGF-β), and platelet-derived growth factor (PDGF). Both TGF-α and EGF act via the EGF receptor, a ligand-inducible tyrosine kinase. The EGF receptor is present on both normal and cancerous cell lines, and in certain cells its transcription is increased by estradiol. A possible mechanism for estradiol function is to increase the expression of the EGF receptor in response to TGF-α and EGF. Estrogens may also promote proliferation of tumor cells by inducing the synthesis of TGF-α and EGF. For example, estradiol induces TGF-α and its mRNA in MCF-7 breast cancer cells, implicating TGF-α as an autocrine growth factor in breast cancer. Overexpression of EGF has been closely associated with poor prognosis in clinical breast cancer and with rapid tumor growth rate in experimental systems.

Insulin-like growth factors have also been implicated in hormonal stimulation of tumor cell growth. The majority of all breast cancer cell lines express mRNA for insulin receptors, IGF-I receptors, and IGF-II receptors. In the breast cancer cell line MCF-7, antibodies to the IGF-I receptor block the mitogenic effect of both IGF-I and IGF-II. Additionally, a 3- to 6-fold induction of IGF-I-like growth factor by estrogen in breast cancer cell lines and secretion of IGF-I related factors is inhibited by antiestrogens. Thus, IGF-I related factors appear to be autocrine growth factors for breast cancer cells.

Estrogens may also block growth factors that would normally inhibit tumor cell growth. For example, TGF-β secretion is inhibited by treatment of MCF-7 breast cancer cells with estrogen, whereas antiestrogens strongly stimulate its secretion. By inhibiting the effects of TGF-β, estrogens may allow unchecked tumor cell growth. The effects of estrogen on TGF-β are dependent on individual cell type; thus, in osteoblast-like osteosarcoma cells, estradiol induces rather than represses production of TGF-β.

Growth factors are not limited to acting in an autocrine fashion. For example, in breast cancer, estrogen-induced PDGF may act in a paracrine manner on fibroblasts and possibly other surrounding tissues. This could result in the production by fibroblasts of mediators such as IGF-I that might further enhance tumor growth. In cancer cells, growth factors and estrogen probably act in concert with other systemic mitogens (e.g., IGF-II) to promote tumor growth.

Two-dimensional gel analysis of protein polypeptide patterns of MCF-7 breast cancer cells support the view that a few, specific polypeptides are regulated by diverse tumorigenic stimuli in MCF-7 cells. Both estrogens and antiestrogens alter the synthesis and/or secretion of several non-growth factor proteins by breast cancer cells, presumably through the estrogen receptor. The role these proteins, which include plasminogen activators and collagenolytic enzymes, play in promoting breast cancer cell growth is not entirely clear.

A particularly intriguing observation is that estrogen induces the cell surface receptor for laminin in MCF-7 breast cancer cells; since the laminin receptor mediates attachment of cells to basement membranes, the induction of this protein in breast cancer cells may contribute to tumor invasiveness. Interestingly, although their action is through the same receptor, estrogens and antiestrogens have differential effects on protein expression in breast cancer. Further characterization of these differentially regulated proteins may provide significant clues as to the mechanisms of action of these important hormones in regulating tumor cell growth.

It has been suggested that the secretion of procathepsin D, a lysosomal acidic protease, may provide a mechanism for the invasiveness of tumor cells. Estrogens stimulate human breast cancer cells to synthesize and secrete procathepsin D more abundantly than normal cells. In endometrial cells, estradiol does not alter the level of cathepsin D produced. Thus, the estrogenic stimulation of cathepsin D appears to be relatively specific for breast cancer cells. In MCF-7 breast cancer cells, cathepsin D is induced by EGF and several other growth factors; the induction by growth factors is indirect, but the induction by estrogens is direct and at the transcriptional level. Cathepsin D can degrade extracellular matrices and proteoglycans. Thus, cathepsin D from breast cancer cells may degrade basement membranes and consequently facilitate tumor invasion when released into an acidic microenvironment. *In vitro* studies have demonstrated that the secreted procathepsin D interacts with the mannose 6-phosphate/IGF-II receptor on breast cancer cells via mannose 6-phosphate signals and displays an autocrine mitogenic activity for breast cancer cells. Clinical studies support the role of cathepsin D by demonstrating that a high level of cathepsin D is an important predictor of earlier relapse.

There is also considerable interest in the role of the pS2 gene in breast cancer. The pS2 mRNA encodes a small 84-amino acid cysteine-rich secretory protein that is regulated at the transcriptional level by estrogens. pS2 is secreted into the medium of MCF-7 breast cancer cells, and its synthesis is induced by estradiol, but not by the antiestrogen tamoxifen. pS2 is not expressed in normal breast tissue and is thought to be an autocrine or paracrine stimulator of breast tumor cell proliferation. It is also induced by several factors including the tumor promoter 12-O-tetradecanoylphobol-13-acetate (TPA), EGF, and the oncogenes *jun* or *ras*. pS2 gene expression is an estrogen-dependent biochemical and immunocytochemical marker in breast cancer; pS2 is expressed in 50% of primary human breast tumors, and its expression correlates with hormonal dependent status.

V. ONCOGENIC POTENTIAL OF STEROID HORMONES AND STEROID HORMONE RECEPTORS

Considerable speculation about the potential oncogenic role of steroid hormone receptors has arisen due to recognition that steroid hormone receptors have structural homology with the avian erythroblastosis viral oncogene v-*erb*-A, which has been shown to transform avian erythrocytes. The human gene c-*erb*-A is a cellular counterpart of the viral oncogene v-*erb*-A and encodes the thyroid hormone receptor. The *erb*-A genes encode a cysteine-rich domain that shows high homology with the zinc finger DNA-binding domain of steroid hormone receptors.

It has been proposed that loss of hormonal dependency of certain tumors might be due to mutated or truncated steroid receptor-like proteins that act constitutively in the regulation of gene transcription in the absence of steroid hormones. A number of estrogen receptor mutations have been uncovered in breast cancer cells. At least some of these mutations give rise to so-called outlaw receptors, receptors that function in the absence of hormone. One type of outlaw receptor is aberrantly active and regulates gene transcription in the absence of estrogen. Such a receptor could have oncogenic potential by promoting breast cancer cell growth, even in the face of hormonal manipulations designed to remove the estrogenic stimulus to cell growth. Another type of outlaw receptor is transcriptionally inactive, but it prevents the func-

tion of the normal estrogen receptor. The implications for this type of defect are important when considering how this aberrant receptor may function during drug treatment. For example, this receptor interferes with the normal estrogen receptor; therefore, cells that would normally respond to the antiestrogen drug tamoxifen are no longer capable of responding and would grow uncontrollably. This type of receptor defect could interfere with the pathway by which an antiestrogen such as tamoxifen inhibits cell growth, resulting in tamoxifen resistance. Evidence is emerging that similar types of outlaw receptors might contribute to the hormone-independent growth of prostatic cancer. A number of androgen receptor mutations have been identified in prostate cancer cells that could generate androgen receptors which are constitutively active in the absence of hormone. Therefore, steroid receptor mutations, like mutations in other important signal transduction pathways, may have important oncogenic potential.

Interest in the potential oncogenic role of steroid hormone receptors has also been stimulated by the possible linkage between the progesterone receptor gene and the gene coding for the human homology of the mouse mammary tumor virus integration site, *int-2*, which surrounds a protooncogene thought to be involved in the development of murine mammary cancers. Both genes map to human chromosome band 11q13. Because these two genes share the same chromosomal location, questions about their possible linkage and about the relationship between the mammary-specific oncogene and the steroid hormone in development growth, and hormone dependence of human cancers have been raised.

Other members of the steroid receptor superfamily, in addition to classic steroid hormone receptors, may contribute to growth regulation in malignant cells. Perhaps the most impressive example is the aberrant expression of the retinoic acid receptor (RAR) in acute promyelocytic leukemia. In this malignancy, the chromosomal translocation t(15;17) fuses RAR with a novel transcription factor, PML, producing a PML–RAR fusion protein. The constitutive activity of this fusion protein appears to block myeloid differentiation, perhaps by acting as a chimeric transcription factor to regulate genes involved in myeloid differentiation. Treatment of acute promyelocytic leukemia patients with retinoic acid induces clinical responses accompanied by leukemia cell differentiation. Hence, it would appear that the t(15;17) translocation places the PML gene product under the control of the RAR ligand-binding domain. A conclusive test of this hypothesis will require identification of PML–RAR target genes crucial for leukemogenesis.

Steroid hormone receptors may also be involved in the pathogenesis of cancer through their interaction with environmental toxins. In addition to the steroid hormone receptors that are members of the steroid receptor superfamily, a closely related receptor belonging to the helix–loop–helix family of transcription factors may also contribute to the pathogenesis of cancer via its interaction with environmental toxins. The aryl hydrocarbon hydroxylase receptor, or the Ah receptor, preferentially binds compounds known to induce microsomal aryl hydrocarbon hydroxylase. These compounds are polycyclic aromatic hydrocarbons (e.g., β-naphthoflavone, 3-methylcholanthrene, benzopyrene, and chlorinated hydrocarbons such as 2,3,7,8-tetrachlorodibenzo-p-dioxin, or TCDD). After binding any of these ligands, the Ah receptor regulates the expression of a number of genes coding for enzymes involved in the metabolism of foreign compounds (cytochrome P450s, glutathione S-transferases, quinone reductases, etc.). The Ah receptor mediates tumor promotion, including epithelial hyperplasia and metaplasia, lymphoid involution, and tetratogenesis, which are characteristic of TCDD exposure. The TCDD-induced thymic hypoplasia in many respects appears to be similar to glucocorticoid-induced atrophy of the thymus. Because the Ah receptor is present in almost every tissue examined, its potential for inducing neoplasia in a variety of tissues is formidable, although the precise role of the Ah receptor in specific tumors remains to be defined.

VI. MECHANISMS OF STEROID HORMONE-INDUCED TUMOR REGRESSION

The tumor regression properties of steroid hormones have been exploited since the early 1900s. It is a conundrum that steroid hormones are implicated not only in promoting tumor cell growth but also in inducing tumor regression.

For example, estradiol binding to the estrogen receptor stimulates the proliferation of breast cancer cells, yet the same receptor when binding the antiestrogen tamoxifen inhibits breast cancer cell growth. Antiestrogen binding sites distinct from the estrogen receptor have been identified in breast cancer cell lines; although these sites selectively bind antiestrogens, they do not appear to function directly to mediate the growth modulation effects of antiestrogens on breast cancer cells. Thus, it has been demonstrated that antiestrogens bind to the estrogen receptor and antagonize the binding of estradiol, although equilibrium binding analysis reveals that the antiestrogen tamoxifen interacts differently with the estrogen receptor than does estradiol. The precise mechanism through which antiestrogens inhibit tumor cell growth has not been defined; antiestrogens appears to act beyond the level of the tumor stem cell and thereby decrease the clonal growth of MCF-7 cells in a soft agar colony assay, consistent with the view that antiestrogens are cytostatic rather than cytotoxic for breast cancer cells. The cytostatic effect of tamoxifen is, at least in part, due to inhibition of growth factor release from tumor cells.

Glucocorticosteroids inhibit the proliferation of lymphoid tumor cells and are actually cytotoxic to lymphoid tumor cells. The ability of this hormone to lyse lymphoid cells is largely responsible for the efficacy of glucocorticoids as therapeutic agents for lymphoid malignancies including non-Hodgkin lymphomas and acute lymphoblastic leukemia. The specific mechanism of glucocorticoid action in lymphoid malignancies has been the subject of intense investigation but remains incompletely understood. However, much has been learned about the cytostatic effect of glucocorticoids from studies of cell lines, such as the P1798 murine lymphoma cell line, that are not lysed by glucocorticoids but whose growth is suppressed by glucocorticoids. In these cells, glucocorticoids disrupt the production of ribosomal RNA, through inhibition of the RNA polymerase I (Pol I) transcription initiation factor. The same effect is seen on the regulation of thymidine kinase. Glucocorticoids appear to have the general property of regulating the synthesis of certain transcription factors. Glucocorticoids also regulate the translation of a certain class of mRNAs, including those that encode ribosomal proteins. In addition, the effect of glucocorticoids on oncogene expression has been investigated. Steady state mRNA levels of c-myc, c-myb, and c-ki-ras are dramatically and rapidly decreased after glucocorticoid treatment of S49 mouse lymphoma cells. In another study, a variety of growth factors and oncogenes were investigated in a human lymphoid leukemia cell line, and only c-myc was found to be regulated by the glucocorticoid hormone dexamethasone.

Lymphoid cells, at immature stages of differentiation, are programmed to undergo an endogenous suicide process on exposure to pharmacological concentrations of glucocorticoids. This cell death program affects many metabolic processes, including inhibition of amino acid incorporation into protein due to a decreased rate of protein synthesis coupled with increased free amino acid pools that result from an accelerated rate of intracellular protein degradation. Glucocorticoid-induced lymphocytolysis in rat thymocytes is blocked by inhibitors of RNA and protein synthesis, suggesting that glucocorticoid regulation of a so-called lysis gene(s) may be the initiating event in glucocorticoid-induced cell death, although specific genes have not been identified. The characteristic morphology of glucocorticoid-induced lymphocytolysis includes nuclear pyknosis which, at the molecular level, is characterized by internucleosomal DNA fragmentation and which appears to precede overt cell death. Human acute lymphoblastic leukemia cells display the same pattern of DNA fragmentation as previously described in mouse lymphoma cell lines and in normal rat thymocytes, suggesting a common mechanism of glucocorticoid-induced lymphocytolysis in different species.

Studies examining androgen withdrawal as it relates to prostate atrophy are beginning to yield interesting results with implications about programmed cell death. Following withdrawal of hormonal stimuli, novel RNAs and proteins are expressed in prostate tissue. One gene, the testosterone repressed prostate message-2 (TRPM-2) is associated with cellular atrophy and death in many rodent tissues. Further characterization of this gene and its product will likely lead to a much better understanding of the events that occur during programmed cell death.

VII. MECHANISMS OF STEROID HORMONE UNRESPONSIVENESS IN TUMOR CELLS

During cancer cell ontogeny, tumor cells that were initially responsive to steroid hormones may become insensitive. This is the case in breast cancer, where the principal limitation to the utility of antiestrogens is the resistance that develops in tumors treated with these agents. Forty percent of patients with estrogen receptor-positive tumors fail to respond to antiestrogens; thus, the presence of estrogen receptors does not necessarily confer estrogen responsiveness. In some cases, tamoxifen resistance may be the result of an estrogen receptor defect. However, the estrogen receptors present in tamoxifen-resistant cells are often not different from those in tamoxifen-sensitive cells, suggesting that resistance to antiestrogens may take place at a step distal to the receptor site.

Hormonal unresponsiveness can result from a low or absent level of estrogen receptor expression in breast cancer cells. Studies have demonstrated that genetic defects may be responsible for decreased estrogen receptor expression in breast cancer cells. A restriction fragment length polymorphism has been identified in the human estrogen receptor gene. This study shows an association between one particular allele and the failure of breast cancer cells to express estrogen receptors. Additional reports have described a frequently occurring estrogen receptor variant that carries two point mutations in the region of the gene encoding the amino-terminal domain of the protein. Analysis of human estrogen receptor mRNA performed on 71 human breast tumors using an RNase protection assay has revealed a detectable mismatch in the RNA coding for the amino-terminal domain of the estrogen receptor. This mutation is associated with low levels of estrogen receptor and thus may have an indirect effect on the success of hormonal therapy. Further studies on the estrogen receptor at a genetic level have demonstrated base pair insertions, deletions, transitions, as well as complete deletion of exons 3, 5, and 7. These exon deletions produce the previously discussed outlaw receptors (see Section V). These mutations produce either dominant-positive receptors (transcriptionally active in the absence of estrogen) or dominant negative receptors (transcriptionally inactive but preventing function of the normal estrogen receptor). These receptor variations may play an important role in the development and treatment of breast cancer.

Glucocorticoid resistance occurs commonly in lymphoid malignancies and frequently limits the success of therapy. Glucocorticoids-mediated lymphocytolysis is contingent on a variety of factors, including the cellular level of glucocorticoid receptors and cAMP-dependent protein kinase activity. The loss of protein kinase activity coincides with a measurable decrease of steroid sensitivity in murine T lymphoma cells. Thus, modulation of the sensitivity of lymphoma cells to steroid hormones may be mediated by cAMP, affecting the level of glucocorticoid receptors as well as the efficiency of the receptor in producing a cytolytic response. The ability of steroid hormones to cross the cell membrane may also be a determinant of glucocorticoid resistance in murine thymoma cells. In addition, a variety of defects in the glucocorticoid receptor have been shown to produce glucocorticoid resistance in mouse lymphoma cell lines. Although the most frequent cause of glucocorticoid resistance is a deficiency of glucocorticoid receptors, in some resistant clones glucocorticoid resistance is due to mutations in the receptor coding sequence that give rise to receptors that function abnormally. Alternative splicing has been the mechanism proposed to be responsible for mutant glucocorticoid receptors being produced in at least one case. In response to glucocorticoid treatment of multiple myeloma, myeloma cells produce glucocorticoid receptors that have been alternatively spliced and no longer respond to glucocorticoids; this aberrant glucocorticoid receptor therefore contributes to resistance of glucocorticoid treatment. Human lymphoid leukemia cells have also been demonstrated to be glucocorticoid resistant because of receptor defects. In certain mouse and human lymphoid lines, glucocorticoid resistance occurs in the presence of a normal complement of functional glucocorticoid receptors. In this case, glucocorticoid resistance has been suggested to be due to a defect(s) at a locus other than the receptor locus. These resistant mutants may have a mutation in the lysis gene (see Section VI), or, alternatively, the lysis gene may be

inactivated during differentiation, possibly through methylation of DNA.

It is important to bear in mind that glucocorticoid resistance may arise *in vivo* by mechanisms different from those *in vitro*. This conclusion stems from work in the P1798 murine lymphoma cell line. P1798 mouse lymphoma cells are functionally haploid. Variants selected for dexamethasone resistance in culture have lost the receptor, whereas selection for resistance to cytolysis *in vivo* is not associated with receptor mutations. Also, cells that are resistant to the cytolytic effects of glucocorticoids *in vivo* may be sensitive to antiproliferative effects of glucocorticoids in culture, whereas cells that are resistant to dexamethasone in culture may undergo cytolysis when treated with dexamethasone *in vivo*. Thus, different mechanisms may be involved in the loss of glucocorticoid responsiveness *in vivo* and *in vitro*. These findings are particularly provocative as we attempt to understand the mechanism of glucocorticoid resistance in acute lymphoblastic leukemia and lymphoma in humans. Thus, *in vitro* assays for glucocorticoid resistance and mechanisms of glucocorticoid resistance *in vitro* may not pertain to the situation *in vivo*.

VIII. USE OF STEROID HORMONE RECEPTORS AS PROGNOSTIC MARKERS

A mechanism for assessing the levels of hormonal receptors in tumor cells has been demonstrated to be a very good indicator for the therapeutic response of tumor cells to steroid hormone treatment. For example, estrogen and progesterone receptors have been investigated extensively as prognostic markers in breast cancer. Biochemical and sensitive immunocytochemical assays to measure receptor levels have been employed and appear to give comparable results. Likewise, the presence of estrogen receptors in breast tumors is of significant prognostic importance. Patients whose tumors display high levels of estrogen receptor have a significantly better prognosis than patients with receptor-negative tumors. Also, the presence of estrogen and progesterone receptors in breast tumors is an important predictor of hormonal responsiveness; patients with advanced breast cancer in whom estrogen receptor status is negative by immunocytochemical assay generally fail to respond to estrogen therapy. Metastatic breast cancer is also predicted by levels of the progesterone receptor, where a high level of receptors is generally indicative of responsiveness to hormone treatment.

The predicative value of receptor levels is not limited to breast cancers, as both estrogen and progesterone receptors are detectable in endometrial adenocarcinoma cells, where the level of these receptors correlates with the degree of cellular differentiation. Immunocytochemical assays of fresh frozen sections of endometrial carcinoma tissue demonstrate considerable heterogeneity in terms of the cellular distribution of estrogen and progesterone receptors. In general, estrogen receptor content is low in tumor tissue compared to normal proliferative or hyperplastic endometrium. Estrogen and progesterone receptors are important prognostic markers in endometrial cancer. There is an inverse correlation between surgical stage and estrogen receptor content of primary tumor specimens. In stage I and II endometrial cancer, estrogen and progesterone receptor status were found to be significant prognostic factors; prognosis was better in patients with tumors positive for estrogen and progesterone receptors than in patients with receptor-negative tumors. The presence of progesterone receptors in biopsy specimens, however, does not necessarily predict a therapeutic response to progesterone therapy; only 60% of cases positive for progesterone receptors respond to progesterone treatment.

In the same manner, the level of glucocorticoid receptors in human acute lymphoblastic leukemia cells varies according to the subtype of leukemia. T-Cell acute lymphoblastic leukemia cells have, on average, fewer glucocorticoid receptors than non-T, non-B cell acute lymphoblastic leukemia cells. Unfortunately, although there is a correlation between the presence of glucocorticoid receptors in human leukemia and lymphoma cells and both *in vitro* and *in vivo* response to treatment with glucocorticoids, the range of glucocorticoid receptors is sufficiently broad and the overlap of receptor levels from responders and nonresponders is so great that measurement of glucocorticoid receptors in acute lymphoblastic leukemia or lymphoma samples has not become a reliable prognostic indicator. Hence, the presence of glucocorticoid receptors in a sample of leukemia cells does not guarantee glucocorticoid responsiveness.

IX. SUMMARY AND CONCLUSIONS

The molecular basis for the effects of steroid hormones and their action through their cognate receptors are beginning to emerge. At the clinical level, the role of steroid hormones in the pathogenesis and treatment of malignancy is now beginning to be understood at the molecular level. As more information is gathered pertaining to the mechanisms involved in steroid hormone interaction with tumor cells, it is likely that this information will lead to new clinical approaches for treatment of cancer.

See Also the Following Articles

BREAST CANCER • CORTICOSTEROIDS • ENDOCRINE TUMORS • ESTROGENS AND ANTIESTROGENS • HORMONAL CARCINOGENESIS • HORMONE RESISTANCE IN PROSTATE CANCER • PANCREATIC CANCER: CELLULAR AND MOLECULAR MECHANISMS

Bibliography

Beato, M. (1989). Gene regulation by steroid hormones. *Cell (Cambridge, Mass.)* **56,** 335–344.

Evans, R. M. (1988). The steroid and thyroid hormone receptor superfamily. *Science* **240,** 889–895.

Graham II, M. L., Dalquist, K. E., and Horowitz, K. B. (1989). Simultaneous measurement of progesterone receptors and DNA indices by flow cytometry: Analysis of breast cancer cell mixtures and genetic instability of the T47D line. *Cancer Res.* **49,** 3943–3949.

Lippman, M. E., and Dickson, R. B. (1989). Mechanisms of growth in normal and malignant breast epithelium. *Rec. Prog. Horm. Res.* **45,** 383–440.

McGuire, W. L., Chamness, G. C., and Fuqua, S. A. W. (1991). Estrogen receptor variants in clinical breast cancer. *Mol. Endocrinol.* **5,** 1571–1577.

O'Malley, B. (1990). The steroid receptor superfamily: More excitement predicted for the future. *Mol. Endocrinol.* **4,** 363–369.

Pratt, W. B. (1993). The role of heat shock proteins in regulating the function, folding, and trafficking of the glucocorticoid receptor. *J. Biol. Chem.* **268,** 21455–21458.

Smith, D. F., and Toft, D. O. (1993). Steroid receptors and their associated proteins. *Mol. Endocrinol.* **7,** 6–11.

Suicide Genes

John C. Morris
National Cancer Institute, Bethesda, Maryland

R. Michael Blaese
ValiGen, Inc., Newtown, Pennsylvania

GLOSSARY

bystander effect (BSE) The ability to kill a greater number of cells in a mixed culture or in a tumor than the fraction of cells expressing the suicide gene. BSE is the result of the transfer of activated prodrug from the cells expressing the suicide gene to cells not expressing the gene.

catalytic constant (K_{cat}) A measure of the efficiency of an enzyme.

cDNA The complementary DNA of a mature spliced mRNA sequence of an expressed gene. It carries the coding sequence of the gene without the introns and is used in place of the larger genomic sequence for gene transfer and expression.

gap junction A highly specialized channel formed between two cells for transfer of small molecules between the cells.

kinase An enzyme that catalyzes the addition of a phosphate moiety to another molecule.

negative selective marker A genetic trait (gene) when expressed, that sensitizes a cell to the toxic effects of a specific drug or class of drugs.

positive selective marker Usually a gene that confers resistance to cells to the toxic effects of a specific drug or class of drugs.

prodrug A typically nontoxic substrate drug that, when added to cells expressing a specific suicide enzyme, is converted into a highly toxic compound, killing the cells.

suicide gene A gene that encodes an enzyme that converts a substrate prodrug into a cytotoxic product.

symporter A cell membrane-associated macromolecular complex that transports specific substrates across a cell membrane.

"Suicide" gene therapy, also known as enzyme-prodrug therapy, involves the transfer of a gene encoding an enzyme into a target tissue, usually a tumor. To confer selectivity, a unique enzyme, usually of viral or bacterial origin, is often used. When the target cells expressing the enzyme are exposed to an ordinarily nontoxic agent known as the prodrug, it is converted into a toxic compound by the enzymatic activity encoded by the transferred gene, killing the cells (Fig. 1). Recombinant viral vectors are the most frequently utilized method of suicide gene transfer; however, direct injection of plasmid DNA and liposomal-mediated gene transfer have also been used. The suicide gene/prodrug paradigm was one of the earliest and is still the most commonly used approach in clinical cancer gene therapy.

I. INTRODUCTION

Early suicide gene systems grew out of efforts to develop cell lines with traits that could be selected by exposure to various agents. The most commonly used selectable traits are positive selectable markers, such as a gene that confers resistance to a toxic antibiotic. A negative selectable marker is a gene whose expression will sensitize cells to a specific drug or class of drugs. Historically, the development of suicide gene systems was an attempt to address fears that random integration of retroviral gene transfer vectors into the host cells could cause insertional mutagenesis and the development of cancers in patients treated with these vectors. Indeed, an early study that used a vector preparation contaminated with recombinant replication-competent retrovirus caused T-cell lymphomas in rhesus macaques. By incorporating a suicide gene into the vector design, if malignant transformation was to occur, the prodrug could be administered to the patient that then would be activated by the suicide gene and eliminate the malignant cells. It was not long before it was recognized that this approach might prove useful as an anticancer therapy.

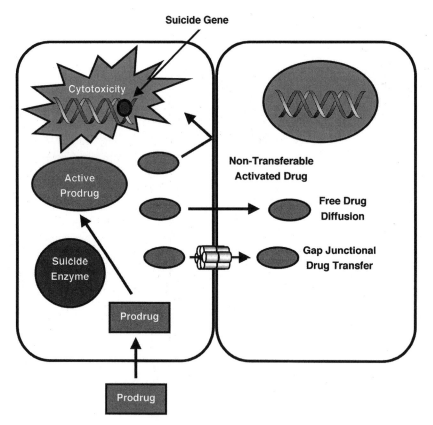

FIGURE 1 Components of a typical suicide gene/prodrug system. A gene is transferred into a cell that encodes a "suicide" enzyme that activates a nontoxic prodrug into a toxic drug at high concentrations, killing the cell. The activated drug may be restricted to the cell expressing the enzyme or it may exhibit a bystander effect by transfer of the activated drug by simple diffusion or through cellular gap junctions to cells lacking the suicide gene.

II. PRINCIPLES OF SUICIDE GENE THERAPY

The basic components of a suicide gene/prodrug system are a gene (cDNA) encoding an enzyme capable of converting an otherwise nontoxic prodrug into a cytotoxic compound, and the prodrug itself. The ideal suicide gene should exhibit certain traits: (1) The expression of the gene itself should cause no toxicity in the absence of the prodrug; (2) the enzyme should have a high catalytic constant (K_{cat}) rapidly activating the prodrug, (3) it should work efficiently at low prodrug concentrations, (4) the gene should encode a relatively low molecular weight protein due to size restrictions of commonly use gene transfer vectors, and (5) the encoded enzyme should be a monomeric protein to avoid having to incorporate more than one coding sequence into the vector or having the appropriate relative expression of each subunit to achieve a functional enzyme. Characteristics of the ideal prodrug include (1) lack of toxicity in the absence of expression of the suicide gene, (2) use of a clinically approved drug such as an antimicrobial, (3) a long half-life of the activated prodrug, and (4) a drug with a "bystander effect" is usually desirable, at least for use in cancer treatment (Fig. 2). The bystander effect (BSE) is the ability of a suicide enzyme/prodrug system to kill a greater fraction of tumor than the number of cells actually expressing the suicide enzyme. The BSE is believed to be due to the transfer of activated prodrug between cells by various mechanisms. Other beneficial characteristics may include cell cycle-specific toxicity to target proliferating (cancer) cells. It has been estimated that the active drug in an enzyme/prodrug system should be at least 100-fold more toxic than the inactive prodrug to achieve an ideal therapeutic index.

III. HERPES SIMPLEX VIRUS THYMIDINE KINASE/GANCICLOVIR

The most common suicide gene in clinical use is the herpes simplex virus type-1 thymidine kinase (HSV-tk). Its use grew out of the recognition that the antiviral nucleoside analogs acyclovir (ACV) and ganciclovir (GCV) selectively kill cells infected with herpes viruses. This selectivity was found to be due to expres-

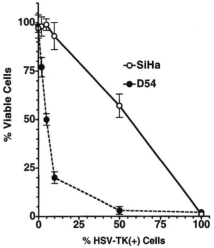

FIGURE 2 The bystander effect (BSE) of the HSV-tk/GCV suicide enzyme/prodrug system. SiHa human cervical cancer cells and D54 astrocytoma cells were infected with a recombinant adenovirus expressing HSV-tk and mixed in varying proportions with nontransduced cells of the same type. After 6 days of incubation in 10 μM GCV, D54 cells show a dramatic decrease in viability disproportionate to the fraction of HSV-tk-positive cells in the coculture. D54 cells express cellular gap junctions allowing the transfer of activated (phosphorylated) GCV between HSV-tk-positive cells and HSV-tk-negative cells. SiHa cells show no enhanced killing beyond the fraction of the population expressing HSV-tk. SiHa cells express few gap junctions.

sion of the viral thymidine kinase. HSV-tk exhibits 200-fold higher activity for the ATP-dependent monophosphorylation of GCV to generate GCV-MP than mammalian thymidine kinase. Native cellular kinases then rapidly catalyze the subsequent di- and triphosphorylation of GCV-MP. When exposed to GCV, mammalian cells expressing HSV-tk rapidly accumulate intracellular GCV phosphate. In contrast, little phosphorylated GCV is found in HSV-tk-negative cell lines. These phosphorylated nucleoside analogs are toxic to proliferating cells by a variety of mechanisms, including inhibition of DNA polymerase, induction of base pair mismatches, and result in DNA fragmentation. Although active in the conversion of ACV and GCV, the thymidine kinase of HSV-2 has not been well studied as a suicide gene system.

The combination of HSV-tk gene transfer and antiviral nucleoside treatment as a potential anticancer strategy was proposed by Moolten after he observed mouse fibroblasts expressing the HSV-tk gene were sensitized to concentrations of GCV 1000-fold lower than wild-type cells and that GCV treatment induced the regression of HSV-tk-transduced sarcomas in mice. He subsequently demonstrated that administration of GCV to transgenic mice expressing HSV-tk under the control of the immunoglobulin promoter resulted in the regression of virally induced lymphomas.

Relatively low levels of HSV-tk expression will sensitize mammalian cells to GCV. Whether intracellular levels HSV-tk exhibit a dose–response effect is controversial. A 10-fold difference in GCV sensitivity was found to correlate with the amount of HSV-tk expression in retroviral-transduced human colon carcinoma cells and rat glioma cells. Cells infected with increasing amounts of an HSV-tk-expressing adenovirus showed increased HSV-tk activity and increased GCV sensitivity. Others have reported little or no dose effect. In a comparison of adenoviral vectors in which HSV-tk expression was driven by either the RSV promoter or the CMV promoter, no difference was found in antitumor activity, despite 20-fold higher levels of HSV-tk expression from the vector with the CMV promoter. The most likely explanation for these conflicting results is that expression of HSV-tk beyond a level that sensitizes cells by 100-fold to GCV does not appear to further enhance cell killing. A prodrug dose effect, however, is clear. Higher doses of GCV result in a greater fractional killing of HSV-tk-expressing cells in culture, as well as increased tumor response rates and survival of animals bearing HSV-tk-positive tumors. Although GCV is the most commonly used prodrug in the system, acyclovir and oral penciclovir are also active and have been used in clinical trials. In addition, the sensitivity of cells to HSV-tk/GCV may also depend on the activity of the other cellular kinases that perform the secondary and tertiary phosphorylations of the drug and the ongoing level of DNA synthesis.

Even the most efficient vectors are only successful in gene transfer to a small minority of cells in a tumor. An early surprising discovery was that not every cell need express HSV-tk in order to kill the majority of cells in a culture or achieve tumor regression in animal models. This phenomenon is termed the bystander effect. Most current evidence suggests that the HSV-tk/GCV enzyme/prodrug system BSE is mediated by the transfer of highly electrostatically charged nondiffusable GCV-phosphate through inter-

cellular gap junctions between cells. Other possible mechanisms include phagocytosis of GCV-phosphate-containing apoptotic vesicles by surrounding tumor cells or the recruitment of an antitumor immune response stimulated by tumor necrosis. Rodent models have demonstrated that treatment of tumors with HSV-tk/GCV can induce antitumor immunity that renders the mice resistant to rechallenge with the same tumor cell line. Immunophenotyping studies show that this response is mediated by $CD8^+$ cytoloytic T cells and natural killer cells.

The HSV-tk/GCV system was the first suicide gene/prodrug system to receive approval for phase I clinical trials and is now the subject of a number of ongoing human gene therapy trials, mostly for treatment of cancer. One of the earliest studies looked at the safety and efficacy of retroviral-mediated HSV-tk gene transfer and GCV administration in patients with recurrent brain tumors. Nineteen lesions in 15 patients underwent CT-guided injection of murine retroviral vector producer cells expressing HSV-tk. One week later, patients began a 14-day course of intravenous GCV. Responses were seen in 6 of 19 treated lesions (5/15 patients). The median duration of response was 6.5 weeks (range, 4–220+ weeks) and all responses were limited to smaller tumors. Gene expression and *in situ* transduction of tumor cells with HSV-tk could be confirmed, but were significantly less than 5% of the tumor cells. Another small trial compared retroviral- to adenoviral-mediated HSV-tk gene transfer and subsequent GCV treatment to patients with primary brain tumors. Patients underwent craniotomy and tumor resection and then had a recombinant adenoviral vector or a retroviral producer cell line expressing HSV-tk injected into the resection margins followed by GCV treatment. Fever and seizures were the major toxicities; however, survival in the adenoviral vector-treated group was significantly longer than the other treatment groups. Results of a randomized phase III trial of patients with newly diagnosed glioblastoma multiforme comparing standard treatment with surgical resection and radiotherapy to standard treatment plus HSV-tk gene transfer and GCV administration have been reported. In this study involving 248 patients, the medium time to progression in the gene therapy group was 180 days compared to 183 days for the standard therapy arm. Overall survival for the gene therapy group was 365 and 354 days in the standard therapy arm, indicating no significant difference in outcome. This study again highlighted the problem of the low levels of gene transfer achieved with current vectors.

A phase I trial of adenoviral-mediated HSV-tk gene transfer and GCV treatment was performed in patients with malignant pleural mesothelioma. Cohorts of patients were treated with increasing doses of vector injected into the affected pleural cavity. Systemic GCV treatment was initiated 24 h later and continued for 2 weeks. Low levels of gene transfer were documented in 11 of 20 patients, and side effects were generally mild and included fever, anemia, skin rash, granulocytopenia, elevation of serum liver enzymes, and transient hypoxemia. No tumor regression was noted in any patient. In another study, 18 patients with locally recurrent prostate cancer were treated in dose-cohort escalation with an adenoviral vector expressing HSV-tk and subsequent GCV. One patient at the highest dose developed thrombocytopenia and hepatotoxicity. Three patients had a 50% decline in serum prostatic-specific antigen levels, suggesting a tumor response.

The HSV-tk/GCV system has been successfully used to remove alloreactive donor lymphocytes in acute graft-versus-host disease (GvHD) in allogeneic bone marrow transplant patients. T-cell-depleted allogeneic bone marrow transplantation as a treatment for leukemia is associated with a higher risk of relapse because of the loss of the graft-versus-leukemia (GvL) effect, as well as an increased incidence of posttransplant Epstein–Barr virus (EBV)-induced lymphoma. Infusions of peripheral blood T lymphocytes derived from the marrow donors have been successful in treating these complications, but at the risk of developing severe or fatal GvHD. There are now several reports on the successful use of HSV-tk transduced allogeneic donor lymphocytes to treat this complication. Patients developing GvHD have the autoreactive donor T cells effectively removed by GCV treatment. The ability to exploit the GvL effect and to prevent transplant-associated lymphoproliferative disease while being able to eliminate immunoreactive donor T cells with the suicide gene/prodrug system represents a significant advance in therapy.

IV. CYTOSINE DEAMINASE/ 5-FLUOROCYTOSINE

Cytosine deaminase (CD) is an inducible enzyme expressed by *Escherichia coli* and certain fungi, not found in mammalian cells, and catalyzes the hydrolyic deamination of cytosine to uracil during times of nutritional stress. CD can also deaminate the antifungal drug 5-fluorocytosine (5FC) to the antineoplastic fluoropyrimidine 5-fluorouracil (5FU). Cellular enzymes convert 5FU to nucleosides by the addition of ribose and deoxyribose. Subsequent phosphorylation generates 5-fluorouridine-5′-triphosphate (5-FUTP), 5-fluorodeoxyuridine-5′-triphosphate (5′FdUTP), and 5-fluoro-2′-deoxyuridine-5′-monophosphate (FdUMP). These compounds irreversibly inhibit the enzyme thymidylate synthase and block both DNA and RNA synthesis, leading to cell death. Most studies of CD have used the *E. coli* enzyme because of its shorter gene sequence (1.3 kb) and greater stability; however, it has been suggested that fungal CD is more active than the bacterial enzyme in the conversion of 5FC. As a prodrug, 5FC has several advantages: (1) it is not deaminated in mammalian cells and therefore has little intrinsic toxicity, (2) oral 5FC is well absorbed, and (3) it is an approved drug with a known clinical profile.

Mammalian cell lines expressing CD convert cytosine to uracil and are killed when exposed to low concentrations of 5FC, whereas the parental cell lines are unaffected. Biochemical analysis of mammalian cells expressing CD incubated with 5FC show measurable intracellular levels of 5FU, inhibition of thymidylate synthase, and formation of RNA adducts. Human cell lines expressing CD are sensitized 100- to 10,000-fold over wild-type cells. WiDr colon carcinoma xenografts in athymic nude mice do not respond to systemic injections of 5FU, but regress after CD gene transfer followed by the administration of 5FC. Unlike the HSV-tk/GCV system, the activity of 5FU is not S phase specific, but does require proliferating cells for its effect. Killing is slower than the HSV-tk/GCV system due to the slower uptake of 5FC by cells compared to GCV. Despite slower cell killing, animal studies comparing CD/5FC to the HSV-tk/GCV system in at least one tumor cell line found CD/5FC to be more active because of its greater BSE. Limitations of the CD/5FC system are the short half-life of 5FU ($t_{1/2}$ ~10–20 min) and the relatively high intracellular concentrations of 5FU required for activity in some tumors.

The prodrug 5FC exhibits a dose–response effect. Higher 5FC concentrations result in greater fractional cell killing of CD-expressing cells. The dose effect of CD gene expression is not as clear and may ultimately depend on the intrinsic sensitivity of the particular cell line to 5FU. Cytotoxicity in sensitive cell lines such as colon, breast, and lung cancer appears to correlate with the degree of CD expression. In less sensitive sarcoma cell lines, a CD dose–response is not clear.

The CD/5FC system exhibits a potent BSE that does not require the expression of gap junctions or cell-to-cell contact. The activated prodrug, 5FU, is a small nonpolar molecule that easily diffuses across cell membranes. In contrast to the HSV-tk/GCV system, where no phosphorylated (activated) GCV is detectable in the media, 5FU can be measured in the conditioned media of CD-expressing cell lines exposed to 5FC. Transfer of cell-free supernatants from CD-expressing cell lines exposed to 5FC to nonexpressing cells causes cytotoxicity, and the BSE of CD/5FC is unaffected in cell lines lacking gap junctions. The magnitude of the CD/5FC BSE is dependent on the intrinsic sensitivity of the cell line to 5FU. Initial studies of this system showed a minimal BSE. This may be a result of the relatively 5FU-resistant sarcoma model used. Studies using sensitive cell lines found a strong BSE with as few as 2% CD-expressing cells in a tumor mass resulting in complete regression of WiDr tumors in athymic nude mice after treatment with 5FC. The CD/5FC system has also been found to sensitize cells to radiotherapy. Experimental expression of CD and 5FC treatment immunized mice against rechallenge by the same tumor cell line. CD/5FC reliably induced immunity against the poorly immunogenic TS/A murine breast cancer in BALB/c mice. Treating with anti-CD8 antibodies could block this "vaccine" response.

Several clinical trials of the CD/5FC system are in progress; however, only one of these studies has been reported. In a phase I trial, 12 women with advanced breast cancer and skin nodules underwent intratumoral injection of a DNA plasmid expressing CD under the transcriptional control of the erbB2 promoter and systemic administration of 5FC. CD expression was demonstrated in 11/12 patients by a variety of methods, and a reduction in tumor volume was noted in 4 patients. No serious toxicity was seen. Trials using adenoviral mediated CD gene transfer into liver metastases and other tumors followed by systemic 5FC are in progress; however, no results have been reported.

V. OTHER SUICIDE GENE/ PRODRUG SYSTEMS

A number of other suicide gene-prodrug systems are currently under investigation (Table I). Most of these systems are incompletely characterized, are in early stages of preclinical development, or lack approved prodrugs, slowing their introduction into clinical trials. What role they will play in clinical suicide gene/prodrug therapy remains to be seen. Some of the better characterized systems are discussed.

A. Carboxylesterase/CPT-11

CPT-11 (irinotecan, 7-ethyl-10-[4-(1-piperidino)-1-piperidino]carbonyloxy-camptothecin), a member of the camptothecin class of topoisomerase I inhibitors, is an active agent in colorectal and other cancers. CPT-11 is converted to its active form (SN38) by a class of enzymes known as carboxylesterases (CEs). CEs are a group of widely distributed isoenzymes important in the metabolism of a number of pharmaceutical agents. CE is overexpressed in many tumors, conferring sensitivity to CPT-11. The local activation of CPT-11 by intestinal CE is believed to account for much of its toxicity. The efficiency of conversion of CPT-11 to its active form SN38 (7-ethyl-10-hydroxycamptothecin) exhibits a high degree of species and isoenzyme specificity. In humans, hepatic carboxylesterase I appears to be the most active enzyme, however, human CE has a relatively low K_{cat}. CEs from several other mammalian species, including rhesus macaque, rabbit, pig, and rat, have significantly higher specific activities for converting CPT-11 to SN-38. Although human and rabbit hepatic CE share more than 80% homology, the rabbit enzyme is 100- to 1000-fold more efficient at converting CPT-11.

TABLE I
Suicide Gene/Prodrug Systems in Clinical Trials and Development

Suicide gene	Source	Prodrug	Activated drug	Bystander effect
Clinical trials				
Thymidine kinase (*tk*)	*herpes simplex* virus-1	Ganciclovir, acyclovir	Ganciclovir, acyclovir monophosphate	Yes, requires gap junctions, ?apoptotic vesicles
Cytosine deaminase (*cd*)	*E. coli*, fungi	5-Fluorocytosine (5FC)	5-Fluorouracil	Yes, simple diffusion
Carboxypeptidase G2	*Pseudomonas*	CMDA	CMDA-mustard	Yes, simple diffusion
CYP 2B1 (cytochrome P450)	Human, rat	Cyclophosphamide, ifosfamide	4-Hydroxycyclophosphamide, 4-hydroxyifosfamide	Yes, simple diffusion
Preclinical trials				
Carboxylesterase	Rabbit	CPT-11 (irinotecan)	SN38	Little or more
CYP 4B1 (cytochrome P450)	Rabbit	2-Aminoanthracene 4-ipomeanol	Unsaturated and furan epoxides	Yes, simple diffusion, but enhanced by cell contact
Deoxycytidine kinase	Human	Cytosine arabinoside (AraC) fludarabine	AraC or fludarabine monophosphate	Weak, via gap junctions?
Guanosine-xanthine phosphoribosyl transferase (*gpt*)	*E. coli*	6-Thioxanthine (6-TX), 6-thioguanine (6-TG)	6-TX or 6-TG monophosphate	Weak to moderate, via gap junctions
Nitroreductase	*E. coli*	CB1954	Hydroxylamine-alkylating agent	Yes, simple diffusion
Purine nucleoside phosphorylase (*DeoD*)	*E. coli*	6-Methylpurine deoxyribosenucleoside	6-Methylpurine	Yes, simple diffusion
Sodium/iodide symporter	Human, rat	Iodine-131	Concentrated iodine-131	Yes, radioactive emissions
Thymidine phosphorylase	*E. coli*	5'-DFUR, tegafur	5-Fluorouracil	Yes, simple diffusion

Human rhabdomyosarcoma cells engineered to express the rabbit CE gene are up to 55-fold more sensitive to CPT-11 than the parental cell line. Mice bearing rhabdomyosarcoma xenografts expressing rabbit hepatic CE were cured of tumor when treated with CPT-11 compared to 0/7 mice with nontransduced tumors. The CE/CPT-11 system exhibits little bystander effect.

B. Carboxypeptidase G2/CMDA

The bacterial enzyme carboxypeptidase G2 (CPG2) is a member of a family of zinc-containing metalloendopeptidases isolated from *Pseudomonas* RS16. It catalyzes the cleavage of amidic, urethanic, and ureidic bonds between a benzene ring and L-glutamic acid. A number of aromatic nitrogen mustard prodrugs are activated by CPG2 to potent alkylating agents. The most commonly used prodrug is 4-([2-chloroethyl][2-mesyloxyethyl]amino)benzyol-L-glutamic acid (CMDA). CPG2 cleaves a glutamic acid moiety from CMDA to generate its benzoic acid-

mustard derivative. Expression of CPG2 sensitizes mammalian cells 95-fold to CMDA. However, unactivated CMDA does not permeate cell membranes and cannot directly enter cells to be activated by intracellular CPG2. To overcome this problem, a cell membrane surface tethered (st) CPG2 enzyme/prodrug system was developed. The stCPG2/CMDA system exhibits a BSE, suggesting the cells are permeable to the activated drug. Other approaches use the CPG2 enzyme conjugated to F(ab')$_2$ fragments of monoclonal antibodies directed against carcinoembryonic antigen (CEA). Treatment with the F(ab')$_2$–anti-CEA–CPG2 conjugate, followed by administration of CMDA, has been shown to be effective against human LoVo colon carcinoma xenografts in athymic nude mice. A phase I pharmacokinetic trial in which an F(ab')$_2$–anti-CEA–CPG2 conjugate was administered to 10 patients with recurrent CEA-positive colorectal cancer, followed by administration of CMDA, was reported. Analysis of tissue and blood samples showed restriction of CPG2 activity to tumor and local prodrug activation.

C. Cytochrome P450 (CYP) Enzymes

Suicide gene/prodrug systems utilizing hepatic microsomal cytochrome P450 enzymes (CYP) to activate a number of different prodrugs are under investigation. Cytochrome P450 is a complex system of isoenzymes with many different substrates that activate the oxazaphosphorine alkylators cyclophosphamide (CP) and ifosfamide (IF). The use of an alkylating agent in an enzyme/prodrug system offers several advantages: (1) cell cycle-independent killing, (2) a low incidence of drug resistance, and (3) a significant difference in cytotoxicity between the prodrug and its activated form. CYP enzymes are expressed primarily in the liver, but may be also expressed in certain cancers, including colon, breast, lung, kidney, and prostate. The isoenzyme CYP 2B1 efficiently activates CP and IF by 4-hydroxylation. The prodrug intermediates 4-hydroxycyclophosphamide (4-HC) and 4-hydroxyifosfamide (4-IF) are rapidly converted into the short-lived bifunctional alkylating agent phosphoramide mustard cross-linking DNA, causing G_2–M arrest and apoptosis. Cells engineered to express CYP 2B1 can be sensitized up to 20-fold to CP and IF. Rats inoculated with CYP 2B1-expressing 9L gliosarcoma cells had complete suppression of tumor growth after treatment with CP, whereas animals injected with wild-type cells developed tumors, despite systemic treatment with CP. Local conversion of CP and IF in tumors to their 4-hydroxy metabolites is more advantageous than hepatic activation of a systemically administered drug because of the short plasma half-lives of these compounds. This system exhibits a moderately strong BSE that appears to be mediated by diffusion of the 4-hydroxy intermediates. A system using the combination of the rabbit CYP 4B1 isoenzyme and 2-aminoanthracene (2-AA) or 4-ipomeanol (4-IM) has been reported. CYP 4B1 selectively converts 2-AA and 4-IM into potent alkylating agents. The activated drugs are highly toxic at very low concentrations and exhibit a powerful BSE with as few as 1% of the cells expressing CYP 4B1.

In a phase I/II trial, 14 patients with inoperable pancreatic cancer were treated with allogeneic cells (293 human embryonic kidney) expressing CYP 2B1 encapsulated in a semipermeable membrane and delivered by angiography to the tumor followed by systemically administered IF. Four tumor regressions were reported, as well as improved median and 1-year survivals when these patients were compared to historical controls. The significance of the improved survival in this small single arm study is uncertain. Twelve adverse events were reported in 7 patients, including cholangitis, gastrointestinal bleeding, a false aneurysm (femoral artery), and a pulmonary embolism that were believed unrelated to the treatment.

D. Deoxycytidine Kinase

Deoxycytidine kinase (dCK) is being investigated as a potential suicide gene based on the observation that responses to the nucleoside analog drugs cytosine arabinoside (AraC), 2-chlorodeoxyadenosine (2CdA), and fludarabine correlate with expression of dCK in the leukemic cells. Deoxycytidine kinase-dependent phosphorylation is the rate-limiting step in the activation of AraC. Phosphorylated AraC, a cytidine analog, is incorporated into replicating DNA, introducing lethal strand breaks. Although AraC is a potent antileukemic agent, it has little activity against most solid tumors. Experimental transfer of the dCK gene into rat glioma cells sensitized them to AraC. However, others have failed to demonstrate increased AraC sensitivity of lung cancer cell lines transduced with the dCK gene. The explanation for these different results may be that AraC sensitivity is not only determined by dCK activity, but also by cellular transporters that concentrate AraC in the cell, as well as other enzymes necessary in the biochemical pathways that activate the drug.

E. Guanosine-Xanthine Phosphoribosyl Transferase (*gpt*)

The *E. coli* guanosine-xanthine phosphoribosyl transferase (*gpt*) gene is unique in that this gene simultaneously confers sensitivity to thioxanthines and resistance to mycophenolic acid, xanthine, and hypoxanthine, allowing both positive and negative selection of cells expressing the gene. Cells are sensitized to 6-thioxanthine (6-TX) and 6-thioguanine (6-TG) by GPT-catalyzed phosphorylation. Retroviral transduction of rat C6 glioma cells with *gpt* increased their sensitivity to 6-TX by 50- to 100-fold. Injection of retroviral vector producer cells expressing *gpt* into intracerebral tumors in athymic nude mice followed by treatment with 6-TX resulted in an 80% reduction in mean tumor volume and improved survival compared to control animals. GPT also activates 6-TG, a drug already in clinical use. Similar to the HSV-tk/GCV system, cell-to-cell contact is required to achieve a BSE because activated 6-TX and 6-TG are phosphorylated and will not freely diffuse between cells.

F. Nitroreductase/CB1954

E. coli nitroreductase (NTR) exhibits a significantly higher catalytic constant (K_{cat}) for the prodrug CB1954 [5-(aziridin-1-yl)-2,4-dinitrobenzamide] than the mammalian homologue DT-diaphorase [NAD(P)H dehydrongenase (quinone)]. NTR is able to reduce CB1954 more than 90-fold faster than DT-diaphorase. The prodrug CB1954, a mustard-like compound, is rapidly converted to a bifunctional hydroxylamine alkylating agent by reduction of its nitro groups. Further reactions with cellular thioesters result in a reactive species that forms DNA interstrand cross-links that are difficult to repair and strand breakage, leading to apoptosis. A flavoprotein with a molecular mass of 24 kDa, NTR requires NADH or NADPH as cofactors. Its mammalian counterpart shares no sequence homology. Cells expressing NTR are sensitized 500- to 2600-fold to CB1954. The onset of cytotoxicity is rapid, occurring after as little as 4 h of exposure to CB1954 *in vitro* and within 24 h *in vivo*. The NTR/CB1954 system is not cell cycle specific. Killing is seen in both actively cycling and quiescent cells. Retroviral- or adenoviral-mediated transfer of the NTR gene followed by CB1954 causes tumor regression and improves the survival of nude mice with human ovarian, pancreatic, hepatocellular, and squamous cell carcinoma xenografts. The NTR/CB1954 system exhibits a strong BSE independent of the expression of cellular gap junctions. The BSE appears to be due to the free diffusion of the 2- and 4-hydroxylamine metabolites and may be seen with as few as 5% NTR-expressing cells. However, significant variability between cell lines has been reported. This is likely due to differences in the intrinsic sensitivities of the cell lines to the activated prodrug.

G. Purine Nucleoside Phosphorylase

The *E. coli* purine nucleoside phosphorylase (PNP) gene (*Deo D*) encodes an enzyme that catalyzes the degradation of the nucleosides inosine, guanosine, and their deoxy analogs by cleavage to the corresponding base. In addition, PNP activates 6-methylpurine-deoxyriboside (6-MeP-dR) to highly toxic 6-methylpurine (6-MeP). 6-MeP inhibits protein, RNA, and DNA synthesis, killing both proliferating and quiescent cells. PNP also activates the antileukemia drug fludarabine. Selective killing of murine B16 melanoma cells exposed to 6-MeP-dR was seen with retroviral transfer of the PNP gene under the control of the tyrosinase promoter. 6-MeP is freely diffusable, and this system exhibits a strong BSE. *In vitro*, as little as 0.1 to 1% of cells expressing PNP are able to kill the majority of tumor cells, and 1% PNP-expressing cells in a tumor improved survival of mice with SKOV-3 ovarian cancer xenografts. PNP also sensitizes a variety of human tumor xenograft models to fludarabine.

H. Thymidine Phosphorylase

The mammalian enzyme thymidine phosphorylase (TP) is identical to the platelet-derived endothelial cell growth factor (PDGF-EC) and catalyzes the reversible phospholytic cleavage of thymidine and deoxyuridine to their respective bases and deoxyribose-1-phosphate. TP also catalyzes the cleavage of several analogs of deoxyuridine, including 5′-deoxy-5-fluorouridine (5′-DFUR) and 1-(tetrahydrofuryl)-5-fluorouracil (tegafur), to produce the anticancer agent 5-fluorouracil (5FU) similar to the cytosine deaminase/5-fluorocytosine system. TP also catalyzes the conversion of 5FU to 5-fluoro-2′-deoxyuridine, the first step in the conversion of 5FU to a deoxynucleotide metabolite (FdUTP) inhibiting DNA synthesis. Murine C26 colorectal carcinoma cells expressing human TP are rendered 10-fold more sensitive to 5FU than wild-type cells. Transfer of the TP gene into human MCF-7 breast cancer cells sensitizes them by 1000-fold to 5′-DFUR. TP has also been shown to enhance the efficacy of the chemotherapy agent, capcitabine (N^4-pentyloxycarbonyl-5′-deoxy-5-fluorocytidine), by also catalyzing its conversion to 5FU. The TP/5-DFUR system exhibits a BSE, with as few as 5% TP-positive cells in the population, reducing the 5′-DFUR median inhibitory concentration (IC_{50}) of MCF-7 cells by more than 50%. Similar to CD, the TP/5′-DFUR system does not require cell-to-cell contact or expression of gap junctions because of the free diffusion of 5FU across the cell membrane.

I. Sodium/Iodide Symporter

While not a true "suicide" enzyme, the gene encoding the thyroid follicular cell sodium/iodide symporter (NIS) has been studied in combination with radioactive iodine for both imaging and as antitumor therapy. NIS is normally expressed in thyroid follicular cells, salivary glands, mammary tissue, and gastric mucosa. NIS facilitates the transport of iodine (I) into thyroid follicles for the production of thyroxine (T_4) and triiodothyronine (T_3). In thyroid tissue, it actively facilitates the accumulation of iodide at concentrations 20- to 40-fold higher than plasma levels. The basis of this approach is that expression of NIS in tumors should allow the local concentration of radioactive ^{131}I to result in tumor exposures of up to 50,000 cGy of ionizing radiation. Both human (hNIS) and rat (rNIS) genes have been cloned and used in this approach. Retroviral transfer of the rNIS gene into human and mouse carcinoma cell lines increased iodine uptake 9- to 35-fold compared to cells transduced with a control vector. Cells expressing rNIS are sensitized to ^{131}I where the viability of control cells is minimally affected. In addition, NIS-expressing tumors in mice could be visualized by scintigraphy by virtue of the ability to concentrate the radioactivity. Similar findings were reported using adenoviral-mediated transfer of the human NIS gene in glioma cell lines. LNCaP human prostate carcinoma cells expressing the hNIS gene under the control of the prostate-specific antigen (PSA) promoter selectively concentrate radioiodine. When animals bearing these tumors were treated with ^{131}I, significant reductions in tumor size were achieved compared to control animals. A problem with the clinical application of the NIS/^{131}I system is that there is no organification pathway in nonthyroid tissue to trap the radioiodine inside of the cells. Intracellular iodine concentrations decline rapidly after a dose. NIS-expressing MCF-7 breast tumors in nude mice are able concentrate more than 16% of a dose of radioiodine; however, less than 1% of the initial dose could be detected in the tumors cells 24 h later. The natural concentrating of iodine in normal thyroid and gastric mucosa also might limit the utility of this approach.

VI. COMBINATION SUICIDE/ PRODRUG GENE THERAPY

The combination of different suicide gene/prodrug systems or the combining of enzyme/prodrug systems with other treatment modalities such as chemotherapy, radiotherapy, or immunotherapy may prove more effective than treatment with individual suicide gene systems and their prodrugs alone. Inhibition of the enzyme thymidylate synthase (TS) decreases the intracellular thymidine pool that competes with GCV for the active site on HSV-tk, increasing the intracellular concentrations of the GCV phosphates. 5FU generated by CD from its prodrug (5FC) is a potent inhibitor of TS and has been shown to increase intracellular pools of phosphorylated GCV. The combination of HSV-tk/GCV and CD/5FC systems was found to enhance responses in a number of preclinical tumor models. This combination approach is under study in a clinical trial using a replication-competent adenovirus expressing an HSV-thymidine kinase-cytosine deaminase fusion gene. Inhibition of TS by exogenously administered 5FU or by tomudex (ZD1694), a TS-specific inhibitor, also synergistically enhances cell killing *in vitro* by GCV and improves tumor response and animal survival in murine models bearing HSV-tk-expressing tumors compared with treatment of GCV alone. As hypothesized, tomudex and 5FU treatment increase intracellular GCV-phosphate pools and enhance incorporation of radiolabeled GCV into cellular DNA in HSV-tk-positive cell lines. The ribonucleotide reductase inhibitor hydroxyurea has been shown to reduce intracellular dGTP pools and increase the level of GCV-triphosphate in cells expressing HSV-tk when exposed to GCV. Cells expressing HSV-tk were sensitized to lower concentrations of GCV and their bystander effect was enhanced. Synergy has been demonstrated between the camptothecin topoisomerase I inhibitor topotecan and the HSV-tk/GCV system. The median effective doses (ED_{50}) of both GCV and topotecan in HSV-tk-expressing colon and ovarian carcinoma cells were significantly lowered by their combination compared to treatment with either drug alone. This approach has been studied in a phase I trial of the combination of adenoviral-mediated HSV-tk gene transfer and GCV administration in combination with topotecan in patients with advanced ovarian cancer.

Combination of the cytochrome P450 CYP 2B1/CP and HSV-tk/GCV systems is a potentially attractive suicide gene combination strategy. CYP 2B1-expressing cells treated with cyclophosphamide accumulate in S phase. Because activated GCV is a S-phase-specific agent, more tumor cells may be sensitized to HSV-tk/GCV by pretreatment with CYP 2B1 and CP. In addition, activated GCV inhibits the repair of CP-induced DNA damage.

See Also the Following Articles

Cationic Lipid-Mediated Gene Therapy • Liposome-Mediated Gene Therapy • Recombination: Mechanisms and Roles in Tumorigenesis • Resistance to Inhibitor Compounds of Thymidine Synthase • Retroviral Vectors

Bibliography

Aghi, M., Chou, T. C., Suling, K., Breakefield, X. O., and Chiocca, E. A. (1999). Multimodal cancer treatment mediated by a replicating oncolytic virus that delivers the oxazaphosphorine/rat cytochrome P450 2B1 and ganciclovir/herpes simplex virus thymidine kinase gene therapies. Cancer Res. **59**, 3861–3865.

Aghi, M., Kramm, C. M., Chou, T. C., Breakefield, X. O., and Chiocca, E. A. (1999). Synergistic anticancer effects of ganciclovir/thymidine kinase and 5-fluorocytosine/cytosine deaminase gene therapies. J Natl Cancer Inst. **91**, 285–286.

Chen, L., and Waxman, D. J. (1995). Intratumoral activation and enhanced chemotherapeutic effect of oxazaphosphorines following cytochrome P-450 gene transfer: Development of a combined chemotherapy/cancer gene therapy strategy. Cancer Res. **55**, 581–589.

Danks, M. K., Morton, C. L., Pawlik, C. A., and Potter, P. M. (1998). Overexpression of a rabbit liver carboxylesterase sensitizes human tumor cells to CPT-11. Cancer Res. **58**, 20–22.

Drabek, D., Guy, J., Craig, R., and Grosveld, F. (1997). The expression of bacterial nitroreductase in transgenic mice results in specific cell killing by the prodrug CB1954. Gene Ther. **4**, 93–100.

Elshami, A. A., Cook, J. W., Amin, K. M., Choi, H., Park, J. Y., Coonrod, L., Sun, J., Molnar-Kimber, K., Wilson, J. M., Kaiser, L. R., and Albelda, S. M. (1997). The effect of promoter strength in adenoviral vectors containing herpes simplex virus thymidine kinase on cancer gene therapy in vitro and in vivo. Cancer Gene Ther. **4**, 213–221.

Freytag, S. O., Rogulski, K. R., Paielli, D. L., Gilbert, J. D., and Kim, J. H. (1998). A novel three-pronged approach to kill cancer cells selectively: Concomitant viral, double suicide gene, and radiotherapy. Hum Gene Ther. **9**, 1323–1333.

Greco, O., and Dachs, G. U. (2001). Gene directed enzyme/prodrug therapy of cancer: Historical appraisal and future prospects. J. Cell Physiol. **187**, 22–36.

Khil, M. S., Kim, J. H., Mullen, C. A., Kim, S. H., and Freytag, S. O. (1996). Radiosensitization by 5-fluorocytosine of human colorectal carcinoma cells in culture transduced with cytosine deaminase gene. Clin. Cancer Res. **2**, 53–57.

Lattime, E. C., and Gerson, S. L. (1999). "Gene Therapy of Cancer." Academic Press, San Diego.

Mandell, R. B., Mandell, L. Z., and Link, C. J. (1999). Radioisotope concentrator gene therapy using the sodium/iodide symporter gene. Cancer Res. **59**, 661–668.

Manome, Y., Wen, P. Y., Dong, Y., Tanaka, T., Mitchell, B. S., Kufe, D. W., and Fine, H. A. (1996). Viral vector transduction of the human deoxycytidine kinase cDNA sensitizes glioma cells to the cytotoxic effects of cytosine arabinoside in vitro and in vivo. Nature Med. **2**, 567–573

Marais, R., Spooner, R. A., Light, Y., Martin, J., and Springer, C. J. (1996). Gene-directed enzyme prodrug therapy with a mustard prodrug/carboxypeptidase G2 combination. Cancer Res. **56**, 4735–4742

Melton, R. G., and Knox, R. J. (1999). "Enzyme-Prodrug Strategies for Cancer Therapy." Kluwer Academic/Plenum, New York.

Moolten, F. L. (1986). Gene therapy: Creating mosaic pattern of drug susceptibility. Mt. Sinai J. Med. **53**, 232.

Moolten, F. L., Wells, J. M., Heyman, R. A., and Evans, R. M. (1990). Lymphoma regression induced by ganciclovir in mice bearing a herpes thymidine kinase transgene. Hum. Gene Ther. **1**, 125–134.

Morris, J. C., Tourraine, R., Wildner, O., and Blaese, R. M. (1996). Suicide genes: Gene therapy applications using enzyme/prodrug strategies. In "The Development of Human Gene Therapy" (T. Friedman, ed.), pp. 477–526. Cold Spring Harbor Laboratory Press, Cold Spring Harbor, NY.

Mroz, P. J., and Moolten, F. L. (1993). Retrovirally transduced Escherichia coli gpt genes combine selectability with chemosensitivity capable of mediating tumor eradication. Hum. Gene Ther. **4**, 589–595.

Mullen, C. A., Kilstrup, M., and Blaese, R. M. (1992). Transfer of the bacterial gene for cytosine deaminase to mammalian cells confers lethal sensitivity to 5-fluorocytosine: A negative selection system. Proc. Natl. Acad. Sci. USA **89**, 33–37.

Niculescu-Duvaz, I., Friedlos, F., Niculescu-Duvaz, D., Davies, L., and Springer, C. J. (1999). Prodrugs for antibody- and gene-directed enzyme prodrug therapies (ADEPT and GDEPT). Anticancer Drug Des. **14**, 517–538.

Pandha, H. S., Martin, L. A., Rigg, A., Hurst, H. C., Stamp, G. W., Sikora, K., and Lemoine, N. R. (1999). Genetic prodrug activation therapy for breast cancer: A phase I clinical trial of erbB-2-directed suicide gene expression. J. Clin. Oncol. **17**, 2180–2189.

Parker, W. B., King, S. A., Allan, P. W., Bennett, L. L., Jr., Secrist, J. A., III, Montgomery, J. A., Gilbert, K. S., Waud, W. R., Wells, A. H., Gillespie, G. Y., and Sorscher, E. J. (1997). In vivo gene therapy of cancer with E. coli purine nucleoside phosphorylase. Hum. Gene Ther. **8**, 1637–1644.

Patterson, A. V., Zhang, H., Moghaddam, A., Bicknell, R., Talbot, D. C., Stratford, I. J., and Harris, A. L. (1995). Increased sensitivity to the prodrug 5'-deoxy-5-fluorouridine and modulation of 5-fluoro-2'-deoxyuridine sensitivity in MCF-7 cells transfected with thymidine phosphorylase. *Br. J. Cancer* **72,** 669–675.

Rainov, N. G. (2000). A phase III clinical evaluation of herpes simplex virus type 1 thymidine kinase and ganciclovir gene therapy as an adjuvant to surgical resection and radiation in adults with previously untreated glioblastoma multiforme. *Hum. Gene Ther.* **11,** 2389–2401.

Ram, Z., Culver, K. W., Oshiro, E. M., Viola, J. J., DeVroom, H. L., Otto, E., Long, Z., Chiang, Y., McGarrity, G. J., Muul, L. M., Katz, D., Blaese, R. M., and Oldfield, E. H. (1997). Therapy of malignant brain tumors by intratumoral implantation of retroviral vector-producing cells. *Nature Med.* **3,** 1354–1361.

Sandmair, A. M., Loimas, S., Puranen, P., Immonen, A., Kossila, M., Puranen, M., Hurskainen, H., Tyynela, K., Turunen, M., Vanninen, R., Lehtolainen, P., Paljarvi, L., Johansson, R., Vapalahti, M., and Yla-Herttuala, S. (2000). Thymidine kinase gene therapy for human malignant glioma, using replication-deficient retroviruses or adenoviruses. *Hum. Gene Ther.* **11,** 2197–2205.

Sterman, D. H., Treat, J., Litzky, L. A., Amin, K. M., Coonrod, L., Molnar-Kimber, K., Recio, A., Knox, L., Wilson, J. M., Albelda, S. M., and Kaiser, L. R. (1998). Adenovirus-mediated herpes simplex virus thymidine kinase/ganciclovir gene therapy in patients with localized malignancy: Results of a phase I clinical trial in malignant mesothelioma. *Hum. Gene Ther.* **9,** 1083–1092.

Wildner, O., Blaese, R. M., and Morris, J. C. (1999). Synergy between the herpes simplex virus tk/ganciclovir prodrug suicide system and the topoisomerase I inhibitor topotecan. *Hum. Gene Ther.* **10,** 2679–2687.

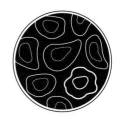

Targeted Toxins

Richard A. Messmann
Edward A. Sausville

National Cancer Institute, Bethesda, Maryland

GLOSSARY

ADP-ribosylation A covalent alteration of certain cellular proteins catalyzed by bacterial toxins such as *Pseudomonas* exotoxin or *Diphtheria* toxin. In the reaction, NAD provides an ADP molecule that becomes covalently linked to the protein synthesis elongation factor E2F, liberating a free nicotinamide.

antibody-dependent enzyme prodrug therapy A strategy in which an antibody conjugated to an enzyme (instead of to a toxin) is administered several hours to several days before a prodrug, which is devoid of intrinsic toxicity but which is converted to a cytotoxic drug under the influence of the cell-bound enzyme; this therefore causes toxicity only at the local site where the antibody–enzyme complex is bound.

chimeric fusion protein toxin A targeted toxin designed so that a growth factor or soluble receptor with high affinity for a potential binding site is expressed in the same read-ing frame with a portion of a toxin molecule. The toxin is generally altered to remove those parts of the toxin molecule responsible for nonspecific binding or toxicity. Single chain immunotoxins may be considered a special case of chimeric fusion protein molecules where the targeting determinant derives from an antibody molecule.

current good manufacturing practices The minimum requirements for the methods to be used in, and the facilities and controls used for, the production, quality control, holding, or distribution of a safe and effective biologic entity or drug product intended for human use.

epitope The three-dimensional "target" recognized by a particular monoclonal antibody. The antigen molecule may contain many different epitopes for different monoclonal antibodies.

immunotoxin A targeted toxin where the targeting domain derives from a monoclonal antibody molecule. The immunotoxin may be synthesized chemically by conjugating the antibody or a fragment of the antibody to the toxin using a chemical linker, or the variable and constant regions of the antibody may be cloned into an expression vector. The resulting synthetic gene now allows the production of a synthetic single chain polypeptide bearing both the heavy and the light chain-derived antigen combining site, fused to a cloned toxin fragment.

Encyclopedia of Cancer, Second Edition
Volume 4

monoclonal antibody An antibody produced from cultured cells, called hybridomas, consisting of a single molecular entity from a single clone of antibody-producing cells. Hybridomas result from the fusion of mouse spleen cells responding to a particular antigen with an immortalized mouse myeloma cell line. This is in contrast to polyclonal antibody preparations obtained from whole serum from animals, which recognize many different parts of the antigen and contain antibody molecules that do not recognize the antigen at all.

***N*-glycosidase** Enzymatic activity present in the A chain of the plant toxins ricin, abrin, and in the single chain ribosome inactivating proteins, gelonin or pokeweed antiviral protein, which catalyzes the removal of a single specific adenine base from the 60S ribosomal subunit, resulting in inhibition of protein synthesis.

targeted toxin A molecule synthesized to contain an intoxicating domain and a targeting domain. The targeting domain binds with high affinity to a cell surface determinant. The intoxicating domain then acts to cause the death of the cell to which the toxin is fixed.

therapeutic index The ratio between beneficial and adverse effects of an agent. In the case of conventionally used antineoplastic agents, the therapeutic index is rather narrow.

vascular leak syndrome A clinical condition characterized by a decrease in serum albumin and an increase of extracellular but not intravascular fluid, resulting in edema of the soft tissues and in severe cases of pulmonary or other organ edema accompanied by hypotension. This can be seen as a result of high doses of exogenously administered cytokines and has been an adverse effect of all targeted toxins containing *Pseudomonas* exotoxin or ricin-based constructs studied to date.

Targeted toxins are a new class of cancer therapeutic agent composed of a tumor selective ligand linked to a polypeptide toxin or, alternatively, conjugated with a "small molecule." The original basis for developing agents of this type was presaged by Ehrlich's concept of antibodies as representing a means to create "magic bullets" for the therapy of human neoplastic disease. Until the production of pure antibodies to single epitopes was feasible, such efforts utilized crude or partially fractionated serum containing antibodies recognizing many different determinants. With the advent of monoclonal antibody technology, where pure molecules directed at particular epitopes can be produced in large quantities from cul-

tured cells, there was a new impetus to define single antibody molecules directed against tumor-specific or tumor-restricted antigens. One obvious advantage of such an agent would be an increase in therapeutic index over conventional cytotoxic antineoplastic therapy. This article serves as a general overview of the current state of targeted toxins, which has matured to the point of certain agents exhibiting early clinical utility, culminating in the licensure of small molecule–antibody conjugates. For a more in-depth analysis, the reader is referred to a number of reviews listed in the bibliography section.

I. INTRODUCTION

Targeted toxins have the basic structure shown in Fig. 1. These molecules contain a high-affinity binding and targeting moiety coupled to some form of toxin, usually a covalently coupled polypeptide toxin. Targeting and toxic moieties may be coupled via a chemical linkage or, alternatively, a single genetically engineered molecule may be produced to contain both targeting and toxic domains. When the targeting component consists of a chemically synthesized or recombinant whole antibody or antibody fragment, the molecule is termed an "immunotoxin." Alternatively, "chimeric fusion protein toxin" contains targeting cytokines, peptide hormones, or growth factors that are most usually recombinantly fused to intoxicating domains. When translated, the sequence produces a single chain molecule.

A general mechanism of action for the most frequently studied targeted toxins involves binding tumor cell receptor or ligand, with subsequent internalization of toxin and inactivation of cytosolic protein synthesis. Alternatively, the targeting ligand can be manufactured to deliver drugs or enzymes capable of converting prodrugs into active molecules directly to the surface of tumor cells.

A number of factors influence the action of targeted toxins. These factors include (1) "residence time" of immunotoxin in circulation as a function of immune and nonimmune clearance mechanisms; (2) depth of penetration into the tumor mass; (3) attachment to tumor cell surface target antigen; (4) uptake and internalization with subsequent endosomal

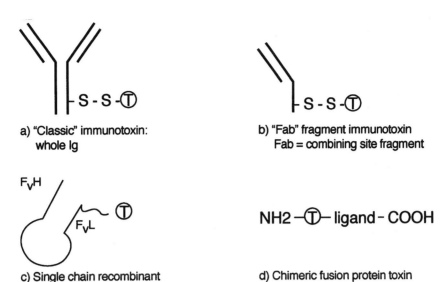

a) "Classic" immunotoxin: whole Ig

b) "Fab" fragment immunotoxin
Fab = combining site fragment

c) Single chain recombinant molecule

d) Chimeric fusion protein toxin

FIGURE 1 Basic structure of targeted toxins. A "classic" immunotoxin (a) consists of a whole immunoglobulin molecule linked by a disulfide (–S-S–) linker to the toxin (T). A F(ab) fragment (b) may be prepared by proteolysis to yield a smaller molecular weight immunotoxin. Alternatively, the variable region from the light chain (FvL) can be cloned adjacent to the variable region of the heavy chain (FvH), joined by linker peptides to each other and to a toxin domain to yield a single chain recombinant toxin (c). The similarity of the recombinant molecule to the original concept of a chimeric fusion protein toxin (d) is apparent, where the toxin domain is expressed by recombinant techniques in the same frame with the ligand, which has high affinity to a cell surface receptor expressed on the neoplastic cell. Both single chain recombinant immunotoxins and chimeric fusion protein toxins must be proteolytically cleaved, and in some cases reduced, in the target cell prior to translocation. A classic and F(ab) immunotoxin must only be reduced prior to translocation of the free toxin.

and endoplasmic reticular processing; (5) proteolysis or cellular metabolism; (6) translocation of immunotoxin into cytoplasm; and (7) dependence of tumor cell on ongoing protein synthesis. Additionally, an "optimized" targeted toxin would exhibit the following general characteristics: (1) the molecule must achieve plasma concentration sufficient for antitumor activity without inducing toxicity at nontumor sites; (2) exhibit ligand-binding specificity that targets receptor/antigen expressed on neoplastic cells without exhibiting adventitious binding to nontumor targets; (3) be subject to clearance mechanisms that allow distribution to tumor tissues before clearance eliminates active drug; (4) easily penetrate tumor, allowing treatment of advanced bulky (> 1 cm) disease; (5) be nonimmunogenic, thereby allowing repeated dosing and maximization of therapeutic benefit; (6) deliver a well-characterized intoxicating mechanism that occurs via an uptake route that is expected to be pre-

sent and functional in tumor cells; (7) not be subject to anticipated mechanisms of resistance; and (8) require a reproducible formulation and manufacturing process. This last point requires further examination. The current good manufacturing practices manufacture of biologic molecules for clinical use requires adherence to stringent regulations maximizing the potential for the reliable production of clinical grade material while minimizing batch-to-batch variability. Optimization and scale-up of production often require labor-intensive efforts that are inherently difficult to achieve and maintain.

II. CLINICAL USE OF TARGETED TOXINS

Several targeted toxin constructs have been produced for clinical evaluation. These targeted toxins have used one of a variety of targeting moieties as listed in Table I.

As with the targeting ligand, the intoxicating component may consist of any one of a number of possibilities that include plant or bacterially derived toxins, RNases, antibody–drug conjugates, or antibody–enzyme prodrug inducers. A brief summary of intoxicating components is as follows.

A. Diphtheria Toxin (DT)

This phage-encoded protein toxin (M_r 61,000), produced by lysogenic strains of the bacterium *Corynebacterium diphtheriae*, consists of three domains (Fig. 2). Upon COOH-terminal domain-mediated binding of target, the hydrophobic middle domain of the toxin translocates an NH_2-terminal ADP-ribosyltransferase intoxicating domain, which catalytically inactivates protein synthesis. Transmembrane transfer of toxin occurs via an acidic endosomal compartment, and subsequent proteolytic cleavage, in the region between the binding and the translocating domain, creates "nicked" toxin. Reduction of a remaining disulfide bond, located between the membrane translocating and receptor-binding domains, occurs intracellularly during the act of cellular intoxication and is necessary for optimum intoxication of the cell.

B. *Pseudomonas* Exotoxin (PE)

This 613 amino acid single chain polypeptide toxin is secreted by *Pseudomonas aeruginosa*, and is similar to DT in that PE consists of three separate domains: an amino-terminal cell-binding domain connected to a COOH-terminal ADP-ribosyltransferase via an intervening translocation domain. Like DT, the ribosyltransferase catalytically inactivates elongation factor 2 (EF2) by the transfer of ADP-ribose to a unique histidine residue in the molecule, thus inactivating protein synthesis in the intoxicated cell. The molecule exists in nature as a single chain species, which is proteolytically cleaved (by a cellular protease) between catalytic and membrane translocating domains during uptake, followed again by reduction of an intramolecular disulfide linkage. Both of these steps are necessary for activity.

C. Ricin

This M_r 64,000 heterodimeric toxin is derived from the seeds of the castor bean, *Ricinus communis*. The toxin consists of two chains, A and B, linked together via a disulfide bond. The A chain possesses *N*-glycosidase activity for a specific adenine–ribose bond in the 60S ribosomal subunit, whereas the B chain binds to mammalian cell surface oligosaccharides. The B chain is removed prior to the creation of toxins utilizing the isolated A chain or, alternatively, the binding site on the B chain can be blocked by covalent linkage to a sugar residue that mimics its endogenous ligand. This results in so-called "blocked ricin." Internalization of the ricin A chain also occurs via a pathway that involves reduction of its disulfide bond linking the A chain to either native B chain or immunoconjugates. The B chain actively synergizes

---

TABLE I
Targeting Moieties Used in Targeted Toxin Constructs[a]

Targeting component	Target	Miscellaneous notes
Antibody: Fab, Fab', F(ab')$_2$	Receptors CD5, CD7, CD19, CD22, CD25, CD30, CD33, CD56, Tf, Lewis^Y antigen, M_r 72,000 and 55,000 antigens, and proteoglycan	
Fv portion of antibody	Lewis^Y, CD22, CD25 antigen and erbB-2 receptor	
Growth factor: TGF-α/EGF, IGF-1, FGF	Growth factor receptors	Growth factor receptors are overexpressed in certain cancers [i.e., epidermal growth factor (EGF) in squamous cell neoplasm] and therefore have inherent appeal as potential targets
Cytokine: IL-2, IL-4, IL-6, GM-CSF	Cytokine receptors	Also overexpressed in certain tumors

[a]Includes antibodies in whole or part, growth factors, and cytokines.

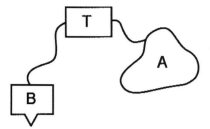

FIGURE 2 Diphtheria toxin is a phage-encoded protein toxin produced by lysogenic strains of the bacterium *Corynebacterium diphtheriae*. The diphtheria toxin is a three domain bacterial exotoxin synthesized as a single polypeptide chain containing an amino-terminal A (active or catalytic) domain, a B (receptor-binding) domain, and a transmembrane (T) domain responsible for membrane insertion and translocation of the A fragment. Proteolytic nicking of the secreted form of the toxin separates the A chain from the B chain.

with the ricin A chain to increase cell killing, and non-B chain-containing targeted toxins have variable efficiencies of uptake. An additional complicating feature in the construction of toxins utilizing the ricin A chain is the existence of carbohydrates that can allow the nonspecific uptake of the ricin A chain into cell types, especially hepatocytes, which exhibit receptors for the carbohydrate residues.

D. Gelonin, Saporin (SO6), and Pokeweed Antiviral Protein (PAP)

These entities also intoxicate the large ribosomal subunit, but differ from ricin in that the toxin is a single chain polypeptide that is resistant to proteolysis and does not contain carbohydrate residues.

E. RNases

A different strategy for the intoxication of targeted cells involves the use of RNases that elicit cell cycle-related mechanisms of cytotoxicity *in vitro*. The use of endogenous human RNase, or the exogenous (but structurally similar) peptide, such as the amphibian enzyme onconase, has the potential advantage of provoking a decreased immunogenic response when compared to plant or bacterially derived toxins.

F. Antibody–Drug Conjugates

Another novel molecular construct involves the direct conjugation of conventional cytotoxic agents to

targeting antibodies. This approach has generated molecules such as antibody-conjugated vinca alkaloids or doxorubicin with reasonable cytotoxic activity *in vitro*. Initial human trials, using anti-Lewis[Y] antibodies coupled to doxorubicin, documented gastrointestinal toxicity as a clinical concern. A different approach would be to couple agents with very little therapeutic index, yet use the antibody to convey an improvement in therapeutic index.

G. Antibody–Dependent Enzyme Prodrug Therapy (ADEPT)

Here, an enzyme that can convert an inert prodrug into, for example, an active antimetabolite or alkylating agent is coupled to an antibody and administered several hours to days before administration of the prodrug (Fig. 3). At local sites of antibody–enzyme binding, the prodrug is converted to an active drug, which, due to its increased concentration in the immediate vicinity of the tumor, has greater access to the tumor. Moreover, the active drug is not generated in normal tissues that have not bound the antibody. Subsequent versions of this approach target a gene to produce the metabolizing moiety in the tumor cell or tumor microenvironment (gene-directed enzyme prodrug therapy, GDEPT).

III. CLINICAL EFFORTS WITH TARGETED TOXINS

A variety of targeted toxins have been evaluated for clinical utility. These studies have helped define the

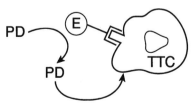

FIGURE 3 Antibody-dependent enzyme prodrug therapy (ADEPT). In this concept, a toxin is not itself targeted, but rather an enzyme (E) with specificity to convert an otherwise nontoxic prodrug (PD) into a toxic drug that achieves high local concentration in the region of the target tumor cell (TTC). The antibody conjugated to the enzyme is administered hours to days prior to the prodrug and remains fixed to the target cell population while the nonbound antibody-enzyme complex is cleared prior to prodrug administration.

current limitations of this form of therapy and, perhaps more importantly, have given invaluable insights into potential strategies to overcome these limitations. Pioneering efforts have resulted in the Food and Drug Administration's recent commercial approval of a targeted toxin for human usage. A brief overview of selected clinical trials using targeted toxins is as follows.

A. Diphtheria Toxin

DAB $_{486}$ interleukin (IL)-2 is a recombinant fusion protein toxin where the binding domain of the DT molecule is replaced by IL-2 to specifically target cells expressing the IL-2 receptor. This entity has been evaluated in clinical trials having exhibited modest antitumor activity and toxicity manifested as elevations in transaminase and creatinine levels. A self-limiting hemolytic–uremic-like syndrome was also observed.

In an effort to produce a DAB construct with increased residence time, the DAB $_{486}$ IL-2 molecule was shortened to produce DAB$_{389}$IL-2 (ONTAK), which exhibits an increased serum half-life over its predecessor. ONTAK is composed of both the transmembrane and catalytic domains of DT recombinantly fused to human IL-2. In a study involving 73 patients with either refractory cutaneous T-cell (CTCL) lymphoma ($n = 35$) or non-Hodgkin's (NHL) lymphoma ($n = 17$), there were five complete (CR) and eight partial (PR) remissions in patients with CTCL with one CR and two PR occurring in NHL. Responding patients expressed IL-2 receptor on tumor cells. ONTAK has recently received FDA approval.

HN66000 (Tf-CRM107) is a Tf-binding site mutant DT. In a recent clinical trial, the toxin was infused interstitially to patients with high-grade gliomas. These patients exhibited a 60% combined partial or complete remission rate with a median survival of responding patients exceeding 1 year.

B. *Pseudomonas* Exotoxin

The first PE immunotoxin (OVB3-PE) was created by conjugation of native PE with whole OVB3, a murine monoclonal antibody directed against ovarian carcinomas. A phase I clinical trial of this entity was halted after unanticipated neurologic toxicity developed due to low-level expression of the determinant on neural tissue.

PE38 is a truncated form of *Pseudomonas* exotoxin where the cell-binding domain is removed and a coupling site is created for cross-linking to suitable targeting agents. The B3-Lys PE 38 (LMB-1) immunotoxin is made by coupling the B3 monoclonal antibody, which reacts with a Lewis^Y antigen present on the surface of many human solid tumors, to recombinantly produced PE 38. When administered as a single intravenous bolus infusion to patients with advanced refractory solid tumors, one patient exhibited a CR lasting 2 months while another patient exhibited a PR lasting 7 months.

In patients with refractory hairy cell leukemia, entirely recombinant anti-TAC (Fv)-PE 38 (LMB-2) displayed antitumor activity in the form of one complete remission lasting 13 months and a decrease in leukemic burden in three additional patients. Partial responses were also noted in patients diagnosed with chronic lymphocytic leukemia, cutaneous T-cell, Hodgkin's, and acute T-cell lymphoma.

A different type of recombinant molecule (BL22) has exhibited antitumor activity in the form of complete responses in patients with hairy cell leukemia and eradication of circulating tumors cells in CLL patients.

C. Ricin

Various methods of attaching ricin toxin to targeting domains have been attempted. First-generation ricin immunotoxins, where ricin A and B chains were linked to immunoglobulin, displayed poor targeting due to the nonspecific uptake mediated by the B chain. Isolated A chains linked to targeting molecules exhibited poor target cell uptake due to the lack of a B chain, and nonspecific uptake into the liver mediated by carbohydrates on the A chain. These shortcomings led to the creation of "blocked ricin," where the B chain is "blocked" by covalent modification of its sugar-binding site. Another strategy resulted in the production of a deglycosylated A chain (dgA), created by the oxidation of ricin A chain's endogenous carbohydrates. Deglycosylated A chain constructs displayed a marked decrease of hepatic uptake and improved overall stability of the construction in the plasma, while retaining facile capacity for reduction of the disulfide linkage between the toxin and antibody once in the intracellular milieu. Two determinants expressed on adult B-cell lymphomas, CD22 and CD 19, have been targeted in a series of clinical studies.

An immunotoxin consisting of dgA linked to the F(ab') fragment of CD22-directed antibody RFB4 was studied in 15 patients in doses administered at 48-h intervals. The $T_{1/2}$ of the toxin was relatively short, in keeping with the small size of the molecule. Partial responses were noted in 38% of patients, lasting 1 to 4 months. While vascular leak syndrome (VLS; see Section IV) was the dominant toxicity, expressive aphasia and rhabdomyolysis were the dose-limiting toxicities.

Clinical responses have also been observed in trials involving immunotoxins consisting of dgA coupled to whole RFB4-dgA (anti-CD22) antibody. One post-transplant patient diagnosed with large B-cell lymphoma exhibited a complete remission that has lasted > 3 years. A phase I trial evaluating the bolus administration of dgA-RFB4 produced five PRs and one CR lasting 30 to 78 days in 26 patients treated. VLS was again the dose-limiting toxicity.

Various dosing schedules have been evaluated in an attempt to ameliorate VLS. These trials indicated that severe toxicity correlated with high levels of immunotoxin achieved at early times after initiation of the infusion. Additionally, the presence of even small numbers of circulating tumor cells correlated with decreased toxicity, with a trend toward increased volume of distribution of the toxin and lower circulating IT concentrations achieved during the infusion.

An 8-day continuous infusion of the combination of RFB4-dgA and HD37-dgA (anti-CD19-dgA) was well tolerated, in doses thus far explored, in patients with circulating tumor cells. However, patients without circulating tumor had unpredictable clinical courses that included two deaths. These patients exhibited a significant potential for association between mortality and (1) a history of either autologous bone marrow or peripheral blood stem cell transplant or (2) a history of radiation therapy. These findings raise the question of whether preexisting endothelial cell damage may predispose ricin-based immunotoxin recipients to an increased risk of toxicity.

A phase II study evaluating adjuvant anti-B4 blocked ricin immunotoxin after autologous bone marrow transplant in patients with minimal residual non-Hodgkin's lymphoma demonstrated the safe administration of the immunotoxin. Although early estimates of disease-free survival were very encouraging, 4-year follow-up data demonstrated continued relapse.

The ricin-containing immunotoxin XMMME-001-RTA targets proteoglycan. In a trial involving 22 patients with metastatic melanoma, one complete response was described, and toxicities included VLS and elevated liver enzyme levels. Virtually all patients developed antimouse or antiricin antibodies.

VLS also occurred during a trial of Mab 260F9 recombinant ricin A chain toxin formed with the antibreast carcinoma cell antibody 260F9. Additionally, a neurologic syndrome consisting of sensorimotor neuropathy complicated this trial. The toxicity was ultimately found to be related to an unsuspected cross-reaction of the antibody with a determinant on Schwann cells.

D. Saporin

Trials using saporin-containing immunotoxins, such as the CD30 directed monoclonal antibody Ber-H2-SO6, have, like the ricin based immunotoxin trials, shown minor clinical responses and predictable toxicity.

E. Antibody–Drug Conjugates

An early phase I study of humanized anti-CD33 calicheamicin immunoconjugate in patients with acute myeloid leukemia sought to selectively ablate leukemic blast cells. Trial results were positive in that leukemia was eliminated in 20% (8/40) of patients, thus indicating a selective ablation of malignant hematopoiesis in some patients with acute myelocytic leukemia (AML). This agent has received FDA approval for the treatment of relapsed adult AML.

IV. CLINICAL ISSUES RELATED TO TARGETED TOXINS

A. Vascular Leak Syndrome

VLS is characterized by increased vascular permeability, decreased serum albumin, and increased extravascular fluid that, if severe, can result in life-threatening pulmonary edema, organ failure, and hypotension. VLS has been observed in trials utilizing PE, DT, ricin, and IL-2 intoxicating moieties. The syndrome manifests itself clinically within 4–6 days of starting targeted toxin therapy. While the etiology of VLS is unknown, it has been shown that an amino acid structural motif that is common to IL-2, dgA, PE, and DT toxins may be responsible for the binding of immunotoxins to endothelial cells with subsequent endothelial cell damage. The structural motif in question is [(x)-aspartic acid-(y)], where x can be leucine, isoleucine, glycine, or valine and y is valine, leucine, or serine.

B. Hemolytic Uremic Syndrome (HUS)

HUS comprises a constellation of clinical symptoms, including renal insufficiency, anemia, and thrombocytopenia. As with VLS, the syndrome is in evidence in certain trials involving ricin toxin, DT, and PE. Additionally, as with VLS, the etiology of this syndrome is unknown.

C. Immunogenicity

Administration of immunotoxin in the presence of antibodies to either the immunoglobulin or to the toxin results in more rapid clearance with lowered plasma concentration of toxin, and the theoretical risk of "serum sickness." These considerations would seem to limit the role of the immunotoxin to that of adjuvant therapy after all the tumor is removed, and for at best one or two courses after the primary therapy. However, the magnitude of an individual immune response is quite variable. Two approaches have been undertaken in an effort to deal with immunogenicity of these constructs. Namely, "humanization" of the antibody, or placement of the mouse-derived antigen recognition region within human "framework" sequences. In the case of toxins, generation of antibodies to the toxin portion would be difficult to avoid. An alternative approach utilizes the administration of novel immune suppressants. In this regard it is noteworthy that patients with B-cell lymphoma, with impaired humoral immunity, can, in some cases, receive multiple courses of an immunotoxin that targets B cells without generation of anti-immunotoxin

antibodies. One approach used to decrease the B-cell mediated immune response was the coadministration of LMB-1 immunotoxin and rituximab (a CD20-targeting human antibody). Results of this effort are pending. A more definitive approach to this problem would be the use of humanized targeting moiety linked to endogenous human-derived intoxicating poisons such as RNases.

V. SUMMARY, PERSPECTIVE, AND FUTURE DIRECTIONS IN TARGETED TOXIN RESEARCH

Certain axioms that should be observed during the development of subsequent generations of immunotoxins include the following:

i. A target antigen or process should be chosen that is as specific for the tumor as possible.
ii. Whenever possible, a "realistic" animal model should be used to demonstrate efficacy and guide dosing (wherein the expression of the target on the tumor is not exaggerated, nor is the target artificially absent from host tissues).
iii. Demonstration of target expression on a particular patient's tumor cells prior to initiating treatment trials in that patient.
iv. Careful documentation of the levels of drug achieved in relation to the clinical features of the patients, especially the bulk of disease and the level of expression of the target in the tumor tissue.

The last point is of importance, as one could conceive of differing maximally tolerated doses in patient groups with, for example, large tumor bulk and abundant antigen expression as compared to tumor with restricted tumor bulk and low levels of expression of target antigen.

The issues of circulating forms of the target antigen (e.g., soluble IL-2 receptors in the face of chimeric fusion protein toxins based on IL-2) or the presence of anti-immunotoxin antibodies (especially if not affecting cellular uptake or toxin function) are more problematic. While it might be reasonably considered that these circumstances would retard the action of the toxin, it is conceivable that the rate of clearance by these mechanisms might not be as rapid as uptake and fixation to high-affinity receptors that could be the basis of a therapeutic effect. Indeed, the DAB series of chimeric fusion protein toxins has been devoid of significant VLS, and these molecules have extraordinarily rapid clearances in comparison to agents based on either ricin or *Pseudomonas* toxins studied to date. One explanation for this result is that the rapid clearance of the DABs may protect the vasculature from toxin-induced damaged that would lead to VLS. Future clinical experiments employing molecules with similar toxins but differing clearances will allow this issue to be satisfactorily addressed.

Another very much unresolved issue is the affinity of the targeting portion of the construct. Very tight binding antibodies may not diffuse satisfactorily even into small tumor masses, whereas antibodies of low affinity have an increased propensity for nontargeted toxicity to occur.

Targeted toxins represent a new class of cancer therapy. The science of targeted toxin delivery has matured to the point where clinical responses have been evident, particularly in the treatment of leukemia and lymphoma. These findings provide impetus for continued development of these novel antitumor agents. However, as noted in the previous edition of this article, this class of agents has not been optimized with respect to either the intoxicating or targeting domains thus far prepared for clinical use. The future of cancer therapy must take into account the biology of the underlying disease if progress is to occur. Targeting toxic moieties through high-affinity binding domains restricted to tumor cells is a rational and seemingly attractive way of using biology to direct the development of novel treatments. The fact that responses have been observed in certain categories of patients treated with initial versions of targeted toxins calls for further development in ways that will capitalize on these experiences.

See Also the Following Articles

ANTIBODY–TOXIN AND GROWTH FACTOR–TOXIN FUSION PROTEINS • ANTI-IDIOTYPIC ANTIBODY VACCINES • MONOCLONAL ANTIBODIES: LEUKEMIA AND LYMPHOMA • RADIOLABELED ANTIBODIES, OVERVIEW

Bibliography

Alexander, R. L., Kucera, G. L., et al. (2000). *In vitro* interleukin-3 binding to leukemia cells predicts cytotoxicity of a *diphtheria* toxin/IL-3 fusion protein. *Bioconjug. Chem.* **11**(4), 564–568.

Barth, S., Huhn, M., et al. (2000). Recombinant anti-CD25 immunotoxin RFT5(SCFV)-ETA' demonstrates successful elimination of disseminated human Hodgkin lymphoma in SCID mice. *Int. J. Cancer* **86**(5), 718–724.

Bernstein, I. D. (2000). Monoclonal antibodies to the myeloid stem cells: Therapeutic implications of CMA-676, a humanized anti-CD33 antibody calicheamicin conjugate. *Leukemia* **14**(3), 474–475.

Desbene, S., Van, H. D., et al. (1999). Application of the ADEPT strategy to the MDR resistance in cancer chemotherapy. *Anticancer Drug Des.* **14**(2), 93–106.

Foss, F. M., Saleh, M. N., et al. (1998). *Diphtheria* toxin fusion proteins. *Curr. Top. Microbiol. Immunol.* **234**, 63–81.

Frankel, A. E., Kreitman, R. J., et al. (2000). Targeted toxins. *Clin. Cancer Res.* **6**(2), 326–334.

Frankel, A. E., Laver, J. H., et al. (1997). Therapy of patients with T-cell lymphomas and leukemias using an anti- CD7 monoclonal antibody-ricin A chain immunotoxin. *Leuk. Lymphoma* **26**(3-4), 287–298.

Frankel, A. E., Lilly, M., et al. (1998). *Diphtheria* toxin fused to granulocyte-macrophage colony-stimulating factor is toxic to blasts from patients with juvenile myelomonocytic leukemia and chronic myelomonocytic leukemia. *Blood* **92**(11), 4279–4786.

Frankel, A. E., McCubrey, J. A., et al. (2000). *Diphtheria* toxin fused to human interleukin-3 is toxic to blasts from patients with myeloid leukemias. *Leukemia* **14**(4), 576–585.

Frankel, A. E., Ramage, J., et al. (2000). Characterization of *diphtheria* fusion proteins targeted to the human interleukin-3 receptor. *Protein Eng.* **13**(8), 575–581.

Iordanov, M. S., Ryabinina, O. P., et al. (2000). Molecular determinants of apoptosis induced by the cytotoxic ribonuclease onconase: Evidence for cytotoxic mechanisms different from inhibition of protein synthesis. *Cancer Res.* **60**(7), 1983–1994.

LeMaistre, C. F., Saleh, M. N., et al. (1998). Phase I trial of a ligand fusion-protein (DAB389IL-2) in lymphomas expressing the receptor for interleukin-2. *Blood* **91**(2), 399–405.

Messmann, R. A., Vitetta, E. S., et al. (2000). A phase I study of combination therapy with immunotoxins IgG-HD37-deglycosylated ricin A chain (dgA) and IgG-RFB4-dgA (Combotox) in patients with refractory CD19(+), CD22(+) B cell lymphoma. *Clin. Cancer Res.* **6**(4), 1302–1313.

Niculescu-Duvaz, I., Friedlos, F., et al. (1999). Prodrugs for antibody- and gene-directed enzyme prodrug therapies (ADEPT and GDEPT). *Anticancer Drug Des.* **14**(6), 517–538.

Pai, L. H., and Pastan, I. (1997). Immunotoxin therapy. *In* "Cancer: Principles and Practice of Oncology" (V. T. DeVita, S. Hellman, and S. A. Rosenberg, eds.), 5th Ed., pp. 3045–3057. Lippincott-Raven, Philadelphia.

Pai, L. H., Wittes, R., *et al.* (1996). Treatment of advanced solid tumors with immunotoxin LMB-1: An antibody linked to *Pseudomonas* exotoxin. *Nature Med.* **2**(3), 350–353.

Saleh, M. N., LeMaistre, C. F., *et al.* (1998). Antitumor activity of DAB389IL-2 fusion toxin in mycosis fungoides. *J. Am. Acad. Dermatol.* **39**(1), 63–73.

Schnell, R., Vitetta, E., *et al.* (1998). Clinical trials with an anti-CD25 ricin A-chain experimental and immunotoxin (RFT5-SMPT-dgA) in Hodgkin's lymphoma. *Leuk. Lymphoma* **30**(5-6), 525–537.

Sievers, E. L., Appelbaum, F. R., *et al.* (1999). Selective ablation of acute myeloid leukemia using antibody-targeted chemotherapy: A phase I study of an anti-CD33 calicheamicin immunoconjugate. *Blood* **93**(11), 3678–3684.

Springer, C. J., and Niculescu-Duvaz, I. (1997). Antibody-directed enzyme prodrug therapy (ADEPT): A review. *Adv. Drug Deliv. Rev.* **26**(2-3), 151–172.

Vitetta, E. S. (2000). Immunotoxins and vascular leak syndrome. *Cancer J. Sci. Am.* **6**(Suppl 3), S218–S224.

Targeted Vectors for Cancer Gene Therapy

Jesús Gómez-Navarro
David T. Curiel
University of Alabama at Birmingham

GLOSSARY

gene therapy An evolving technique used to treat inherited and acquired diseases. The medical procedure involves replacing, manipulating, or supplementing nonfunctional genes with therapeutic genes.

targeted virus A virus that has been modified by genetic or chemical means to direct it toward, or away from, a certain population of cells.

targeting A strategy to limit the vector-mediated gene transfer and expression to a certain population of cells. The targeted cells usually share the same histology (e.g., prostate) or physiology (highly proliferative, malignant transformation).

transcriptional targeting A targeting strategy based on limiting the expression of transferred genes to cells that have a particular regulatory sequence, or promoter, acti-

vated. An example is the delivery of toxin genes under the control of the α-fetoprotein promoter, which is activated in hepatocarcinoma cells.

transductional targeting A targeting strategy based on limiting the binding capacity of the vector system exclusively, or preferentially, to the cell surface of target cells.

vector An agent, such as a virus or a small piece of DNA called a plasmid, that carries a modified or foreign gene. When used in gene therapy, a vector delivers the desired gene to a targeted cell.

T he genetic fingerprint associated with malignant transformation and progression, consisting of a myriad of acquired genetic lesions, is now being identified rapidly and precisely in a large variety of human cancers. Armed with this knowledge of the molecular anatomy of the cancer cell, gene therapy has emerged as a rational method of therapeutic, and possibly preventive, intervention against cancer targeted at the level of cellular gene expression.

I. WHY TARGETED VECTORS ARE NEEDED FOR CANCER GENE THERAPY

Gene therapy attempts to alter the cancerous pathophysiologic state by delivering nucleic acids into tumoral or normal cells. The expression of transferred genes may achieve a desired effect on the cellular phenotype. Based on this concept, a number of strategies have been developed to accomplish cancer gene therapy. These approaches include (i) mutation compensation, (ii) molecular chemotherapy, (iii) genetic immunopotentiation, and (iv) viral oncolysis. For mutation compensation, gene therapy techniques are designed to correct the molecular lesions that are etiologic of malignant transformation or to avoid the contribution to the malignant growth by tumor-supporting nonmalignant stromal cells. For molecular chemotherapy, methods have been developed to achieve selective delivery or expression of a toxin gene in cancer, or stromal cells, to induce their eradication or, alternatively, to increase their sensitivity to concomitant chemotherapy or radiotherapy. Also, attempts are made to deliver genetic sequences that protect normal bone marrow cells from the toxic effects of standard chemotherapeutic drugs, thus allowing the administration of higher drug doses without reaching otherwise limiting myelosuppression. Genetic immunopotentiation strategies attempt to achieve active immunization against tumor-associated antigens by gene transfer methodologies. Both tumor cells and cellular components of the immune system have been genetically modified to this end. Viral oncolysis is a means to induce tumor cell eradication by exploiting the lytic life cycle of replication-competent viruses.

Of note, each of these approaches has been rapidly translated into human gene therapy clinical trials. Importantly, a number of critical requirements, however, have been made apparent in these studies that preclude the full realization of the promise of gene therapy. The development of targeted vectors is directed by, and is aimed to overcome, each of these limitations, as follows.

A. Mutation Compensation Requires Enhancing Gene Transfer

Both the replacement of tumor suppressor genes and the blockade of oncogenes mostly modulate intracellular responses. Thus, nearly every tumor cell might have to be targeted for these approaches to be clinically effective. The current state of development of gene therapy vectors, both viral and nonviral, makes this feat unachievable within nontoxic margins of vector dose. Surprisingly, gene transfer of certain genes, such as p53, has been followed by tumor responses that exceed by far the amount of genetically modified tumor cells, suggesting that a "bystander effect" is being induced. Despite this encouraging observation, breakthrough developments in vector technology are still needed to dramatically increase the efficiency of gene transfer currently achievable. The recent development of genetically modified vectors with enhanced infectivity and of replicative vectors is an exciting step toward that end (Fig. 1).

B. Molecular Chemotherapy Demands Selectivity

With all its promise, molecular chemotherapy also bears some practical limitations. To date, the strategy of molecular chemotherapy has been mainly used in locoregional disease models to overcome the lack of vector systems that deliver toxic genes selectively into target cells. In these *in situ* schemas, a vector encoding the toxin gene is administered intratumorally or into an anatomic compartment containing the tumor mass. The goals of this delivery method are (1) to achieve high local vector concentration in order to favor tumor transduction and (2) to limit vector dissemination to avoid untoward toxicity. As mentioned, however, transduction efficiencies of presently available vectors are inadequate; even in closed compartments, such as intrapleural and intraperitoneal cavities, it has not been possible to modify a sufficient number of tumor cells to achieve a clinically relevant tumoral response. Furthermore, increasing the dose of the viral vector to obtain transduction of a larger fraction of the tumor cells has been associated with limiting regional toxicity, both in model animals and in humans. Thus, the small therapeutic index of currently available vectors in the context of *in situ* administration is a critical limiting factor for the purposes of gene therapy of cancer.

C. Genetic Immunopotentiation Requires Broadening the Viral Tropism

The main theoretical advantage of the genetic immunopotentiation approach is the possibility of en-

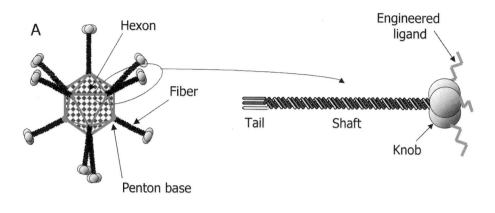

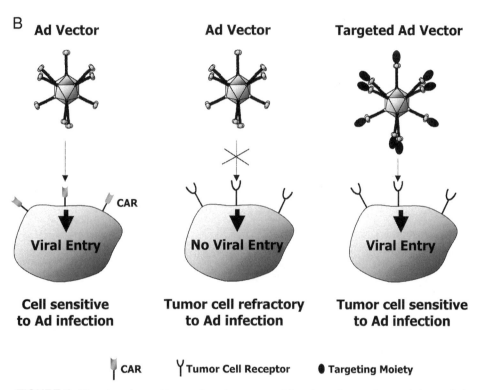

FIGURE 1 Targeting of recombinant adenovirus vectors. Adenoviruses have a characteristic morphology consisting of an icosahedral shell composed of 20 equilateral triangular faces and 12 vertices. The protein coat (capsid) consists of hexon subunits and penton subunits at each vertex. A fiber with a knob at the end projects from each penton; this fiber is involved in the process of attachment of the virus particle to the host cell. Genetic modifications into the knob (A) endow the fiber with new binding capacities that enable the virus to attach to alternate cellular receptors, thus either augmenting gene transfer efficiency (when the new receptors are more abundant) or making the gene transfer more selective (when the receptors are present preferentially in the target cells) (B).

listing physiological mechanisms for a potentially vast amplification of the therapeutic maneuver, e.g., inducing a systemic cytotoxic T lymphocyte-mediated reaction against the tumor. In this regard, it was expected that even modest levels of gene transfer would be followed by clonal expansion and systemic spread of antitumoral effector immune cells and mediators. Thus, efficiency of gene transfer would be not essential, given the relatively low amounts of cells and gene products needed to obtain a potentially powerful response from the immune system. In truth, the level of gene transfer into tumor and immune effector cells observed clinically has indeed been poor, and the results obtained by tumor immunotherapy in humans have also been in general very modest. Of note, a better definition of viral cell entry mechanisms and of cell receptors in target tumor or immune system cells is rapidly accruing (Fig. 2). Thus, the evaluation of novel means to augment the efficiency and spectrum of infectivity of gene transfer vectors into these cells, and to favorably modulate their phenotype, is in order.

D. Viral Oncolysis Demands Selective Replication in the Tumor and Ample Lateral Spread

For this strategy to be clinically applicable, viral replication should spare nontumoral cells and be nearly universal within the tumor cell population. The latter condition requires that the ideal viral agent would possess the capacity to efficiently infect target cells *in situ* and to spread laterally after replication. Both specifications demand a degree of efficiency and selectivity in

cell infection that is over and above the capacities of the viruses clinically tested to date. An increasing understanding of the biology of viral entry into the cell is available, however, thus permitting the evaluation of a variety of approaches for viral targeting that might satisfy the aforementioned requirements.

E. The Treatment of Disseminated Neoplasms Requires Targeting the Tumor and Bypassing Several Physiological Barriers

A majority of cancer patients are diagnosed when their tumors have already disseminated systemically. The use of gene therapy strategies targeted directly against the tumor would then require that the vector system is capable, after intravascular administration, of both systemic distribution into the multiple organ sites that harbor cancer foci and of efficient and selective gene delivery into target cancer cells thereafter. Although a reasonable understanding of the na-

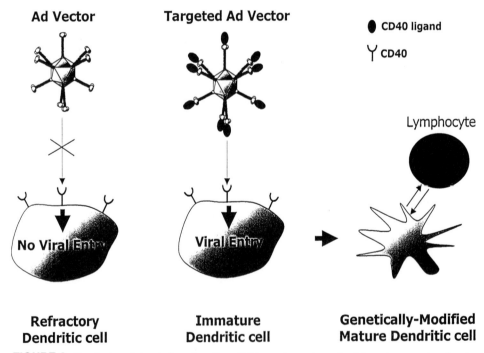

FIGURE 2 Broadening of the viral tropism. Cross-linking and genetic methods have been employed to insert the ligand of the CD40 molecule into the viral knob. Such a targeted viral vector has an increased capacity to infect otherwise refractory dendritic cells, which express CD40 in their surface, and to thus trigger cell maturation. As a consequence, dendritic cells genetically modified in this manner have an enhanced efficacy for vaccination.

tive determinants of viral tropism at the cellular level exists (see later), a scarcity of information is, however, apparent regarding the determinants of vector efficacy at the entire organism level, which seem in fact distinct from the former. The physical properties and stability of viral particles in the presence of the complement, their sequestration by cells of the mononuclear phagocytic system, including liver Kupffer cells, and the structure of the vascular endothelium and dynamics of vascular egression are all being analyzed in this context. Certainly, a more complete understanding of these and related immunological factors (neutralizing antibodies and cellular immune response) may allow developing targeting strategies and, thus, progressing in the utilization of viral vectors *in vivo*.

II. MODALITIES OF VECTOR TARGETING

Targeted gene therapy for cancer can be accomplished at different levels. In one approach, the spatial distribution of the vector is restricted by virtue of the maneuver used for its administration into the body, which physically confines the vector into a site or cavity. In addition, targeting can be based on exploiting the distinctive physiology of solid tumors. Alternatively, the tumor cell can be targeted at the level of transduction to achieve the selective delivery of the therapeutic gene. This involves the derivation of a vector that binds selectively to the target cancer cell. Finally, the therapeutic gene can be placed under the control of tumor-specific transcriptional regulatory sequences that are activated in tumor cells but not in normal cells and therefore target expression selectively to the tumor cell (Table I). Of note, as mentioned earlier, these modifications of viral vectors are implemented not only for restricting the host range, but also for enhancing the capacity for gene transfer to certain cells and for extending the types of cells that can be infected effectively.

A. Physical Targeting

The feasibility of the first human clinical trials of gene therapy was predicated on the capacity to efficiently infect T cells with recombinant retroviral vec-

tors. This was made possible only by removing the target cells from the patient, appropriately maintaining and modifying genetically the cells in the test tube, and by later infusing them back into the patient. In this case, cell targeting was obtained by cell isolation. Unfortunately, this approach is useful only with sessile cells, when the cells are aimed for generating an immune response or when the cells secrete a therapeutic product. In another early example of physical targeting, plasmid DNA encoding the costimulatory gene B7 was injected directly into melanoma nodules to generate an antitumoral immune response. This method of gene delivery, however, is inefficient for most purposes and does not precisely spare nontumor cells from gene transfer. These two means of targeting, albeit rudimentary, have proved the most effective to date.

More recently, attempts have been made to increase the delivered vector inoculum by confining the vector administration to closed anatomical compartments, such as the pleural and peritoneal cavities, frequently affected by malignancies of regional distribution. The levels of gene transfer achieved with retroviral and adenoviral vectors in several clinical trials in mesothelioma and ovarian cancer have been insufficient to translate into clinically relevant effects. In addition, infusion of vectors into the vasculature of target organs has been explored, mainly as a means to allow delivery of higher vector doses and, thus, to increase efficiency while simultaneously decreasing the exposure of nontarget tissues to the vector. In fact, vector-associated toxicities have been prohibiting in animal models and humans, such as those seen after intrahepatic artery infusion of adenoviral vector, thus revealing a small therapeutic index. These observations highlight the need of vector tropism modifications, perhaps via exploitation of the tumor physiology and via improved vector design.

B. Targeting Strategies Exploiting Tumor Physiology

1. Tumor Cells Divide in a Background of Quiescent Cells

The physiology of solid tumors at the microenvironmental level provides a unique target for making cancer treatment more selective. Early in the development

TABLE I
Vector Targeting Strategies

Basis of the targeting maneuver	Modality	Example[a]
Physical delivery	*In vitro* gene transfer	Infection of T lymphocytes with a retrovirus encoding adenosine deaminase
	Intraarterial infusion	VEGF plasmid infused in coronary arteries
	Intratumoral injection	HLA-B7 DNA–liposome complexes injected into melanoma nodules
	Intraperitoneal infusion	Adenovirus encoding thymidine kinase followed by intravenous ganciclovir
	Intrapleural infusion	Adenovirus encoding thymidine kinase followed by intravenous ganciclovir
Tumor physiology	Dividing versus nondividing cells	Treatment of brain tumors using intratumoral transduction with a retrovirus encoding the thymidine kinase gene and intravenous ganciclovir
	Tumor hypoxia	Regulation of therapeutic gene with promoter containing a hypoxia responsive element[b]
	Tumor vasculature	Angiogenic endothelial cells avidly bind and internalize cationic liposomes and liposome–DNA complexes[b]
	Lower apoptosis threshold	Adenovirus encoding proapoptotic Bax induces tumor cell cytotoxicity and radiosensitization without apparent toxicity in normal cells[b]
Cell-specific surface factors (transduction)	Cross-linker-based targeting	Fab–FGF2 conjugates bind to the adenoviral fiber knob and to FGF2 tumor cell surface receptors, thus allowing an increased therapeutic ratio *in vivo*[b]
	Genetic targeting	RGD peptide engineered into the Hl loop of the adenovirus knob allows targeting avβ3 and avβ5 integrin receptors[b]
Cell-specific regulators of gene expression (transcription)	Tissue-targeted expression	The PSA promoter controls the expression of replication-enabling viral vector genes, thus allowing prostate-specific viral replication and oncolysis
	Disease-targeted expression	The endothelin-1 promoter, activated in growing endothelium, can direct the expression of a therapeutic gene to areas of angiogenesis[b]
	Externally regulated expression	A radio-inducible suicide gene (EGR-tk) can be constructed by cloning the early growth response (Egr)-1 promoter upstream of the herpes simplex virus thymidine kinase (HSV-tk) gene[b]

[a]PSA, prostate specific antigen; RGD, tripeptide Arg-Gly-Asp.
[b]Animal models only.

of vector systems, virologists observed the dependence of retroviral infection on cell division and proposed to exploit this feature to selectively deliver genes into the dividing tumor cells, surrounded by quiescent nontumor cells. Unfortunately, although feasible with highly proliferative murine tumor models, this approach is suboptimal for human tumors in which the fraction of actively dividing tumor cells is usually less than 20% at any given time point. In addition, all other viral vectors in current use do not require cells to divide for gene transfer and transgene expression to occur, thus limiting the value of exploiting this aspect of tumor biology for targeting purposes.

Viral vectors have been engineered for allowing their selective replication in tumor cells. In some cases, the cell phenotype that determines the desired selectivity is associated with cell proliferation. This fact, for the reason mentioned earlier, might restrict the replication and compromise the potency of such replicative viral vectors. It would seem preferable that, for the sake of potency, selective replication is engineered based on more widespread, nearly universal tumor cell traits.

2. The Tumor Microenvironment Is Hypoxic

Regions of hypoxia and necrosis within solid tumors present opportunities for targeted, tumor-selective gene therapy. For example, hypoxia induces the transcription of certain genes, such as vascular endothelial growth factor (VEGF) and erythropoietin, via the activity of hypoxia responsive elements (HRE) located at the 3′ flanking region of those genes. Gene therapy strategies have been evaluated whereby hypoxia induces the transcription of a prodrug-activating enzyme gene controlled by a HRE. These hypoxia-inducible vectors have been shown to indeed drive focal transgene expression in murine tumor models. It remains to be seen, however, whether hypoxia can be exploited in the microenvironment of human tumors in which a typically smaller growth fraction and perhaps a more heterogeneous distribution of hypoxic foci will impose more challenging conditions for efficient targeting.

Gene therapy strategies could similarly be designed to exploit tumor necrosis. In this regard, certain species of anaerobic bacteria of the genus *Clostridium* can selectively germinate and grow in hypoxic/necrotic regions of solid tumors after the intravenous injection of spores. Thus, it might prove possible to exploit clostridia as gene therapy vectors engineered to express therapeutic genes, e.g., a prodrug-activating enzyme. Studies in murine tumor models suggest the feasibility of this concept.

3. The Tumor Vasculature Is Aberrant

Tumors require constant new vessel growth to maintain their local progression, invasion, and metastasis. The resulting vasculature, however, develops structural and physiological abnormalities that render the vessels leaky and the blood circulation sluggish and irregular. These characteristics determine obstacles for many therapeutic interventions, but also offer some opportunities. For instance, increased vascular permeability, due to incomplete endothelial cell and basal membrane lining, has been shown to allow the targeting of anticancer drugs into tumors via small, sterically stabilized (stealth) liposomes with prolonged bioavailability. Alternatively, angiogenic endothelial cells have been shown to avidly bind and internalize cationic liposomes and liposome–DNA complexes (but not other types of liposomes), thus raising the possibility of using liposomes to deliver therapeutic genes selectively to the endothelium at areas of angiogenesis rather than to the tumor or interstitial cells. This would possibly be used to exert an antiangiogenic effect, and an antitumoral outcome would conceivably ensue.

4. Carcinogenic Transformation Is Associated with a Lower Threshold for Apoptosis

Tumor cells are characterized by a lower threshold than normal cells for undergoing apoptosis after exposure to certain proapoptotic stimuli. Although not yet fully understood, this differential sensitivity offers a potential therapeutic window for gene-based proapoptotic interventions. Given the ubiquity of the numerous cellular proteins involved in regulating apoptotic pathways, however, highly selective activation of the lethal processes in cancer cells might still be a critical requirement of therapeutic maneuvers. In that case, targeted gene transfer, as described later, could restrict the expression of proapoptotic genes to the tumor cells.

C. Transductional (Cell Surface) Targeting

Attempts to modulate the binding of vectors to cell surface receptors have consisted most frequently on modifying viral vectors, given their generally higher gene transfer efficiency. In this regard, the ability to alter viral-binding tropism has followed the increasing understanding of the basic biology of viral entry. Thus, knowledge on retrovirus cell entry led to the first maneuvers for viral vector targeting using recombinant retrovirus, rapidly following for analogous strategies with recombinant adenovirus and later with adeno-associated virus, herpesvirus, and others as soon as the corresponding viral entry biology has been defined.

1. Biology of Viral Entry into Target Cells

In general, viral entry into target cells occurs in three phases. First, viruses adsorb to a receptor in the cell surface. Adsorption occurs via molecular interactions of viral surface proteins with molecules in the plasma membrane of the cell. This process proceeds as well at 37°C and at 4°C. For example, the surface subunit of the lentivirus envelope glycoprotein binds to CD4 and the chemokine receptors; herpes simplex virus envelope glycoproteins bind to heparan sulfate and to a tumor necrosis factor receptor; and the adenoviral carboxy-terminal knob domain of the fiber binds to the coxsackievirus and adenovirus receptor, CAR. Second, viruses penetrate through or fuse with the cell membrane and are uncoated as they enter the cytoplasm. This process is energy dependent, occurs optimally at 37°C but not at 4°C, and is frequently initiated during adsorption by the interaction of viral surface proteins with cellular receptors. For example, internalization of the adenovirus virion is potentiated by the interaction of Arg-Gly-Asp (RGD) peptide sequences in the penton base with secondary host cell receptors, the integrins $\alpha_v\beta_3$ and $\alpha_v\beta_5$. This interaction induces receptor aggregation, which usually triggers a biochemical signal followed by internalization through an endocytic process that involves clathrin-coated pits. Thus, the virus is brought into endosomes in the cytoplasm. Third, in many instances, uncoating of the virus progresses when the pH of the endosome decreases, thus inducing further biochemical interactions of the viral surface with the endosome membrane, which ultimately lead to release of the viral capsid contents into the cytoplasm.

An important characteristic of viral entry from the targeting standpoint is the level of interdependence of the molecules involved in the steps just described. In effect, the participation of distinct molecules during binding and internalization allows modulating the former without disturbing the second. In this regard, retargeting of adenoviral vectors has been facilitated by the fact that the entry of adenovirus into susceptible cells requires two sets of molecules acting autonomously at two sequential steps, as mentioned previously. Thus, targeting maneuvers need only to assure the initial binding step. After anchoring has occurred, which can be determined by binding of the targeted vector with receptors other than CAR, internalization rapidly follows. However, targeting of retroviruses has been hampered by the participation in viral entry of a single molecular complex of the viral envelope containing multiple domains. As a consequence, most attempts to modify binding have been followed by a parallel dramatic loss of internalization efficiency.

The particular mechanisms whereby viruses enter into human cells are very diverse, as are the targeting strategies and the hurdles encountered for modifying entry of the derived vectors into cells. Based on the aforementioned facts, two main strategies have been evaluated for modifying the binding and entry of viral vectors into target cells. These include (i) the use of bifunctional cross-linkers that bind both to the viral vector and to a specific surface receptor in target cells and (ii) the genetic modification of the viral superficial proteins (Table II).

TABLE II
Transductional (Surface) Targeting

Targeting strategy	Modality	Example (vector—applications)[a]
Cross-linker-based targeting	Immunological	Ad—Fab portion of antiadenoviral knob antibody chemically linked to ligand, e.g., Fab–folate conjugates for targeting into ovarian cancer cells
		Ad—Bispecific single chain antibodies that bind to Ad knob and to EGF receptor
Genetic targeting	Modification of viral coat proteins	Retro—insertion of erythropoietin in env protein
		Ad—insertion of RGD ligand in HI loop and in carboxy terminus
		HSV—insertion of erythropoietin in envelope protein
		AAV—CD34 and bispecific Fab$_2$ antibody
		Sindbis and HCG
	Ablation of binding	Ad—mutations of knob and penton base ablate binding into natural receptors, CAR, and integrins
	Pseudotyping	Retro—replace the coat proteins of the vector with the coat proteins of another virus endowed with desired tropism
	Hybrids	Ad—substitution of the fiber with an artificial structure that possesses alternate targeting ligands
		Ad—construction of vectors with mulitple fibers of distinct binding properties
Combination of cross-linker and genetic targeting	Biotin–avidin based	Several vectors—biotinylation of viral coat or envelope proteins, which can be facilitated by genetically engineering biotin acceptor tags; allows combination with targeting moieties complexed with avidin
		Retro—display Ig-binding domain on vector as genetic fusion with coat protein; use mAb to cross-link vector with targeted cell

[a]Ad, adenovirus; CAR, coxsackie and adenovirus receptor; Ig, immunoglobulin; retro, retrovirus.

2. Cross-Linker-Based (Immunological) Targeting

Targeting by using bifunctional cross-linkers has been reported for adenoviral vectors. We have shown that it is possible to redirect adenoviral infection by employing the Fab fragment of a neutralizing antiknob monoclonal antibody (mAb) chemically conjugated to a cell-specific ligand. When complexed with preformed adenoviral vector particles, the bispecific conjugate simultaneously ablates endogenous viral tropism and introduces novel tropism, thereby resulting in a truly targeted adenoviral vector. We have employed a number of targeting ligands, including folate, basic fibroblast growth factor, and an antibody directed against the epidermal growth factor receptor. In this manner, it has been demonstrated that tropism-modified adenoviral vectors can infect cells that are refractory to transduction by the native vector; that tropism-modified adenoviral vectors can enhance gene transfer to target cells; and that this enhancement in infection can be translated into a therapeutic benefit *in vivo*. Others have similarly retargeted adenoviral vectors by means of bispecific antibodies comprising a monoclonal antibody to an epitope engineered in the penton base and a monoclonal antibody to a cell surface receptor. The cross-linker approach to the generation of tropism-modified adenoviral vectors suffers, however, from a number of limitations. In particular, because the targeting ligand is not covalently coupled to the adenovirus particle, there is the potential for the bispecific conjugate to become dissociated from the vector *in vivo*. Production and scale-up of the conjugates may also hamper the widespread clinical application of the strategy. The production of recombinant fusion proteins containing binding domains to the viral vector and to a cell ligand is a more feasible approach and might advance cross-linker-based strategies to practical implementation. Two examples are fusion proteins containing two antibody fragments, or diabodies, and the fusion of the soluble adenovirus CAR receptor with a variety of cell ligands.

3. Genetic Targeting

The drawbacks inherent in any strategy to redirect adenovirus tropism by complexing the vector parti-cles with bispecific targeting conjugates could be avoided by the direct genetic engineering of viral capsid proteins to contain cell-targeting ligands. In this regard, the carboxy terminus of the adenovirus fiber protein can be modified to incorporate targeting motifs with specificity for cellular receptors. In an alternative approach, we have also reported that targeting ligands can be incorporated within the so-called HI loop of the fiber knob. Adenoviral vectors, which have been engineered to incorporate either a polylysine motif at the carboxy terminus of the fiber or an RGD motif at the carboxy terminus or in the HI loop, have demonstrated a significantly enhanced infection of cancer cell lines and primary tumor cells that express low levels of the primary adenovirus receptor. Thus, these genetic modifications to the fiber protein have resulted in expanded tropism by successfully redirecting adenovirus binding to alternative cellular receptors.

The next challenge will be to employ genetic methods to engineer adenoviral vectors with restricted specificity for a single target cell type. In addition to recognizing novel receptors, such vectors should also lack the ability to bind to the native primary adenovirus receptor. This indeed has been accomplished by site-directed mutagenesis of the fiber knob domain to eliminate the cell-binding site. An important consequence of the ablation of native adenovirus tropism is that it will not be possible to propagate these vectors on standard cell lines that express the fiber receptor. However, we have developed a novel artificial primary receptor that can be recognized by adenovirus vectors that fail to bind the native fiber receptor. This technology should be useful in the propagation of genetically modified, truly targeted adenoviral vectors.

As said before, and in contrast to adenoviruses, retroviruses employ a single envelope glycoprotein to accomplish both binding to the cellular receptor and the subsequent step of membrane fusion. As a consequence, modification of retroviral tropism has proven problematic, with few reports of modified envelope proteins that retain these two functions of binding and fusion such that efficient delivery can be achieved. A number of molecules, including single chain antibodies, growth factors, and cytokines, have been genetically incorporated into the retroviral envelope glycoprotein, whereupon they confer novel binding specificities into the engineered viral particles. However, some of these surface-displayed polypeptides failed to mediate retroviral infection; rather, they proved inhibitory to gene delivery by the modified vectors. In an elegant approach to overcome this obstacle, a protease cleavage site has been incorporated into the design of the retargeted vector. Thus, upon contact with proteases expressed on the surface of the target cell, the inhibitory polypeptide is cleaved from the viral surface, thereby restoring infectivity. To date, tropism-modified retroviral vectors have suffered from significantly lower viral titers than parental vectors and it is therefore not yet proven possible to employ targeted retroviruses *in vivo*.

4. Target Definition

A key factor in any transductional targeting schema is the availability of appropriate specific molecules on the target cells that can be exploited as specific anchor receptors. To date, proof of principle has been accomplished with a limited range of targeting moieties chosen for their ability to bind to the relatively short list of previously identified cellular receptors. However, a number of groups have described systems that employ high-throughput screening of phage libraries for identifying molecules, including peptides and single chain antibodies, which bind to specific cell types, both *in vitro* and *in vivo*. Of note, this powerful new technology allows the rapid isolation and screening of potential tumor-specific or tumor vasculature-specific ligands without requiring that the target of the ligand be identified. This approach has already permitted the derivation of cell surface-targeted adenoviral vectors for enhanced gene transfer, currently being tested for cancer gene therapy.

D. Transcriptional Targeting

In contrast to surface targeting, which attempts to augment the specificity of gene transfer but, importantly, also seeks to expand vector tropism and to enhance its overall efficiency, transcriptional targeting has been applied mostly for restricting the expression of transgenes to target cells. Thus, it has found wide application in the area of molecular chemotherapy, where tumor- or tissue-specific regulatory sequences have been employed to limit the expression of

prodrug-converting enzymes specifically to the target cancer cells and dispensable homotypic cells (Table III). In the same vein, more recently, transcriptional targeting is being used to "untarget" the expression of transgenes from nontarget organs that are unduly sensitive to the effect of the transferred gene. For example, it may be desirable to minimize the expression of thymidine kinase in the liver, where it induces a limiting toxicity in animal models after intraperitoneal and intrahepatic vector administration. In both cases, by limiting the transgene expression to tissues of a particular type, cycling and angiogenic tissues, or transformed cells, and by diminishing the expression

TABLE III
Transcriptional (Promoter) Targeting

Promoters	Organ or condition of expression
Tissue-specific promoters	
α-Fetoprotein	Hepatoma
β-Casein	Breast
Calcineurin α	Neuroblastoma, glioblastoma
Carcinoembryonic antigen	Colon, lung
DF3/MUC	Breast
erbB-2	Breast, pancreas, gastric
HSV-LAT	Neuroblastoma, glioblastoma
Ig heavy and light chain	B-cell leukemia and lymphoma
Myelin basic protein	Glioblastoma
Osteocalcin	Osteosarcoma
Prostate-specific antigen	Prostate
sis	Osteosarcoma or chondrosarcoma
Secretory leukoprotease inhibitor	Colon, lung, breast, bladder, oropharyngeal, ovarian, endometrial
Synapsin 1	Neuroblastoma, glioblastoma
Tyrosinase	Melanoma
Tyrosinase-related protein 1	Melanoma
Disease-associated promoters	
COX-2	Tumor cells
Cyclin A	Proliferation
Endoglin	Angiogenesis
Endothelin-1 promoter	Ischemia
E2F-1	Proliferation
E-selectin	Angiogenesis
Glucose response protein 78	Acidic, anoxic, glucose-starved tumor tissue
Hypoxia response element	Hypoxia
L-Plastin	Tumor cells
Midkine	Tumor cells
Myc–Max responsive element	Lung
Phosphoglycerate kinase promoter	Hypoxia

in other normal tissues, a net increase in the therapeutic index may be achieved.

1. Tissue-Target Expression

Tumor markers have been used in the clinic extensively for diagnostic purposes. Many were early on considered by vector engineers to represent attractive candidate gene promoters (Table III). Thus, transcriptionally targeted adenoviral vectors expressing the toxin gene thymidine kinase under the control of the tumor-specific promoter α-fetoprotein and prostate-specific antigen were employed in molecular chemotherapy approaches to hepatocellular and prostate carcinoma, respectively. The selective expression of the therapeutic gene in the target tumors suggests that transcriptionally targeted adenoviral vectors would be of clinical utility in other diseases. However, it has been reported that certain tumor-specific regulatory elements lose their specificity in the context of an adenoviral vector genome. "Insulator" elements are being engineered in vector genomes that are able to restrict back the expression of the transgene to the desired tissues. Further limitations come from the prohibitively large size of many regulatory sequences, which exceed the capacity of certain current vectors. However, novel gene transfer systems with larger capacity are being developed and could be employed to overcome this limitation—these vectors include gutless adenoviral vectors and recombinant herpes virus.

2. Disease-Targeted Expression

A number of genes are overexpressed in cells with high metabolic and proliferating activity. These include not only genes activated in the tumor cells, but also those genes in the stromal cells that, induced by the tumor microenvironment milieu, contribute to sustaining locally tumor progression, such as genes regulating angiogenesis, invasion, and metastasis (Table III).

3. Externally Regulated Expression

Certain promoters can be activated regionally by the application of conventional cancer therapies such as radiation or, systemically, by drugs such as derivatives of tetracycline and steroids. In both cases, these systems allow to superimpose the timing of expression as an additional level of control in the expression of targeted genes. Further development of the technology seems, however, contingent upon the availability of adequate surface and transcriptional targeting systems.

4. Promoter Definition

High-throughput screening of phage display libraries promises to define organ- and tumor-specific ligands. In a technological breakthrough of similar potential, the rapid and precise definition of genes overexpressed and underexpressed in tumor versus normal tissues, and of the corresponding regulatory promoter sequences, is being revolutionized with other high-throughput techniques, including microarrays and serial analysis of gene expression (SAGE). For instance, based on this last method, most transcripts in tumor and normal cells can be quantitated and compared, defining gene expression profiles with a potential value that seems hard to overestimate in the current context.

III. FUTURE DIRECTIONS

To date, targeted gene therapy has been attempted most frequently by employing either transductional targeting or transcriptional targeting alone. However, it is immediately possible to enhance the overall level of gene transfer specificity by combining the complementary approaches of transductional and transcriptional targeting, each of which might be imperfect or "leaky" by itself. It is also readily possible to enhance the potency and stringency of each targeting strategy by combining several of its modalities, such as deriving "cocktail" approaches that simultaneously exploit the genetic and immunological targeting maneuvers against a variety of tumor cell targets or by adding dual promoters. It is very possible, however, that major advances in the field will come from the application of the high-throughput technologies mentioned earlier, which will allow to define targeting moieties and gene expression regulatory sequences of utmost relevance and precision, at scale. Together with a better understanding of the factors determining vector distribution at the entire organism level, the predictable development of targeted vector systems seems to put paradigmatic, targetable, and injectable vectors at our fingertips.

Acknowledgments

We appreciate the secretarial support of Connie H. Weldon. Our work cited in this manuscript was conducted at the Gene Therapy Center, University of Alabama at Birmingham, and was supported by the following grants: NIH N01 CO-97110, United States Department of Defense PC 970193, United States Department of Defense PC 991018, and grants from the Juvenile Diabetes Foundation, the CapCURE Foundation, and the Cancer Treatment Research Foundation.

See Also the Following Articles

ADENO-ASSOCIATED VIRUS: A VECTOR FOR HIGH-EFFICIENCY GENE TRANSDUCTION • ANTIBODIES IN THE GENE THERAPY OF CANCER • CATIONIC LIPID-MEDIATED GENE THERAPY • GENE THERAPY VECTORS, SAFETY CONSIDERATIONS • HYPOXIA AND DRUG RESISTANCE • P53 GENE THERAPY • REPLICATION-SPECIFIC VIRUSES FOR CANCER TREATMENT • RETROVIRAL VECTORS • TRANSGENIC MICE IN CANCER RESEARCH

Bibliography

Brown, K. C. (2000). New approaches for cell-specific targeting: Identification of cell-selective peptides from combinatorial libraries. *Curr. Opin. Chem. Biol.* **4,** 16–21.

Curiel, D. T. (1999). Strategies to adapt adenoviral vectors for targeted delivery. *Ann. N. Y. Acad. Sci.* **886,** 158–171.

Fechner, H., Haack, A., Wang, H., Wang, X., Eizema, K., Pauschinger, M., Schoemaker, R., Veghel, R., Houtsmuller, A., Schultheiss, H. P., Lamers, J., and Poller, W. (1999). Expression of coxsackie adenovirus receptor and alphav-integrin does not correlate with adenovector targeting in vivo indicating anatomical vector barriers. *Gene Ther.* **6,** 1520–1535.

Gomez-Navarro, J., Curiel, D. T., and Douglas, J. T. (1999). Gene therapy for cancer. *Eur. J. Cancer* **35,** 2039–2057.

Nettelbeck, D. M., Jerome, V., and Muller, R. (2000). Gene therapy: Designer promoters for tumour targeting. *Trends Genet.* **16,** 174–181.

Peng, K. W. (1999). Strategies for targeting therapeutic gene delivery. *Mol. Med. Today* **5,** 448–453.

Russell, S. J., and Cosset, F. L. (1999). Modifying the host range properties of retroviral vectors. *J. Gene Med.* **1,** 300–311.

Wickham, T. J. (2000). Targeting adenovirus. *Gene Ther.* **7,** 110–114.

Taxol and Other Molecules That Interact with Microtubules

George A. Orr
Lifeng He
Susan Band Horwitz

Albert Einstein College of Medicine, New York, New York

GLOSSARY

microtubule A major component of the eukaryotic cytoskeleton. A hollow cylindrical polymer formed primarily by the self-association of α,β-tubulin heterodimers. The cylinder is composed of 13 protofilaments with an overall diameter of 25 nm.

microtubule-associated proteins Proteins associated with microtubules and persist with tubulin during purification by assembly–disassembly.

mitosis The process of separation and segregation of replicated chromosomes.

Taxol An antitumor drug of natural product origin that stabilizes microtubules and inhibits eukaryotic cell division.

tubulin A highly conserved protein consisting of two major subunits, α and β, each $\sim$50,000 Da.

Taxol has demonstrated activity in human malignancies and has been approved by the Food and Drug Administration (FDA) for the treatment of ovarian, breast, and nonsmall cell lung carcinomas and, in addition, for Kaposi's sarcoma. Taxol is currently undergoing clinical trials as a single agent and in combination with other drugs for the treatment of a variety of other cancers, including head and neck and bladder.

I. INTRODUCTION

Taxol has an unusual chemical structure (Fig. 1) and mechanism of action. The interaction of the drug with

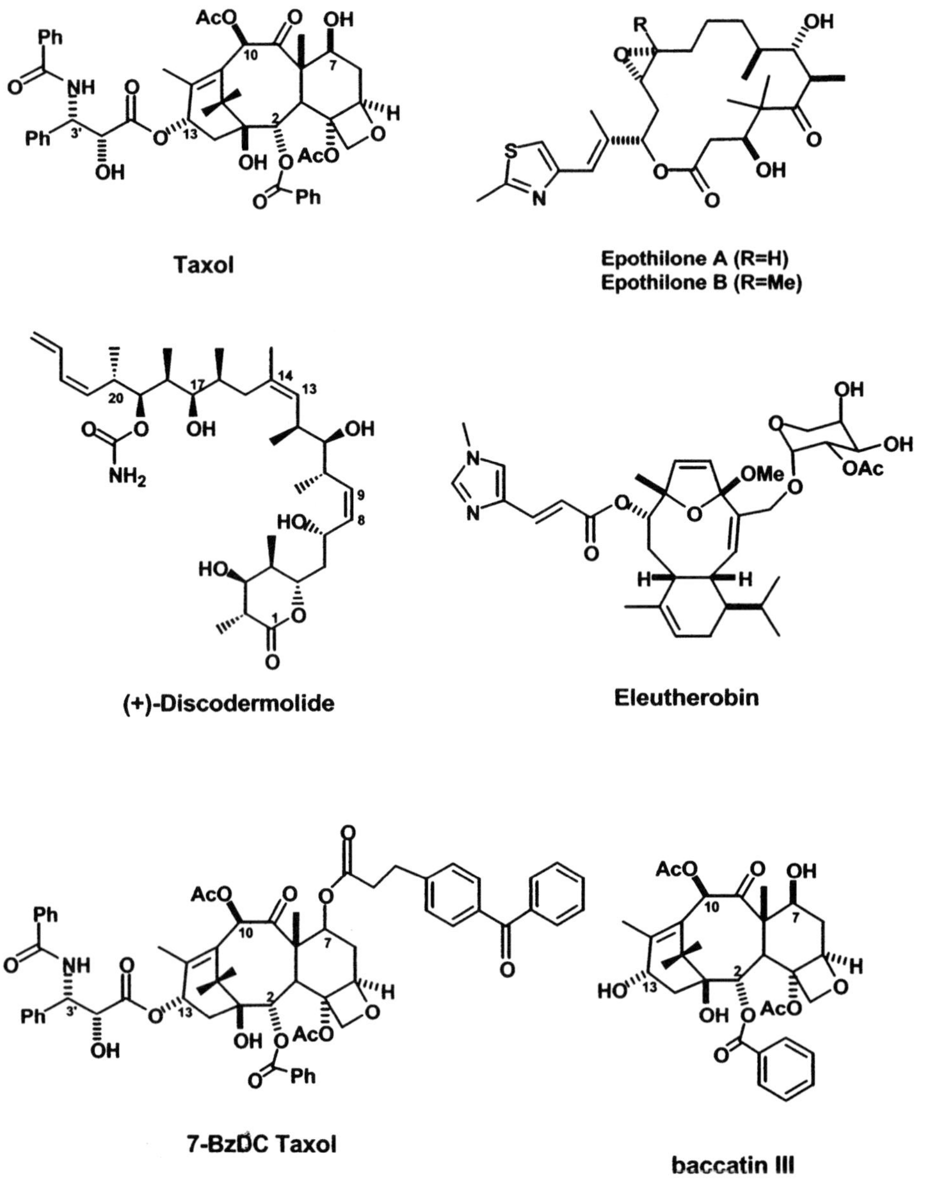

FIGURE 1 Structure of Taxol, 7-BzDC Taxol, baccatin III, epothilones A and B, eleutherobin, and discodermolide.

its cellular target, the microtubule polymer, represents a novel mechanism for an antitumor agent. Additional natural products, the epothilones, eleutherobin, and discodermolide, have been identified whose mechanism of action is similar to that of Taxol. An understanding of how these drugs interact with the microtubule system will further our knowledge of the structure and function of this important cytoskeletal system and should add impetus to the development of rationally designed antitumor agents that interact with and disrupt the function of microtubules.

II. EFFECTS OF TAXOL *IN VITRO*

Our laboratory was the first to examine the mechanism of action of Taxol, and although it became obvious that the drug was an antimitotic agent, it was also clear that Taxol was not a typical antimitotic drug such as colchicine or the *vinca* alkaloids. These latter drugs have binding sites on the tubulin dimer, whereas Taxol binds only to a tubulin oligomer or polymer. There is no evidence that Taxol can bind to the tubulin dimer. Taxol has a unique mechanism of action in that even today it is the only drug approved by the FDA known to interact exclusively with a polymer form of tubulin. *In vitro*, Taxol enhances the polymerization of tubulin, and those microtubules formed in the presence of drug possess unusual stability and resist depolymerization by cold temperature, dilution, and Ca^{2+} (Fig. 2). The drug is able to polymerize tubulin in the absence of GTP, which under normal conditions is an absolute requirement for microtubule polymerization. The interaction of Taxol with a normal microtubule instantly conveys stability to the polymer. The drug binds to the β-tubulin subunit in microtubules specifically and reversibly with a stoichiometry, relative to the tubulin heterodimer, approaching one. Binding is reversible, as unlabeled Taxol can displace [³H]Taxol from polymerized microtubules. Taxol is mechanistically distinct from other antimitotic drugs, such as the *vinca* alkaloids and colchicine, which disrupt microtubule assembly by virtue of their ability to bind to the free tubulin heterodimers.

In vitro, Taxol alters the kinetics of microtubule assembly. A typical microtubule assembly progress curve as measured by turbidity is shown in Fig. 3. In the absence of Taxol there is a characteristic 3- to 4-min lag phase prior to any observable increase in turbidity (a measure of polymer mass). In the presence of Taxol the lag phase is eliminated and the usual sigmoidal progress curve becomes hyperbolic. The overall effect of Taxol is to decrease the critical concentration of microtubule protein necessary for microtubule assembly. At a Taxol concentration of 5 μM, the critical concentration of tubulin required for assembly decreases by a factor of 20 from 0.2 to less than 0.01 mg protein/ml. Furthermore, electron microscopic examination revealed that microtubules polymerized in the presence of Taxol were considerably shorter (1.4 ± 0.7 mm). This would suggest that Taxol acts by increasing the number of nucleation events at the start of microtubule assembly. Under the correct conditions, vinblastine or colchicine can inhibit Taxol induced assembly if added prior to Taxol. However, this is probably due to an inhibition of assembly by these agents, resulting in a decrease in the number of microtubules, the target for Taxol action.

III. EFFECTS OF TAXOL ON CELLS

Microtubules are an essential component of eukaryotic cells and are required for cell division, cell motility, maintenance of cell shape, and organelle transport. At low drug concentrations, Taxol suppresses microtubule dynamics. The ability of Taxol to alter

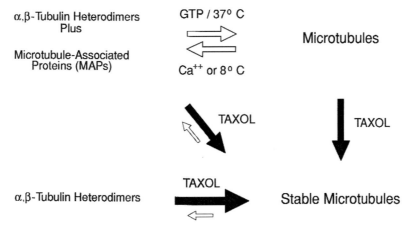

FIGURE 2 Taxol alters the normal equilibrium between soluble tubulin heterodimers and polymerized microtubules.

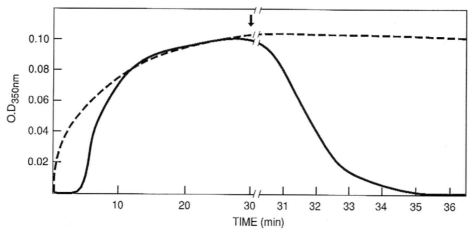

FIGURE 3 Effect of Taxol on the kinetics of calf brain microtubule polymerization and depolymerization. Microtubule polymerization was measured by turbidity in a final volume of 1.0 ml at 37 °C. The assay mixture contained 1 mM EGTA, 0.5 mM MgCl$_2$, 1 mM GTP, 0.1 M 2-[N-morpholino]ethane sulfonic acid (MES) at pH 6.6, and 1 mg/ml microtubule protein. Solid line, control; dashed line, 10 μM Taxol. The arrow indicates a shift in temperature from 37 to 8 °C. From Schiff and Horwitz (1981).

the dynamic equilibrium between tubulin heterodimers and the microtubule polymer would be expected to disrupt normal cellular functions in which microtubules are involved. Taxol has been found to be a potent inhibitor of eukaryotic cell replication, causing a block in the late G$_2$/M phase of the cell cycle. After DNA replication during the S phase, centrioles separate and migrate to opposite poles of the cell. Each forms a spindle aster that serves to organize and align the duplicate chromosomes prior to cell division. Treatment of HeLa cells with low concentrations of Taxol (0.25 μM) for 18 h established that all cells had a tetraploid DNA content as measured by flow microfluorometry. The addition of Taxol to synchronized HeLa cells at the beginning of S phase did not alter progress through this phase of the cell cycle. The effects of low concentrations of Taxol on DNA, RNA, and protein synthesis are negligible. Taxol has also been found to cause alterations in cell shape and movement, and these effects also are believed to be mediated via disruption of the microtubule:tubulin dimer equilibrium.

As viewed by immunofluorescence (Fig. 4) and electron microscopy, Taxol-treated cells exhibit an unusual interphase microtubule cytoskeleton. Treated cells, in addition to maintaining their cytoplasmic microtubules, also develop prominent bundles of microtubules often aligned in parallel. These bundles

are diagnostic of Taxol treatment and are a consequence of a Taxol-induced reorganization of the microtubule cytoskeleton. Taxol-induced bundles are extremely stable and are not depolymerized by antimitotic agents (e.g., colchicine) or by cold. When cells are depleted of ATP, no bundle formation is observed, even though Taxol does bind to and stabilize the microtubules. This suggests that Taxol-induced bundle formation is a two-step process and that the second step requires an intact cell with normal levels of ATP. In human leukemic cell lines, after treatment with clinically relevant concentrations of Taxol, both microtubule bundles and abnormal spindle asters are observed.

All of the experimental evidence available suggests that a primary cellular target for Taxol in cells is the microtubule. Specific binding of [^{3}H]Taxol to cells saturates in a concentration-dependent manner. Pretreatment of cells with colchicine, which resulted in depolymerization of cellular microtubules, inhibited [^{3}H]Taxol binding. Erythrocytes, which lack tubulin, exhibited no specific drug-binding activity. However, Taxol may interact with other cellular targets, in addition to the tubulin/microtubule system, although it is not clear if such functions of Taxol relate to its therapeutic activity. For example, the effects of Taxol on the induction of tumor necrosis factor (TNF-α) gene expression, on tyrosine and serine phosphoryla-

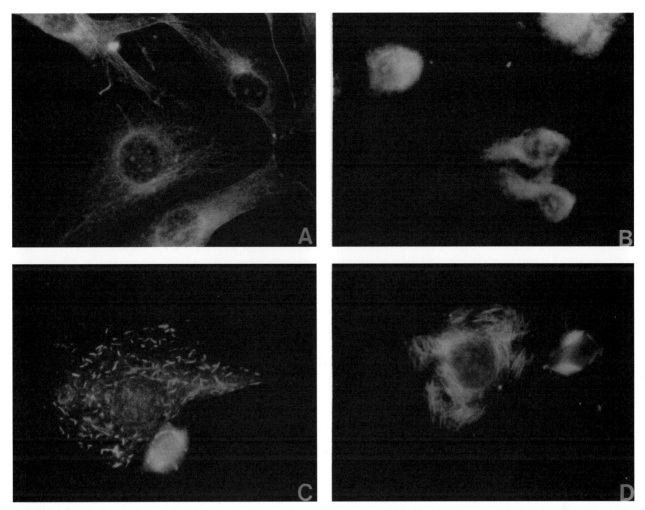

FIGURE 4 Indirect tubulin immunofluorescence of mouse 3T6 cells after treatment with colchicine, vinblastine, or Taxol at 37 °C. A, control; B, 30 μM colchicine for 60 min; C, 30 μM vinblastine for 60 min; and D, 30 μM Taxol for 240 min. From Manfredi and Horwitz (1984), with permission.

tion of Shc, and on formation of a Shc/Grb-2 complex in the murine cell line, RAW 264.7, and in A549 human lung cells have been examined in our laboratory. Structure–activity relationship (SAR) studies using Taxol and related taxanes demonstrated that the effects of Taxol on TNF-α gene expression are distinct from its known cytotoxic properties that are related to the ability of the drug to stabilize microtubules. Some of these activities are obvious only at concentrations of drug that are greater than those needed to observe microtubule stabilization. CD18 is also a cellular target for Taxol in murine macrophages. In other studies using phage-displayed peptides, Bcl-2 has been identified as a Taxol-binding protein. Hsps

of the 70- and 90-kDa families, as well as LPS, are targets for Taxol. This provides a rationale for the Taxol, LPS-like mediated activation of murine macrophages.

IV. BINDING SITE FOR TAXOL IN THE MICROTUBULE

Although it was clear that Taxol was capable of stabilizing normal microtubules, thereby indicating that there was a binding site on the polymer for the drug, there was essentially no information on the nature of this binding site. This represented a major deficiency in our knowledge of the mechanism of action of Taxol.

In the absence of a high-resolution structure of tubulin, we decided to use photoaffinity labeling, a powerful method, to address the nature of the interaction between Taxol and its target protein. Initially, direct photoaffinity-labeling studies demonstrated that Taxol binds specifically to the β subunit of tubulin. However, the low extent of photoincorporation precluded a detailed analysis of the Taxol binding site. The availability of a series of Taxol analogs bearing photoreactive groups at defined positions around the taxane nucleus afforded the opportunity to define sites of interaction between the drug and tubulin. These photoaffinity-labeling studies, using analogs with photoreactive groups at the C-2, C-3′, or C-7 positions, also identified definitively the β-tubulin subunit as the site of specific photoincorporation. Studies with [³H]3′-(*p*-azidobenzamido)Taxol, where the arylazide was incorporated into the C-13 side chain, resulted in the isolation of a photolabeled peptide containing amino acid residues 1–31 in β-tubulin. Studies with [³H]2-(*m*-azidobenzoyl)Taxol, where the photoreactive group was attached to the B ring of the taxoid nucleus, demonstrated that a peptide containing amino acid residues 217–233 of β-tubulin is involved in Taxol binding. Finally, when a benzophenone (BzDC) substituent was attached to the C-7 hydroxyl group of the C ring, specific photocross-linking to Arg₂₈₂ was observed.

Nogales and collaborators have succeeded, by electron crystallography, in obtaining a model of the α/β-tubulin dimer fitted to a 3.7-Å density map. In their structure, obtained using zinc-induced tubulin sheets, the Taxotere binding site was located at one side of the β-tubulin monomer that is believed to reside in the microtubule lumen. Although the tubulin structure is derived from an unnatural polymer, there is good agreement between the binding site as determined by photoaffinity labeling and electron crystallography. With the definition of two binding domains obtained through photoaffinity-labeling studies using arylazide analogs plus identification of Arg₂₈₂ in β-tubulin as the site of photoincorporation of [³H]7-BzDC-Taxol, we have been able to envision a qualitative model for the binding of Taxol to β-tubulin. We have looked at Taxol-containing nitrenes at the *para* position of the C-3′ benzamido (labeling residues β 1–31) and the *meta* position of the C-2 benzoyl moieties (labeling residues β 217–233), and the BzDC

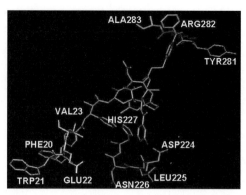

FIGURE 5 A composite model for the interaction of β-tubulin with Taxol-containing nitrenes at the *para* position of the C-3′ benzamido and the *meta* position of the C-2 benzoyl moieties, and the BzDC group at the C-7 position. The close proximity of the C-7 BzDC moiety to Arg₂₈₂, of the nitrene at the *meta* position of the C-2 benzoyl moiety to His₂₂₇, and of the nitrene at the *para* position of the C-3′ benzamido moiety to Val₂₃ is in excellent agreement with the photoaffinity-labeling studies. From Rao *et al*. (1999), with permission.

group at the C-7 position (labeling β-Arg₂₈₂), as a composite model for defining the three Taxol–tubulin contacts (Fig. 5). The nitrene on the C-3′ benzamido moiety is close to Val23 in good agreement with the photoaffinity-labeling result (close to the domain it photolabels, β 1–31), as well as the tubulin crystal structure. This structure is in clear agreement with photoaffinity-labeling results and strongly suggests that Taxol interacts with cellular microtubules as depicted in the molecular model that has been described. The benzophenone oxygen atom of the 7-BzDC moiety can be located at ~3 Å distance from the α carbon of the β-Arg₂₈₂. Moreover, in its energy-minimized conformation based on the Taxotere X-ray structure, the nitrene moiety at the *meta* position of the C-2-benzoyl moiety is clearly close to the domain it photolabels (β 217–233) and approaches the imidazole ring of His227 that may be the site of photoincorporation (Fig. 5).

V. STRUCTURE–FUNCTION STUDIES

Taxol was originally isolated from the bark of the Pacific yew (*Taxus brevifolia*), which is native to the ecologically threatened old-growth forests of the Pacific Northwest. However, Taxol is present in minute quantities in bark and it required approximately 3 kg of bark to isolate 300 mg of pure drug. Harvesting of bark also resulted in destruction of the tree. Drug availability was an initial problem in the development of Taxol as a chemotherapeutic agent. This has been overcome due to the semisynthesis of Taxol from more readily available precursors such as 10-deacetyl baccatin III. This precursor can be isolated from the needles of a variety of *Taxus* species (~3 g of 10-deacetyl baccatin III/3 kg of leaves) and converted to Taxol in reasonable yield. Because the needles regenerate, they provide a continuous source of the precursor.

The hydrophobic nature of Taxol and its limited solubility in water delayed and made difficult its pharmacological formulation. Presently Taxol is formulated in a polyethoxylated castor oil (Cremphor EL) containing 50% ethanol. When Taxol was first introduced into clinical trials, there were serious hypersensitivity reactions reported in humans that may have been related to the Cremphor EL vehicle. These anaphylactoid reactions have been largely overcome by a premedication regimen including antihistamines, corticosteroids, and histamine H_2 receptor antagonists and altered drug delivery. Nevertheless, the availability of Taxol analogs with increased solubility in H_2O and retention of antitumor activity would be highly desirable.

Considerable efforts have been made to define the structure–activity profile of Taxol in order to design more potent and possibly more water-soluble Taxol analogs. These studies have also provided insights into the chemical nature, both structural and stereochemical, of the Taxol–microtubule interaction. Evaluation of the structure–activity relationships for Taxol has used two principal assays: (1) cytotoxicity toward tumor cell lines and (2) enhancement of microtubule assembly *in vitro* in the absence of GTP.

Taxol is a complex diterpenoid consisting of a taxane ring system fused to a four-membered oxetane ring and an ester side chain at C-13 of the Taxol A-ring (Fig. 1). Structure–activity studies have revealed that modifications to C-7, C-9, and C-10 are tolerated. For example, 7-OH can be esterified, epimerized, or even removed without significant loss of activity. However, studies indicate that the size of the substituent at this position may influence polymerization activity. We have found that the presence of the bulky BzDC substituent at this position results in a Taxol analog that cannot enhance the polymerization of microtubules, but can, however, stabilize GTP-induced microtubules against depolymerization by cold temperatures. A possible explanation is that the analog may be able to bind to small oligomers, but the presence of the bulky C-7 substituent prevents tubulin dimers from adding to these stabilized nucleation centers. In agreement with this idea, the loop containing Arg_{282}, the M loop, has been shown to be involved in lateral interactions between protofilaments.

The C-2 benzoyl, the oxetane D-ring, and the A-ring side chain are all important determinants for both cytotoxicity and stabilization of microtubules exhibited by Taxol. The presence of substituents on the C-2 benzoyl group can have profound effects on the biological activity of these Taxol analogs. A series of *para-* and *meta*-substituted 2-benzoyl analogs of Taxol have been synthesized and exhibit radically different biological activities from each other and from Taxol. All the *para*-substituted analogs were considerably less cytotoxic than Taxol. In contrast, the *meta*-substituted analogs were significantly more toxic than Taxol in the P-388 murine leukemia cell line. In some cases, cytotoxicities of 700- to 800-fold greater than that of Taxol were observed. In the *in vitro* microtubule assembly assay, all the *meta*-substituted analogs were more active than Taxol, whereas the *para*-substituted analogs were less active. The A-ring side chain has long been considered absolutely essential for biological activity. Baccatin III, which lacks the A-ring side chain, is not cytotoxic and is totally inactive in an *in vitro* microtubule assembly assay. We have found, however, that 2-m-azido baccatin III, a Taxol analog lacking the C-13 side chain but with a *meta* azido benzoyl group at the C-2 position, possesses all of the activities that are characteristic of Taxol. It promotes microtubule assembly in the absence of GTP, stabilizes microtubules, and competitively inhibits the binding of [^{3}H]Taxol to the microtubule protein. The compound is cytotoxic and arrests cells at the mitotic phase of the cell cycle. Although 2-m-azido baccatin III is less potent than Taxol, the fact that it is biologically active reveals valuable information on the binding of Taxol to tubulin. Binding of the C-2 benzoyl ring and C-13 side chains serve as "anchors" to secure and enhance the binding of the taxane ring. Removal of either side chain results in loss of microtubule stabilization. In the case of 2-m-azido Taxol, the binding of the C-2 side chain led to an increase in activity compared to Taxol. For

2-m-azido baccatin III, the presence of the *meta* azido group partially compensated for the loss of the C-13 side chain and increased the binding affinity of the compound. Binding of the C-2 side chain is quite specific because an azido at the *para* position is inactive and actually inhibits the interaction of Taxol with the microtubule.

VI. INTERACTION OF OTHER NATURAL PRODUCTS WITH MICROTUBULES

Two factors, namely the low aqueous solubility of Taxol and the development of clinical drug resistance, have led to a search for new compounds that may have a greater or comparable efficacy relative to Taxol. Several natural products all with unique structures unrelated to that of Taxol have been reported to have similar mechanisms of action as Taxol (Fig. 1). Epothilones A and B, isolated from a *Myxobacterium* fermentation broth, also were found to induce tubulin polymerization, arrest cells in mitosis, and cause the formation of microtubule bundles. Epothilone B was reported to be more potent than Taxol and epothilone A in promoting microtubule assembly *in vitro*. The epothilones are 30 times more water soluble than Taxol. Structure–activity studies with epothilones have demonstrated that the acyl region (C1-C8) is essential for Taxol-like activity. Most importantly, the epothilones retained sensitivity in P-glycoprotein-expressing cells that were resistant to Taxol. Discodermolide was isolated from a marine sponge and reported to induce the assembly of microtubules *in vitro* more rapidly than Taxol and to cause mitotic arrest and microtubule bundling. Discodermolide has been predicted to be 100-fold more water soluble than Taxol and is not a substrate for P-glycoprotein. Interestingly, the combination of Taxol and discodermolide exhibited a synergistic cytotoxic interaction in human carcinoma cell lines. A fourth microtubule-stabilizing agent, eleutherobin, has been isolated from a marine soft coral and shown to have activity comparable to that of Taxol. Structure–activity analysis of eleutherobin analogs concluded that the C8 urocanic acid moiety is required for Taxol-like activity. Eleutherobin displayed cross-resistance in MDR cell lines, an effect that was reversible by ve-

rapamil, suggesting that eleutherobin is a substrate of P-glycoprotein. It is their distinct chemical structures and improved aqueous solubility that will influence their therapeutic activity based on the pharmacokinetics, bioavailability, and metabolism of each drug.

VII. COMMON PHARMACOPHORE FOR TAXOL AND OTHER MICROTUBULE-STABILIZING DRUGS

Several common pharmacophore models for Taxol and the epothilones have been proposed. Early common pharmacophore models were proposed based on the comparison of the chemical structures of Taxol and the epothilones. In 2000, Fojo and collaborators proposed two possible common pharmacophore models using β-tubulin mutations identified in epothilone-resistant cells as an indirect indication for the binding of the epothilones to β-tubulin. Because the mutations found in the epothilone-resistant cells, β274 and β282, were located near the taxane binding site in β-tubulin, they proposed that the macrolide ring of the epothilones mimics the taxane ring. Due to the lack of accurate information on the binding of the epothilone molecule in β-tubulin, they were unable to identify the orientation of the thiazole side chain and therefore proposed two alternative models: in model I, the thiazole side chain was matched with the C-2 side chain of Taxol, whereas in model II, the thiazole side chain was superimposed with the C-13 side chain of Taxol. Our observation that the C-13 side chain is not an absolute requirement for biological activity in a taxane molecule has enabled us to develop a new common pharmacophore model between Taxol and epothilone. We proposed a model in which the thiazole side chain of epothilone corresponds to the C-2 side chain of 2-m-azido baccatin III and the macrolide ring system overlaps with the taxane ring system (Fig. 6). This model is essentially equivalent to model I described by Fojo and colleagues. Based on this model, alterations to the thiazole ring system may influence biological activity, as has been observed with the 2-benzoyl group of Taxol. In fact, replacement of the thiazole with a phenyl group, shortening the linker between C-15 and the thiazole ring, depletion of the thiazole ring, or bulky substituents on the

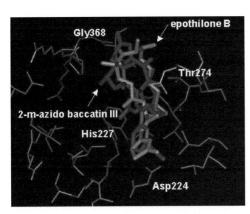

FIGURE 6 Common pharmacophore model for epothilone B and 2-m-azido-baccatin III. Epothilone B and 2-m-azido baccatin III are superimposed to show their structural similarities. From He *et al.* (2000), with permission.

thiazole ring all resulted in significant decreases in biological activity. Considering this model in the context of the structure–activity research data available on eleutherobin, where we have reported that removal of the C-8 urocanic acid group resulted in a complete loss of activity, we proposed that the 14-membered fused ring system in eleutherobin, like the macrolide ring of the epothilones, overlays with the taxane ring of Taxol and that the urocanic acid side chain, like the thiazole side chain of the epothilones, mimics the C-2 side chain of Taxol. These similarities among Taxol, the epothilones, and eleutherobin may allow them all to bind at the same or overlapping binding sites in β-tubulin on the microtubule.

See Also the Following Articles

MAP Kinase Modules in Signaling • Vinca Alkaloids and Epipodophyllotoxins

Bibliography

Burkhart, C. A., Berman, J. W., Swindell, C. S., and Horwitz, S. B. (1994). Relationship between the structure of taxol and other taxanes on induction of tumor necrosis factor-alpha gene expression and cytotoxicity, *Cancer Res.* **54,** 5779–5782.

Derry, W. B., Wilson, L., and Jordan, M. A. (1995). Substoichiometric binding of taxol suppresses microtubule dynamics. *Biochemistry* **34,** 2203–2211.

Giannakakou, P., Gussio, R., Nogales, E., Downing, K. H., Zaharevitz, D., Bollbuck, B., Poy, G., Sackett, D., Nicolaou, K. C., and Fojo, T. (2000). A common pharmacophore for

epothilone and taxanes: molecular basis for drug resistance conferred by tubulin mutations in human cancer cells. *Proc. Natl. Acad. Sci. USA* **97,** 2904–2909.

He, L., Jagtap, P. G., Kingston, D. G., Shen, H. J., Orr, G. A., and Horwitz, S. B. (2000). A common pharmacophore for Taxol and the epothilones based on the biological activity of a taxane molecule lacking a C-13 side chain. *Biochemistry* **39,** 3972–3978.

Manfiedi, J. J., and Horwitz, S. B. (1984). *Pharmacol. Ther.* **25,** 83–125.

Martello, L. A., McDaid, H. M., Regl, D. L., Yang, C. P., Meng, D., Pettus, T. R., Kaufman, M. D., Arimoto, H., Danishefsky, S. J., Smith, A. B., III, and Horwitz, S. B. (2000). Taxol and discodermolide represent a synergistic drug combination in human carcinoma cell lines. *Clin. Cancer Res.* **6,** 1978–1987.

Nogales, E., Wolf, S. G., and Downing, K. H. (1998). Structure of the alpha beta tubulin dimer by electron crystallography. *Nature* **391,** 199–203.

Parness, J., and Horwitz, S. B. (1981). Taxol binds to polymerized tubulin in vitro. *J. Cell Biol.* **91,** 479–487.

Rao, S., He, L., Chakravarty, S., Ojima, I., Orr, G. A., and Horwitz, S. B. (1999). Characterization of the Taxol binding site on the microtubule: Identification of Arg(282) in beta-tubulin as the site of photoincorporation of a 7-benzophenone analogue of taxol. *J. Biol. Chem.* **274,** 37990–37994.

Rao, S., Orr, G. A., Chaudhary, A. G., Kingston, D. G., and Horwitz, S. B. (1995). Characterization of the taxol binding site on the microtubule: 2-(m-Azidobenzoyl)Taxol photolabels a peptide (amino acids 217-231) of beta- tubulin. *J. Biol. Chem.* **270,** 20235–20238.

Rodi, D. J., Janes, R. W., Sanganee, H. J., Holton, R. A., Wallace, B. A., and Makowski, L. (1999). Screening of a library of phage-displayed peptides identifies human bcl-2 as a taxol-binding protein. *J. Mol. Biol.* **285,** 197–203.

Rowinsky, E. K. (1997). The development and clinical utility of the taxane class of antimicrotubule chemotherapy agents. *Annu. Rev. Med.* **48,** 353–374.

Schiff, P. B., Fant, J., and Horwitz, S. B. (1979). Promotion of microtubule assembly in vitro by taxol. *Nature* **277,** 665–667.

Schiff, P. B. and Horwitz, S. B. (1980). Taxol stabilizes microtubules in mouse fibroblast cells. *Proc. Natl. Acad. Sci. USA* **77,** 1561–1565.

Schiff, P. B., and Horwitz, S. B. (1981). "Molecular Actions and Targets for Cancer Chemotherapeutic Agents" (A. Sartorelli, J. S. Lago, and J. R. Bertino, eds.), p. 483. Academic Press, New York.

Snyder, J. P., Nettles, J. H., Cornett, B., Downing, K. H., and Nogales, E. (2001). The binding conformation of taxol in beta-tubulin: A model based on electron crystallographic density. *Proc. Natl. Acad. Sci. USA* **98,** 5312–5316.

Su, D.-S., Balog, A., Meng, D., Bertinato, P., Danishefsky, S. J., Zheng, Y.-H., Chou, T.-C., He, L., and Horwitz, S. B.(1997). Structure-activity relationships of the epothilones and the first in vivo comparison with Paclitaxel. *Agnew. Chem. Int. Ed. Engl.* **36,** 2093–2096.

T Cells against Tumors

Peter S. Goedegebuure
David C. Linehan
Timothy J. Eberlein
Washington University School of Medicine, St. Louis, Missouri

I. Introduction
II. Tumor-Reactive T cells
III. Tumor-Associated Antigens
IV. Summary

GLOSSARY

anergy A state of temporary T-cell unresponsiveness induced by a lack of costimulation.

antigen A molecule that induces a lymphocyte-mediated immune response.

antigen-presenting cell A cell that is highly specialized to process antigens and present peptide fragments on the surface for lymphocyte activation.

antigen processing Degradation of proteins into peptides that will bind to MHC molecules. The peptide–MHC complex is transported to the surface for presentation to T cells.

cytokine A polypeptide regulates the behavior of other cells, including cell growth. Cytokines produced by lymphocytes are called lymphokines.

major histocompatibility complex (MHC) Cluster of genes that are highly polymorphic. The MHC comprises class I molecules that present peptides generated in the cytosol to $CD8^+$ T cells, and class II molecules that present peptides from cytosolic compartments to $CD4^+$ T cells.

protooncogene A normal gene that, by alteration, produces a product that potentiates the transformation of a normal cell into a tumor cell.

signal transduction Progression of a signal through a series of sequential biochemical reactions.

T-cell receptor A receptor complex on T lymphocytes for antigen binding.

tolerance Failure to respond to an antigen.

Humans have a number of different types of immune cells at their disposal to effectively deal with transformed cells and foreign invaders such as viruses and other microorganisms. An important function of T lymphocytes in this process known as immune surveillance is to recognize and destroy transformed or infected body cells. The T cells circulate through the body, mainly through the bloodstream and lymphatics, and infiltrate tissues, thereby surveying the body. Expression of tumor-associated antigens on tumor cells permits T cells to recognize, bind, and destroy tumor cells.

I. INTRODUCTION

A. Tumor-Specific Rejection Antigens

More than 40 years ago, conclusive evidence was provided for the existence of tumor-specific rejection antigens that conferred immunity to tumor. These experiments in inbred mice involved transplantation of methyl cholantrene (MCA)-induced sarcomas. Tumor-inoculated mice from which the tumor was excised rejected a second inoculum of the same tumor. In contrast, untreated mice or mice that were inoculated with normal tissue from the original tumor-bearing mouse did not reject a tumor inoculum. Later experiments showed that rejection of tumors was not unique to MCA-induced tumors, as immunity could also be induced with other tumors induced by chemical or physical carcinogens, such as UV light-induced tumors. These experiments led to the postulation that tumor-specific antigens were expressed on the tumors that were referred to as transplantation antigens or rejection antigens.

B. Role of T Cells against Tumors

In subsequent years, it became apparent that immunity against transplanted tumors is primarily mediated by T lymphocytes. When tumor cells were mixed with lymph node cells from immunized mice before inoculation, significant inhibition of tumor growth was observed. Similar experiments yielding similar results were performed with spleen cells and peritoneal cells from immunized mice. Subsequently, investigators demonstrated that adoptive transfer of T cells from immunized mice before tumor inoculation could protect mice from tumor growth. More conclusive evidence for T-cell-mediated eradication of syngeneic tumors was obtained in the early 1970s. Adoptive transfer of murine immune spleen cells mixed with syngeneic plasma tumor cells protected against tumor growth. However, immune spleen cells depleted of T cells prior to mixing with tumor cells did not provide protection, whereas depletion of B cells had no effect on the antitumor efficacy.

Although human tumors differ from the experimental tumors used in mice, Thomas postulated that the outgrowth of tumors is immunologically con-

trolled. Building on this hypothesis, Burnet introduced the immune surveillance theory in 1970. Burnet postulated that the development of T-cell-mediated immunity during evolution was specific for the elimination of transformed cells and that T cells continuously survey the body and eliminate those cells that underwent cancerous transformations (Fig. 1). In subsequent years, the idea of immune surveillance was largely abandoned when experiments in nude mice showed that they were not more susceptible to chemically induced tumors. However, the finding that nude mice are not completely devoid of functional T cells and observations that interferon (IFN)-γ and perforin are involved in the prevention of tumors in mice have renewed interest in the immune surveillance theory. A direct role for lymphocytes and IFN-γ in tumor suppression has been demonstrated by Schreiber and colleagues. It has become apparent

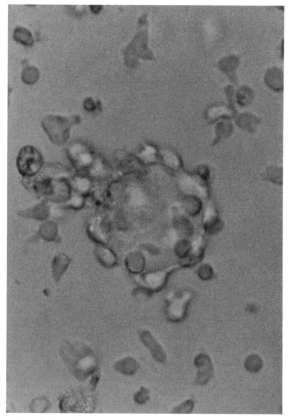

FIGURE 1. Multiple T cells attacking a single tumor cell (center) in a tissue culture flask (x400). T cells were cocultured with irradiated autologous melanoma cells in the presence of IL-2.

that T cells are efficient at eliminating virus-induced malignancies, but the response to chemical or physical carcinogen-induced tumors is much weaker. The difference in response is primarily related in the nature of the antigen, as will be discussed later. Because T cells discriminate self from nonself, transformed cells need to undergo phenotypic changes before T cells can be activated. The initiation phase of tumor development is characterized by a series of genetic changes that occur in sequence. The genetic changes may, however, not lead to activation of T cells. Several mechanisms for T-cell unresponsiveness have been postulated: early genetic changes may not sufficiently alter the transformed cell to be recognized by T cells or tumor cells expressing tumor antigens may induce tolerance because the T cells do not receive the proper costimulatory signals (see later). Finally, resistance to immune responses may be acquired during tumor development, such as downregulation of antigen expression and/or antigen processing and expression of immunosuppressive factors.

The relatively poor T-cell response to nonvirus-induced tumors does not mean that T cells play no role in the elimination of cancerous transformations induced by chemical or physical carcinogens. In clinical studies performed in the 1980s, objective clinical responses, including complete remissions, were observed in patients with metastatic melanoma after adoptive transfer of the lymphokine interleukin (IL)2 or autologous T cells expanded *ex vivo* in IL-2 administered with IL-2. Since then, numerous clinical trials have been performed emphasizing T-cell antitumor responses. Progress in molecular biology techniques helped identify tumor-specific antigens in common cancers that confer T-cell-mediated tumor immunity. In fact, some of these antigens form the basis of newly developed tumor vaccines and other immune-based therapies that are currently ongoing.

C. How Do Tumor Cells Stimulate T Cells?

The far majority of T lymphocytes express a cell surface receptor, antigen receptor, or T cell receptor (TcR) that binds to a molecular complex consisting of an antigenic peptide bound to a molecule of the major histocompatibility complex (MHC) on the

antigen-presenting cell (APC) (Fig. 2). The peptides are derived either from cellular proteins (endogenous antigens) or from extracellular proteins (exogenous antigens) after proteolytic degradation. The function of the MHC complex is to present peptides to T cells; MHC class I molecules bind peptides in the endoplasmic reticulum, usually endogenously derived peptides, whereas MHC class II molecules bind peptides in endosomal compartments, usually exogenously derived peptides. Fairly recently, however, evidence was found for presentation of exogenous antigens, including tumor antigens by MHC class I on professional APC, referred to as cross-priming. It is not clear how

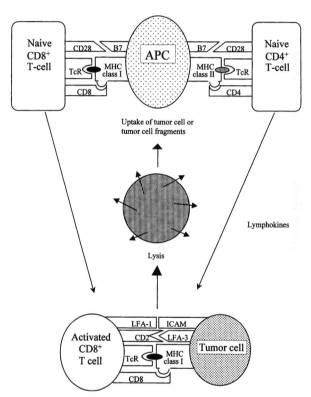

FIGURE 2. Schematic overview of the general activation pathways of tumor-specific CD4+ and CD8+ T cells. Antigen-presenting cells (APC) take up apoptotic tumor cells or tumor cell fragments and, after intracellular processing of proteins by proteolytic enzymes, present peptides by both MHC class I and II molecules on the cell surface. Naive CD8+ and CD4+ T cells recognize tumor antigen presented by MHC class I and II molecules, respectively, and, when costimulatory signals are provided, become activated. Activated CD4+ T cells secrete lymphokines that regulate activated CD8+ T cells, but do not interact with tumor cells that lack expression of MHC class II molecules. CD8+ T cells can directly interact with MHC class I-expressing tumor cells and lyse the tumor cells upon recognition.

certain exogenous antigens access the cytosol and the MHC class I presentation pathway and what the frequency is of this alternative pathway. While the TcR interacts with the MHC/antigen complex, CD4 or CD8 coreceptors on the T cell simultaneously interact with the same antigen-presenting MHC class II or I molecule, respectively.

D. Costimulation of T Cells

The specific interaction between a T cell and the MHC/antigen complex is an essential part of the two-signal requirement for T-cell activation introduced in the late 1980s. Accordingly, antigen-stimulated T cells require a second signal to become fully activated. The costimulatory signals are provided by molecules on the T-cell surface that bind to their respective ligands on the APC. Some of the best described T cell–APC costimulatory interactions are CD11a/CD18 (LFA-1), which binds to CD54 (ICAM-1) or CD102 (ICAM-2); CD2, which binds to CD58 (LFA-3); and CD28, which binds to CD80 (B7.1) or CD86 (B7.2). The latter interaction is essential for the stimulation of naïve T cells, but not of activated T cells (Fig. 2). In general, costimulatory molecules are responsible for cell–cell adhesion and transduce costimulatory signals. Lack of costimulation leads to the induction of tolerance or anergy. After the initial cell–cell contact, the TcR checks the MHC/antigen complexes on the APC for matching. If the TcR recognizes the MHC/antigen complex, a signal is transduced through the TcR/CD3 complex and the T cell is activated. If the TcR does not find a complementary MHC/antigen complex, the T cell and APC dissociate.

Tumor cells generally express MHC class I molecules that may present tumor antigens and thereby directly stimulate CD8$^+$ T cells. Tumors other than those of hematopoietic origin usually do not express MHC class II and, as such, do not directly stimulate CD4$^+$ T cells. However, professional APCs, such as macrophages and dendritic cells, can take up tumor cell fragments or apoptotic tumor cells and present tumor antigens by both MHC class I and II.

E. T-Cell Activation Pathway

The TcR of most T cells consists of an αβ protein chain heterodimer associated with the CD3 mole-

cule, which consists of protein chains γ, δ, and ε and a ζ homodimer (Fig. 3). The three CD3 chains each contain one and the ζ chains each contain three copies of intracytoplasmic motifs termed immunoreceptor tyrosine-based activation motifs (ITAMs). Each motif consists of paired tyrosine and leucine/isoleucine residues in a precise topological orientation. Engagement of the TcR with the MHC/antigen induces phosphorylation of the tyrosine residues in a process that also involves nonreceptor tyrosine kinases belonging to the Src and Syk/ZAP (ζ-associated protein)-70 families. A fully phosphorylated TcR/CD3 complex recruits as many as 10 ZAP-70 molecules that subsequently become phosphorylated, which stimulates ZAP-70 kinase activity. This leads to the phosphorylation of phospholipase Cγ1 and, subsequently, to the generation of second messengers that further the signal and eventually regulate the transcription of genes. In contrast, suboptimal stimulation of the TcR may phosphorylate only part of the ITAMs, resulting in incomplete or lack of phosphorylation of ZAP-70. When ZAP-70 is insufficiently activated, the T cell may not exert one or more of its basic functions, such as clonal expansion, secretion of cytokines, migration, or cytolytic activity.

II. TUMOR-REACTIVE T CELLS

Tumor-reactive T cells can be derived from various sources: primary solid tumors usually contain tumor-infiltrating lymphocytes (TIL); malignant fluids, such as pleural fluid or ascites, contain tumor-associated lymphocytes (TAL); lymph nodes; peripheral blood; and the spleen. Current purification techniques yield high (>95%) purities of T cells, even from solid tumor tissue. Intuitively, one would expect the highest frequency of tumor-reactive T cells among TIL because they are in the closest proximity to antigen-presenting tumor cells. Supporting this hypothesis is the observation made in the mid-1980s that the adoptive transfer of TIL to syngeneic tumor-bearing mice induced a higher antitumor efficacy than the transfer of similar numbers of splenocytes. However, more and more scientists currently think that in human, peripheral blood is a better source for tumor-reactive T cells than the tumor itself because of immunosup-

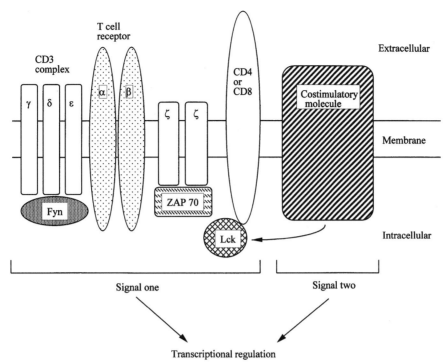

FIGURE 3. Schematic overview of the two-signal requirement for T-cell activation. Signal one is provided through binding of TcR molecules to MHC/antigen complexes, which leads to the phosphorylation of immunoreceptor tyrosine-based activation motifs on CD3 chains with help from TcR/CD3-associated protein-tyrosine kinases (fyn, lck). Costimulatory molecules transduce signal two, which, combined with signal one, leads to T-cell activation.

pressive mechanisms active in the tumor environment, including those that lead to T-cell death.

Within the T-cell population, both TcRαβ and TcRγδ T cells can exert antitumor activity. TcRγδ T cells comprise only 1–10% of the lymphocytes in peripheral blood in normal individuals. Recognition of target cells by TcRγδ cells is not restricted by MHC molecules. Studies suggest that TcRγδ cells are triggered when elevated levels of endogenous self-antigens are expressed on cells. However, TcRγδ T cells only rarely infiltrate tumors and their role as antitumor effector cells *in vivo* is not clear.

A. TcRαβ/CD4$^+$ T Cells

One of the primary functions of CD4$^+$ T cells is to provide helper activity for other immune cells. The helper activity is mediated through cell–cell contact or in the form of lymphokines that are released by CD4$^+$ T cells and bind specific receptors on other cells (see Fig. 2). Three main subsets of CD4$^+$

T helper (Th) cells based on lymphokine secretion profiles have been defined, originally in mice and later in humans: Th1 cells that produce IL-2, IFN-γ, and TNF-β among others, and consequently support the development of a cellular immune response; Th2 cells that produce IL-4, IL-5, IL-6, IL-10, and IL-13, and are essential for the development of a humoral response; and Th0 cells (Table I). In mice, Th0 cells are considered progenitor cells that mature into either Th1 or Th2 cells. In humans, however, Th0 cells seem a fully differentiated subset of CD4$^+$ Th cells based on the analysis of individual Th clones. Th0 cells produce IL-2, IL-4, and IFNγ and, as such, could theoretically support both cellular and humoral responses. Because of the dominance of CD4$^+$ T cells over CD8$^+$ T cells in the peripheral blood, an important parameter for the effectiveness of a CTL-mediated immune response is the ratio of Th1/Th2. For example, a shift from Th1 toward Th2 cells means a decreased availability of IL-2 and IFNγ and increased levels of IL-4 and IL-10. In a tumor

TABLE I
Classification of CD4⁺ and CD8⁺ T Cells

Subsets		Cytokine profile	Primary function
CD4	Th0	IL-2, IL-4, IL-6, IL-10, IL-13, IFN-γ, TNF-β	Th1, Th2 precursor?
	Th1	IL-2, IFN-γ, TNF-β	T-cell help
	Th2	IL-4, IL-5, IL-6, IL-10, IL-13	B-cell help
	Tr	IL-4, IL-10, IL-13, TGF-β	Maintenance of self-tolerance
CD8	Tc0	IL-2, IL-4, IFN-γ	Tc precursor?
	Tc1	IL-2, IFN-γ, TNF-β	Killing
	Tc2	IL-4, IL-5, IL-10	Killing

environment in which IL-2-dependent CTL are required for tumor eradication, the presence of a dominant Th1 subset is essential. Direct cloning experiments of CD4⁺ TIL from patients with renal cell carcinoma and subsequent analysis of the cytokine patterns demonstrated that over 80% of the CD4⁺ TIL were Th2. In contrast, identical experiments using CD4+ TIL from melanoma patients showed that only 19% were Th2 and the remainder were IL-2-producing Th0 and Th1 clones. These findings illustrate the disproportionate availability of helper cytokines for CTL in each of the tumors, which happens to be consistent with the higher response rate to T-cell-mediated immune therapy in melanoma compared to renal cell carcinoma.

In addition to CD4⁺ helper T lymphocytes, regulatory T lymphocytes exist (Tr). In the past, regulatory T cells have also been referred to as suppressor cells. Several different mechanisms of suppression have been noted, including the secretion of immunosuppressive cytokines, such as IL-4, IL-10, IL-13, and TGFβ, and cell contact-mediated suppression. Tr cells are essential for the maintenance of peripheral tolerance by suppressing autoreactive T cells. Because most tumor antigens appear to be derived from self-antigens, autoreactive T cells include tumor-reactive T cells. Tr cells are not confined to a particular lymphocyte subset as defined by lineage or phenotypic markers. Most common are CD4⁺CD25⁺ (IL2 receptor α chain) T cells, but other CD4⁺ Tr and CD8+ Tr have been described as well. A Tr with an unusual phenotype is the natural killer T (NKT) cell. First described in the mid-1980s in the mouse, NKT cells are TCRαβ⁺ T cells that share some characteristics with NK cells. NKT cells recognize glycolipid antigens presented by the MHC class I-like molecule CD1d and produce large amounts of Th1 cytokines, such as IFNγ and TNF, and Th2 cytokines, such as IL-4 and IL-10. Because of this, the proposed role of NKT cells ranges from suppression of autoimmunity to tumor rejection. Experimental evidence has been found for both roles and these results have ensured continued debate.

B. Tumor-Specific CD4⁺ T Cells

Increasing evidence indicates that optimal antitumor responses require the participation of both CD4⁺ and CD8⁺ T cells. In addition to being essential for the priming of an immune response, CD4⁺ T cells are important for the maintenance of a CD8⁺ memory response and CD8⁺ T-cell survival. Relatively few MHC class II-restricted tumor antigens have been identified. Similar to MHC class I-restricted antigens, the group of MHC class II-restricted antigens includes nonmutated self-antigens as well as mutated antigens. Cell-mediated cytotoxicity by CD4⁺ T cells is associated with Th1 cells, but not with Th2 cells, and occurs primarily through the binding of T-cell surface Fas ligand (FasL) to the apoptosis-inducing molecule Fas on Fas-expressing tumor cells. Antigen activation of T cells leads to an increase of cell surface expression of FasL to permit binding and elimination of cells with elevated expression levels of Fas. Some CD4⁺ T cells may kill via granule exocytosis, but this pathway is of minor significance. Cytotoxic CD4⁺ T cells have been identified in peripheral blood and in tumors such as melanoma, breast, and ovarian and in renal cell carcinoma. However, because only few tumors of nonhematopoietic origin express MHC class II molecules, tumor reduction in patients is primarily mediated by MHC class I-restricted CD8⁺ T cells.

C. TcRαβ/CD8⁺ T Cells

The primary function of activated CD8⁺ T cells is to lyse target cells. CD8+ T cells recognize antigenic peptides presented by MHC class I molecules and can therefore directly interact with tumor cells. Naïve CD8⁺ T cells, however, are dependent on CD28-mediated costimulation for activation and cannot interact with tumors of nonhematopoietic origin that do not express the CD28 ligands CD80 or CD86. Instead, professional APC stimulate naïve CD8⁺ T cells through cross-priming (Fig. 2). Once CD8⁺ T cells are activated, interaction with targets cells is independent of the expression of CD80/CD86 on the target cell. Expression of costimulatory or adhesion molecules such as ICAM and LFA3 is, however, essential; lack of expression of these molecules is a documented escape mechanism of tumor cells from immune surveillance.

CD8⁺ T cytotoxic (Tc) cells are derived from Tc0 precursor cells and can be subdivided into Tc1 and Tc2, similar to CD4⁺ T cells (Table I). Tc1 and Tc2 have similar functions: both are cytotoxic via secretion of pore-forming molecules, such as perforin, or through Fas-mediated killing. They also induce similar levels of DTH responses. However, Tc1 and Tc2 secrete different cytokines and as such act through different mechanisms: Tc1 cells secrete IL-2, IFNγ, and TNFα, whereas Tc2 cells secrete IL-4, IL-5, IL-10, and IL-13. Just as there is a balance between Th1 and Th2 during an ongoing immune response, there is a balance between Tc1 and Tc2. Imbalance of the Tc1/Tc2 ratio because of expansion of the Tc2 population has been associated with the progression of viral disease, such as HIV infection, and cancer. Most tumor-specific CD8⁺ T cells secrete IFN-γ and can therefore be classified as Tc1.

III. TUMOR-ASSOCIATED ANTIGENS

Tumor-specific T cells, primarily CD8⁺ T cells, have been identified in many types of solid tumors and have been instrumental for the identification of tumor-derived antigenic peptides. Advances in molecular biology techniques since the early 1990s have resulted in a rapidly growing list of tumor antigens that can induce activation of specific T cells. Most of the TAA are nonmutated peptides derived from shared tissue-specific differentiation antigens or shared tumor-specific antigens; only a small number of unique or mutated antigens have presently been identified (Table II). A shared antigen means that a T cell specific for a particular MHC/antigen complex potentially recognizes all tumors that express the same MHC/antigen complex, even when the tumors are of different histologic types. For example, the Her2/neu-derived peptide p654-662 presented by HLA-A2.1 was found to be a tumor antigen in carcinomas of the breast, ovary, and pancreas, nonsmall cell lung carcinoma, renal cell carcinoma, and gastric cancer.

A. Antigens Derived from Normal Proteins

Like many other tumor antigens, the Her2/neu-derived p654-662 is not mutated and, as such, is a self-peptide. Nonetheless, circulating CD8⁺ T cells specific for this peptide have been isolated from normal individuals as well as from patients. The presence of potentially autoreactive T cells indicates that elimination of these cells during T-cell development did not occur. The T-cell repertoire is shaped in the thymus by positive and negative selection: positive selection for T cells recognizing self-MHC, followed by negative selection of T cells that are potentially autoreactive because of recognition of self-MHC plus self-peptide. However, not all self-peptides are presented in the thymus and thus not all potentially autoreactive T cells are deleted, as evidenced by the wide spectrum of autoimmune diseases. In general, however, these cells are tolerized in peripheral tissues when they encounter self-antigen because of the absence of costimulation. Alternatively, it is possible

TABLE II
Tumor Antigens

Type	Examples	
	Tumor	Antigen
Shared		
Tissue specific	Melanoma	gp100, MART-1
Tumor specific	Melanoma	MAGE-1, MAGE-3
Ubiquitous	Ovarian/breast/pancreas	Her2-neu, MUC-1
Unique/mutated	Melanoma	CDK4, MUM-1

that self-antigens are ignored by T cells able to recognize these antigens because their expression level does not reach the threshold level required for T-cell activation. This phenomenon is referred to as immunological ignorance. Ignorance differs from tolerance where the density of antigen surpasses the required threshold level, but binding to TcRs on the T cell results in clonal deletion or inactivation. Immunological ignorance may be overcome when the density of antigen is increased, as is the case for many self-antigens that are overexpressed on tumor cells. An example of such an antigen is the earlier mentioned p654-662 of the protooncogene Her2/neu, which is overexpressed in many epithelial tumors. It is not entirely clear how tolerance to self-antigens is broken, but several theories have been proposed. According to one theory, some tumor antigens are not presented in the thymus even though they are self-antigens and thus there was no negative selection against these antigens. Another conceivable explanation is that tolerized T cells become activated when self-antigens are encountered in the presence of costimulation. This may occur when tumor cells or tumor cell fragments are processed by APC and peptides are presented by MHC molecules on the cell surface (Fig. 2).

The identification of tumor antigens as mostly self-antigens has important consequences for the design of T-cell-mediated immune therapies because of the potential to develop autoimmune disease. Even though tumor-specific T cells recognizing a self-antigen generally bind with a low affinity, they may cross-react with normal tissue expressing the same antigen. The best documented example is the development of vitiligo in patients with malignant melanoma that were vaccinated with antigens derived from melanosomal proteins involved in the synthesis of melanin. Development of vitiligo has been found to be correlated with clinical responses to immunochemotherapy.

B. Viral, Mutated, and Altered Self-Antigens

Tumor antigens that are nonself generally induce strong T-cell responses. This category includes viral antigens such as Epstein–Barr virus-derived antigens, mutated antigens, and altered self. Even though the far majority of adults are EBV positive, immunocompetent individuals do not develop EBV-associated malignant lymphomas. An example of altered self antigens are chromosomal transformations that may create new antigens such as in soft tissue sarcomas or idiotypic determinants associated with B-cell lymphomas. Studies with idiotypic protein vaccination in patients with residual lymphoma suggest that tumor-specific T cells can be induced that significantly prolong disease-free survival.

IV. SUMMARY

During the past decade, numerous tumor-specific antigens have been identified on human tumors, some of which have been implicated as rejection antigens. Elimination of tumor cells and induction of immunity are primarily mediated by the various types of T lymphocytes. Tumor progression has been associated with an imbalance between $CD4^+$ Th1/Th2 and $CD8^+$ Tc1/Tc2 ratios, as well as with the presence of regulatory T cells, suggesting that various types of T cells are involved in the eradication of tumor cells. Tumor-specific T cells can be detected in most cancer patients. However, immunologic unresponsiveness is often observed because of T-cell tolerance or ignorance. Additionally, acquired resistance of the tumor to T cells plays an important role in some tumors.

See Also the Following Articles

CELL-MEDIATED IMMUNITY TO CANCER • EPSTEIN-BARR VIRUS • HIV • IMMUNE DEFICIENCY: OPPORTUNISTIC TUMORS • MOLECULAR BASIS OF TUMOR IMMUNITY • NEOPLASMS IN ACQUIRED IMMUNODEFICIENCY SYNDROME • T CELLS AND THEIR EFFECTOR FUNCTIONS • TUMOR ANTIGENS • TUMOR CELL MOTILITY AND INVASION

Bibliography

Old, L. J., Boyse, E. A., Clarke, D. A., and Carswell, E. A. (1962). Antigenic properties of chemically induced tumors. *Ann. NY Acad. Sci.* **101**, 80.

Pardoll, D. M. (1998). Cancer vaccines. *Nature Med.* **4**, 525.

Prehn, R. T., and Main, J. M. (1957). Immunity to methylcholanthrene-induced sarcomas. *J. Natl. Cancer Inst.* **18**, 769.

Rouse, B. T., Rollinghoff, M., and Warner, N. L. (1972). Anti-θ serum-induced suppression of the cellular transfer of tumor-specific immunity to a syngeneic plasma cell tumor. *Nature New Biol.* **238,** 116.

Schwartz, R. H. (1990). A cell culture model for T lymphocyte clonal anergy. *Science* **248,** 1349.

Shankaran, V., Ikeda, H., Bruce, A. T., White, J. M., Swanson, P. E., Old, L. J., and Schreiber, R. D. (2001). IFNγ and lymphocytes prevent primary tumor development and shape tumor immunogenicity. *Nature* **410,** 1107.

Wang, R. F. (1999). Human tumor antigens: Implications for cancer vaccine development. *J. Mol. Med.* **77,** 640.

T Cells and Their Effector Functions

Ruben C. Fragoso
Michael Wei-Chih Su

Harvard Medical School and Dana Farber Cancer Institute

Steven J. Burakoff

Skirball Institute of Biomolecular Medicine and New York University Cancer Institute

GLOSSARY

antigen-presenting cells (APC) Cells that can process protein antigen into peptide fragments and present them at the cell surface in association with MHC molecules where they can be recognized by T cells. Some specialized APCs express both MHC class I molecules and MHC class II molecules. Examples of these specialized APCs include B cells, macrophages, and dendritic cells.

CD4/CD8 Surface receptors expressed on T cells. They are referred to as coreceptors because they simultaneously bind the same MHC molecule as the TCR to deliver a robust activation signal to the T cell. Most mature T cells express either CD4 or CD8 but not both. CD4 binds to MHC class II and CD8 binds to MHC class I. Cells that are single positive for CD4 usually produce cytokines and are referred to as helper T cells, whereas those T cells that are single positive for CD8 lyse virally infected cell or malignantly transformed cells and are referred to as cytolytic T cells.

cytokines Proteins that are secreted by immune cells and usually cross talk with other immune cells. Cytokines include interleukins, interferons, and tumor necrosis factors.

cytolytic T cells A subset of mature T cells that express the CD8 but not the CD4 coreceptor. The main function of these cells is to lyse cells that have been infected with pathogen or have undergone malignant transformation. Unlike helper T cells, cytolytic T cells survey peptide antigen loaded onto MHC class I molecules.

helper T cells A subset of mature T cells that express the CD4 but not the CD8 coreceptor. Functionally, these cells produce cytokines that either help recruit more leukocytes or help other specialized cells, such as B cells and macrophages, to perform their function. These cells survey peptide antigen loaded onto MHC class II molecules.

immunotherapy Manipulation of the method of antigen delivery to optimize the activation of the immune system for the destruction of tumor cells. This could be accomplished by modifying the formulation of cancer vaccines or the immunogenicity of cells associated with antigen presentation.

major histocompatibility complex (MHC) Surface proteins responsible for presenting peptides to T cells. Two types of MHC molecules are involved in peptide presentation. MHC class I molecules are involved in presenting peptides that originate within the cell. This class is expressed on virtually all nucleated cells. Cytolytic T cells recognize peptide in the context of MHC class I. MHC class II molecules are involved in presenting peptides that originate outside the cell. MHC class II molecules are expressed on specialized APCs. Helper T cells recognize peptide in the context of MHC class II.

T-cell receptor (TCR) A heterodimeric cell surface antigen receptor expressed on T cells. The TCR imparts to the T cell its unique antigen specificity. T cells express either an αβ TCR or a γδ TCR but not both. TCRs, specifically αβ TCRs, recognize peptide fragments bound to MHC molecules on the surface of APCs. Other TCRs, particularly γδ TCRs, recognize nonpeptide moities or nonprocessed protein antigen on the surface of APCs.

thymocytes T-cell precursors within the thymus that are undergoing development or have just completed the developmental process. When development is completed they exit the thymus as mature T cells.

tumor-specific antigen (TSA) Unique protein products expressed by tumor cells that potentially can be processed and presented in association with the syngeneic or self-MHC molecules to elicit an immune response.

T he immune system employs various strategies to ward off or keep at bay a virtual universe of foreign pathogens, as well as to destroy malignantly transformed cells. Some of these strategies are carried out by specific classes of cells. T cells play a central role as exemplified by those individuals whose T cells have been destroyed or diminished by the AIDS-causing virus. The collective group of T cells is composed of several T-cell classes. Some T cells are involved in screening cells for intracellular infection or malignant transformation, whereas others are involved in regulating other immune cells in surveying for and destroying pathogens. This article discusses the effector functions of T cells, as well as the developmental processes leading to the generation of the different T-cell classes that can discriminate between self and nonself. In addition, it discusses how some pathogens or malignant cells try to thwart T cells.

I. INTRODUCTION

The immune system consists of innate and adaptive branches of immunity. T cells represent one arm of the adaptive branch, i.e., the cellular arm of the immune system responsible for generating specific immunity against foreign pathogens; B cells represent the other arm, the humoral arm, cells that produce antibodies. There are two broad categories of T cells and they can simply be differentiated by the composition of their T-cell receptor (TCR). T cells are of either αβ or γδ T-cell lineage. T cells can further be categorized into subgroups and their developmental state gauged by assessing the expression of several essential surface molecules that include CD3, CD4, and CD8, in addition to the TCR. T cells perform varied physiological functions that include cell-mediated cytolysis and secretion of cytokines that regulate other cells. The more studied and better understood group of T cells are the αβ T cells found in the vasculature, lymph nodes, and spleen. They are primarily either $CD4^+CD8^-$ or $CD4^-CD8^+$ and are referred to as single positive (SP) T cells. CD4 SP T cells are involved in extracellular immune surveillance and are commonly referred to as helper T cells. CD8 SP T cells are involved in intracellular immune surveillance and are usually referred to as cytolytic T cells/lymphocytes (CTLs). Both types of SP T cells, however, derive from common precursors in the thymus, the primary site of T-cell production.

T-cell receptors are those surface molecules that impart to the cell its unique antigen specificity. The TCR is a heterodimer composed of a TCR α and TCR β chain (αβ TCR) or a TCR δ chain and TCR γ chain (γδ TCR). T cells express one or the other type of TCR but not both. Associated with the TCR is the invariant CD3 complex, which acts primarily as the signaling machinery for the TCR. The CD3 complex consists of several proteins that are transmembrane but primarily cytoplasmic and contain critical tyrosine residues. These tyrosine residues can be phosphorylated and used to recruit other signaling molecules to the complex. The other two highly relevant surface molecules are the coreceptors CD4 and CD8. They act in concert with the TCR to activate the cell. The CD4 coreceptor is believed to act as a monomer, whereas the CD8 coreceptor is known to be a dimer. The CD8 coreceptor, however, can be a homodimer consisting of two CD8α chains or a heterodimer consisting of a CD8α and CD8β chain. Which CD8 dimer is expressed by the T cell depends on which T-cell subgroup it belongs to.

II. T-CELL MATURATION

A. αβ T-Cell Development

The thymus, as already mentioned, is the primary production site for T cells. Immature T cells within the thymus are referred to as thymocytes. The thymus is a bilobed mediastinal structure positioned immediately superior to the heart. It is at its largest prior to puberty, after which it begins to involute. The thymus

is like a "bag" of stromal cells filled with thymocytes. These stromal cells include epithelial cells of endodermal and ectodermal origin. Additionally, bone marrow-derived dendritic and macrophage cells play critical roles in the thymus. All these cells are important because they contain the ligands and produce the factors that guide thymocyte development and translocation through the thymus. The thymus can be divided into three morphological regions: subcapsular, cortical, and medullar. Different groups of epithelial cells can be found in each of the three different regions. Each region is associated with a certain stage of thymocyte development.

T-cell development in the thymus follows both a spatial and a sequential mode of development (Fig. 1). That is, the most primitive cells are found at the subcapsular region of the thymus and are CD3⁻CD4⁻CD8⁻. They are referred to as triple negative (TN) thymocytes or double negative (DN; with respect to CD4 and CD8) thymocytes. This population accounts for about 5% of total thymocytes. Besides entering the γδ T-cell lineage and the αβ T-cell

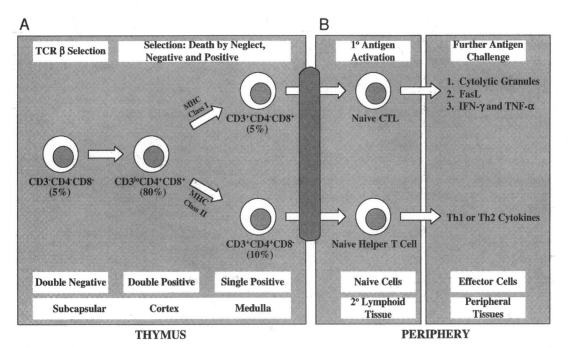

FIGURE 1 (A) T-cell development in the thymus follows a sequential mode of development. The most immature T-cell precursors are found in the subcapsular region. Thymocytes that are further along in development are closer to the medulla. Thymocytes that are positively selected will mature into single positive T cells that leave through the medulla as naive T cells. (B) Naive T cells must first be activated in secondary lymphoid tissue prior to mediating any effector functions. Once that happens, they can survey peripheral tissues where if reencounter with antigen occurs, they can mediate their effector functions according to their T-cell lineage.

lineage, these early precursors have the potential to develop into the natural killer (NK) cell, dendritic cell (DC), or B-cell lineage. Development of DN thymocytes can further be gauged by the sequential expression of two other surface markers: CD44 and CD25. The earliest precursor is CD44$^+$CD25$^-$ followed by CD44$^+$CD25$^+$, CD44$^-$CD25$^+$, and CD44$^-$CD25$^-$ expression in that order. At the CD44loCD25$^+$ stage, a critical event occurs: the TCR β chain alleles undergo rearrangement. This germline DNA rearrangement is presumably unique for each precursor cell and each allele. Rearrangement continues until a productive rearrangement occurs leading to a TCR β chain being expressed at the cell surface. This event results in allelic exclusion, in which the other β chain allele is silenced from further rearrangement so that only one uniquely rearranged allele is expressed on that cell. Many cells, however, fail to productively rearrange their TCR β alleles. Those cells die. The ones that manage to express a TCR β chain (along with CD3) at the surface begin to proliferate and enter the next phase of development—a process referred to as β selection. They provide a pool of cells expressing a common TCR β chain to which a unique TCR α chain will be added to provide each cell with its own unique antigen specificity, referred to as a clone.

In the next phase of development, thymocytes begin to further upregulate CD3 expression along with CD4 and the CD8αβ heterodimer. Rearrangement of the TCR α alleles is already underway. They pass through a transient immature single positive stage (ISP), where only one of the two coreceptors is expressed (in most mice strains it is CD8). The next critical phase is the triple positive stage (TP), or more commonly referred to as the double positive (DP; CD4$^+$CD8$^+$) stage. This population accounts for about 80% of all thymocytes. They express an intermediate level of CD3 and an αβ TCR. This population is phenotypically TCR/CD3loCD4$^+$CD8$^+$. Cells at this stage are primarily found in the cortex of the thymus. This large pool of cells provides a diverse TCR repertoire from which cells that have useful TCRs will be selected to mature and ultimately leave the thymus to populate the periphery. Prior to this, however, cells must go through a developmental stage that leads them to be either CD4 SP (helper T cells)

or CD8 SP (cytolytic T cells). CD4 and CD8 coreceptors are critical at this point for development to mature T cells as are molecules from the major histocompatibility complex (MHC).

There are two important types of MHC molecules: MHC class II molecules and MHC class I molecules. MHC class II molecules are expressed only on certain cells, most of which are bone marrow-derived cells, and MHC class I molecules are expressed on virtually all nucleated cells. The job of MHC molecules is to present to TCRs peptides generated from degraded proteins (discussed later). Both MHC molecules, from a TCR perspective, have a similar shape resembling a hot dog in a bun where the hot dog is the peptide and the bun the MHC. A critical difference between MHC classes is the source of peptide: MHC class II molecules present extracellular derived peptides and MHC class I molecules present intracellular derived peptides. CD4 binds to MHC class II molecules and CD8 binds to MHC class I molecules (Fig. 2). An individual DP thymocyte is selected into the CD4 SP lineage if its TCR and CD4 simultaneously engage

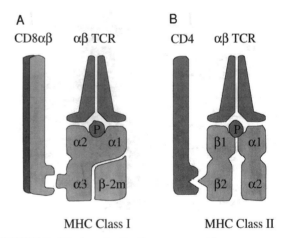

FIGURE 2 The basis for T-cell recognition of foreign antigen results from the T cell's TCR interaction with peptide loaded on MHC molecules on the surface of an APC. Selection processes in the thymus select for those TCRs that have weak affinity for self-peptide on MHC molecules but have the potential to robustly cross-react with a foreign peptide on MHC molecules that results in activation of the T cell. Recognition occurs when the TCR and coreceptor simultaneously engage the same peptide MHC complex. In the case of cytolytic T cells (A) they recognize MHC class I molecules, and in the case of helper T cells (B) they recognize MHC class II molecules. The coreceptors, CD8 and CD4, bind nonpolymorphic regions of the MHC molecule, whereas the TCR interacts with both MHC and its bound peptide (labeled P).

MHC class II molecules and into the CD8 SP lineage if its TCR and CD8 simultaneously engage MHC class I molecules. Exactly how the whole selection process occurs is still not well understood.

Several events, however, are clear regarding thymocyte development. First, CD4 and CD8 are essential for the efficient selection of thymocytes into their respective lineages. If a coreceptor is deficient, then there is a severe impairment in the generation of SP T cells expressing that coreceptor. Likewise, if MHC molecules are deficient, then SP cells selected by those MHC molecules are deficient. What still remains poorly understood is the identity of the endogenously derived peptides (self-peptides) used by MHC molecules for thymocyte development. Also, it is not well understood what different signals are generated by the coreceptors to drive cells into either SP lineage. Several models have been proposed to try and explain how DP thymocytes make the lineage commitment to be either CD4 SP or CD8 SP T cells. In the stochastic model, DP thymocytes at random commit to a SP lineage and turn off the nonselected coreceptor. If the expressed coreceptor and TCR can still simultaneously engage a MHC molecule, then the thymocyte will receive signals to further mature along the lineage pathway of the expressed coreceptor. In the instructive model, if the TCR engages MHC class I molecules, then CD8 will also bind, resulting in instructive signals to the thymocyte to pursue development along the CD8 SP lineage. Likewise, if CD4 and TCR engage MHC class II molecules, then instructive signals toward the CD4 SP lineage result. Another model is the strength of signal hypothesis. In this case, if the coreceptor and TCR result in a very potent signal upon MHC engagement, then the cell pursues a CD4 SP pathway. If the signal is weaker, then the thymocyte pursues a CD8 SP pathway. In this model, the signal is thought to be primarily generated by a tyrosine kinase termed Lck. Lck is responsible for phosphorylating CD3 tyrosine residues and other molecules that are subsequently recruited to the CD3 complex. Both CD4 and CD8 bind Lck, but CD4 binds substantially more Lck than CD8. Hence, coreceptor interactions involving CD4 during thymocyte development are thought to involve stronger Lck activity relative to CD8. This difference in signal strength is thought to somehow be processed

by developing thymocytes. Ultimately, however, DP thymocytes will be selected into either the CD4 or the CD8 SP lineage.

Mature SP T cells are located in the medulla of the thymus and it is from here that they will exit to the periphery. CD4 SP T cells represent roughly 10% of all thymocytes, whereas CD8 SP T cells represent 5% of all thymocytes. Phenotypically mature SP T cells express a high level of TCR/CD3, unlike the lower TCR/CD3 levels in the DP thymocytes. Hence, mature T cells exit into the periphery as SP TCR/CD3hi T cells. The end result of thymic development is a pool of self-tolerant CD4 SP and CD8 SP T cells.

B. Generation of TCR Diversity and Thymic Education

The main purpose of development in the thymus is to give rise to a population of mature T cells that have a diverse TCR repertoire with T-cell clones that are tolerant to self but capable of responding to foreign antigens. However, a heavy price is paid both in the generation of diversity and in selection of self-tolerant TCRs. The immune system employs a combinatorial approach to generate diversity. Each germline TCR allele is divided into regions. They can include V(ariable), D(iversity), J(oining), and C(onstant) regions. Further, each region can contain multiple coding segments of which any could be used to combine with a coding segment of another region. For example, a productive TCR β allele will contain rearranged DNA where VDJC coding segments have been joined together (the TCR α allele contains no D segments and only one C segment). The extent of combinatorial diversity depends on the number of V coding segments available as well as the number of D, J, and C coding segments available. Further diversity is generated by other mechanisms when the DNA coding segments are cleaved and religated. Enzymatic processes during this event introduce extra noncoded nucleotides to the DNA ends prior to religation, generating further diversity at the coding segment junctions. This diversity is important because it increases the likelihood of generating T cells that can recognize a wide range of foreign antigens that include those expressed on pathogens and malignantly transformed cells. Finally, the pairing of a β chain to an α chain to generate a TCR also generates diversity. It is estimated that the theoretical TCR diversity that can be generated by these mechanisms is upward of 10^{18} T cell clones. The cost for having these mechanisms to generate diversity is that many of the DNA rearrangements are out of frame, and hence, no TCR chain is produced. Thymocytes that fail to generate TCR β or α chains do not receive further maturational signals and die. The expression of a TCR is essential for survival because it is only through TCR interacting with self-peptide:MHC that a clone can receive survival signals for further development. This same interaction forms the basis for T-cell recognition of pathogens and malignant cells in peripheral immune surveillance. That is, the TCR of a clone interacts with foreign peptide bound to self-MHC with sufficient affinity to activate the cell.

It is estimated that only a few percent of αβ TCR DP thymocytes will actually survive the developmental process and exit the thymus. The unique TCR expressed by a clone has one of three fates. First, the TCR may be useless. That is, it does not recognize either type of MHC class with any appreciable affinity. Such a TCR would be useless in peripheral immune surveillance. These clones do not receive any maturational signals and so die—referred to as "death by neglect." The majority of thymocytes fall into this category. The second fate is that a TCR may recognize a self-peptide:MHC ligand extremely well. This TCR would be detrimental in the periphery. MHC molecules present peptides that are generated from the host's own germline encoded proteins. Presumably, if the TCR of a clone recognizes self-peptides during development and survives, then it can encounter self-peptides in the periphery. Such a situation could lead to an autoimmune reaction. A clone bearing a TCR falling into this category receives a signal to die; it undergoes "negative selection." The third fate of a TCR is that it weakly recognizes a self-peptide:MHC ligand. This TCR could potentially be useful in the periphery. The idea is that in the process of peripheral immune surveillance, only foreign-peptide:MHC ligands can generate a high enough affinity that can activate these T cells with low affinity for self-peptides. Clones bearing TCRs in this category receive signals for further development into SP cells; they undergo "positive selection." Cells that

exit the thymus have been thymically "educated" to be self-tolerant and are termed naive T cells because they have not yet encountered foreign antigen. It is important to stress that it is those T cells that have been positively selected that have the capacity to be activated by cross-reacting with foreign peptide:MHC ligands. Collectively, these cells form the diverse self-tolerant repertoire that helps protect the host from foreign pathogens or transformed cells.

C. Other TCR-Bearing Cells

The other class of T cells, γδ T cells, also develop in the thymus. Their developmental progression is less clear. γδ T cells are thought to arise in waves early in thymic ontogeny. Each wave expresses an invariant TCR due to the preferential expression of specific V_γ and V_δ coding segments with no junctional diversity. Also, each wave seems to home to a particular location, primarily to skin and mucosal tissues. However, the development of αβ T cells quickly predominates and supersedes that of γδ T cells that then continue to develop at low levels in the thymus. The branch point for development is at the TN stage. They commence TCR rearrangement at the same time that TCR β chain rearrangement begins. How TN precursors choose which T-cell lineage to develop into is not known. Peripheral γδ T cells are primarily CD8⁻CD4⁻ but some express the CD8α homodimer.

Further heterogeneity of T-cell subsets exists. For example, the collective group of lymphocytes that reside within the mucosa in contact with epithelial cells (intraepithelial lymphocytes, IELs) includes T cells of both γδ and αβ TCR lineages. αβ T cells are CD8⁺CD4⁺, CD8⁻CD4⁺, or CD8⁺CD4⁻, where CD8 can be either a hetero- or a homodimer. γδ T cells are CD8⁻CD4⁻ or CD8⁺CD4⁻. Although most development occurs intrathymically, some development may occur extrathymically for IELs.

D. Activation of Naive T Cells

Naive SP T cells in the periphery are incapable of mediating any effector functions because they have not yet been exposed to foreign antigen (Fig. 1B). Antigen recognition for naive SP T cells occurs in secondary lymphoid tissues such as lymph nodes (and spleen). Naive SP T cells have homing receptors that direct them to lymph nodes. Antigen is transported to the lymph node via the afferent lymphatic vessels primarily by Langerhan cells. Langerhan cells become dendritic cells in the lymph node. The antigen is processed and presented on MHC molecules by these DCs. Successful activation of a T cell will result if two signals are received. The first signal occurs via the TCR and CD4 or CD8 coreceptor, and the second is a costimulatory signal delivered to the cell through the CD28 receptor. If the T cell only receives a signal via the TCR, the cell may apoptose or become anergic, i.e., it is unresponsive to subsequent antigen encounters. Dendritic cells are potent antigen-presenting cells (APCs) frequently termed professional APCs because they express antigen on MHC molecules and constitutively express the CD28 ligand, B7, to provide the second signal. Activated B cells and macrophages also express B7 and can serve as professional APCs. The need for a costimulatory signal is hypothesized to be a mechanism for generating peripheral tolerance. APCs are activated when they encounter foreign antigen and will then express B7. The outcome of the TCR interacting with the MHC of the APC then depends on whether B7 is present on that APC. If B7 is not present, the T cell is probably detecting self-antigen and it must be killed or anergized to prevent an unwanted response. If B7 is present, then foreign antigen is being detected and the T cell should be activated.

Once a T cell is activated, it begins to clonally expand. Clonally expanded cells leave the lymph node as effector cells or memory cells. They will no longer home to lymph nodes, but rather gain the capacity to enter peripheral tissues by expressing specific homing receptors. These cells can be reactivated by antigen at various sites. Effector cells can immediately respond to antigen, whereas memory cells serve as a reservoir to rapidly elicit effector functions upon future antigenic challenge.

III. ANTIGEN RECOGNITION AND EFFECTOR FUNCTIONS OF CD8 SINGLE POSITIVE T CELLS

As mentioned, MHC class I molecules are expressed on all nucleated cells. The susceptibility of nucleated cells to viral infection or malignant transformation requires that their cytoplasmic contents be monitored for viral or malignant cell protein in order to target them for lysis. The TCR restriction to MHC class I molecules generated during development dictates that CD8 SP T cells will survey peptides that are derived from the cytoplasm of potential target cells. The polymorphic nature of MHC genes in general, as well as the multiple MHC alleles codominantly expressed in each host, helps maximize the presentation of intracellular proteins to CD8 SP T cells. The mechanism of MHC class I peptide presentation is important for CD8 SP T-cell activation and subsequent effector functions.

A. MHC Class I Antigen Presentation

Class I MHC molecules are pivotal for the transport of intracellular peptides to the cell surface, thereby providing the immune system with a snapshot of the proteins synthesized endogenously. Endogenous proteins can be self-encoded, e.g., metabolic enzymes or acquired from a foreign source, e.g., viral pathogens. Structurally, MHC class I molecules are the heterodimer of a polymorphic α chain bound noncovalently to a common β_2-microglobulin chain (β_2M; Fig. 2A). An antigenic peptide of about 8–10 amino acids in length is also an integral part of the MHC molecule that confers structural stability to the complex. The MHC α chain is further organized into three distinct domains: α1, α2, and α3. The α1 and α2 domains together form the peptide-binding cleft where they interact extensively with the bound peptides. Therefore, in order to accommodate a wide range of foreign peptides that the MHC molecule might encounter, genes encoding the α1 and α2 domains are highly polymorphic. In contrast, the α3 domain and β_2M are not in direct contact with the antigenic peptide or TCR, and their sequences share remarkable conservation. The relatively invariant nature of the α3 domain is apparently necessary for its binding to a constant region on the CD8 coreceptor on T cells. This interaction augments T-cell responses by increasing the half-lives of the interaction between TCR and peptide–MHC complexes.

The processing of antigens into peptides that can be presented in the cleft of class I MHC molecules is the result of several cellular processes involving various organelles and molecular chaperones. The initial step is the generation of peptide fragments from the proteins in the cytoplasm. This is mediated by the proteolytic cleavage of proteins destined for degradation by the proteasomes. Peptide fragments generated by this process may be protected from degradation by molecular chaperones called heat shock proteins (HSPs) and then delivered to a dedicated transporter protein called TAP (transporters associated with antigen processing) for the translocation of peptides into the lumen of the endoplasmic reticulum (ER), where partially folded class I MHC molecules reside. ER resident molecular chaperones assist in the sequential assembly of MHC α chains with β_2M prior to the acquisition of peptides from TAP. MHC molecules stabilized by the peptide cargo adopt a mature conformation that dissociates from TAP to follow the secretory pathway for export to the cell surface. Once the MHC molecules are anchored on the cell membrane, T cells can interact with the MHC molecules and their bound antigens. Thus, the ability for MHC to process and present the antigenic peptides in a context that can be recognized by T cells is critical to the survival of the host.

Given the pivotal role of antigenic peptides in the activation of T-cell responses, viruses have evolved elaborate mechanisms for circumventing the effectiveness of antigen processing and presentation. For example, the herpes simplex viruses (HSV)-1 and -2 encode proteins that can interfere with TAP-mediated peptide transport into the ER, which then results in the retention and degradation of class I MHC molecules. Another example is the product of UL18 from human cytomegalovirus (HCMV), which downregulates the surface expression of class I MHC molecules by the binding and sequestration of the cellular pool of β_2M that otherwise would be available to the endogenous class I MHC. Additionally, HCMV-encoded US2 and US11 can reverse the transport of newly synthesized MHC α chains from ER to the cytosol for degradation. Another protein known to interfere with MHC presentation is the Nef viral protein encoded by the human immunodeficiency virus (HIV). Expression of the Nef viral product alone can induce the internalization of surface class I MHC molecules for degradation in endosomal vesicles.

B. CD8 SP T-Cell Effector Functions

Activated CD8 SP CTLs can directly damage the target cells by using at least three distinct effector functions: (1) release of preformed granules harboring toxic substances, e.g., perforin, granzymes, and granulysin, (2) triggering of programmed cell death, or apoptosis, by the engagement of Fas receptor with Fas ligand (FasL), and (3) secretion of cytokines such as tumor necrosis factor (TNF)-α and interferon (IFN)-γ. Among these mechanisms, perforin degranulation appears to be the predominant pathway used for cytolysis. Named after its ability to perforate the cytoplasmic membrane, perforin is structurally homologous to the terminal components of the complement pathway that make up the membrane attack complex. In the presence of calcium ion, perforin polymerizes in the lipid membrane of target cells, forming discrete transmembrane channels that ultimately lead to osmotic lysis. Perforin is also needed to facilitate the entry of another important constituent of the granule, granzyme B (GrmB). GrmB is capable of activating proapoptotic cysteine protease aspases, or caspases. In turn, these caspases unleash self-destructive cleavage of endogenous substrates, including poly(ADP-ribose) polymerase (PARP), a known DNA repair enzyme, and lamin B, a structural constituent of the nuclear membrane. GrmB can also bypass the caspases and directly cleave the nuclear substrates involved in apoptosis, such as DNA-PKcs and NuMA. Finally, granulysin, a bacteriocidal agent, has also been identified in the granules of CD8 SP CTLs. Granulysin contributes to the resistance against a variety of microbial pathogens, such as *Listeria*, *Chlamydia*, and *Mycobacteria*. In macrophages infected with *Mycobacterium tuberculosis*, the combination of granulysin and perforin can potently destroy the macrophage, as well as *M. tuberculosis*.

Fas is a member of the TNF receptor family (TNFR1, DR3, DR4, and DR5) expressed on many cell types, including CD4 and CD8 SP T cells. The engagement of Fas receptor on target cells leads to apoptosis that is dependent on the activation of caspases. It is known that the delivery of Fas-mediated apoptosis requires the *de novo* synthesis of FasL on T cells, hence Fas-mediated cell death is not readily detectable until 8–12 h after T-cell activation. This is in contrast to perforin, which predominates the killing that occurs within hours and usually minutes after target cell engagement. The cytoplasmic tail of Fas receptors contains a protein modular domain termed the death domain (DD). Upon receptor oligomerization by FasL, the DD region of Fas receptor recruits a cytosolic adaptor molecule, FADD, which in turn binds to procaspase 8 to form the death-inducing signaling complex (DISC). The procaspase-8 recruited to the DISC undergoes further modification by autocleavage to yield a catalytically active subunit that proceeds to activate downstream caspases -3, -6, and -7. These caspases ultimately culminate in the cleavage of the inhibitor of caspase-activated DNase (ICAD), thereby liberating an active DNase to induce DNA fragmentation and apoptosis.

The evolutionary pressure exerted by the host immune system on viral pathogens has led to the emergence of survival strategies that the viruses use to thwart Fas-mediated cell death. As an example, the cytokine response modifier (CrmA) gene encoded by cowpox virus is a protease inhibitor that can render caspases enzymatically inert. A second mechanism is the blockade of the recruitment of caspase-8 to FADD by viral FLICE inhibitory proteins (vFLIPs), which are encoded by several herpes viruses and poxvirus. Finally, the engagement of Fas by FasL can be blocked by soluble decoy receptors (e.g., DcR3) that can bind to the FasL expressed on T cells and prevent the engagement of Fas.

While the *coup de gras* delivered by the exocytosis of granular contents or the engagement of Fas receptor requires intimate cellular contact, soluble factors such as cytokines and chemokines obviate this necessity and provide alternative strategies to dealing with intracellular pathogens. Interferon-γ released by T lymphocytes has been shown to enhance the killing of intracellular microbes in macrophages through the increased expression of inducible nitric oxide synthetase (iNOS) and the production of reactive radicals. In addition, IFNs and TNF factors suppress the overall viral replication and transcription by turning on interferon-inducible genes, such as the double-stranded RNA-activated protein kinase (PKR). TNF-α can also induce caspase-dependent apoptosis analogous to the triggering of Fas receptor. Finally, chemokines such as MIF-1α and MIF-1β secreted by CTLs can impair HIV infection by competing for viral coreceptors. Chemokines can also recruit other inflammatory cells and potentiate the proliferation and cytokine secretion by other lymphocytes.

IV. ANTIGEN RECOGNITION AND EFFECTOR FUNCTIONS OF CD4 SINGLE POSITIVE T CELLS

MHC class II molecules are expressed by bone marrow-derived cells such as B cells and dendritic cells and may be induced by IFN-γ to be expressed in cell types such as macrophages and endothelial cells. CD4 SP T cells only recognize antigen presented by MHC class II molecules; thus they are termed MHC class II restricted. CD4 SP cell effector functions primarily consist of cytokine production that enhances leukocyte recruitment and "helps" other leukocytes perform specific functions, including macrophages, B cells, and CD8 SP T cells. Naive CD4 SP cells that encounter antigen and are activated further differentiate into one of two subgroups that can be distinguished by their cytokine production profile.

A. MHC Class II Antigen Presentation

MHC class II molecules consist of two chains: an α and a β chain (Fig. 2B). Both chains are glycosylated and are noncovalently associated. Each chain is divided into two domains. α1 and β1 domains collectively form the peptide-binding cleft. The overall topology is similar to that of the MHC class I molecule. The bound peptide is similarly nestled, although structural differences between MHC classes allow MHC class II molecules to bind and present significantly longer peptides. α2 and β2 domains form Ig domains and are conserved, unlike the α1 and β1 segments, which are polymorphic. CD4 binds to the β2 domain, analogous to how CD8 binds the α3 domain on a MHC class I molecule. As in the case for MHC class I molecules, multiple loci encoding both chains exist for MHC class II molecules. However, further heterogeneity exists for MHC class II molecules because an α chain from one locus may pair with a β chain of another locus.

In the ER, each MHC class II molecule is bound by one invariant chain (Ii). Significantly, the Ii chain occupies the peptide-binding cleft, preventing the aberrant loading of the MHC class II molecule with a cytoplasmic-derived peptide. Further, Ii trimers serve to direct MHC class II complexes into exocytic vesicles through the golgi. These vesicles then fuse with endocytic and lysosomal vesicles carrying extracellular protein. This results in a MHC class II compartment vesicle, referred to as a MIIC vesicle. Prior to fusion, however, within the endocytic and lysosomal vesicles, a combination of low pH and proteases degrades the extracellular proteins to peptide fragments of varying lengths. Those same mechanisms degrade the Ii in the MIIC vesicle. Ii is reduced to a MHC class II bound peptide, termed class II-associated invariant chain peptide (CLIP). Other MHC class II-like molecules present in the vesicle remove CLIP and allow for foreign peptides to bind. Only those MHC molecules with a bound foreign peptide reach the cell surface.

B. CD4 SP T-Cell Effector Functions

Naive CD4 SP T cells can differentiate into polarized subsets of helper T cells (Th1 or Th2) as defined by the patterns of cytokines produced. Th1-mediated responses are typically dominated by IFN-γ and interleukin (IL)-12, which are cytokines considered necessary for the activation of cells involved in cell-mediated immunity, such as macrophages, NK cells, and CD8 SP T cells. Therefore, a Th1-polarized immune response is effective against intracellular pathogens that are dealt with by these cell types, such as M. tuberculosis. In contrast, a Th2 subset of T cells produces IL-4, IL-5, IL-10, and IL-13 cytokines, which promote the functions of eosinophils and augment the production of IgE. Thus, a Th2 coordinated response is effective against extracellular pathogens such as parasites and is often associated with the pathogenesis of allergic inflammation.

The cytokine milieu is a major determinant of the developmental fates adopted by naive T cells. The differentiation of Th1 cells is dependent on IL-12 and IFN-γ released by NK cells and macrophages. In contrast, the Th2 subset requires IL-4 from mast cells or NK1.1 CD4 SP T cells. These cytokines activate a distinct family of signal transducers and activators of transcription (STAT) molecules in naive T cells to coordinate the polarization of Th subsets. Additionally, the potency, dose, and route of entry of antigens, as well as the quality of antigen-presenting cells during T-cell priming, appear to also influence Th differentiation. Finally, cytokines necessary for polarization of one subset of Th cells appear to also antagonize the development of the other. Thus, while IFN-γ supports Th1 responses, it actively suppresses Th2 cell growth at the same time. Conversely, the combination of IL-4 and IL-10 suppresses Th1 development and may also serve to limit tissue injury that is often associated with Th1 cell-mediated immunity.

1. Th1 T Cells

A classical Th1-mediated response is delayed-type hypersensitivity (DTH), which is commonly seen in patients sensitized to the purified protein derivatives of M. tuberculosis in a tuberculin skin test. The DTH reaction is typically characterized by the infiltration of T cells and macrophages into the tissues exposed to M. tuberculosis. IL-12 produced by macrophages that have encountered these microbes skews the development of naive CD4 SP T cells toward the Th1 subset, which, in turn, releases IFN-γ to activate the bacteriocidal functions of macrophages. The Th1 subset has also been implicated in the pathogenesis of inflammatory autoimmune disorders such as rheumatoid arthritis.

2. Th2 T Cells

Th2 cells promote IgE production and eosinophil function, which are the key players in the pathogenesis of allergic inflammation and immunity against parasitic infections. Cytokines such as IL-4 and IL-5 released by Th2 cells stimulate, respectively, B-cell switching to the production of IgE antibody and activation of eosinophils. The coordinate actions of these effector mechanisms result in heightened immunity against, for example, helminthic parasites, which can be coated with IgE and destroyed by the toxic granular contents of eosinophils.

The balance between Th1 and Th2 cells may serve to determine the outcome of an infection. The Th1-mediated response is an effective deterrent for the protozoan parasite *Leishmania major*. In strains of mice with a genetic predisposition to mount predominantly Th2 responses, infection by *L. major* results in a severe cutaneous and systemic disease that cannot be eliminated effectively. In contrast, if mice were vaccinized with leishmania antigens coadministered with IL-12 to induce a Th1 response, the mice are protected from subsequent challenges with *L. major*. In an analogous manner, responses to *Mycobacterium leprae* in humans can have two sharply different outcomes depending on the polarization of Th cells. In lepromatous leprosy, a Th2-dominated response can result in diffuse and destructive lesions due to an ineffective response against *M. leprae* antigens. In contrast, patients who develop a strong Th1-mediated immunity have a less destructive disease called tuberculoid leprosy.

V. γδ T CELLS AND INTRAEPITHELIAL LYMPHOCYTES

The exact functions of intraepithelial lymphocytes, which includes γδ T cells, remain undefined but are thought to include T-cell subsets that have the following properties: Th1 and Th2 cytokine production, cytolysis, and suppression of other immune cells. It is also not quite clear how these cells are activated. For example, γδ T cells, some of which lack CD4 and CD8, have been shown to be activated by nonpeptide moities. However, other studies have shown that γδ T cells can be activated by protein that has not been processed and presented in the context of MHC. These antigens are presented by MHC-like molecules that are distinct from those classic MHC molecules involved in peptide presentation.

VI. TUMOR IMMUNOLOGY

The concept of immunosurveillance stipulates that a physiological function of the immune system is to eradicate cells that have undergone malignant transformation. However, most malignant tumors found *in vivo* are weak to nonimmunogenic. Often tumor antigens are difficult to detect or are presented without a costimulatory signal. It is also not uncommon to find tumors adopting strategies to thwart the immune response, e.g., by the downmodulation of class I MHC molecules. Recent approaches of immunolog-

ical intervention have focused on rendering tumors susceptible to the effector functions of the immune system.

A. Tumor Antigens

Most malignant tumors are poorly immunogenic because self-peptides rather than the elusive tumor antigens occupy the majority of their surface MHC molecules. Nonetheless, a number of tumor-specific antigens (TSAs) can still be recognized by CD8 SP CTLs isolated from regional lymph nodes or the peripheral blood of cancer patients, giving rise to the possibility that T cells, when stimulated under optimal conditions, may reject the tumor burden. TSAs identified to date can be classified into two categories based on their pattern of expression: (1) shared TSAs are found in the same as well as different types of cancer cells from different individuals and (2) unique TSAs are found only in a particular cancer cell line from a specific patient. The understanding of the precise nature of TSAs is important for the design of vaccines to accelerate tumor regression by the immune system, an approach termed immunotherapy.

Cellular protooncogenes and tumor suppressor genes are often mutated in cells with a malignant phenotype. Alterations of these genes by point mutation, deletion, chromosomal translocation, or viral gene insertion may generate unique neoantigens expressed by the tumors, thus hypothetically these neoantigens are possible candidates for immunotherapy. For example, point mutants of the small GTP-binding proteins Ras or the p53 tumor suppressor genes have been identified as targets of CTLs in colorectal and lung cancer. Other potential vaccine candidates are the self-proteins that are overexpressed or aberrantly expressed in tumor cells. An example of this type of TSA is the tyrosinase enzyme that is expressed by melanocytes for melanin biosynthesis. The antigens from tyrosinase can be seen by T cells from melanoma patients. Other differentiation antigens from melanocytes, such as MART-1 or Melan-A, have also been reported to represent dominant T-cell epitopes, as is the product of the melanoma antigen (MAGE) family of genes that are normally expressed in testicular germ cells or placental trophoblasts. For unknown reasons, MAGE genes are reexpressed in a large number of human melanomas and unrelated cancers. Finally, oncogenic viruses may express viral proteins that are processed and presented by MHC molecules and therefore function as tumor antigens. Studies have revealed that human papilloma virus (HPV) is associated with cervical carcinomas and penile cancer. In particular, the oncogenic E6 and E7 proteins from HPV are found in transformed tissues, and their peptides can be presented by MHC antigens and may result in the tumor being targeted for immune destruction. Epstein–Barr virus is another oncogenic virus often associated with Burkitt's lymphoma, nasopharyngeal carcinoma, and posttransplant lymphoproliferative disorders.

B. T-Cell Responses to Tumors

The principal mechanism of tumor destruction is the release of perforin/granzymes by CD8 SP CTLs. The importance of perforin is demonstrated in mice by ablation of the gene that encodes perforin. These mice develop spontaneous malignancies in the lymphoid compartment at a higher frequency. Alternatively, Fas receptor engagement can also induce apoptosis of susceptible tumor cell lines. Finally, cytokines such as IFN-γ may stimulate NK cells and macrophages to participate in the killing of tumor cells. IFN-γ can also increase the efficacy of antigen processing and presentation of MHC molecules to T cells. The combination of TNF-α and IFN-γ can also enhance the sensitivity of tumor vasculature to undergo apoptosis, in particular the rich capillary beds of the angiogenic blood vessels that supply tumor cells the nutrients required to sustain a rapid rate of cell division.

C. Mechanisms of Tumor Escape

Experimental tumors can often be ignored or be unrecognized despite a robust, antigen-specific response to other foreign antigens. The downregulation of tumor antigens or components of the class I/II MHC processing pathway in tumors may accomplish this. Because most malignant cells are genetically unstable, the genes encoding the structural components of MHC molecules, such as MHC α chain, $\beta_2 M$, or TAP, may be lost so that these tumor cells are invisible to T cells. Likewise, class II MHC presentation of tumor antigens can be disrupted by the deletion of HLA-

DM, a molecule that facilitates the loading of antigenic peptides onto the class II MHC molecules, or by mutation of the transcriptional activator, CIITA, which is necessary for the optimal expression of class II MHC molecules. Alternatively, malignant cells can also protect themselves from destruction by displaying the Fas ligand on their cell surface, giving them the ability to destroy tumor-specific T cells that express Fas. Other soluble factors, such as transforming growth factor β (TGF-β), can be released by tumor cells to antagonize the proliferation of lymphocytes and also promote the formation of stroma that supports tumor growth. Finally, most tumor tissues do not express costimulatory molecules and therefore upon contact they can anergize tumor-specific T cells.

D. Immunotherapy for Tumors

Because most tumors are not particularly immunogenic, novel approaches for stimulating T cells have turned to the use of professional antigen-presenting cells like dendritic cells to express the tumor antigen. Bone marrow-derived DC are capable of inducing and sustaining the activation of immune responses by expressing high levels of adhesion molecules, as well as costimulatory molecules such as B7 (CD28/86). Because the engagement of TCR must take place concurrently with the ligation of CD28, one of the approaches to immunotherapy has focused on the expression of B7 molecules in tumors. Also, intact DCs transfected with genes encoding tumor antigens or pulsed with synthetic or acid-eluted peptides from tumor cells have been used to induce tumor regression. Autologous DCs have been used as a fusion partner for cancer cells to create heterokaryons that retain the expression of both tumor antigens and costimulatory molecules. Immunogenenicity can also be boosted by fusion of, for example, allogeneic DC with human renal carcinoma, which has been reported to be effective in the treatment of metastatic disease.

CTLA-4, a homologue of CD28, is expressed on T cells after activation. CTLA-4 is thought to compete with CD28 for the binding of B7 and to deliver a negative signal for the downmodulation of T-cell responses. The cytoplasmic tail of CTLA-4 interacts with a tyrosine phosphatase, SHP-2, and upon B7 engagement the complex is recruited to the proximity of

CD3ζ to diminish signals initiated by the TCR/CD3 complex. Therefore, the blockade of the CTLA-4/B7 interaction might terminate the inhibitory signal and restore an active immune response. This hypothesis is supported by observations that anti-CTLA-4 antibodies administered to mice can promote the rejection of a wide variety of tumors of different tissue origins. However, for many poorly immunogenic tumors, CTLA-4 blockade alone is insufficient to confer a complete protection against tumor growth.

Another approach to alter the microenvironment of tumor sites is to transfect tumor cells with cytokine genes. Tumors engineered to express cytokines such as IL-2, IL-4, IFN-γ, and GM-CSF (granulocyte-monocyte colony-stimulating factor) have been shown to stimulate antigen-specific T-cell immunity to protect the animal against subsequent challenges with unmodified tumor cells. Thus, the production of cytokines in the tumor microenvironment may augment the priming and recruitment of T cells. Cytokines can also be used to expand lymphocytes *in vitro* and then return them intravenously to the patient. For example, lymphokine activated killer cells harvested from peripheral blood can be expanded *in vitro* with recombinant IL-2 and reinjected into patients to induce the regression of solid tumors. Similarly, tumor-infiltrating lymphocytes harvested from tumor explants can be expanded with high doses of IL-2 and adoptively transferred into patients.

Besides vaccination with tumor antigens, purified heat shock proteins derived from tumor tissues may also induce antitumor responses, as HSP is one of the molecular chaperones for peptides generated in the cytosol and a rich source for protein antigens. *In vitro*, dendritic cells have been shown to internalize purified HSP, e.g., gp96, and represent its peptide antigens in the context of class I MHC molecules. Preliminary results from several pilot studies suggest that HSP vaccination as an adjuvant therapy can enhance immunity against human malignancies.

VII. SUMMARY

The bulk of T-cell development occurs in the thymus where common progenitor T cells give rise to different classes of T cells. The best understood group of T cells are the αβ T cells that populate the vasculature, lymph nodes, and spleen. The thymic developmental process selects those T cells that are tolerant to self but can recognize and respond to foreign antigens. The two principal classes are CTLs and helper T cells. CTLs, which survey peptide antigen on MHC class I molecules, can destroy target cells using cytotoxic granules, FasL, and TNF-α and IFN-γ. Helper T cells, which survey peptide antigen on MHC class II molecules, produce specific cytokines based on whether they are Th1 or Th2 cells. Key aspects about T-cell antigen recognition and the requirements for T-cell activation are becoming better understood. It is hoped that with an increasing understanding of T cells that better vaccines can be generated and that immunotherapies for cancer may become a reality.

See Also the Following Articles

CELL-MEDIATED IMMUNITY TO CANCER • CYTOKINES • HIV • IMMUNE DEFICIENCY: OPPORTUNISTIC TUMORS • MOLECULAR BASIS OF TUMOR IMMUNITY • NEOPLASMS IN ACQUIRED IMMUNODEFICIENCY SYNDROME • T CELLS AGAINST TUMORS • TUMOR ANTIGENS • TUMOR CELL MOTILITY AND INVASION

Bibliography

Abbas, A. K., Lichtman, A. H., and Pober, J. S. (2000). "Cellular and Molecular Immunology," 4th Ed. Saunders, Philadelphia.

Benjamini, E., Coico, R., and Sunshine, G. (2000). "Immunology: A Short Course," 4th Ed. Wiley-Liss, New York.

Benoist, C., and Mathis, D. (1999). T-lymphocyte differentiation and biology. In "Fundamental Immunology" (W. E. Paul, ed.), 4th Ed., p. 367. Lippincott-Raven, Philadelphia.

Henkart, P. A. (1999). Cytotoxic T lymphocytes. In "Fundamental Immunology" (W. E. Paul, ed.), 4th Ed., p. 1021. Lippincott-Raven, Philadelphia.

Henkart, P. A. (2000). Overview of cytotoxic lymphocyte effector mechanisms. In "Cytotoxic Cells" (M. V. Sitkovsky, and P. A. Henkart, eds.), p. 111. Lippincott Williams & Wilkins, Philadelphia.

Janeway, C. A., Travers, P., Walport, M., and Capra, J. D. (1999). "Immunobiology: The Immune System in Health and Disease," 4th Ed. Elsevier Science, New York.

Kisielow, P., and Von Boehmer, H. (1995). Develoment and selection of T cells: Facts and puzzles. *Adv. Immunol.* **58**, 87–209.

McGhee, J. R., and Kiyono, H. (1999). The mucosal immune system. In "Fundamental Immunology" (W. E. Paul, ed.), 4th Ed., p. 909. Lippincott-Raven, Philadelphia.

Robbins, P. F., Wang, R.-F., and Rosenberg, S. A. (2000). Overview of cytotoxic lymphocyte effector mechanisms. In "Cytotoxic Cells" (M. V. Sitkovsky, and P. A. Henkart, eds.), p. 363. Lippincott Williams & Wilkins, Philadelphia.

Telomeres and Telomerase

Tej Krishan Pandita
Columbia University, New York

GLOSSARY

telomerase A ribonuclear reverse transcriptase that maintains telomere length through the addition of TTAGGG repeats.

telomere fusions Also known as chromosome end-to-end associations and are commonly observed at metaphase.

telomeres Protective caps that stabilize chromosome ends and prevent them from being recognized as double-strand breaks by the cellular surveillance systems that monitor genomic damage.

terminal restriction fragment length Size of the most distal restriction fragments of chromosomes. They are composed of TTAGGG repeats, as well as some subtelomeric sequences, and are commonly used to assess telomere length.

Telomeres are a specialized DNA–protein complex at the ends of linear chromosomes. They are essential for the proper maintenance of chromosomes and may play a role in aging and cancer. Telomerases are specialized reverse transcriptases involved in the synthesis of telomeres in most organisms. They are very interesting DNA polymerases in that they carry RNA template within them. Biochemical and genetic studies have established an association between telomere maintenance and cellular transformation. The loss or shortening of telomeres in telomerase-negative somatic cells has been linked with genomic instability and carcinogenesis. Reactivation of telomerase stabilizes telomeres and allows continued cell growth. Telomerase levels remain very low in most human somatic cell populations with only a few exceptions. In most transformed cell populations, up-regulation of telomerase is required for immortality, and telomerase activity is detected in most human tumors. Based on the fact that telomerase plays such a fundamental role in cell transformation and tumorigenesis, it is believed that therapeutic manipulations to modulate telomere stability and telomerase levels therefore hold promise for future potentially novel cancer treatments.

I. INTRODUCTION

Herman J. Muller coined the term telomere, which means literally end part, coming from the two Greek roots, telos (meaning "end") and meros (meaning "part"). The molecular biology of telomeres began in 1978 with a report describing telomere repeat sequences from the rDNA of *Tetrahymena thermophila*. Since then, telomeric repeat sequences have been determined for a great variety of species, including humans. Telomeres are essential genetic elements that stabilize the natural ends of linear eukaryotic chromosomes. The ends of the linear DNA duplex cannot be fully replicated by conventional DNA polymerases, which utilize an RNA primer to initiate DNA synthesis; this can lead to the problem that extreme terminal sequences will not be represented on the 5' end of one daughter DNA strand after removal of a terminal RNA primer. In the absence of a mechanism to overcome this end replication problem, organisms would fail to pass their complete genetic complement from generation to generation. Telomerase, a reverse transcriptase with a tightly associated RNA that serves as a template, synthesizes telomeric repeat DNA sequences. It has been suggested that the telomere–telomerase system represents an adaptation of organisms with a prolonged life span to avoid malignant tumors at the expense of cellular dysfunctions associated with the aged phenotype. An important recent discovery has been the observation that about 85% tumors are positive for telomerase activity. This article describes (1) the structure and function of telomeres and telomerase and (2) their role in the development of cancer.

II. TELOMERES

Telomeres are a substructure of all eukaryotic chromosomes that is essential for their stability. The most essential function of telomeres is to prevent chromosomes from fusing with one another. They are involved in nuclear architecture, in chromosome localization, and in repression of the expression of adjacent genes.

A. Telomere Structure

Human telomeres consist of thousands of base pairs of TTAGGG repeats and an unknown number of proteins. The telomeres of human somatic cells range greatly in length, depending on the type of tissue and the person's age. The TTAGGG repeat array of most human telomeres ranges in size from 5 to 15 kb. However, some human telomeres seem to contain 20–30 kb of TTAGGG repeats. TTAGGG repeats are oriented such that the G+T-rich strand extends toward the 3' ends of each chromosome and are of variable length. Several causes could lead to such variation: (1) Physical maps of subtelomeric DNA are variable; (2) the telomeric array at each chromosome end is heterogeneous; and (3) all human chromosome ends lose telomeric repeats during development and cellular proliferation. Two methods are used to determine the size of telomeres. The first method measures what is called the terminal restriction fragment length and involves digestion of DNA with frequently cutting restriction enzymes, e.g., *Rsa*I and *Hin*fI, and analyzing the digested DNA on agarose gels. The length of the resulting telomeric fragments is measured in genomic blots after hybridization with TTAGGG as a probe (Fig. 1). This procedure cannot determine the telomere length of an individual chromosome and may be affected by subtelomeric sequences resistant to digestion. To overcome this problem, quantitative *in situ* hybridization coupled with enhanced chromatin spreading methods have helped to reveal the actual length of telomeric repeat arrays at individual chromosome ends.

Biochemical studies have revealed that termini of human telomeres carry single-stranded TTAGGG repeats, called G-strand overhangs, that appear to be present in all cells irrespective of the presence of

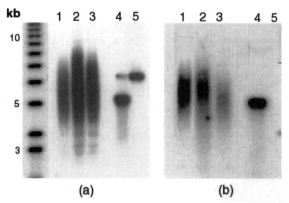

FIGURE 1 Measurement of telomere length and detection of single strand extension of the G-rich strand by Southern hybridization shown for three isogenic cell types [14-3-3σ$^{+/+}$, 14-3-3σ$^{+/-}$, and 14-3-3σ$^{-/-}$ colorectal cells (HCT116)]. Lane 1, DNA from 14-3-3σ$^{+/-}$; lane 2, DNA from 14-3-3σ$^{+/+}$; lane 3, DNA from 14-3-3σ$^{-/-}$; lane 4, denatured plasmid DNA (ssDNA) containing telomeric repeats (positive control); and lane 5, ds plasmid as a negative control (only lights up once the DNA is denatured, as seen only in a. M, molecular weight markers. (a) Genomic blotting analysis of telomeric length was determined using a denatured gel. Genomic DNA was digested with restriction enzymes *Hin*fI and *Rsa*I and hybridized with telomere repeat probes. Note that no difference in mean telomere length was found among the three different cell types. (b) A nondenaturing hybridization to genomic DNA digested with restriction enzymes *Hin*fI and *Rsa*I. This method allows visualization of G-strand overhangs of telomeres. Note the difference in the signal intensity in the nondenatured gel between 14-3-3σ$^{+/+}$ and 14-3-3σ$^{-/-}$ cells.

telomerase (Fig. 1). The average size of G-rich overhangs is 130–210 bases in length. The disruption of a G-strand overhang disrupts telomere function. Therefore, this overhang is important for telomere stability.

The conformation of telomeric DNA may be different from that of B-DNA because telomeric DNA is rich in G bases. Structural studies of G-rich oligonucleotides have shown that such molecules can form four stranded structures called G quartets. Some models for telomere functions have been drawn showing a linear configuration of telomeres at their ends. However, electron microscope analysis of telomeres has revealed that the chromosome ends form a higher order structure called the "T" loop (the free 3' end of the G overhang is tucked back inside the double-stranded DNA, forming a "T" loop). Cells where the chromosomes were known to have long telomeres contained larger "T" loops than those that had short telomeres. T loops may protect telomeres by physically stitching the potentially vulnerable single-stranded G-strand

terminus back into the double-stranded telomere sequence, several kilobases internal to the terminus.

B. Telomere Function

Fluorescent *in situ* hybridization studies have demonstrated that telomeres contain TTAGGG repeat sequences (Fig. 2) and that such sequences are required for telomere function. The minimal length of TTAGGG repeat arrays required for proper function of human telomeres is not yet known. Human cells use shortening of telomeres with each cell division to count the number of cell divisions they have undergone, and stop dividing after about 80 doublings. In humans, a critical shortening of telomeres has been related to cellular senescence and oncogenesis. Telomeres in somatic human cells shorten by 50–200 bp per cell division. Once average telomere length reaches 5–7 kb, cells enter an irreversible state of arrested growth. Programmed telomere shortening in normal human cells is considered a tumor suppressor mechanism that limits the growth potential of premalignant cells. Several different mechanisms have been proposed for how telomere shortening may lead to senescence. Telomeres that are too short to mask their ends from the DNA damage-sensing machinery may signal a checkpoint arrest. This results in activation of the p53-dependent damage checkpoint, which induces growth arrest of the cells. Alternatively, silent senescence genes could become activated by the removal of heterochromatic regions. Although the effects of telomere position on gene expression are a well-established phenomenon in yeast. It has been recently demonstrated in human cells.

Unlike double strand breaks, telomeric DNA does not activate DNA damage checkpoint proteins, such as ATM and its downstream effectors. Telomeres also do not serve as substrates for repair enzymes because of their compaction in a special structure. Because the maintenance of telomeres is essential for long-term cell proliferation, regulation of their length has been a key focus of research on tumorigenesis.

The length of a telomere is only one determinant of whether it is sufficiently long to function as a cap, stabilizing the chromosome end. Several lines of evidence converge on the notion that for telomere length regulation and other telomere functions, the very few

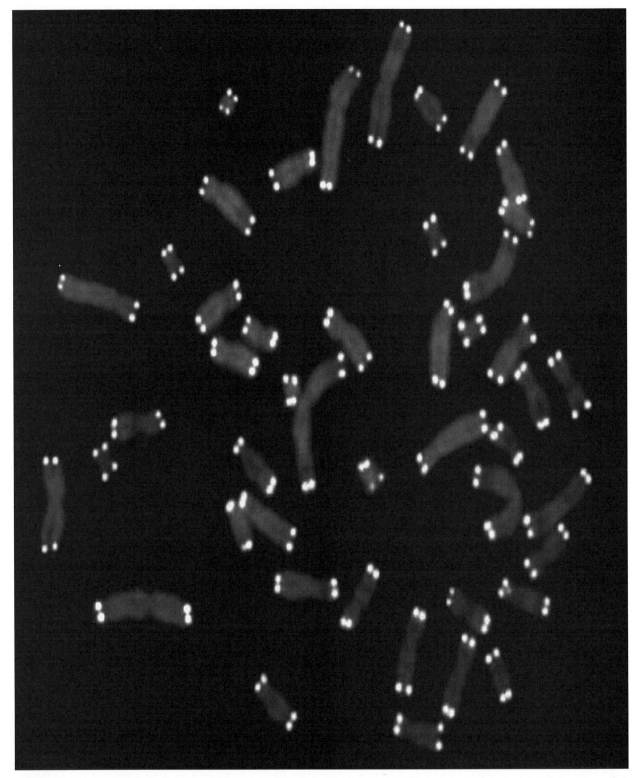

FIGURE 2   Human metaphase showing telomeres as detected by fluorescent *in situ* hybridization using a telomeric probe. Telomeres are at the end of each chromosome and look like red colored caps. See color insert in Volume 1.

last repeats at the tip of the telomeres are the most crucial.

C. Telomere Fusions

Telomeres shorten as a function of age in cells derived from normal human blood, skin, and colonic mucosa. As mentioned earlier, this shortening of telomeres results in a loss of telomere function. Such a loss could result in telomeric fusions, which could either involve single chromatids or double chromatids and can occur between sister chromatids or between chromatids of different chromosomes. Telomere fusions are seen at metaphase, and with the use of premature chromosome condensation technology, they have been observed in the G1 and G2 phase of the cell cycle. Occasionally, telomeric associations could lead to a bridge formation at anaphase and thus to genomic instability, gene amplification, and tumorigenesis. Tumor karyotypes display many changes, such as loss of heterozygosity, chromosome rearrangements, and gene amplification. The nature of most of the other abnormalities seen, such as deleted chromosomes and chromosomes with additional unidentifiable material, is consistent with their being formed as a result of breakage of the dicentric fused chromosomes at telophase. Increased telomeric associations, seen at metaphase, have been reported in cells derived from tumor tissues, senescent cells, the Thiberge Weissenbach syndrome, ataxia telangiectasia individuals, and following viral infections. The rate of telomeric association varies from cell line to cell line and from passage to passage, but there is no particular pattern to the variations. It is still unclear what the major factors are that influence chromosome end-to-end associations.

D. Telomere Proteins

Mammalian telomeres are hidden from the cellular DNA repair machinery that would normally treat the ends of a linear DNA molecule as a broken strand that needs to be repaired. Growing evidence suggests that both the shielding of telomeric ends and their elongation by telomerase are dependent on telomere-binding proteins. Mammalian telomeres are packaged in telomere-specific chromatin. Human cell lines have their telomeric tracts attached to the nuclear matrix, which is a proteinaceous subnuclear fraction. Telomere proteins comprise a class of structural proteins that bind sequence specifically to telomeric DNA. Several human telomere-binding proteins have been identified, such as TRF1 or PIN2, TRF2, TIN2, Tankyrase, and Ku70/80. Some of these bind to TTAGGG repeats *in vitro* irrespective of the presence of a DNA terminus, properties that are consistent with their presence along the ends of chromosomes. Telomere-binding proteins (TRF) are ubiquitously expressed. Some have an N-terminal acidic domain, a TRF-specific DNA-binding motif, and a C-terminal Myb type domain. For instance, TRF1 has been implicated in the regulation of telomere length. This protein is a negative regulator of telomere length maintenance because the inhibition of TRF1 results in telomere elongation (long telomeres) and overexpression results in a gradual shortening of telomeres. Another regulator of telomere length in human cells is TIN2. This protein shares no homology with known genes, interacts with TRF1 *in vitro*, and colocalizes with TRF1 in nuclei and metaphase chromosomes. Mutations in *TIN2* also lead to the elongation of human telomeres. TRF2 interacts with hRap1 and Mre11/Rad50/Nbs1/DNA repair complex. TRF2 has been shown to protect the chromosomes from end-to-end fusions. Furthermore, TRF2 is involved in the formation or stabilization of T loops.

Studies have shown that genes involved in DNA damage sensing and repair could influence the function of telomere repeat binding factors. One such gene is *ATM* (ataxia telangiectasia mutated), which mediates the disease ataxia telangiectasia (A-T). ATM is a protein kinase involved in the control of cell cycle progression, processing of DNA damage, and maintenance of genomic stability. Because of the homology of *ATM* to *TEL1* mutants of yeast (such mutants have defective telomere maintenance), it has been suggested that mutations in *ATM* could lead to defective telomere maintenance. Cells derived from A-T patients show a prominent defect at chromosome ends in the form of telomeric associations, seen at G1, G2, and metaphase. Inactivation of the *ATM* gene product influences the frequency of chromosome end-to-end associations and telomere length. This could be because the ATM protein influences interactions between telomeres and the nuclear matrix, and the alterations in the telomere nuclear matrix interactions could influence telomere maintenance. Patients with A-T are prone to develop cancer, and the *ATM* gene influences telomere metabolism. Therefore, genes involved in the signaling pathway associated with ATM may have a role in maintaining telomeres.

Other proteins known to influence telomere stability are poly(ADP-ribose) polymerase (PARP), c-Abl, 14-3-3σ, ku, hnRNP, etc. Mice with inactivated PARP have short telomeres as compared to wild-type controls. Similarly, chromosomes of a mouse cell line with inactivated hnRNP A1 also display short telomeres. Cells with mutations in *c-Abl* have been found to have large telomeres. Inactivation of 14-3-3σ fails to promote G2 arrest following DNA damage, which correlates with a loss of telomeres in a telomerase-independent manner. Curiously, this protein is not expressed in many primary breast tumors cells.

III. TELOMERES IN TUMOR CELLS

A marked reduction in telomere size is seen in somatic cells as compared to germ cells from the same individual. Like telomeres in normal somatic cells, telomeres of tumor precursor cells appear to undergo progressive telomere shortening. Short telomeres have been reported in several tumor cells, but there are some tumors with very long telomeres. Because telomeres in tumor cells are shorter than the cells of adjacent normal tissue, in some instances, telomere shortening appears to occur in the early stages of tumorigenesis. The shortening of telomeres in tumors has been reported for Wilms' tumor, breast, colon, and several other human tumor types. Telomere length differs widely between various types of human cancer cells, although, in general, cancer cells have more stable telomeres than normal somatic cells, presumably because telomerase adds back telomeric nucleotides that are lost during each cell division. Most of these tumors have lost 3–5 kb of TTAGGG repeats. Telomeric reduction may act as an oncogenic event. However, some tumors, e.g., renal carcinoma, appear to have lost minimal amounts of telomeric DNA. Many primary and metastatic human tumors appear to have short telomeres, and the average length of TTAGGG repeats in some tumor cells is about 3 kb per chromosome.

IV. TELOMERASE

Eukaryotic DNA polymerases are unable to synthesize in the 3′-5′ direction or start chains *de novo*, leading to the problem that extreme terminal sequences will not be replicated. This could lead to loss of the 5′ end of one daughter DNA strand. To counter this problem, a special type of DNA polymerase related to reverse transcriptase and called telomerase is found in eukaryotes. Telomerase is capable of extending the 3′ end of the G-rich strand of the telomeric repeats and continue lagging C-rich strand synthesis to complete the replication of chromosomal ends, thus compensating for the shortening that otherwise occurs. In immortalized and germline cells, telomeres can be maintained by telomerase. However, there are reports that telomeres in certain immortal cells might be maintained by alternative mechanisms that are independent of telomerase.

The telomerase enzyme is a ribonucleoprotein complex with two components required for core activity *in vitro*: telomerase RNA (TR) and a telomerase reverse transcriptase protein (TERT). In addition to the RNA and TERT components, the telomerase complex contains several other proteins. In humans, the foldsome proteins hsp 90 and p23 and three telomerase RNA-binding proteins, dysterin, L22, and hStau, are each associated with telomerase activity in cell extract. The enzyme has been partially characterized and was shown *in vitro* to be able to polymerize TTAGGG sequences. Telomerase recognizes the G-rich strand of an existing telomere repeat sequence and, in the absence of a complementary DNA strand, synthesizes a new copy of the repeat using its internal RNA as a template. Using a standard biochemical method, the detection of telomerase activity was first demonstrated in crude HeLa cell extracts. A sensitive and simple technique, termed telomeric repeat amplification protocol (TRAP), is used for the detection of telomerase activity. With the TRAP or a TRAP-ELISA assay, telomerase activity has been detected in ~85% of human cancers, but not in most somatic cells, with a few exceptions that include proliferative stem cells. The difference in telomerase activity between normal and cancer cells therefore makes telomerase a useful marker for cancer detection.

Cells with telomerase activity have positive nuclear signals for hTERT protein, whereas cells without telomerase do not. In most normal epithelial tissues, hTERT expression is limited to stem cells and their immediate descendants. The immunolocalization of hTERT in specimens of adult cancers reveal that the level of telomerase activity mainly depends on the number of tumor cells in a specimen. In cancers with high telomerase activity, hTERT is detected by immunostaining in almost all cells, whereas cancers with low telomerase activity have fewer hTERT-positive cells. The signal intensity per nucleus of hTERT-positive cells does not differ substantially between tumors with various levels of telomerase activity, suggesting that the relative telomerase activity of tissue specimens from cancer patients may be a surrogate indicator of overall tumor burden.

A. Telomerase Activation

Normal human somatic cells have a finite life span *in vitro* and retire into senescence after a predictable number of divisions. Cellular senescence is triggered by the activation of two interdependent mechanisms. One induces irreversible cell cycle exit involving the activation of two tumor suppressor genes, p53 and pRb, and the proper time point is indicated by a critical shortening of chromosomal ends due to the end-replication problem of DNA synthesis. A second occurs when telomeres are so short that massive end-fusion events prevent further replication. Development of a malignant cancer cell is only possible when both mechanisms are circumvented. In addition, the majority of human cancers and tumor cell lines contain active telomerase. While the hTR subunit of telomerase is present in almost all human cells, this is not the case for a human telomerase reverse transcriptase protein. Thus, telomerase activity has been shown to correlate more closely with the expression status of the telomerase catalytic subunit gene *hTERT*. Ectopic expression of hTERT in telomerase-negative cells results in reconstitution of telomerase activity, elongation of telomeres, and extension of cellular life span.

Telomerase is activated by different pathways, which are under intense investigation. It is also worth mentioning that telomerase activity may be a better indicator of tumorigenicity than simply telomere length, as the latter does not often correlate with tumor stage. Evidence shows that the regulation of telomerase is multifactorial, involving telomerase gene expression, posttranslational protein–protein interactions, and protein phosphorylation. The human pappillomavirus (HPV) oncogene and c-MYC can directly upregulate telomerase in some cell types. Two viral genes, E6 and E7, which are involved in the etiology of human cervical cancer, immortalize primary cells in culture. These cells also gain telomerase activity. E6 was the first gene shown to induce telomerase activity directly in preimmortal cells. However, the expression of E7 did not activate telomerase activity. Expression of the MYC oncogene in primary human epithelial cells that lack telomerase activity leads to telomerase activation. Levels of MYC are known to correlate with cell proliferation and thus possibly the continous MYC expression is necessary for telomerase activation. MYC is a downstream target of the SRC, YES, and FYN kinase pathways. Because MYC is upregulated during early T-cell activation, this suggests that telomerase activation could occur through the SRC kinase to MYC to hTERT promoter. However, there could be alternative pathways, as some cells deficient in MYC have also been found to be positive for telomerase activity.

While many aspects of the regulation of telomerase activity are not yet clear, it is thought to be executed primarily through the transcriptional control of hTERT. Studies have shown that the catalytic subunit of telomerase associates directly with the c-Abl protein tyrosine kinase. c-Abl phosphorylates hTERT and inhibits its activity. The functional significance of the c-Abl-hTERT interaction is supported further by the demonstration that cells deficient in c-Abl function exhibit telomere lengthening.

Interestingly, telomerase activity has been detected in most human cancer cells but not in most normal cells from the same patients. Some of the cancer cells have short but stable telomeres. These observations suggest that progression of the malignant state depends on continued telomerase activity and that telomerase could be a target for new therapeutic approaches to cancer treatment. Telomerase activation preceded oncogenic transformation in some human cell types, yet was lacking in other transformed cells.

B. Telomerase Activity as a Measure for Monitoring Curability of Tumor Cells

As mentioned earlier, telomerase activity is frequently associated with the malignant phenotype and could be a useful monitor of chemo- or radiotherapeutic efficacy and an early predictor of outcome. Several lines of evidence support a link among cellular differentiation, cell killing, and telomerase activity. Because radiotherapy plays a key role in the treatment of many tumors, telomerase activity could be determined after (or during) radiotherapy. Studies found a dose-dependent decrease in telomerase activity that was proportional to cell killing and tumor regression after ionizing radiation treatment.

V. CONCLUSION AND PERSPECTIVES

Telomere biology is important in human cancer. Tumor cells need a mechanism to maintain telomeres if they are going to divide indefinitely, and telomerase solves this problem. Therefore, telomerase represents a promising anticancer drug target. It is unclear at present what is the optimum means of targeting this complex ribonucleoprotein and its associated telomeric DNA and binding proteins: various strategies are actively being explored. At least some of the molecular components that form the catalytic core of this ribonucleoprotein enzyme have been identified in humans. The stage is now set for chemists to develop telomerase inhibitors, which hold promise as cancer chemotherapeutic agents. Some data (e.g., 2-5A antisense against telomeric RNA, targeting TRF2, introduction of dominant-negative hTERT into cells) have raised doubts about the previous presumption of a requirement for prolonged enzyme inhibition with gradual telomere erosion, especially in tumor cells with relatively short telomeres. Highly potent and selective *in vivo* inhibitors are required to validate the target and address these critical issues. Peptide nucleic acids (PNAs) that inhibit telomerase have

demonstrated that unexpected regions of the enzyme can serve as targets for inhibitors. Alternatively, cationic porphyrins, capable of interacting with guanine quadruplex (G4) telomeric folds, inhibit telomerase activity in human tumor cells. The antisense approaches directed at hTERT also show promise for telomerase inhibition. Finally, would inhibition of the enzyme in the classical sense, which requires a lag phase before any detrimental effects on cells, be a reasonable strategy in patients with a large tumor burden? Probably in such situations use of telomerase inhibitors would be used as an adjuvant treatment in combination with radiation treatment, surgery, and chemotherapy. It is possible that telomerase inhibitors could be used following standard therapies in which there is no clinical evidence of disease to treat possible micrometastases and thus prevent cancer relapse. The question will arise what will be the effects of telomerase inhibition on normal hematopoietic and germ cells? Such a question will be answered when drugs are moved into clinical trials.

See Also the Following Articles

Ataxia Telangiectasia Syndrome • c-myc Protooncogene • Lung Cancer: Molecular and Cellular Abnormalities • Ovarian Cancer: Molecular and Cell Abnormalities • Ribozymes and Their Applications • Senescence, Cellular

Bibliography

Bacchetti, S., and Wynford-Thomas D. (1997). Telomeres and telomerase in cancer: Special issue. *Eur. J. Cancer* **33,** 703.

Blackburn, E. H., and Greider, C. W. (1995). "Telomeres." Cold Spring Harbor Laboratory Press, Cold Spring Harbor, NY.

Greider, C. W. (1999). Telomerase activation one step on the road to cancer. *Trends Genet.* **15,** 109.

Griffith, J. D., Comeau, L., Rosenfield, S., Stansel, R. M., Bianchi, A., Moss, H., and de Lange, T. (1999). Mammalian telomeres end in a large duplex loop. *Cell* **97,** 503.

McClintock, B. (1941). The stability of broken ends of chromosomes of *Zea mays. Genetics* **26,** 234.

McElligott, R., and Wellinger, R. J. (1997). The terminal DNA structure of mammalian chromosomes. *EMBO J.* **16,** 3704.

Muller, H. J. (1938). The making of chromosomes. *Collect. Net* **8,** 182.

Nugent, C. I., and Lundbald, V. (1998), The telomerase reverse transcriptase: Components and regulation. *Genes Dev.* **12,** 1073.

Sawant, S. G., Gregoire, V., Dhar, S., Umbricht, C. B., Cvilic, S., Sukumar, S., and Pandita, T. K. (1999). Telomerase activity as a measure for monitoring radiocurability of tumor cells. *FASEB J.* **13,** 1047.

Shay, J. W. (1999). At the end of the millennium, a view of the end. *Nature Genet.* **23,** 382.

Shay, J. W, and Wright, W. E. (1999). Mutant dyskerin ends relationship with telomerase. *Science* **286,** 2284.

Smilenov, L. B., Dhar, S., and Pandita, T. K. (1999). Altered telomere nuclear matrix interactions and nucleosomal peri-odicity in ataxia telangiectasia cells before and after ionizing radiation treatment. *Mol. Cell. Biol.* **19,** 6963.

Vaziri, H., and Benchimol, S. (1998). Reconstitution of telomerase activity in normal human cells leads to elongation of telomeres and extended replicative life span. *Curr. Bio.* **8,** 279.

Wright, W. E., and Shay J. W. (1992), Telomere positional effects and the regulation of cellular senescence. *Trends Genet.* **8,** 193.

Zakian, V. A. (1997). Life and cancer without telomerase. *Cell* **91,** 1.

Testicular Cancer

Robert Amato

Baylor College of Medicine, Houston, Texas

I. Epidemiology and Etiology
II. Pathology and Natural History
III. Diagnosis
IV. Staging and Treatment
V. Conclusions

GLOSSARY

seminoma The most common germ cell tumor, accounting for approximately 45% of testicular cancers and believed to arise from primordial germ cells that have distinct clinical and pathologic features.

teratoma A common component of mixed germ cell tumors but in its pure form only represents 2 to 3% of all testicular malignancies.

Most testicular tumors are malignant and of germ cell origin. They constitute only 1% of cancers in males overall but are the most common malignant neoplasm in men aged 15 to 35 years. Testicular cancers frequently present at an early stage, are very sensitive to chemotherapy, and are variably sensitive to

radiotherapy. These tumors are highly curable, and the success in treating testicular cancer has turned the focus of many studies to reducing toxicity in selected good prognosis patients and identifying poor prognosis patients who require more aggressive treatment. This article reviews the epidemiology, etiology, pathology, diagnosis, and treatment of testicular cancers.

I. EPIDEMIOLOGY AND ETIOLOGY

In 2001, an estimated 7000 new cases of testicular cancer will be diagnosed in the United States, with an associated 350 deaths. This represents an incidence of 2.1 cases per 100,000 males. Testicular cancer is most common in white males, who have an incidence more than four times that of black males. The risk is highest in northern Europe. For example, in Denmark, the incidence is reported to be 6.3 per 100,000 males.

Several conditions have been associated with testis cancer. Abnormal testicular development and descent are strongly associated with cancer; males with cryptorchidism are 10 to 40 times more likely than males with normal testes to develop testicular carcinoma. The risk appears to be greater if the testis is retained in the abdomen rather than in the inguinal canal. Surgical placement of the undescended testis into the scrotum before the age of 6 years reduces the risk, but not to a normal level. The higher temperature the undescended testis is exposed to in cryptorchidism was held to play a role in the development of testicular cancer, but epidemiologic studies have not supported this hypothesis. In patients with unilateral cryptorchidism, 25% of testis cancers occur in the normally descended testis.

Testicular feminization syndromes have been shown to increase the risk of cancer in the gonads by 40 times, and these tumors are often bilateral. Herniorrhaphy before age 15 years, exposure to diethylstilbestrol early in gestational life, disorders of sexual differentiation, and infertility constitute other risk factors. In addition, trauma, torsion of the testis, testicular atrophy from mumps, orchitis, radiation, and exposure to dimethylformamide during leather tanning are possible risk factors.

II. PATHOLOGY AND NATURAL HISTORY

Testicular cancer is a general term for several distinct but related neoplasms. The most commonly used classification in the United States is a modified version of the system described by Dixon and Moore in 1952 (Table 1). Germ cell neoplasms account for nearly 93% of all primary testicular malignancies. Testicular lymphomas represent about 4 to 5% of testicular cancers, and sex cord stromal tumors make up nearly 3%. A few other rare tumors are occasionally seen.

A. Carcinoma *in Situ* (CIS)

Carcinoma *in situ* was originally perceived as a curiosity. Alhough not malignant, it is now recognized as an important precursor to testicular cancer. In one study, the incidence of progression to invasive cancer was estimated to be 70% at 7 years. In this study, no cases of regression were noted. In 75 to 99% of tes-

TABLE I
Pathologic Classification of
Testicular Malignancies

Germinal neoplasms
1. Carcinoma *in situ*
2. Seminoma
    a. Classic
    b. Spermatic
3. Embryonal carcinoma
4. Yolk sac tumor (endodermal sinus tumor)
5. Choriocarcinoma
6. Teratoma
    a. Mature
    b. Immature
    c. With malignant transformation
7. Mixed
Nongerminal neoplasms
1. Sex cord stromal tumor
    a. Leydig cell tumor
    b. Sertoli cell tumor
    c. Granulosa thecal cell tumor
2. Gonadoblastoma
3. Lymphomas and leukemias
4. Rhabdomyosarcoma
5. Other rare tumors and tumorous conditions
    a. Carcinoid
    b. Adenocarcinoma of the rete testis
    c. Epidermoid cyst
    d. Malacoplakia
Metastatic neoplasms

ticular cancers, CIS is found adjacent to the tumor. It is unclear whether all germ cell tumors go through this stage, but it must be regarded as a preinvasive lesion and not ignored.

B. Seminoma

Pure seminoma is the most common germ cell tumor and accounts for approximately 45% of testicular cancers. The distinction between seminoma and nonseminoma is important because the natural histories of these tumor types and their responses to treatment modalities differ, and hence so do appropriate treatment strategies.

Seminomas are believed to arise from primordial germ cells and have distinct clinical and pathologic features. The metastatic potential is low, and most patients present with early stage disease. Overall, 75% present with stage I disease, 20% with stage II disease, and 5% with stage III or IV disease. Seminoma is generally divided into two types: classic seminoma, which accounts for about 90% of cases, and spermatic seminoma, which accounts for the rest.

Classic seminoma typically presents in the fourth or fifth decade as an enlarging, painless testicular mass, and 2% of the time, bilateral disease is present. The pattern of spread is predominantly via the lymphatics to the paraaortic lymph nodes and then to the mediastinal and supraclavicular lymph nodes. Hematogenous dissemination to lung, liver, bone, and adrenals occurs, but is generally a late finding.

Low levels of β-human chorionic gonadotropin (β-hCG) are seen in 10 to 25% of pure seminomas, but this characteristic does not appear to influence prognosis. Seminomas do not secrete α-fetoprotein (AFP), and an elevated AFP level should alert the clinician to the presence of nonseminomatous elements.

Anaplastic seminoma used to be regarded as a separate category because it appears more aggressive under a microscope and tends to present at a later stage. However, when compared with classic seminoma on a stage-for-stage basis, the prognosis is no worse. For this reason, it is no longer regarded as a distinct entity and is included with the classic variant.

Spermatic seminoma accounts for about 10% of seminomas. It differs from classic seminoma in that it typically appears after the age of 60 years, is bilateral 10% of the time, and has an extremely indolent course. Metastases are rare, and the prognosis is excellent.

C. Nonseminomatous Germ Cell Tumors

Nonseminomatous germ cell tumors are a heterogeneous group of tumors that are grouped in the same category largely because they are frequently found together. It is difficult to generalize about their collective behavior, so each will be discussed separately, but it should be remembered that several or all of the histologic types discussed may be present in the same patient. Nonseminomatous tumors that contain elements of seminoma are also common, behave like nonseminomas, and should be treated as such.

1. Embryonal Carcinoma

Embryonal carcinoma is the second most common testicular malignancy and, in its pure form, accounts for 15 to 30% of nonseminomatous germ cell tumors. It occurs most commonly in the second decade of life and is rare after the fifth decade. It is not found in infants or children. One-third of patients present with metastases to the paraaortic lymph nodes, lungs, or liver. This tumor secretes both AFP and β-hCG. Placental alkaline phosphatase and cytokeratin are usually elevated, but the carcinoembryonic antigen (CEA) generally is not.

2. Yolk Sac Carcinoma (Endodermal Sinus Tumor)

Yolk sac carcinoma is the most common testicular neoplasm in children, accounting for 75% of testicular tumors in this population. It is associated with an excellent prognosis. It is rare in its pure form in adults but is frequently seen next to other germ cell elements. When it does appear as pure yolk sac carcinoma in adults, it is a virulent neoplasm. It typically spreads via the lymphatics, but has hematogenous dissemination. It has particular affinity for metastasis to the liver. AFP levels are generally elevated, whereas β-hCG levels are not.

3. Choriocarcinoma

Choriocarcinoma is extremely rare in its pure form, accounting for fewer than 1% of all testicular tumors, but is commonly found as a component of other testis tumors. This is the most aggressive variant in adults, with early hematogenous and lymphatic spread. The poor prognosis of these patients is probably related to the typically larger volume of disease at presentation rather than an intrinsic resistance to treatment. This tumor secretes high levels of β-hCG but normal levels of AFP.

4. Teratoma

Teratoma is a common component of mixed germ cell tumors but in its pure form only represents 2 to 3% of all testicular malignancies. It has been referred to as benign in the past because, technically, no malignant tissue exists in these terminally differentiated tumors. Degeneration to a malignant form, however, is observed, and patients have died of associated metastases. Younger patients tend to have more mature tumors and older patients more immature forms. These tumors do not respond to chemotherapy and can manifest as an enlarging mass during chemotherapy in a serologically responding tumor. Surgery is the only effective therapy. Teratomas can secrete both β-hCG and, more typically, AFP, although usually neither is elevated.

5. Mature Teratoma

All three germ cell elements (endoderm, mesoderm, and ectoderm) are presenting mature forms of teratoma, and elements such as skin, bone, teeth, and hair can sometimes be seen.

6. Immature Teratoma

Immature tumors contain tissues that cannot be recognized as normal elements. The immaturity of the teratoma has not been shown to be an indicator of biologic aggressiveness. This behavior appears to be more related to the age of the patient, with aggressive disease more common in older patients

7. Teratoma with Malignant Transformation

A variant of teratoma containing malignant nongerm cell elements, presumably derived from somatic tissue within the teratoma, has been described. The presence of malignant nongerm cell elements at diagnosis or after induction chemotherapy implies a poor prognosis. Teratomas have been demonstrated to degenerate into a variety of poor prognosis malignancies, including sarcomas, adenocarcinomas. and neuroepitheliomas. Acute myelogenous leukemia (AML) also occurs in patients with a history of teratomas. Patients with one of these tumors who have had a germ cell malignancy in the past should be evaluated for a duplication on the short arm of chromosome 12p, or i(12p).

This duplication is a good indicator that the tumor is of germcell origin. Limited success has been reported using platinum-based chemotherapy.

D. Sex Cord Stromal Tumors

1. Leydig (Interstitial) Cell Tumors

Leydig cell tumors account for 1 to 3% of all testicular neoplasms. They can appear at any age, but the median age at which they develop is 60 years. Leydig cells secrete both androgens and estrogens, and the clinical symptoms are usually related to endocrine abnormalities. Testicular swelling, gynecomastia, and decreased libido are common in patients with these tumors. Only 7 to 10% metastasize.

2. Sertoli Cell Tumors

Fewer than 1% of testicular neoplasms are Sertoli cell tumors. They can occur at any age, but 30% appear in the first decade of life. Patients generally present with a scrotal mass and sometimes have gynecomastia. Only about 10% of these tumors are malignant and, as with Leydig cell tumors, the primary treatment is surgical.

3. Granulosa Cell Tumor

Granulosa cell tumors have two distinct types: juvenile and adult. The juvenile variety is the most frequently seen nongerm cell testicular tumor in infants, and no malignant behavior has been reported in this type. The adult form is the least common of the sex cord stromal tumors.

4. Gonadoblastomas

Gonadoblastoma is a mixed germ cell and sex cord tumor that generally occurs in dysgenetic gonads or undescended testes during the teenage years. It is bilateral about 30% of the time. These tumors are clinically benign, but pathologic analysis reveals that they are accompanied by foci of malignant germ cell tumors in 10 to 50% of cases. The prognosis varies and appears to depend on the other germ cell components present and their extent of invasion. For patients with pure gonadoblastoma, the outcome is excellent.

E. Lymphomas and Leukemias

Primary malignant lymphomas of the testis are uncommon, accounting for only 5% of all testicular neoplasms. Lymphoma involves the testis more commonly as a late manifestation of disseminated disease. This occurs in about 20% of all cases of lymphoma. It is important to note that the frequency of primary testicular lymphoma increases with age, and in patients over 60 years old it is the most common malignant tumor of the testis.

Leukemic infiltration of the testis usually occurs when the disease is disseminated; it can be detected in autopsy in up to 5% of patients with acute leukemia and 30% of patients with chronic leukemia. Testicular involvement is especially common among children with acute lymphoblastic leukemia who have had relapses after therapy.

F. Rhabdomyosarcomas

Rhabdomyosarcoma is the most common sarcoma in children and can originate in the testis. Ninety-five percent of these patients present with a scrotal mass. The testicular parenchyma is rarely involved, but the tumor is common in the spermatic cord and paratesticular tissue. After surgery, local recurrences are frequent, and the pelvic lymph nodes are a common site of metastases.

G. Metastatic Neoplasms

Testicular metastases occur in 2.5% of men with malignant tumors. The most common primary sites are the prostate, lung, skin (melanoma), colon, and kidney.

H. Extragonadal Germ Cell Tumors

Extragonadal germ cell tumors account for about 2 to 4% of all germ cell tumors. They can be seminomas or nonseminomas and generally occur in midline structures in the retroperitoneum, mediastinum, or pineal gland. Historically, it was felt that extragonadal nonseminomas had a worse prognosis than tumors arising in the testis. This is certainly true for those arising in the mediastinum. However, data indicate that nonseminomas arising in the retroperitoneum behave similarly to comparably sized stage II nonseminomas in the testis.

Extragonadal seminomas, regardless of their origin, do no worse than testicular seminomas of similar stage. Many, if not most, germ cell tumors arising in the retroperitoneum originate in the testis, so patients with retroperitoneal tumors should all be evaluated for an occult testicular malignancy. At least 40% will have an occult testis tumor or carcinoma *in situ*. This is not the case for germ cell tumors arising in the mediastinum; testicular biopsies for individuals with such tumors are not indicated.

III. DIAGNOSIS

Testicular cancer is the most common malignancy in young males and frequently occurs during a crucial developmental period of their lives. For a variety of psychological, social, and educational reasons, the average delay in diagnosis after symptoms appear is 4 to 6 months. There are no early symptoms. About 65% of patients present with painless swelling or a nodule in one gonad. In another 20%, the testicular enlargement is painful because of bleeding or infarction in the tumor, and acute pain in a patient with a cryptorchid testis suggests torsion of a hidden mass. About 10% of patients present with symptoms from metastases, such as lumbar back pain, gastrointestinal disturbance, respiratory symptoms, or a neck mass. Gynecomastia is seen in about 5% of patients and occasionally infertility is the initial complaint. Exophthalmos and skin metastases can be the first manifestations of choriocarcinoma.

The physical examination should include bimanual examination of the testes. The normal testis has an even consistency, is freely movable, and is separable from the epididymis. Any nodule or firm fixed area or mass is suggestive of disease, and testicular cancer must be considered until this possibility is disproved.

Differential diagnosis includes testicular torsion, epididymitis, epididymal orchitis, hydrocele, hernia, hematoma, or spermatocele. High-resolution ultrasonography is a rapid, reliable tool for excluding the possibility of hydrocele or epididymitis when a tumor is suspected. It can also demonstrate whether the mass is intratesticular or extratesticular. If it is extratesticular and does not involve the tunica albuginea, then conservative treatment can be elected. A suspected testicular tumor should be surgically explored and biopsied through an inguinal incision. Careful histologic examination will establish the diagnosis. Transscrotal biopsy is contraindicated because it alters the lymphatic drainage and, if a malignancy is found, a more extensive surgical procedure is required to remove the primary tumor. After the diagnosis is made, clinical tests to stage the patient are performed. These include a computed tomography (CT) scan of the abdomen and pelvis, chest X-ray and β-hCG, AFP, lactate dehydrogenase (LDH), and sometimes placental alkaline phosphatase. If clinically indicated, a magnetic resonance imaging (MRI) or CT scan of the brain and a bone scan may be done.

The diagnosis and staging evaluations for extragonadal germ cell tumors are similar to those for testicular tumors. Those with a retroperitoneal presentation should be explored for an occult testicular primary, which is frequently present. Again, with a mediastinal tumor this is not indicated.

A. Tumor Markers and Cytogenetic Abnormalities

Our ability to accurately diagnose, stage tumors, monitor response to treatment, and assess patients for early relapse has been greatly facilitated with the identification of tumor markers. These markers can be divided into three categories: (1) serum proteins, such as β-hCG, AFP, placental alkaline phosphatase, and LDH; (2) cytogenetic or chromosomal markers, such as i(12p); and (3) molecular markers, including oncogenes and tumor suppressor genes. Serum protein markers are the best studied and the most clinically relevant to date.

β-hCG, first detected in 1930 in the urine of patients with advanced choriocarcinoma, was the first tumor marker associated with testis cancer. Subsequent refinements in our ability to measure β-hCG have taken us from detecting it only occasionally in advanced disease to precisely measuring it in patients who have no observable tumor. The β-hCG protein is composed of two subunits, α and β, and modern assays measure only the β portion. β-hCG is elevated in 40 to 50% of patients with testis cancer, including all patients with choriocarcinoma, approximately 80% of patients with embryonal carcinoma, and 10 to 25% of patients with pure seminoma. The degree of elevation has some correlation with the volume of disease, and recurrent elevation is an excellent marker of early relapse. β-hCG has a half-life of 24 to 36 h, and, after surgery, levels should fall in accordance with this half-life. If they do not, residual disease is likely present.

When using β-hCG to monitor the response to chemotherapy, a 90% decrease every 21 days should be seen. Less steep declines are associated with the emergence of drug resistance and a poorer outcome. It is important to note that some β-hCG assays cross-react with luteinizing hormone (LH). When the treatment has resulted in testicular atrophy, the LH can be substantially elevated. If a falsely elevated β-hCG level is suspected, a single 200-mg injection of testosterone cypionate can be given and the β-hCG level rechecked after 2 weeks. β-hCG can also be increased in patients who use tobacco or marijuana, and this possibility should be looked into if a minor elevation persists.

α-Fetoprotein was detected in adult germ cell tumors in 1974. It is an abundant serum-binding protein in the fetus, but only minimal amounts of AFP are normally detectable in individuals more than 1 year old. Fifty to 70% of patients with testis cancer have elevations of AFP, which are most often seen in patients who have elements of embryonal or yolk sac carcinomal and occasionally seen in patients with teratoma, but not seen in patients with pure choriocarcinoma or pure seminoma. Seminoma with an elevated AFP behaves like nonseminoma and should be treated as such.

High levels of AFP correlate with bulky disease and, after treatment, rising levels are a good marker for early recurrence. Because of the long half-life (5–7 days) of AFP, its occasional production by teratomas, its frequent sequestration inside cysts, and the variety of benign liver conditions that can cause it to be elevated, caution should be used when monitoring its rate of decline to assess response to therapy.

1. LDH

Levels of LDH and, in particular, its isoenzyme, are elevated in approximately 80% of patients with advanced testis cancer. Although not as specific as β-hCG or AFP, LDH in some patients is the only elevated marker, so it can have clinical utility. High levels correlate with tumor burden, risk for relapse, and a poorer survival.

2. Placental Alkaline Phosphatase

Placental alkaline phosphatase is the fetal isoenzyme of adult alkaline phosphatase. It is detectable in 30 to 50% of patients with stage I seminoma and in nearly 100% of patients with advanced seminoma, but is less commonly elevated in nonseminomatous tumors. Clinical experience with this marker is more limited than with β-hCG, AFP, or LDH, but when it is elevated, it can be useful in following the course of seminoma. Smoking can cause false elevations of this marker; thus, in patients who smoke, placental alkaline phosphatase monitoring is less reliable.

3. Cytogenetics and Molecular Markers

Cytogenetic abnormalities in testicular tumors are beginning to be explored. Detailed karyotypic analysis has revealed nonrandom changes in chromosomes 1, 5, 6, 7, 9, 11, 12, 16, 17, 21, 22, and X. Of these, a duplication on the short arm of i(12p) is the best studied and the most characteristic. This marker was present in one or more copies in approximately 89% of seminomas and 81% of nonseminomas studied. Most of the remaining patients had other abnormalities involving the i(12p) chromosome. The i(12p) marker is also observed in extragonadal germ cell tumors and occasionally in ovarian dysgerminomas, but is rare in other tumors. It is a highly specific marker for germ cell tumors and a useful diagnostic tool in cancers of unknown origin.

How i(12p) participates in the development of testis cancer is unknown. The oncogene *c-ki-ras* 2 resides on the short arm of chromosome 12, but amplification of this gene as a transforming event has been difficult to show. Other oncogenes and their products have been investigated, but as yet their significance and roles in the pathogenesis of testis cancer remain to be demonstrated.

In summary, β-hCG, AFP, LDH, and placental alkaline phosphatase have been shown to be of value in diagnosis by identifying patients who have histologic types other that those reported, in staging by identifying patients with a high tumor volume that is not readily radiographically apparent, in monitoring response to treatment, and in detecting relapse early, when it is most curable. The presence of i(12p) is useful in identifying tumors of unknown origin. Molecular markers are at present still research tools but ultimately are expected to yield improved diagnostic and therapeutic strategies, as well as provide a much better understanding of these diseases.

IV. STAGING AND TREATMENT

A. Carcinoma *in Situ*

Carcinoma *in situ* is known to be a preinvasive lesion, and detecting and treating it early in patients at risk for testicular carcinoma could potentially prevent cancer development. The only reliable way to diagnose CIS is with a surgical biopsy after puberty.

The likelihood of eventually developing a testicular tumor where CIS is present is extremely high, so screening is useful in groups at high risk of developing CIS. Estimates of individuals with increased risk show that men with a unilateral testicular tumor have a 6% incidence of CIS in the other testis, and men with a history of cryptorchidism have a 2 to 3% incidence of CIS. In patients with extragonadal germ cell tumors of the retroperitoneum, the incidence is greater than 40%, and in intersex patients, as well as individuals with gonadal dysgenesis, a greater than 25% incidence has been reported.

Orchiectomy is the treatment of choice in patients in whom one testis is normal and the other contains CIS. In men who have had a previous unilateral orchiectomy and now have CIS in the remaining testis, 20 Gy of radiation given in 10 doses of 2 Gy is sufficient to eradicate the CIS and still maintain adequate endogenous testosterone. Fertility does not appear to be compromised by this degree of radiation, but men with a history of testicular cancer in one testis and CIS in the other frequently have impaired spermatogenesis prior to any therapy.

Screening is only recommended for patients with a history of unilateral testis cancer, extragonadal germ cell tumors of retroperitoneal origin, or gonadal dysgenesis and for intersex patients. In patients with a history of cryptorchidism, a testicular biopsy can be considered. Newer methods that involve examining the semen are being developed that may expand the designation of reasonable candidates for screening.

B. Seminoma

The treatment of seminoma is gratifying to the oncologist because the disease is quite curable. The expected overall survival is approximately 97%. This tumor is quite radiosensitive as well as very chemosensitive. Seminoma is relatively indolent and follows a predictable pattern of progression. It starts in the testis and spreads via the paraaortic lymph nodes to the mediastinal nodes and then the supraclavicular nodes. It rarely metastasizes to distant organs such as the lungs or bones without first being seen at nodal sites. Overall, 75% of patients present with stage I disease (confined to the testis), 20% with stage II disease, and fewer than 5% with stage III or IV disease.

The International Germ Cell Consensus Classification for seminoma has been developed (Table II). The initial considerations when planning treatment are to confirm that the tumor is truly a pure seminoma and to determine its stage. Careful review of the histologic and pathologic features is mandatory. The AFP level must be normal for the tumor to be considered a pure seminoma; β-hCG and LDH levels should also be tested. The initial staging evaluation should include a chest X ray, CT of the abdomen and pelvis, bone scan if symptoms indicate, and CT or MRI of the brain if neurologic symptoms are present.

1. Stage I Treatment

Treatment of stage I seminoma is somewhat controversial. The paraaortic lymph nodes are involved in approximately 15% of clinical stage I cases, and standard treatment has been orchiectomy plus radiotherapy to the paraaortic nodes as well as the ipsilateral common iliac and external iliac nodes. If there has been a previous inguinal surgery or if an advanced local primary has invaded the scrotal skin, there is an increased risk of pelvic node spread, and the radiotherapy field is extended to include the ipsilateral inguinofemoral node region.

The standard dose of radiation, 25 to 40 Gy, results in a disease-free survival of 98 to 99%. A dose of 40 Gy has not been shown to be more effective than 25 Gy so the lower dose should be used. Side effects of radiation include dyspepsia in 6% of patients and frank peptic ulceration in 3%. The effects on fertility are unclear, but most patients experience a decrease in sperm count that usually resolves in 3 years. The relative risk of developing a second cancer within the irradiated field seems to be increased, but this effect does not become evident until 15 years after treatment. Because salvage treatment in seminoma is so successful and most patients with stage I seminoma patients are cured with their initial surgery, close surveillance after orchiectomy is being reported as a viable option to radiation to reduce short- and long-term toxicity. The advantage of this approach is that it avoids radiation in the 85% of patients who are cured with orchiectomy. The disadvantage is that those who relapse will have an increased tumor volume and may be more difficult to cure.

Results in 583 patients treated with orchiectomy alone and followed by investigators from the Princess Margaret Hospital, the Royal Marsden Hospital, and the Danish National Study are encouraging. At 3 years, the rate of relapse was 15.5%, with a median time to relapse of 12 to 15 months. The relapses were treated with salvage radiation or chemotherapy. Only 2 of the original 583 patients (0.3%) died with disease, producing a 99.7% disease-free survival.

2. Stage II Treatment

The treatment strategy for stage II prognosis disease differs with the size of the involved abdominal lymph

TABLE II
International Germ Cell Consensus Classification for Seminoma[a]

Characteristic	Good prognosis	Intermediate prognosis	Poor prognosis
Primary site	Any	Any	No patients are poor prognosis
Metastatic sites	and no NPVM	and no NPVM	
STM	and no NPVM	and NPVM	
AFP	N1	N1	
HCG	Any	Any	
LDH	Any	Any	
Seminoma patients	90%	10%	
PFS at 5 years	82%	67%	
OS at 5 years	86%	72%	

[a]NPVM, nonpulmonary visceral metastases; STM, serum tumor markers; PFS, progression-free survival; OS, overall survival.

nodes. Historically, radiotherapy was used for all stage II patients and is still the treatment of choice for early stage II disease (abdominal masses less than 5 cm).

The usual dose is 36 Gy, which yields a disease-free survival of about 95%. Mason and Kearsley, in a review of the literature, found that the risk of relapse in stage II disease was directly related to tumor bulk. Abdominal masses between 5 and 10 cm had a risk of relapse of 8%, and for masses greater than 10 cm, the risk of relapse increased to 35%. Prophylactic irradiation to the mediastinum for abdominal masses smaller than 10 cm should be avoided because this strategy does not appear to improve survival but does cause an excess of cardiac, pulmonary, and marrow toxic effects.

There is no consensus on the optimal treatment for abdominal masses between 5 and 10 cm in diameter. The kidneys generally tolerate only 15 to 20 Gy of fractionated radiotherapy, and with tumors greater than 5 cm, there is frequently a significant amount of tumor overlying the kidneys. For this reason, some centers now recommend chemotherapy for all tumors greater then 5 cm. If, however, the tumor is less than 10 cm and the kidneys are not in the field of radiation, then radiotherapy is still a good choice. Stage II disease with an abdominal mass larger than 10 cm is treated with chemotherapy similar to that used for stage III disease.

3. Stage III Treatment

The development of effective chemotherapy for advanced seminoma has lagged behind that for nonseminoma, in part because advanced seminoma is so uncommon. In the era before platinum drugs, responses to chemotherapy were common but cures were not. Platinum-based therapy has dramatically improved our ability to cure advanced-stage seminoma.

In 1974, the activity of cisplatin (Platinol) in germ cell tumors was first reported, and this agent quickly became the backbone of testicular chemotherapy regimens. Improved results with the PVB [cisplatin, vinblastine, and bleomycin (Blenoxane)] regimen were first reported in 1981 and subsequently confirmed in a larger multicenter trial. The most common variations on this regimen are the BEP [bleomycin, etoposide (VePesid), and cisplatin] regimen, in which etoposide is substituted for vinblastine, and the VIP

[vinblastine, ifosfamide (Ifex), cisplatin] regimen in which ifosfamide is used in place of bleomycin. These have yielded comparable disease-free survivals, ranging from 75 to 85%.

The combination of cisplatin and etoposide has been shown to be at least as effective as other standard regimens with less toxicity, and it is now the standard in some institutions. The role of bleomycin in the treatmnent of seminoma is uncertain. The drug appears to add little benefit, and the high frequency of fatal pulmonary side effects among patients with pure seminoma suggests that this population may have a unique sensitivity to bleomycin.

A somewhat different approach employs the use of sequential weekly cisplatin and cyclophosphamide (Cytoxan). In one study, this combination resulted in a 92% long-term continuous disease-free survival. In another group of patients, cisplatin alone and carboplatin (Paraplatin) alone were less successful, but a high proportion of these patients did respond to cisplatin-based salvage regimens. In 1992, a cure rate of 97% was reported with the combination of carboplatin, ifosfamide, and selective consolidation with alternating noncross-resistant chemotherapy agents. Substituting cytoxan for ifosfamide with carboplatin has resulted in a 97% durable complete response rate.

4. Residual Mass

A residual mass can be detected after chemotherapy for bulky metastatic seminoma in one-half to two-thirds of cases. Attempts to resect these masses have often revealed only densely fibrotic tissue that is adherent to major blood vessels, and severe operative and postoperative complications have been reported. The relationship between the size of a residual mass and whether it contains viable tumor is unclear, with some studies showing that a mass greater than 3 cm correlates with residual disease and other studies not demonstrating this relationship. A practical policy is to monitor these masses closely and administer radiotherapy to those that do not continue to shrink.

C. Nonseminomatous Germ Cell Tumors

The natural history of nonseminomatous germ cell tumors tends to be less indolent and less predictable than that of seminomas. Nonseminomas have a greater likelihood of dissemination via the blood to distant sites, sometimes while bypassing the retroperitoneal lymphatics. Although nonseminomas (except for teratomas) are probably equally as chemosensitive as seminomas, they are less radiosensitive. As a result of these differences, the staging, treatment, and follow-up recommendations for nonseminoma are somewhat different from those for seminoma.

The International Germ Cell Consensus Classification staging system for nonseminomas tumors has been developed (Table III).

1. Stage I Treatment

Clinical stage I tumors represent approximately 50% of all nonseminomatous germ cell tumors. About 30% of these patients will relapse with occult metastatic disease if not given some form of adjuvant therapy. A number of treatment approaches for stage I nonseminoma have been tried, but there is no consensus on which is best. These approaches have included (1) retroperitoneal lymph node dissection (RPLND) after orchiectomy, (2) close surveillance after orchiectomy (no adjuvant therapy), (3) adjuvant chemotherapy for all patients or for selected individuals with adverse prognostic features, (4) RPLND and adjuvant chemotherapy for pathologic stage II patients, and (5) adjuvant radiotherapy.

Most of these approaches have their advocates, but adjuvant radiotherapy has fallen out of favor. Nonseminomas are less radiosensitive than seminomas,

and side effects from the increased doses of radiation required to treat nonseminomas are prohibitive. Also, nonseminoma is more likely than seminoma to relapse outside the radiation ports.

Proponents of RPLND for all stage I nonseminomas list the following advantages: This technique provides more accurate staging, it may be curative in 60 to 75% of cases with early evidence of nodal metastases, and it can provide an indication for immediate adjuvant chemotherapy in cases with more extensive nodal disease. The disadvantages of the procedure include the following: Retrograde ejaculation occurs in most patients who undergo traditional RPLND and in 10 to 15% of patients who have a nerve-sparing RPLND, even when performed by experienced urologists. A major surgery is performed in the 70% of patients who were already cured by orchiectomy alone, and the rate of relapse in patients who undergo RPLND is only decreased from 30% to about 12%. Most of these relapses, however, occur in the lungs and are generally easily managed with chemotherapy.

Another approach, surveillance after orchiectomy, was introduced at the Royal Marsden Hospital in 1979 and is currently the recommended treatment for most clinical stage I patients in Europe and some centers in the United States. In 1993, Sternberg reported on 1337 patients culled from published studies who were not given RPLND or other adjuvant therapy. The median follow-up was 40 months, and the relapse rate was 28% with a median time to relapse of

---

TABLE III
International Germ Cell Consensus Classification
for Nonseminomatous Germ Cell Tumors

Characteristic	Good prognosis	Intermediate prognosis	Poor prognosis
Primary site	Testis or RP	Testis or RP	Mediastinal OR
Metastatic sites	No NPVM	No NPVM	NPVM
STM	and all of	and any of	or any of
AFP	<1000 ng/ml	≥1000≤10,000 ng/ml	<10,000 ng/ml
HCG	<1000 ng/ml	≥1000≤10,000 ng/ml	<10,000 ng/ml
LDH	<1.5 × uln	≥1.5≤10 × uln	<10 × uln
NSGCT patients	56%	28%	16%
PFS 5 years	89%	75%	41%
OS at 5 years	92%	80%	48%

RP, retroperitoneal; NPVM, nonpulmonary visceral metastases; uln, upper limit of normal; STM, serum tumor marker; NSGCT, nonseminomatous germ cell tumor; PFS, progression-free survival; OS, overall survival.

5 to 6 months. The rate of complete remission with chemotherapy after recurrence and the overall survival were 99%. Adjuvant chemotherapy after orchiectomy with two cycles of chemotherapy, either for all patients or for selected high-risk patients, is another choice. This option is only beginning to be studied so there are few data on this topic. The extremely high rate of cure with observation and chemotherapy at recurrence makes it difficult to justify giving adjuvant chemotherapy to all patients. However, if a group with a sufficient risk of developing metastatic disease could be identified and if these patients could be cured with less chemotherapy and less associated toxicity, then it would be a reasonable option.

The Medical Research Council reported on a group of 259 patients, of which 61 were felt to have a greater than 50% chance of relapse. This assessment was based on the presence of three or all of the following four factors: tumor invasion of the testicular veins, tumor invasion of the testicular lymphatics, the presence of undifferentiated cells, or the absence of yolk sac elements. These high-risk patients were given two cycles of adjuvant BEP chemotherapy, and after a median followup of 18 months, no relapses have been seen.

In summary, none of the treatment options just described have been conclusively shown to be superior, and the best choice for a given patient will likely depend on the resources and experience of the treating institution as well as the preferences and reliability of the individual.

2. Stage II Treatment

The optimal management of stage II nonseminomas is no more settled than for stage I disease, but fortunately, several good options exist. Stage IIC (unresectable) should be treated with chemotherapy similar to that recommended for good prognosis stage III patients. However, for stages IIA and IIB, the decision of whether to treat initially with chemotherapy or with RPLND with or without adjuvant chemotherapy is unsettled. In Europe and in a few centers in the United States, primary chemotherapy for stage II patients is becoming the standard. However, most large cancer centers in the United States still recommend that patients with resectable stage II disease be treated with RPLND first.

Drawing conclusions from the literature is challenging because comparative trials are not available, and it is likely that neither option is superior in every situation. The expected cure rate with either treatment is greater than 95%, and aggressive therapy is not likely to affect this rate significantly. Thus, the goal is to maintain this cure rate while minimizing morbidity. Opinions vary as to whether chemotherapy or RPLND is more toxic, but it is obvious that surgery and full-course chemotherapy together are associated with greater morbidity than either approach alone. The goal, therefore, is to select the therapy that is most likely to be curative by itself.

The traditional approach for stage IIA and IIB disease has been RPLND. The rationale is that it is effective therapy and the most accurate method of staging. In a large prospective trial reported by the Testicular Cancer Intergroup Study, the risk of recurrence after RPLND without adjuvant chemotherapy was 40% for patients with N1 disease using TNM staging, 55% for patients with N2A disease, and 60% for patients with stage N2B disease. These results agree with those of other retrospective series in that about 50% of patients with pathologic stage II disease relapse after RPLND. The risk of recurrence after RPLND correlates with the degree of nodal involvement. When lymph nodes are larger than 3 cm, the risk of relapse rises to greater than 70% (Table IV).

Patients who are treated initially with RPLND can either receive two cycles of adjuvant chemotherapy or be observed closely and, if relapse occurs, receive three to four cycles of chemotherapy and possibly a second surgery. The advantage of observation is that it avoids any chemotherapy in the 50% of patients who are cured with their surgery alone. The disadvantage is that more chemotherapy is required if a relapse occurs and a second surgery could be indicated should a residual mass remain after this treatment. Because the toxicity of bleomycin and cisplatin is cumulative, two cycles of chemotherapy are significantly less toxic than three or four.

In the Testicular Cancer Intergroup Study, greater chemotherapy-related toxicity was seen in the group assigned to observation with chemotherapy at relapse than in the group treated initially with adjuvant chemotherapy. However, fewer patients in the observation arm required chemotherapy. Which therapy is

Tumor status	Regional lymph node status	Metastasis status
T2: Confined to body of testis	N0: No nodes involved	M1: Supradiaphragmatic or extralymphatic involvement
T2: Extending through the tunica albica	N1: Microscopic only	
T3: Involving the rete testis or epididymis	N2A: Largest node ≤2 cm and ≥6 involved nodes	
T4: Involving the scrotal wall	N3: Nodal extension into adjacent structures	
	N4: Gross tumor following retroperitoneal lymph node dissection	

[a]The T value does not affect (enter into) stage but is of some prognostic value in stage 1 disease.

selected should be based on the patient's risk factors for recurrence. Individuals with risk factors such as vascular or lymphatic invasion in the primary or abdominal lymph nodes larger than 3 cm should probably receive two cycles of adjuvant chemotherapy. If these factors are not present, then close observation is a reasonable option.

A more recent approach to the management of stage IIA and stage IIB disease is to treat with three to four cycles of chemotherapy initially and to reserve RPLND for radiographically persistent retroperitoneal disease. Several studies have shown the feasibility of this approach. Although most of these studies included patients with stage IIC disease, the complete remission rates were between 95 and 100%. However, to achieve a complete remission, 15 to 30% of the patients required an RPLND because of a residual mass. In studies of this approach with sufficient follow-up, the overall survival is comparable to that obtained with primary RPLND.

The advantages of primary chemotherapy vs RPLND alone are that a major surgery is avoided in 70 to 85% of the patients and that less compliance in returning for follow-up is required from the patient because the incidence of relapse is much less. Also, nerve-sparing RPLND cannot generally be done in this setting and, as a result, absent or retrograde ejaculation occurs in 70 to 80% of the patients undergoing RPLND. The disadvantages are that every patient receives three to four cycles of chemotherapy, rather than only the 50% of patients who eventually relapse after surgery, and that 15 to 30% of the patients who receive primary chemotherapy will still require RPLND for a residual mass.

In choosing appropriate therapy, the importance of histologic type in the primary tumor site is becoming more clear. If embryonal carcinoma without teratoma predominates, then initial treatment with chemotherapy is appropriate because residual abdominal masses are uncommon, and this tumor frequently recurs in the lungs, making patients treated with RPLND alone at high risk of recurrence. If teratoma is present, then there is a high likelihood that a residual mass will remain in patients treated with primary chemotherapy and a RPLND will be needed anyway. Such patients would probably benefit most from initial treatment with a RPLND. At RPLND, if only minimal disease is found, then surgery alone is likely sufficient and observation is appropriate. If lymph nodes larger than 3 cm are found or if the primary had a predominant embryonal component in addition to teratoma, then adjuvant chemotherapy is indicated. The best predictor of who will relapse is the response to initial therapy as manifested by the rate of all of AFP and β-hCG.

Standard salvage chemotherapy uses new agents in combination with cisplatin to treat patients at conventional or moderately increased doses. More aggressive treatment involves either increasing the frequency and number of cycles of chemotherapy or administering very high doses of chemotherapy with bone marrow rescue.

The conventional approach for patients with a first relapse is to use salvage chemotherapy. Approximately 25 to 30% of patients treated in this manner will achieve a durable complete remission. The prognosis is much worse for those who fail to achieve a complete remission at initial therapy. Only about 7% of these will be cured with standard salvage treatment.

The most common salvage regimens used are PVbI (cisplatin, vinblastine, ifosfamide) for patients who relapse after BEP and PEI (cisplatin, etoposide, ifosfamide) for patients who relapse after PVB.

For patients who do not respond to standard salvage therapy and possibly for those who do not achieve a complete remission with initial therapy, high-dose chemotherapy with bone marrow support is another approach. A review of the literature indicates that between 8 and 20% of these patients can still achieve a durable complete remission. In some of these studies, however, follow-up was short and a selection bias was likely present. This remission rate is far from ideal, but in this setting it is the best evaluated option so far.

New strategies are being developed that involve novel chemotherapeutic agents, alternation of noncross-resistant courses as short a time frame as possible, induction with two or more courses of standard salvage chemotherapy followed by high-dose chemotherapy with bone marrow support, and two or more courses of high-dose chemotherapy with bone marrow rescue.

V. CONCLUSIONS

The treatment of testicular neoplasms is both rewarding and challenging, rewarding because of its high cure rate and challenging because knowing which therapies to select and how to use them requires a thorough understanding of the literature and the disease. It is also challenging because patients with testis cancer frequently require aggressive treatment to provide the best opportunity for cure, yet expert management to avoid unnecessary morbidity and mortality. There are still many improvements to be made in finding ways to reduce both short-term and long-term toxicity as well as in the area of salvage treatment.

See Also the Following Articles

BLADDER CANCER: ANATOMY AND EVALUATION • COLORECTAL CANCER: MOLECULAR AND CELLULAR ABNORMALITIES • GERM CELL TUMORS • PROSTATE CANCER • STEROID HORMONES AND HORMONE RECEPTORS

Bibliography

Begent, R. H. J., Newlands, E. S., and Rustin, G. J. S. (1983). Further advances in the management of malignant teratomas of the testis and other sites. *Lancet* **1**, 948–951.

Bosl, G., Cirricione, C., Geller, N., *et al.* (1983). Serum tumor markers in patients with metastatic germ cell tumors of the testis: A 10-year experience. *Am. J. Med.* **75**, 29–35.

Dixon, F. J., and Moore, R. A. (1952). Tumors of the male sex organs. *In* "Atlas of Tumor Pathology." Armed Forces Institute of Pathology, Washington, DC.

Einhorn, L. H., and Donohue, J. (1977). Cis-diamminedichlorplatinum, vinblastine and bleomycin combination chemotherapy in disseminatied testicular cancer. *Ann. Intern. Med.* **87**, 293–298.

Higby, D. J., Wallace, H. J., Albert, D. J., *et al.* (1974). Diamminodichloroplatinum II: A phase I study showing response in testicular and other tumors. *Cancer* **33**, 1219–1225.

International Germ Cell Cancer Collaborative Group (1997). International germ cell consensus classification: A prognostic factor-based staging for metastatic germ cell cancers. *J. Clin. Oncol.* **15**, 594–603.

Mead, G. M., Stenning, S. P., Parkinson, M. C., *et al.* (1992). The second Medical Research Council study of prognostic factors in nonseminomatous germ cell tumors. *J. Clin. Oncol.* **10**, 85–94.

Sternberg, C. N. (1993). Role of primary chemotherapy in stage I and low-volume stage II nonseminomatous germ-cell testis tumors. *Urol. Clin. North. Am.* **20**, 93–103.

Williams, S. D., Birch, R., Irvin, L., *et al.* (1987). Disseminated germ cell tumors: Chemotherapy with cisplatin plus bleomycin plus either vinblastine or etoposide. *N. Engl. J. Med.* **316**, 1435–1440.

TGFβ Signaling Mechanisms

Nicole T. Liberati
Xiao-Fan Wang
Duke University Medical Center

GLOSSARY

BMP Bone morphogenic protein.
CamKII Calmodulin-dependent protein kinase II.
EGF Epidermal growth factor.
IFNγ Interferon gamma.
JNK Jun N-terminal kinase.
MAPK Mitogen activated protein kinase.
TGFβ Transforming growth factor beta.
TNFα Tumor necrosis factor alpha.

Few cytokines affect as many cellular functions as the TGFβ peptide hormones. Proliferation, extracellular matrix deposition, gene expression, differentiation, and morphogensis make up just a small sample of the many cellular processes influenced by TGFβ signaling. Reflecting the relevance of TGFβ signaling to overall tissue homeostasis, a number of different pathologies are associated with mutations in the TGFβ signaling pathway. For instance, 100% of pancreatic cancers and 83% of colon cancers harbor mutations affecting at least one component of the TGFβ signaling pathway. Unveiling the mechanisms that underlie TGFβ signaling, therefore, will provide targets for therapeutic intervention.

I. INTRODUCTION

To produce its many biological effects, TGFβ relies on what has been called a simple "signaling engine." This evolutionarily conserved signaling unit is remarkable in that it relies on only three key components: the TGFβ ligand, its receptors, and the Smad family of transcription factors (Fig. 1A). Multiple levels of specificity modulate the activity of each component to produce the diverse range of cellular effects elicited by TGFβ. This article follows the TGFβ signaling pathway from the outside of the cell, through the cytosol and into the nucleus. At each step of the pathway, the many modes of regulation that impose upon each component of the TGFβ signaling engine are summarized. An explosion of the field in recent years puts a comprehensive summary out of the scope of one review. For this reason, specific focus is put on the mammalian pathway and its related pathologies.

II. TRANSFORMING GROWTH FACTOR β (TGFβ) LIGANDS

Five structurally related molecules constitute the transforming growth factor β ligand family. Members of the TGFβ family (TGFβ1, 2, 3, 4, and 5) share significant amino acid sequence identity (64–82%), including nine conserved cysteine residues. Six of the nine invariant cysteines participate in intramolecular disulfide bonds to form the unique structure known as the "cysteine knot." A fourth disulfide bond forms an intermolecular bridge between two TGFβ peptides to produce a TGFβ dimer.

Secreted TGFβ1 dimers are noncovalently bound to a propeptide, the TGFβ latency-associated protein (LAP). LAP is linked to one of several large glycoproteins known as latent TGFβ-binding proteins (LTBPs). Together, the TGFβ1 dimer, LAP, and LTBP constitute the latent form of the ligand. The latent complex may play important roles in targeting and concentrating the TGFβ signal to specific regions within tissues. Various proteins, including matrix metalloproteinase-2 and -9, mannose 6-phosphate receptor, members of the plasminogen activation cascade, and thrompospondin-1, have been implicated in ligand activation. The precise mechanistic contribution of each factor to ligand activation is unclear, but is known to involve the dissociation of TGFβ dimers from LAP.

TGFβs are members of an extended superfamily of peptide hormones that regulate several distinct biological processes. Superfamily members share structural similarities, including conserved cysteine residues, but have less than 40% amino acid identity

in common with TGFβ. However, all superfamily members, including TGFβs, signal through heteromeric complexes of type I and type II serine-threonine receptor kinases (Fig. 1B).

III. TGFβ RECEPTORS

A heteromeric signaling complex on the cell surface transduces the TGFβ signal into the cell. The membrane-anchored type II serine/threonine receptor kinase binds activated TGFβ at the cell surface. Upon engagement, the transmembrane type I serine/threonine receptor kinase is recruited by the ligand-bound type II receptor to form the multiprotein surface signaling complex. Within the receptor complex, the type II receptor phosphorylates a glycine/serine-rich region of the type I receptor known as the GS box, thereby activating the type I receptor kinase. All known cellular effects of TGFβ are dependent on type I receptor kinase activity. The ubiquitous expression of type I and type II receptors is consistent with the ability of TGFβ to elicit biological responses from a number of cell types and tissues.

Two accessory TGFβ receptors have also been identified. Betaglycan (also known as type III TGFβ receptor) and endoglin promote the association of ligand with the type II receptor. Betaglycan is a transmembrane protein that lacks a recognizable intracellular signaling domain but facilitates TGFβ2 signaling through the type I/type II receptor signaling complex. In the cardiac primordium, betaglycan expression is necessary and sufficient for endothelial cells to undergo epithelial mesenchymal transformation in response to TGFβ2. Endoglin is a membrane-bound glycoprotein, specifically expressed by endothelial cells that bind TGFβ1 and TGFβ3. Although the mechanistic contribution of endoglin in TGFβ signaling is poorly understood, its importance to tissue homeostasis is revealed genetically in patients diagnosed with the vascular disease hereditary hemorrhagic telangiectasia. People with this disease frequently harbor mutations that inactivate or reduce endoglin levels as described in Section X.

A multitude of receptor-binding proteins have also been identified. They include FKBP12, STRAP, TRIP-1, and the B-α regulatory subunit of the protein

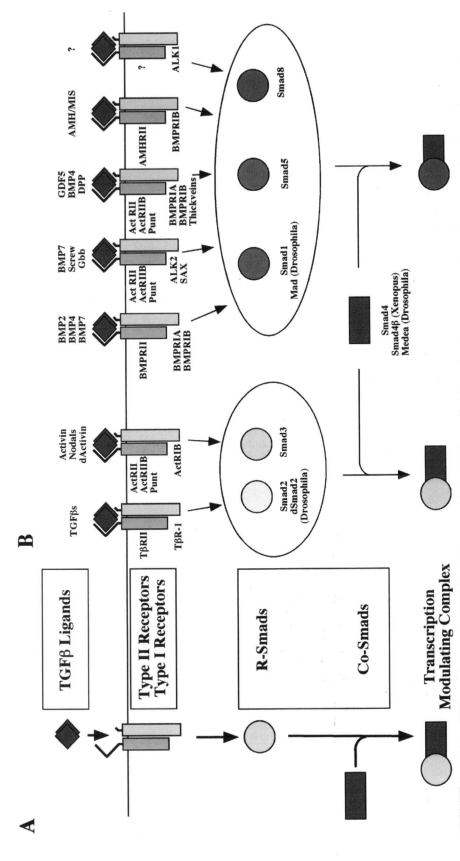

FIGURE 1 (A) The TGFβ signaling engine. TGFβ ligand dimers employ the TGFβ type II and type I receptors to initiate the signaling pathway. Ligand activation stimulates serine phosphorylation of R-Smads through the intracellular serine/threonine kinase domain of the type I receptor. R-Smad phosphorylation promotes R-Smads–Co-Smad heterodimerization and the entry of activated Smad multimers into the nucleus. TGFβ-induced transcriptional modulation is carried out by nuclear Smad complexes. (B) The TGFβ signaling engine is conserved across the TGFβ superfamily of ligands. Each superfamily member signals through a specific set of type II receptors, type I receptors, and Smads to produce different transcription-modulating Smad complexes. Adapted from Massagué et al. (2000).

phosphatase 2A (PP2A). Although most of these interactions are regulated by TGFβ, their functional contributions to TGFβ signaling are just beginning to be elucidated.

IV. SMADS: INTRACELLULAR EFFECTORS OF TGFβ SIGNALING

Inside the cell, the TGFβ signal is relayed by members of the Smad family of proteins. Structurally, these proteins share two highly conserved globular domains—mad homology domains 1 and 2 (MH1 and MH2)—linked together by a proline-rich sequence (Fig. 2). Receptor activated Smads, or R-Smads, serve as the direct substrates of the type I receptor kinase. Specifically, Smad2 and Smad3 are recognized by TGFβ, activin, and nodal type I receptors. Smad1, Smad5, and Smad8, however, serve as substrates for BMP and GDF type I receptors (Fig. 1). Phosphorylation of the SSxS motif at the very carboxy terminus of the MH2 domain by the receptor kinase relieves the inhibitory effect of an intramolecular interaction between the MH1 and MH2 domains and results in R-Smad activation.

Upon phosphorylation at C-terminal serines, R-Smads gain the capacity to associate with a different functional subgroup of the structurally conserved Smad protein family, the Co-Smads. Members of this group, which include the mammalian Co-Smad, Smad4, lack the C-terminal SSxS motif and are not phosphorylated by the receptor. In the basal state, Smad4 exists as a stable homotrimer through intermolecular interactions between key residues in its MH2 domain. Upon ligand stimulation, Smad4 binds to R-Smads activated by either TGFβ or other TGFβ family members. Heteromeric complex formation between activated R-Smads and Smad4 permits the entry of Smad4 into the nucleus.

In addition to the formation of heterodimers with Smad4 in response to ligand, Smad2 and Smad3 also form homomers and heteromers with each other upon ligand activation. Thus, ligand stimulation may induce the production of a variety of different Smad complexes that may contain Smad4, each able to en-

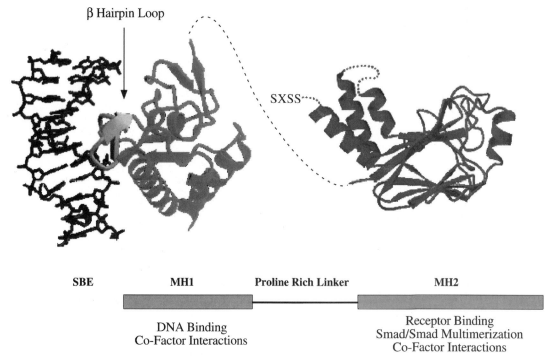

FIGURE 2 Smad crystal structures of MH1 and MH2 domains. Crystal structures of the Smad3 MH1 domain bound to the SBE and the MH2 domain of Smad4. These globular domains are linked by a less structured proline-rich linker sequence. The β-hairpin loop DNA-binding motif and the SSXS site of inducible phosphorylation by the type I receptor are noted. Documented molecular interactions with each domain are also noted. Structures reprinted by permission from *Nature* **388**, 87–93, © 1997 Macmillan Magazines Ltd.

ter the nucleus. As a result, a mixture of very different Smad complexes may localize to the nucleus in response to ligand.

Important mechanisms for the regulation of R-Smad activation lie in the cytoplasm. For example, the phosphatidylinositol-3-phosphate-binding protein SARA may potentiate the complex formation of Smad2 with the type I receptor at the intracellular face of cell membranes. Cytoplasmic Smad2 and Smad3 also associate with the microtubule component of the cytoskeleton, and TGFβ treatment induces the release of Smad2/3 from microtubules. The extent to which these interactions impact Smad signaling remains largely unknown.

V. TGFβ SIGNALING WITHIN THE NUCLEUS

A. DNA Binding

Although Smads contain no previously characterized DNA-binding motif, Smad4 directly binds a bipartite sequence within concatamerized TPA response elements from the collagenase promoter. Consistent with this result, an oligonucleotide library screen identified a similar palindromic sequence of 5′-GTCTAGAC-3′, known as the Smad-binding element (SBE), that associates with Smad3 and Smad4 and confers TGFβ responsiveness to nonresponsive promoters. The crystal structure of the MH1 domain of Smad3 bound to DNA demonstrates that residues within the β-hairpin loop of Smad3 bind the major groove of the short 5′-AGTAT GTCTAGAC TGA-3′ duplex (Fig. 2). Further evidence supporting the importance of the β-hairpin in the association of Smads and DNA comes from studies of Smad2. Smad2, which does not bind DNA, contains a 30 amino acid insert sequence just upstream of the β-hairpin. An alternative splice variant of Smad2 that lacks this insert possesses an affinity for DNA similar to that of Smad3, suggesting that the insert sequence inhibits the association of the β-hairpin with DNA.

B. Association with Transcriptional Cofactors

The affinity of the Smad3 MH1 domain for its binding site is weak, in the 10^{-7} M range. Furthermore,

the nearly equal affinities of Smad1 and Smad3 for the SBE do not allow for selective transcriptional activation by either BMP or TGFβ. For these reasons, it is thought that in addition to the presence of Smad DNA-binding elements within an endogenous promoter, Smad transcriptional responses are specified by individual promoter contexts. Cooperation of Smads with other promoter-bound transcription factors may target ligand-specific Smad-mediated transcriptional regulation of a particular gene. Supporting this notion, a multitude of Smad-binding transcription factors have been identified. These Smad-associated proteins can be categorized into three transcriptional subgroups: Smad coactivators, Smad corepressors, or constitutive repressors that are inactivated by the Smads (Table I).

Coactivators of Smad transcription include many DNA-binding transcription factors, as well as the chromatin remodeling enzymes, p300/CBP and P/CAF histone acetyltransferases. Similarly, both DNA-binding factors and factors that associate with histone deacetylase, HDAC1, such as ski/Sno oncoproteins and TGIF, serve as corepressors of Smad transcription. In addition, proteins such as Hoxc-8, found to associate with Smads, may potentiate the ability of Smads to derepress transcription. In this instance, Smads activate the transcription of a particular gene by inactivating a constitutive repressor that is associated with the gene. The interactions of Smads with various cofactors are likely to prove critical for different cellular effects that allow TGFβ to maintain normal tissue homeostasis and function. Supporting this notion, mutations in AML-3 (Runx2/PEBP2/CBFA1) associated with cleidocranial dysplasia inhibit its interaction with Smad4. Future work will identify the contribution of Smad transcriptional cofactors to different physiological effects of TGFβ.

VI. SIGNAL INTENSITY PRODUCES DIFFERENT TRANSCRIPTIONAL OUTCOMES

The intensity of TGFβ signaling may be altered by the number of ligand molecules bound to type II receptors at the cell surface. In a cell autonomous manner, activin occupation of approximately 100 receptors induces transcription of the *Xenopus* gene, Xbrachyury (Xbra), in *Xenopus* blastula cells. A switch

TABLE I
Smad Transcriptional Cofactors

	Cofactor	Functions	DNA recognition sequence	DNA-binding motif	Associated Smads[a]	Smad+ cofactor gene targets
Coactivators	FAST-1	Mediates activin-induced transcription	TGT(G/T)(T/G)ATT	Winged helix	S2/S3/S4	Nodal, lefty-2, XMix.2, Xgsc
	Jun	General transcriptional coactivator	TGACTCA	Basic leucine zipper	S1/S2, S3/S4/S5	c-fos, cJun, TGFβ1
	ATF-2	General transcriptional coactivator	TGACGTCA	Basic leucine zipper	S3/S4	Fibronectin
	TFE3	Regulates B-cell activation	CACGTG	Basic helix loop helix	S3/S4	PAI-1, Smad7
	SP-1	General transcriptional coactivator	G-rich and G(T/C)ACC	Zinc finger	S2/S3/S4	p15, p21, Col1A2, Smad7, β5 integrin, PAI-1,
	HNF-4	Regulates hepatocyte function	GGTCT	Zinc finger	S3/S4	ApoCIII
	VDR	Mediates vitamin D-induced transcription	GGGTCAxxxGGGTGA	Zinc finger + CTE	S3	Osteopontin
	Lef1	Mediates Wnt-induced transcription	GGGATTTCACC	HMG box	S2/S3/S4	Xtwn
	AML1,2,3	Regulates IgA class switching and osteoblast differentiation	TGT/cGGT	Runt domain	S33/S4	IgCα, IgA,
	OAZ	Induces Xenopus ventral mesoderm development	BMP response element in Xvent.2 promoter	Zinc finger	S1/S4	Xvent-2
	p300 and P/CAF	Histone acetyltransferases	—	—	S1/S2/S3/S4	PAI-1, type I collagen, others
Corepressors	c-ski/SnoN	Associates with histone deacetylase	Indirectly to SBE	—	S2/S3/S4	JunB, PAI-1, c-myc?
	TGIF	Associates with histone deacetylase	TGTCA	Homeodomain	S2/S3	PAI-1
	Snip-1	Inhibits S4-p/300 association	—	—	S1/S2/S4	Xgsc
	Schnurri	Blocks Brinker transcription	?	Zinc finger?	MAD	Brinker
Inhibited repressors	Hoxc-8	Represses osteopontin expression	TAAT	Homeodomain	S1	Osteopontin
	SIP1	Represses Xbra expression	CACCT	Zinc finger	S1/S2/S5	?
	Evi-1	Hematopoietic cell transformation?	GACAAGATA	Zinc finger	S3	?

[a] S1, Smad1; S2, Smad2; S3, Smad3; S4, Smad4.

to occupation of approximately 300 receptors with a higher concentration of ligand results in the expression of Xgoosecoid (Xgsc) and Xeomes while Xbra expression is turned off. Cells overexpressing functional type II receptors shift the gene expression pattern with the occupation of the same absolute numbers of occupied receptors (100 and 300). A shift from Xbra to Xgsc gene expression also correlates with a three-fold difference in the amount of Smad2 protein in the nucleus of cells injected with Smad2 RNA. Together, this work suggests that the absolute number of ligand-bound receptors has a linear relationship with the amount of Smad2 protein that enters the nucleus. Data also suggest that alterations in the number of Smad molecules in the nucleus, induced by different ligand concentrations, may elicit different transcriptional outcomes. Further studies are necessary to define the relationship among ligand concentration, the amount of endogenous Smads in the nucleus, and the resulting transcriptional program in mammalian tissues to understand the impact of changing ligand concentrations on physiological outcomes.

VII. TURNING OFF THE TGFβ SIGNAL

To ensure that TGFβ signaling takes place in a temporally and biologically appropriate manner, several mechanisms exist to specifically inactivate the TGFβ signal.

A. I-Smads

Members of the inhibitory Smad (I-Smad) subgroup of the Smad protein family include Smad6 and Smad7. These proteins compete with R-Smads for access to the activated type I receptor. In this way, I-Smads block R-Smad nuclear entry and TGFβ transcriptional induction. Smad6 preferentially blocks R-Smad activation by BMP, whereas Smad7 inhibits R-Smad activation by TGFβ, activin, and BMP. Revealing the physiological significance of I-Smad function, homozygous-null Smad6 mice have multiple cardiovascular defects, the most apparent being ossification of the aorta, indicative of hyperactive BMP signaling.

B. BAMBI

Similarly, the transmembrane protein BAMBI relies on a competition mechanism to inhibit TGFβ signaling. BAMBI forms heterodimers with type I receptors to interfere with receptor signaling and participates in a negative feedback loop with the BMP signaling pathway in *Xenopus*. The human gene product, nma, is closely related to BAMBI and was originally identified to its reduced expression levels in metastatic versus nonmetastatic melanoma lines. The role of BAMBI/nma in TGFβ signaling pathways in mature organisms remains unknown.

C. R-Smad Degradation

Beyond competitive binding mechanisms, the TGFβ signal is also dampened by targeted degradation of the Smads. Members of the HECT family of E3 ubiquitin ligases (Smurf1 and Smurf2) and members of the UbcH5 family of ubiquitin ligases bind and ubiquitinate ligand-activated Smads, targeting the Smads for degradation by the proteosome. Indicating the pathological relevance of these findings, tumor-derived mutants of Smad2 and Smad4 that contain a missense mutation in the MH1 domain at a conserved arginine are degraded more quickly than wild-type forms.

VIII. CROSS TALK WITH OTHER SIGNALING PATHWAYS

Given the pleiotrophic nature of the cellular effects induced by TGFβ, it is not unexpected that other signal transduction pathways impinge on TGFβ signaling. Innumerable studies demonstrating instances of such interplay (Fig. 3) reveal that Smads frequently serve as platforms for cross talk with the TGFβ signaling pathway. Smad activation by the type I receptor, Smad nuclear entry, and the transcriptional activity of Smad-containing DNA complexes are Smad functions that have repeatedly been shown to be modulated by these pathways. Signals that impinge on Smad activity include the interferon-γ (IFN-γ), tumor necrosis factor α (TNFα), bone morphogenic protein (BMP), epidermal growth factor (EGF), Vitamin D, and Wnt pathways, as well as TGFβ itself.

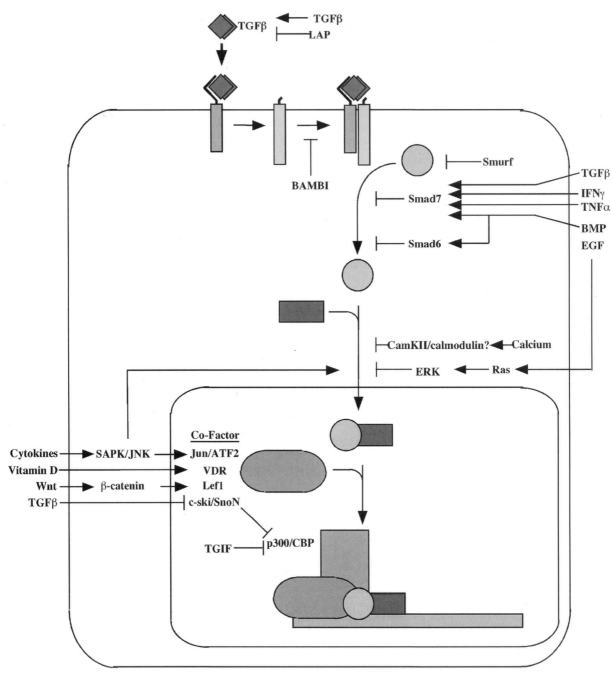

FIGURE 3 Cross talk with the TGFβ signaling pathway. Smads provide a platform for the integration of various signals with the TGFβ pathway. Inhibition of Smad activation is induced through the induction of I-Smads by TGFβ, IFNγ, TNFα, and BMP. Smad nuclear entry is inhibited by EGF-activated ERK and calcium-activated CamKII, but induced by mitogen-stimulated JNK. The activation of Smad cofactors by mitogens, vitamin D, and Wnt activates Smad-mediated transcription. TGFβ-induced degradation of c-ski and SnoN relieves the repressive effect of these proteins on Smad-activated transcription.

IX. TGFβ-MODULATED GENES

With genes being added to the roster of TGFβ transcriptional targets almost daily, an all-inclusive list is nearly impossible. This section presents a partial list of the extensive number of genes regulated by TGFβ, categorized into several functional subgroups that include cell cycle regulation, extracellular matrix production, and autoregulation.

TGFβ-induced cell cycle arrest at the G1–S phase of the cell cycle is brought about by two mechanisms: the inhibition of cyclin-dependent kinase (CDKs) activity and the downregulation of c-myc. In many cell types, the production of CDK inhibitors (CDKIs), p15 or p21, is significantly induced by TGFβ. CDK inactivation by these proteins results in the hypophosphorylation of the Rb tumor suppressor family and inhibition of S-phase gene expression, thereby halting cell cycle progression. Rapid downregulation of c-myc transcription in response to TGFβ is generally observed in cells that are sensitive to the antiproliferative effects of TGFβ. Exogenous expression of c-myc blocks the induction of either p15 or p21, indicating that downregulation of c-myc may be necessary for CDKI induction by TGFβ.

Generally, TGFβ induces the expression of extracellular matrix proteins and inhibits the degradation of these deposited proteins. Various collagens (including collagen I and collagen IV), basement membrane proteins (laminin, entactin, perlecan), and interstitial matrix proteins (fibronectin, osteopontin, thrombospondin, elastin, and decorin) are induced by TGFβ in a cell type specific manner. Maintaining the deposited matrix, TGFβ downregulates the expression of several matrix-degrading metalloproteinases (including collagenases MMP-1 and -8 and the stromelysin MMP-3) and upregulates the expression of inhibitors of these metalloproteinases, known as TIMPs. The nature of the matrix induced by TGFβ is likely to depend on the tissue type and the biological state of the tissue (i.e., developing tissue versus the healing tissue of a wound).

TGFβ regulates the activity of its own signaling pathway to form both positive and negative regulatory feedback loops. TGFβ1 promotes its own signaling through autoinduction of its own expression in various cell types. In contrast, the expression of I-Smads, Smad6 and Smad7, is also induced by TGFβ treatment. The mechanisms that underlie a possible integration of these opposing feedback loops are completely unknown, but may allow TGFβ to balance the effects of its signaling pathway under changing biological circumstances.

Many other genes are regulated by the TGFβ signaling pathway. The transcriptional expression of different surface adhesion molecules such as E-cadherin, various integrins, and surfactant protein B is altered by TGFβ. The expression of various immediate early genes, including the AP-1 members c-Jun and JunB, is also regulated by TGFβ at the level of transcription. The transcription of soluble molecules such as connective tissue growth factor, clusterin (ApoJ), and Fas ligand are modulated by TGFβ signaling. The established importance of TGFβ signaling on specific cellular functions with no known target genes responsible for these effects indicates that many more direct targets of the TGFβ signaling pathway will be identified in the future.

X. TGFβ AND HUMAN DISEASE

Revealing the significance of TGFβ signaling to normal tissue development and function, alterations in the TGFβ signaling pathway are associated with cancer, fibrosis, the vascular disease hereditary hemorrhagic telangiectasia, artherosclerosis, and other pathologies.

Mutations affecting the function or the expression of the TGFβ type II receptor, type I receptor, Smad2, and Smad4 have been discovered in human cancers. Smad4, originally identified as DPC for deleted in pancreatic cancer, is more frequently mutated with 50% of pancreatic cancers and 30% of colorectal carcinomas containing mutations in Smad4. Deletion or mutation of both Smad4 alleles is often found in these cancers, establishing Smad4 as a bona fide tumor suppressor. Supporting an antiproliferative role for TGFβ signaling, the expression of several oncoproteins (ras, myc, E1A, p53, c-ski, and SnoN) can overcome TGFβ-mediated growth inhibition.

Although matrix deposition is critical for its promotion of wound healing, this cellular response to

TGFβ can have pathological results when unchecked. Circulating TGFβ levels are found in patients with various pathological fibroses, such as nephritis, hepatic fibrosis, pulmonary fibrosis, systemic sclerosis, myelofibrosis, Crohn's disease, eosinophilia–myalgia syndrome, and proliferative vitreoretinopathy. Polymorphisms in the TGFβ1 gene have been linked to increased TGFβ1 production in humans and the development of fibrotic lung disease.

As previously mentioned, mutations in two genes, endoglin and ALK-1 (a member of the TGFβ type I receptor family), are genetically linked to hereditary hemorrhagic telangiectasia, a disease characterized by telangiectasias of the skin, recurrent epistaxis, gastrointestinal bleeding, and nuerologic sequelae due to arteriovenous malformations in the central nervous system and lungs. Clonal populations of cells derived from atherosclerotic lesions contain mutations leading to either low expression levels or inactive forms of the TGFβ type II receptor. Thus, genetic alterations of the TGFβ signaling pathway may contribute to artherosclerosis.

XI. CONCLUDING REMARKS

Through a seemingly simple linear signaling pathway (from ligand to receptors to Smad to target gene), TGFβ has a hand in multiple physiological events. Signaling intensity fluctuations, cross talk with other signaling pathways, and a repertoire of promoter-bound transcription factors on a particular Smad target gene change the TGFβ signaling engine, modifying its signal. In this way, a cellular outcome is produced that reflects the temporal, spatial, and biological context of the TGFβ-bound cell. Macroscopically, the summation of these integrated cellular activities on millions of TGFβ responsive cells permits TGFβ to regulate more global biological events of a particular tissue or organ that are linked to the pathological outcomes of defective TGFβ signaling. Future work will reveal mechanisms involved in the orchestration of numerous TGFβ-induced cellular activities to produce these events. These studies, in turn, will facilitate therapeutic targeting of the TGFβ pathway.

See Also the Following Articles

Cytokines • Integrin Receptor Signaling Pathways • Interferons: Cellular and Molecular Biology of Their Actions • Kinase-Regulated Signal Transduction Pathways • MAP Kinase Modules in Signaling • Signal Transduction Mechanisms Initiated by Receptor Tyrosine Kinases • Tumor Necrosis Factor • Wnt Signaling

Bibliography

Blobe, G. C., Schiemann, W. P., *et al.* (2000). Role of transforming growth factor beta in human disease. *N. Engl. J. Med.* **342,** 1350–1358.

Branton, M. H., and Kopp, J. B. (1999). TGF-beta and fibrosis. *Microbes Infect.* **1,** 1349–1365.

Datto, M., and Wang, X. F. (2000). The Smads: transcriptional regulation and mouse models. *Cytokine Growth Factor Rev.* **11,** 37–48.

Gurdon, J. B., Dyson, S., *et al.* (1998). Cells' perception of position in a concentration gradient. *Cell* **95,** 159–162.

Kawabata, M., Imamura, T., *et al.* (1999). Intracellular signaling of the TGF-beta superfamily by Smad proteins. *Ann N. Y. Acad. Sci.* **886,** 73–82.

Massagué, J., and Blain, S. W., *et al.* (2000). TGFb signaling in growth control, cancer, and heritable disorders. *Cell* **103,** 295–309.

Massagué, J., and Chen, Y. G. (2000). Controlling TGF-beta signaling. *Genes Dev.* **14,** 627–644.

Miyazono, K. (2000). TGF-beta signaling by Smad proteins. *Cytokine Growth Factor Rev.* **11,** 15–22.

Mulder, K. M. (2000). Role of Ras and Mapks in TGFβ signaling. *Cytokine Growth Factor Rev.* **11,** 23–35.

Murphy-Ullrich, J. E., and Poczatek, M. (2000). Activation of latent TGF-beta by thrombospondin-1: Mechanisms and physiology. *Cytokine Growth Factor Rev.* **11,** 59–69.

Shi, Y., Hata, A., *et al.* (1997). A structural basis for mutational inactivation of the tumour suppressor Smad4. *Nature* **388,** 87–93.

Shi, Y., Wang, Y. F., *et al.* (1998). Crystal structure of a Smad MH1 domain bound to DNA: Insights on DNA binding in TGF-beta signaling. *Cell* **94,** 585–594.

ten Dijke, P., Miyazono, K., *et al.* (2000). Signaling inputs converge on nuclear effectors in TGF-beta signaling. *Trends Biochem. Sci.* **25,** 64–70.

Wrana, J. L., and Attisano, L. (2000). The Smad pathway. *Cytokine Growth Factor Rev.* **11,** 5–13.

Zimmerman, C. M., and Padgett, R. W. (2000). Transforming growth factor beta signaling mediators and modulators. *Gene* **249,** 17–30.

Thyroid Cancer

Wendy J. Mack
Susan Preston-Martin
University of Southern California

I. Histology and Survival
II. International and Ethnic Comparisons
III. Age and Gender
IV. Secular Trends
V. Risk Factors for Thyroid Cancer

GLOSSARY

adenoma A benign tumor arising from epithelial cells.

goiter An enlargement of the thyroid gland.

goitrogen A substance that inhibits the production of thyroid hormones and produces goiters.

hyperthyroid Disease state defined by abnormally high level of thyroid hormones.

hypothyroid Disease state defined by abnormally low levels of thyroid hormones.

iodine A trace chemical element required for the synthesis of thyroid hormones.

ionizing radiation Radiation energy, including X rays and γ rays, that will dislodge electrons from atoms.

radioiodine Radioactive iodide often used in medical diagnostic tests.

thyroid stimulating hormone Hormone produced in the pituitary gland. It stimulates synthesis and secretion of thyroid hormones in the thyroid gland. It also stimulates growth of the thyroid gland itself.

thyroiditis An inflammation of the thyroid gland.

Cancer of the thyroid is a relatively rare cancer that comprises approximately 1% of all cancers in the United States.

I. HISTOLOGY AND SURVIVAL

There are four primary histologic types of thyroid cancer. Papillary and follicular cancers arise from the thyroid follicular cells and occur primarily in young to middle-aged women. Anaplastic cancers also arise from follicular cells and occur primarily in the elderly. Medullary cancers arise from the parafollicular cells of the thyroid. In the United States between 1988 and 1992, the distribution by histology was 79% papillary, 14% follicular, 3% medullary, and 1% anaplastic. Survival after a diagnosis of thyroid cancer varies by histology. The probability of surviving for at least 10 years after diagnosis is 98% for papillary, 92% for follicular, and 80% for medullary, but only 13% for anaplastic thyroid cancer. The distribution of thyroid cancer by histology varies across the world. Higher rates of follicular and anaplastic thyroid cancers occur in geographic areas that are locally deficient in iodine, and rates of papillary thyroid cancer are reported to be higher in geographic areas that are relatively rich in iodine.

II. INTERNATIONAL AND ETHNIC COMPARISONS

Age-adjusted annual incidence rates of thyroid cancer vary around the world and across ethnic groups, from a low of around 0.5 per 100,000 to a high of around 25 per 100,000. Among the United States white population, the average age-adjusted incidence rate is 2.5 per 100,000 in males and 6.5 per 100,000 in females. U.S. Latino and other Latino populations have incidence rates that are roughly equivalent to the U.S. white population. Lower incidence rates occur in African-American populations, in certain Asian populations (India, China), and in the United Kingdom. Populations with relatively high incidence rates are Iceland (6.1 per 100,000 in males and 9.8 per 100,000 in females), the Philippines (2.9 per 100,000 in males and 8.7 per 100,000 in females), Filipino immigrant populations in areas such as Los Angeles and Hawaii, and all other ethnic groups in Hawaii. The highest thyroid cancer rates in the world

are found in Filipino women living in Hawaii (5.1 per 100,000 in males and 25.5 per 100,000 in females).

III. AGE AND GENDER

Figure 1 displays the incidence of thyroid cancer in the United States by age and gender. In childhood, thyroid cancer incidence is extremely low for both sexes. In females, rates increase rapidly between ages 15 and 40. After this, thyroid cancer rates remain relatively stable in women, and male rates continue to rise up to older ages. Age-adjusted incidence rates for thyroid cancer are two- to threefold higher in females than in males. The excess thyroid cancer rate in females tends to be highest between the ages of 15 to 55. In the elderly, male and female incidence rates are roughly equal. The higher thyroid cancer rates among females occur for papillary, follicular, and medullary cancers. There is no clear gender difference in rates of anaplastic thyroid cancer.

IV. SECULAR TRENDS

During the 1900s, small increases in thyroid cancer incidence rates have been noted throughout the world. The increase over time has occurred primarily for papillary thyroid cancer. Part of the increase in incidence is due to the use of more sophisticated technology to image and diagnose thyroid tumors and to increased attention to identification and diagnosis of

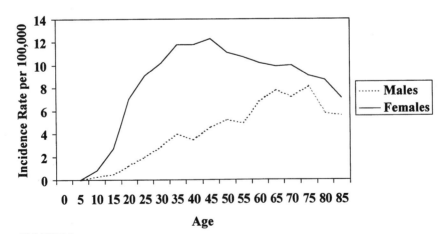

FIGURE 1 Age-specific thyroid cancer incidence rates by gender: U.S. Surveillance, Epidemiology, and End Results (SEER) program: 1988–1992.

thyroid cancer. In addition, the methods used to classify thyroid tumors changed in the 1970s, which resulted in certain follicular thyroid cancers being classified as papillary thyroid cancer. It has been hypothesized, but not clearly proven, that another portion of the observed increases result from the use of radiation treatment for certain childhood medical conditions (such as tinea capitis, enlarged thymus, and acne). Radiation treatments to the head and neck area for such conditions were practiced widely in the United States from the 1920s to the 1950s. In support of this hypothesis, analyses of U.S. thyroid cancer data show that increases in thyroid cancer incidence are limited to populations of persons born before 1950 (who would have had the opportunity to be treated with radiation). However, radiation therapies were not common in Europe, where increases in incidence have also been observed.

V. RISK FACTORS FOR THYROID CANCER

One of the strongest and most consistent exposure relationships observed in the epidemiology of cancer is the association between exposure to ionizing radiation and the subsequent increase in risk of thyroid cancer. Other than ionizing radiation, our current knowledge of other risk factors for thyroid cancer is limited. Epidemiological investigations for risk factors other than radiation are guided by the hypothesis that alterations in the levels of hormones, which influence the thyroid gland, may influence the development of thyroid cancer. For example, thyroid-stimulating hormone (TSH) promotes thyroid growth, and in laboratory animals, chronic elevations in TSH produced through a variety of mechanisms lead to excessive thyroid growth and thyroid tumors. Investigations have therefore tended to focus on exposures and conditions that might influence these hormones or have direct effects on the thyroid gland.

A. Radiation

An increased rate of thyroid cancer has been demonstrated in a number of cohorts of persons who were exposed to external ionizing radiation, and the increase in thyroid cancer risk associated with external radiation is among the highest of all radiation-related cancers. These cohorts include survivors of the atomic bombs in Japan and groups receiving radiation (X-ray) treatments for certain medical conditions, including tinea capitis, enlarged tonsils, enlarged thymus gland, and other (nonthyroid) cancer. The association of external ionizing radiation to thyroid cancer risk is strongly affected by the age at which the radiation exposure occurred. Children are much more vulnerable to the effects of ionizing radiation on the thyroid. In a pooled analysis of a number of cohorts exposed to ionizing radiation, there was little increase in thyroid cancer risk if radiation exposures occurred after age 20. The effects of ionizing radiation on the risk of thyroid cancer are seen long after the exposure occurred. In the pooled analysis, the elevated thyroid cancer risk was still evident (although appearing to plateau) up to 40 years after the radiation exposure had occurred. Few epidemiological studies have examined the association of lower dose diagnostic radiography with thyroid cancer. Results of these studies are inconsistent, and whether thyroid cancer risk is influenced by these lower radiation doses characteristic of diagnostic radiography remains a question for further research.

Relative to the firmly established relationship between high-dose external radiation and thyroid cancer, the literature regarding exposure to radioiodine (I^{131}) and risk of thyroid cancer is less clear. There is no clear evidence that exposure to radioiodine for diagnostic or therapeutic purposes increases thyroid cancer risk. Increases in thyroid cancers and other thyroid diseases have, however, been noted in cohorts exposed to nuclear fallout associated with aboveground nuclear testing and nuclear reactor accidents.

B. Benign Thyroid Disease

A number of epidemiological investigations conducted throughout the world have consistently shown that the risk of thyroid cancer is much higher among persons who have a past history of certain thyroid conditions, particularly conditions that involve excess growth of the thyroid gland. These thyroid conditions include goiter, benign thyroid nodules or adenomas, thyroid enlargement in adolescence, and thyroiditis. Hyperthyroidism has been inconsistently associated with thyroid cancer, and hypothyroid conditions are in general not associated with the later development of thyroid cancer. Radiation treatments to the head and neck in childhood increase the risk of benign thyroid adenomas as well as thyroid cancer. Part of the relationship of hyperplastic thyroid conditions with thyroid cancer is likely due to the fact that persons with thyroid conditions may undergo more medical surveillance and routine thyroid examinations, which would make it more likely that they would have a thyroid cancer detected, regardless of whether they were experiencing symptoms. Benign thyroid nodules or adenomas may in fact be a precursor condition to thyroid cancer. This would in part explain the very high relative risks associated with these conditions.

C. Reproductive Factors

Many epidemiological investigations of thyroid cancer have focused on reproductive history among females because of the highly elevated thyroid cancer incidence in women of reproductive age relative to males. Thyroid-related hormone levels and the thyroid gland itself are affected by reproductive events. The volume of the thyroid gland varies throughout the menstrual cycle and increases in pregnancy. Levels of TSH and human chorionic gonadotropin (hCG) increase in pregnancy, and hCG may directly stimulate the thyroid with TSH-like activity during pregnancy.

Most reproductive variables studied, including a history of irregular menstruation, number of births or pregnancies, occurrence of a natural menopause, and age at menopause, are in general not associated with thyroid cancer. Reproductive factors that have been found with some consistency, and in a pooled analysis of several case-control studies, to increase the risk of thyroid cancer risk in women include a later age at menarche, a history of infertility, occurrence of a miscarriage in the first pregnancy, a later age at first birth, and the occurrence of a surgical menopause (hysterectomy with removal of ovaries). However, these reproductive factors convey only a mild increase in thyroid cancer risk.

An open research question in this area regards the possible interaction between reproductive events and radiation exposures. Two case-control studies found

that the thyroid cancer risk associated with diagnostic X rays and radiation treatments is higher in women who had multiple pregnancies. These findings could be explained by elevated levels of TSH and hCG occurring in pregnancy, which might promote cellular proliferation and replication of cellular mutations caused by an earlier radiation exposure. This hypothesis, however, remains to be proven.

D. Exogenous Hormones

Epidemiological studies have also focused on women's use of hormones, such as oral contraceptives and post-menopausal estrogens, to explain the female excess of thyroid cancer. TSH levels are slightly elevated among women who use oral contraceptives. While some studies have reported a slightly elevated risk of thyroid cancer in women who use oral contraceptives, others have found no association. There is also no clear relationship by duration of use of oral contraceptives. Estrogens and other hormones used to relieve post-menopausal symptoms are also not related to thyroid cancer. In a few studies, the use of lactation suppressants is associated with a moderately elevated risk of thyroid cancer.

E. Diet

Epidemiological studies of diet and thyroid cancer have focused on the potential role of iodine-rich seafoods and goitrogenic vegetables. Both excesses and deficits of iodine are related to thyroid cancer. Similarly, both iodine excess and iodine deficiency may lead to elevations in TSH. Although it is hypothesized that eating large amounts of seafoods rich in iodine will increase the risk of thyroid cancer, epidemiological studies conducted throughout the world have shown remarkably inconsistent findings. While some studies do find an increased risk of thyroid cancer associated with consuming high amounts of seafood, other studies report no association or even a decrease in thyroid cancer risk.

Epidemiological studies of vegetable consumption have focused on cruciferous vegetables (such as cauliflower and broccoli) because they contain thioglucosides, which can form goitrogens. By blocking iodine uptake and synthesis of thyroid hormones, goitrogens can cause the pituitary gland to increase secretion of TSH. Animals fed large amounts of such goitrogens develop thyroid cancer. However, human consumption of dietary goitrogens is normally too low to expect that the effect seen in these animal studies will translate to human populations. In certain rare populations that do eat a large amount of goitrogens and also live in geographic areas that are deficient in iodine, increased TSH levels and abnormal thyroid conditions are found. Consistent with this observation, a case-control study reported that a higher consumption of cruciferous vegetables increased thyroid cancer risk only among persons who had lived in iodine-deficient areas where goiter was endemic. Far more epidemiological studies report a decreased risk associated with cruciferous and other vegetables. Most epidemiological studies of diet have not examined risk according to residence in iodine-rich versus iodine-poor areas.

Dairy products can be a major source of dietary iodine if the animal source was fed iodine-supplemented foods. Butter and cheese, but not yogurt and milk, were found to increase the risk of thyroid cancer in case-control studies. The association with milk products may be limited to subjects who had lived in iodine-deficient areas of endemic goiter.

F. Body Size

Several epidemiological studies report that body size and weight gain increase the risk of thyroid cancer. Thyroid volume increases with higher body weight. When analyzed by gender, most studies find this relationship with increased body weight in women; the association of higher body weight and thyroid cancer risk in men is not as clear. In a pooled analysis of several case-control studies, women and men who were taller had a mildly increased risk of thyroid cancer. In this same pooled analysis, a higher body weight assessed at the time of diagnosis was related to a mild increase in thyroid cancer risk in women, but not in men.

G. Familial Aggregation and Molecular Genetics

Many epidemiological studies find an increased risk of thyroid cancer in persons with family members who have had thyroid diseases or thyroid cancers. The multiple endocrine neoplasia (MEN) type 2 syndrome is an inherited autosomal-dominant disorder. Approximately 20–25% of all medullary thyroid cancers occur as a defining disorder in all three of the MEN subtypes (MEN 2A, MEN 2B, and familial medullary thyroid cancer). There is no clear pattern of genetic inheritance for other types of thyroid cancer or for the remaining 75% of medullary thyroid cancers.

Activation mutations of the ret protooncogene have been found in the MEN 2 syndromes (specific germline mutations) and in nonfamilial medullary and papillary thyroid cancers (somatic mutations and rearrangements). Specific rearrangements of the ret protooncogene found in papillary cancer were particularly prevalent among pediatric thyroid cancer cases diagnosed after the Chernobyl nuclear reactor accident. Both mutations and rearrangements of this gene lead to oncogenic activity. Mutations of the ras oncogene are found in follicular thyroid cancers. Mutations of the p53 tumor suppressor gene are highly prevalent in undifferentiated (anaplastic) thyroid cancer, but not in the papillary and follicular thyroid cancers.

H. Occupation

Relatively few studies have investigated the role of occupational or specific chemical exposures in relation to thyroid cancer. Cohort studies that examine thyroid cancer rates in a specific exposed group are difficult to conduct because of the very low incidence rates of thyroid cancer. Occupations found in repeated epidemiological studies to carry a higher than expected rate of thyroid cancer include X-ray technicians and other medical technicians who may have occupational radiation exposure (including dentists and dental assistants, and laboratory technicians).

I. Residence

Around the world, it is reported that rates of follicular thyroid cancer are higher in iodine-deficient areas characterized by endemic goiter. Rates of papillary thyroid cancer may be higher in iodine-rich areas. In iodine-deficient areas that were supplemented with iodine in the water, some studies reported increases in the rates of papillary thyroid cancer; other studies did not find this increase. In case-control studies, a history of residence in areas characterized by endemic goiter increases the risk for both papillary and follicular thyroid cancers. As noted earlier, residence in iodine-deficient areas may also increase thyroid cancer risk among persons who consume large amounts of goitrogens.

J. Smoking

Epidemiological studies examining cigarette smoking have fairly consistently shown a mild decrease in the risk of thyroid cancer. Because many of the epidemiological studies have been conducted among women, this result has been reported more often in women than in men.

See Also the Following Articles

BLADDER CANCER: EPIDEMIOLOGY • ENDOCRINE TUMORS • KIDNEY, EPIDEMIOLOGY • LIVER CANCER: ETIOLOGY AND PREVENTION • PANCREATIC CANCER: CELLULAR AND MOLECULAR MECHANISMS • PROSTATE CANCER • TOBACCO CARCINOGENESIS

Bibliography

Dal Maso, L., La Vecchia, C., Franceschi, S., Preston-Martin, S., Ron, E., Levi, F., Mack, W., Mark, S. D., McTiernan, A., Kolonel, L., Mabuchi, K., Jin, F., Wingren, G., Galanti, M. R., Hallquist, A., Glattre, E., Lund, E., Linos, D., and Negri, E. (2000). A pooled analysis of thyroid cancer studies. V. Anthropometric factors. *Cancer Causes Control* **11,** 137–144.

Franceschi, S., Preston-Martin, S., Dal Maso, L., Negri, E., La Vecchia, C., Mack, W. J., McTiernan, A., Kolonel, L., Mark, S. D., Mabuchi, K., Jin, F., Wingren, G., Galanti, R., Hallquist, A., Glattre, E., Lund, E., Levi, F., Linos, D., and Ron, E. (1999). A pooled analysis of case-control studies of thyroid cancer. IV. Benign thyroid diseases. *Cancer Causes Control* **10,** 583–595.

Gilliland, F. D., Hunt, W. C., Morris, D. M., and Key, C. R. (1997). Prognostic factors for thyroid carcinoma: A population-based study of 15,698 cases from the Surveillance, Epidemiology and End Results (SEER) Program 1973–1991. *Cancer* **79,** 564–573.

La Vecchia, C., Ron, E., Franceschi, S., Dal Maso, L., Mark, S. D., Chatenoud, L., Braga, C., Preston-Martin, S., McTiernan, A., Kolonel, L., Mabuchi, K., Jin, F., Wingren, G., Galanti, M. R., Hallquist, A., Lund, E., Levi, F., Linos, D., and Negri, E. (1999). A pooled analysis of case-control studies of thyroid cancer. III. Oral contraceptives, menopausal replacement therapy and other female hormones. *Cancer Causes Control* **10,** 157–166.

Negri, E., Dal Maso, L., Ron, E., La Vecchia, C., Mark, S. D., Preston-Martin, S., McTiernan, A., Kolonel, L., Yoshimoto, Y., Jin, F., Wingren, G., Galanti, M. R., Hardell, L., Glattre, E., Lund, E., Levi, F., Linos, D., Braga, C., and Franceschi, S. (1999). A pooled analysis of case-control studies of thyroid cancer. II. Menstrual and reproductive factors. *Cancer Causes Control* **10,** 143–155.

Parkin, D. M., Whelan, S. L., Ferlay, J., Raymond, L., and Young, J. (eds) (1997). "Cancer Incidence in Five Continents," Vol. VII. IARC Scientific Publications, Lyon.

Ron, E. (1996). Thyroid cancer. *In* "Cancer Epidemiology and Prevention" (D. Schottenfeld, and J. F. Fraumeni, Jr., eds.), pp. 1000–1021, Oxford Univ. Press, New York.

Ron, E., Lubin, J. H., Shore, R. E., Mabuchi, K., Modan, B., Pottern, L. M., Schneider, A. B., Tucker, M. A., and Boice, J. D., Jr. (1995). Thyroid cancer after exposure to external radiation: A pooled analysis of seven studies. *Radiat. Res.* **141,** 259–277.

Schneider, A. B., and Robbins, J. (1998). Ionizing radiation and thyroid cancer. *In* "Thyroid Cancer" (J. A. Fagin, ed.), pp. 27–58, Kluwer Academic, Norwell, MA.

TLS–CHOP in Myxoid Liposarcoma

Marc Ladanyi
Cristina R. Antonescu

Memorial Sloan-Kettering Cancer Center

GLOSSARY

C/EBP family Group of homologous CCAAT/enhancer-binding proteins, including C/EBPα, C/EBPβ, C/EBPδ, and C/EBPζ, involved in preadipocyte differentiation.

endoplasmic reticulum stress Impairment of protein folding within the endoplasmic reticulum.

liposarcoma Malignant tumor of fatty tissue.

myxoid Denotes the presence of mucoid intercellular matrix, similar to primitive mesenchymal tissue.

translin Endogenous DNA-binding protein found to bind some specific sequences at recombination hotspots; may mediate or facilitate heterologous recombination.

Certain liposarcomas contain a specific fusion of the *TLS* and *CHOP* genes, producing an oncogenic protein that functions primarily as an aberrant tran-scription factor. The analysis of this fusion oncogene is yielding insights not only into these uncommon tumors, but also into the normal functions of the two fusion partners and into normal adipogenesis.

I. BACKGROUND

Liposarcoma is one of the most common soft tissue tumors in adults. Among liposarcomas, the most common subtype of liposarcoma is myxoid liposarcoma, accounting for more than half of the cases. It occurs predominantly in the soft tissue of the extremities in young adults. Formation and function of the *TLS–CHOP* fusion oncogene in myxoid liposarcomas follow a pattern observed in certain sarcomas characterized by specific recurrent chromosomal translocations. These translocations produce highly specific gene fusions. Genes rearranged by these translocations encode two general types of proteins, transcription factors and RNA-binding proteins (*TLS, EWS*). Due biological consequence of the involvement of RNA-binding proteins (TLS and EWS) in these fusions is that their N-terminal domain can function as a strong transactivation domain and that their promoters are constitutively activated, as described in further detail later. Clinically, given the remarkable prevalence and specificity of different gene fusions in selected sarcomas, they have come to define these entities. Thus, the detection of the *TLS–CHOP* fusion can be used as a diagnostic test for myxoid liposarcoma.

II. DISCOVERY AND STRUCTURAL ASPECTS

In the 1980s, the work of several groups established that t(12;16)(q13;p11) was detectable in more than 90% of cases of myxoid liposarcoma, including both lower grade (pure myxoid) and higher grade (myxoid/round cell and pure round cell) forms of myxoid liposarcoma. In 1992, the rearrangement of the previously identified transcription factor gene *CHOP* at 12q13 in myxoid liposarcomas with t(12;16)(q13;p11) was described. The following year, two independent groups isolated the fusion partner, which they designated *TLS* (for translocated in liposarcoma) or *FUS* (for fusion), respectively. *TLS* is a novel gene most closely related to *EWS*, suggesting that the two genes may have originated from a common ancestor gene. At the protein level, TLS and EWS show >50% amino acid identity, especially in the carboxy-terminal region containing the RNA-binding domains. It is therefore interesting to note that in approximately 2% of myxoid liposarcoma, a variant chromosomal translocation has been described, t(12;22), in which *CHOP* fuses instead with *EWS*. The clinical and pathologic specificity of the association of *TLS–CHOP* (and *EWS–CHOP*) with myxoid liposarcoma has been fully confirmed.

Three major types of *TLS–CHOP* fusion transcripts types have been reported in myxoid liposarcoma, a result of variability of the *TLS* portion of the chimeric transcripts. These are generated through splicing of exons 5, 7, or 8 of *TLS* to exon 2 of *CHOP* and are referred to as type I (7-2), type II (5-2), and type III (8-2). Thus, exons 1 to 5 of *TLS* are invariably present in the tumor-associated fusion gene. All three types of fusions produce in-frame transcripts. So far,

no obvious clinical or molecular correlates of this fusion variability have been identified.

The genomic structure of the human *TLS* gene is well described. It consists of 15 exons located within 11 kb. The translocation breakpoint region of *TLS* corresponds to a region delimited by introns 5 to 8 of approximately 3.9 kb. The *CHOP* gene consists of 4 exons, spanning about 4 kb on band 12q13. Most breakpoints are upstream of exon 2, but rare cases may have breaks in the second intron. Breaks upstream of exon 1 result in fusion transcripts in which exon 1 is spliced out due to lack of a 5′ splice acceptor site.

Sequence analysis of the genomic breakpoints in *TLS* and *CHOP* in t(12;16) suggest the involvement of Translin and topoisomerase II in the process of translocation. Indeed, Translin has been shown to bind to sequences adjacent to the breakpoints of the *TLS* and *CHOP* genes in liposarcomas.

III. FUNCTIONAL ASPECTS AND MOUSE MODELS

The *CHOP* gene (C/EBP homologous protein, also called C/EBPζ) encodes a leucine zipper transcription factor important in adipocyte differentiation and growth arrest. *CHOP* was also separately isolated as a growth arrest and DNA-damage-inducible gene, *GADD153*. Indeed, forced overexpression of the protein results in growth arrest. *CHOP* is normally expressed at very low levels in most cells, including adipocytes; however, it is markedly activated primarily by perturbations that induce endoplasmic reticulum (ER) stress. Specifically, in response to ER stress, CHOP is thought to activate a gene expression program, of which the component targets genes are just beginning to be identified.

TLS is a ubiquitously expressed protein that binds RNA through a C-terminal domain with a distinct RNA recognition motif (RRM) surrounded by Arg-Gly-Gly (RGG) repeats. TLS is involved in nucleo-cytoplasmic shuttling, possibly reflecting a role in chaperoning mRNA or pre-mRNA. It also interacts with components of the basal transcriptional machinery. Its amino-terminal sequences appear to harbor a strong transcriptional activation domain, which functions as an essential transforming domain within TLS–CHOP in myxoid liposarcoma and within TLS–ERG in some acute myeloid leukemias.

In TLS–CHOP, the amino-terminal portion of TLS is joined to the entire CHOP coding region. In addition, CHOP exon 2, normally untranslated, is included in the open reading frame. TLS–CHOP dimerizes stably with C/EBPβ, and the leucine zipper domain of CHOP is necessary for transformation, implying an oncogenically crucial role for dimerization with C/EBP. Expression of the TLS–CHOP fusion gene in NIH/3T3 cells allows anchorage-independent growth in soft agar, loss of contact inhibition, and tumor formation in nude mice. In contrast to native CHOP, TLS–CHOP does not induce growth arrest at the G1/S checkpoint in NIH/3T3 cells and inhibits the cell cycle effects of native CHOP.

Transformation of preadipocytes by TLS–CHOP may reflect the multifaceted effects of the fusion on expression pattern, protein localization, transactivation potential, dominant-negative effects, and target specificity. First, the TLS promoter region confers strong and stable expression to the chimeric protein, in contrast to the tightly regulated expression of CHOP. Second, TLS–CHOP shows a different nuclear localization pattern compared to CHOP. Third, the amino-terminal-transactivating domain of TLS converts TLS–CHOP into an accentuated form of CHOP. Fourth, the retained CHOP leucine zipper domain mediates heterodimerization with C/EBP family members and thus possible dominant-negative functions, as these TLS–CHOP–C/EBP complexes may not bind classic C/EBP sites. Fifth, the amino-terminal portion of TLS seems to provide an additional effector domain, which confers novel target specificities to TLS–CHOP. This is suggested by studies that show that the amino-terminal portion of TLS contributes more than a strong "generic" transcriptional activation domain to the chimeric protein because other types of activation domains cannot fully substitute in transformation assays, whereas the amino-terminal domain of the related EWS can. The critical contribution of the TLS portion to TLS–CHOP-mediated oncogenesis has now also been confirmed in a mouse model of myxoid liopsarcoma (see below).

Two groups have used different approaches to identify TLS–CHOP downstream targets. These targets include a novel secreted protein (designated DOL54) also transiently expressed in normal adipocytic differentiation, as well as a set of neurodevelopmental transcripts and some novel genes.

Two groups have published TLS knockouts, with slightly different phenotypes. One set of TLS-null mice displayed male sterility and enhanced radiation sensitivity, whereas another set showed defective B lymphocyte development and activation, high levels of chromosomal instability, and perinatal death. Despite their phenotypic disparities (which may reflect differences in the host strains used), both models indicate an important role for TLS in genome maintenance and stability. CHOP knockout mice, although born at the expected frequency and phenotypically normal, are defective in the apoptotic response to ER stress.

A transgenic mouse model of myxoid liposarcoma using a TLS–CHOP transgene driven by the elongation factor 1 (EF1) promoter has been produced. The resulting tumors were similar to human myxoid liposarcoma at the morphologic and molecular genetic levels. Interestingly, no other tumor types were observed in these transgenic mice, supporting the oncogenic specificity of TLS–CHOP for the adipocytic lineage. Using a transgene driven by the same EF1 promoter, similar mice transgenic for intact CHOP did not develop liposarcomas.

See Also the Following Articles

ALL-1 • EWS/ETS Fusion Genes • PAX3–FKHR and PAX7–FKHR Gene Fusions in Alveolar Rhabdomyosarcoma • RUNX/CBF Transcription Factors

Bibliography

Aman, P., Panagopoulos, I., Lassen, C., Fioretos, T., Mencinger, M., Toresson, H., Hoglund, M., Forster, A., Rabbitts, T. H., Ron, D., Mandahl, N., and Mitelman, F. (1996). *Genomics* **37,** 1–8.

Aman, P., Ron, D., Mandahl, N., Fioretos, T., Heim, S., Arheden, K., Willen, H., Rydholm, A., and Mitelman, F. (1992). *Genes Chromosome Cancer* **5,** 278–285.

Antonescu, C. R., Elahi, A., Humphrey, M., Lui, M. Y., Healey, J. H., Brennan, M. F., Woodruff, J. M., Jhanwar, S. C., and Ladanyi, M. (2000). *J. Mol. Diagnost.* **2,** 132–138.

Antonescu, C. R., Tschernyavsky, S. J., Decuseara, R., Leung, D. H., Woodruff, J. M., Brennan, M. F., Bridge, J. A., Neff, J. R., Goldblum, J. R., and Ladanyi, M. (2001). *Clin. Cancer Res.* **7,** 3977–3987.

Barone, M. V., Crozat, A., Tabaee, A., Philipson, L., and Ron, D. (1994). *Genes Dev.* **8,** 453–464.

Bertolotti, A., Lutz, Y., Heard, D. J., Chambon, P., and Tora, L. (1996). *EMBO J.* **15,** 5022–5031.

Crozat, A., Aman, P., Mandahl, N., and Ron, D. (1993). *Nature* **363,** 640–644.

Darlington, G. J., Ross, S. E., and MacDougald, O. A. (1998). *J. Biol. Chem.* **273,** 30057–30060.

Hicks, G. G., Singh, N., Nashabi, A., Mai, S., Bozek, G., Klewes, L., Arapovic, D., White, E. K., Koury, M. J., Oltz, E. M., Van Kaer, L., and Ruley, H. E. (2000). *Nature Genet.* **24,** 175–179.

Hosaka, T., Kanoe, H., Nakayama, T., Murakami, H., Yamamoto, H., Nakamata, T., Tsuboyama, T., Oka, M., Kasai, M., Sasaki, M. S., Nakamura, T., and Toguchida, J. (2000). *Oncogene* **19,** 5821–5825.

Kanoe, H., Nakayama, T., Hosaka, T., Murakami, H., Yamamoto, H., Nakashima, Y., Tsuboyama, T. N. T., Ron, D., Sasaki, M. S., and Toguchida, J. (1999). *Oncogene* **18,** 721–729.

Kuroda, M., Ishida, T., Horiuchi, H., Kida, N., Uozaki, H., Takeuchi, H., Tsuji, K., Imamura, T., Mori, S., Machinami, R., *et al.* (1995). *Am. J. Pathol.* **147,** 1221–1227.

Kuroda, M., Ishida, T., Takanashi, M., Satoh, M., Machinami, R., and Watanabe, T. (1997). *Am. J. Pathol.* **151,** 735–744.

Kuroda, M., Sok, J., Webb, L., Baechtold, H., Urano, F., Yin, Y., Chung, P., de Rooij, D. G., Akhmedov, A., Ashley, T., and Ron, D. (2000). *EMBO J.* **19,** 453–462.

Kuroda, M., Wang, X., Sok, J., Yin, Y., Chung, P., Giannotti, J. W., Jacobs, K. A., Fitz, L. J., Murtha-Riel, P., Turner, K. J., and Ron, D. (1999). *Proc. Natl. Acad. Sci. USA* **96,** 5025–5030.

Morohoshi, F., Ootsuka, Y., Arai, K., Ichikawa, H., Mitani, S., Munakata, N., and Ohki, M. (1998). *Gene* **221,** 191–198.

Panagopoulos, I., Hoglund, M., Mertens, F., Mandahl, N., Mitelman, F., and Aman, P. (1996). *Oncogene* **12,** 489–494.

Panagopoulos, I., Mandahl, N., Ron, D., Hoglund, M., Nilbert, M., Mertens, F., Mitelman, F., and Aman, P. (1994). *Cancer Res.* **54,** 6500–6503.

Park, J. S., Luethy, J. D., Wang, M. G., Fargnoli, J., Fornace, A. J. J., McBride, O. W., and Holbrook, N. J. (1992). *Gene* **116,** 259–267.

Perez-Losada, J., Pintado, B., Gutierrez-Adan, A., Flores, T., Banares-Gonzalez, B., del Campo, J. C., Martin-Martin, J. F., Battaner, E., and Sanchez-Garcia, I. (2000a). *Oncogene* **19,** 2413–2422.

Perez-Losada, J., Sanchez-Martin, M., Rodriguez-Garcia, M. A., Perez-Mancera, P. A., Pintado, B., Flores, T., Battaner, E., and Sanchez-Garcia, I. (2000b). *Oncogene* **19,** 6015–6022.

Prasad, D. D., Ouchida, M., Lee, L., Rao, V. N., and Reddy, E. S. (1994). *Oncogene* **9,** 3717–3729.

Rabbitts, T. H., Forster, A., Larson, R., and Nathan, P. (1993). *Nature Genet.* **4,** 175–180.

Ron, D. (1997). *Curr. Top. Microbiol. Immunol.* **220,** 131–142.

Ron, D., and Habener, J. F. (1992). *Genes Dev.* **6,** 439–453.

Thelin-Jarnum, S., Lassen, C., Panagopoulos, I., Mandahl, N., and Aman, P. (1999). *Int. J. Cancer* **83,** 30–33.

Wang, X. Z., Kuroda, M., Sok, J., Batchvarova, N., Kimmel, R., Chung, P., Zinszner, H., and Ron, D. (1998). *EMBO J.* **17,** 3619–3630.

Zinszner, H., Albalat, R., and Ron, D. (1994). *Genes Dev.* **8,** 2513–2526.

Zinszner, H., Kuroda, M., Wang, X., Batchvarova, N., Lightfoot, R. T., Remotti, H., Stevens, J. L., and Ron, D. (1998). *Genes Dev.* **12,** 982–995.

Zinszner, H., Sok, J., Immanuel, D., Yin, Y., and Ron, D. (1997). *J. Cell Sci.* **110,** 1741–1750.

Tobacco Carcinogenesis

Stephen S. Hecht
University of Minnesota Cancer Center

GLOSSARY

carcinogen Any compound that is capable of inducing tumors in laboratory animals or humans.

DNA adduct A covalent binding product formed between a chemical and DNA.

metabolic activation Process by which a carcinogen is converted to a more reactive form that can bind to DNA.

metabolic detoxification Process by which a carcinogen is converted to a form that is excreted without reacting with DNA.

nitrosamines Compounds having a nitroso group bound to the nitrogen of a secondary amine.

polycyclic aromatic hydrocarbons A group of compounds consisting of more than two condensed benzene rings, generally formed in the incomplete combustion of organic matter.

Tobacco carcinogenesis is the process by which tobacco products and their constituents interact with cells to cause cancer. Cigarettes are the main tobacco product worldwide. Manufactured cigarettes are available in all countries, but in some areas of the world, roll-your-own cigarettes are still popular. Other smoked products include *kreteks*, clove-flavored cigarettes popular in Indonesia, and "sticks" which are smoked in Papua, New Guinea. *Bidis*, a small amount of tobacco wrapped in *temburni* leaf and tied with a string, are very popular in India and neighboring areas and have recently taken hold in the United States. Cigars are presently increasing in popularity, and pipes are still used. A substantial amount of tobacco is consumed worldwide in the form of smokeless tobacco products. These include chewing tobacco, dry snuff used for nasal inhalation, moist snuff, which is placed between the cheek and gum, a popular practice in Scandinavia and North America, and *pan* or betel quid, a product used extensively in India. All products are complex mixtures of defined compounds, many of which are capable of inducing tumors. The compounds that induce tumors are called carcinogens. The study of cancer induction by tobacco products and their constituents results in the elucidation of mechanisms by which many of the common human cancers develop.

I. INTRODUCTION

Due to the addictive power of nicotine, worldwide tobacco use is staggering. According to estimates by the World Health Organization, there are about 1100 million smokers in the world, representing approximately one-third of the global population aged 15 years or higher. China alone has approximately 300 million smokers, about the same number as in all developed countries combined. Globally, about 47% of men and 12% of women smoke. Smoking prevalence varies widely by country. For example, in Korea, 68% of men smoke daily, while the corresponding figure for Sweden is 22%. Among women, the highest smoking prevalence is in Denmark, where 37% of women smoke, while in many Asian and developing countries, prevalence is reported to be less than 10%. Although smoking prevalence is lower in the less developed countries in general, it is expected that this will increase markedly as smoking takes hold and larger numbers of young smokers grow older.

Tobacco in all forms was consumed to the extent of 6.5 billion kg annually in the period 1990–1992, and there were six trillion cigarettes sold. It does not appear that tobacco use will disappear in the near future.

Worldwide, smoking is estimated to have caused about 1.05 million cancer deaths in 1990. About 30% of all cancer death in developed countries is caused by smoking. The corresponding figure for developing countries is 13%. Lung cancer is the dominant malignancy caused by smoking, with 514,000 lung cancer deaths attributed to smoking in developed countries in 1995. Smoking is also an important cause of bladder cancer, cancer of the renal pelvis, oral cancer, oropharyngeal cancer, hypopharyngeal cancer, laryngeal cancer, esophageal cancer, and pancreatic cancer. Other cancers that may be caused by smoking include renal adenocarcinoma, cancer of the cervix, myeloid leukemia, colon cancer, and stomach cancer. In the United States, about 30% of all cancer death is caused by smoking, similar to worldwide estimates for developed countries.

Lung cancer was rare at the beginning of the 20th century. However, the incidence and death rates increased as smoking became more popular. In the United States, the lung cancer death rate in 1930 for men was 4.9 per 100,000. By 1990, this had increased to 75.6 per 100,000. The lung cancer death rate can be shown to parallel the curves for cigarette smoking prevalence, with an approximate 20-year lag time. In 1964, the first Surgeon General's report on the health consequences of cigarette smoking was published. Following this landmark report, smoking prevalence began to decrease in the United States, but there has been no change since 1990. There are still 47 million adult smokers in the United States.

Unburned tobacco is a cause of oral cavity cancer. The annual mortality from tobacco chewing in south Asia, where it is used primarily in the form of betel quid, is estimated to be of the order of 50,000 deaths per year. Oral cavity cancer is the leading cancer killer in India. Snuff dipping, as practiced in North America, is an accepted cause of oral cavity cancer as well. The prevalence of snuff dipping has increased markedly in recent years in the United States, especially among young males.

II. TUMOR INDUCTION IN LABORATORY ANIMALS

One goal of scientists studying tobacco carcinogenesis has been to replicate in laboratory animals the effects of tobacco products that are observed in humans. This has been challenging for a variety of reasons, which can be summarized simply: laboratory animals will not voluntarily use tobacco products the way humans do.

The International Agency for Research on Cancer has reviewed and summarized this work. According to their conclusions, experimental studies evaluating the ability of cigarette smoke and its condensate to cause cancer in laboratory animals have collectively demonstrated that there is sufficient evidence that inhalation of tobacco smoke, as well as topical application of tobacco smoke condensate, causes cancer in experimental animals. The Syrian golden hamster has been the model of choice for inhalation studies of cigarette smoke because it has a low background incidence of spontaneous pulmonary tumors and little interfering respiratory infection. Inhalation of cigarette smoke has repeatedly caused carcinomas in the larynx of hamsters and this model system has been widely applied. It is the most reliable model for induction of tumors by inhalation of cigarette smoke. Studies in mice, rats, and dogs have been less frequent.

According to the International Agency for Research on Cancer, there are a number of operational problems inherent in inhalation studies of cigarette smoke. The smoke must be delivered in a standardized fashion and this has been accomplished in different ways. Both whole body exposure and nose-only exposure designs have been used. Generally, a 2-s puff from a burning cigarette is diluted with air and forced into the chamber. Animals will undergo avoidance reactions and will not inhale the smoke. Thus, the dose to the lung is less than in humans, which partially explains the occurrence of larynx tumors rather than lung tumors in hamsters. Unlike humans, rodents are obligatory nose breathers. Their nasal passages are more complex than those of humans, thereby affecting particle deposition in the respiratory tract. Tobacco smoke is irritating and toxic, creating further problems in inhalation studies with rodents.

Inhalation studies have reproducibly demonstrated that cigarette smoke, especially its particulate phase, causes laryngeal carcinomas in hamsters. Some experiments with mice resulted in low incidences of lung tumors, in tests of both mainstream smoke and environmental tobacco smoke. Evidence shows that gas phase components of cigarette smoke may be tumorigenic in mice. Respiratory tract tumors were produced in one long-term exposure of rats to cigarette smoke. Studies in rabbits and dogs were equivocal. Treatment-related tumors other than those of the respiratory tract have not been consistently observed.

Cigarette smoke condensate (CSC) has been tested extensively for tumor induction. CSC is produced by passing smoke through cold traps. The material in the traps is recovered by washing with a volatile solvent, which is then evaporated. Some volatile and semi-volatile constituents may be lost during this process. CSC is roughly equivalent to cigarette total particulate matter (TPM), the material collected on a glass fiber filter that has had smoke drawn through it. The term "tar," which is often used in official reports on cigarette brands, is equivalent to TPM but without nicotine and water.

CSC generation and collection techniques have been standardized. CSC has been widely tested for carcinogenicity in mouse skin. Consistently, CSC induces benign and malignant skin tumors in mice. This bioassay has been employed to evaluate the carcinogenic activities of cigarettes of different designs and to investigate subfractions of CSC. Mouse skin studies led to the identification of carcinogenic polycyclic aromatic hydrocarbons in cigarette smoke. The overall carcinogenic effect of CSC on mouse skin appears to depend on the composite interaction of tumor initiators and enhancing factors, such as tumor promoters and cocarcinogens.

Many studies have evaluated tumor induction in rodents by extracts of unburned tobacco. Although some positive results have been obtained, there is presently no widely accepted and reproducible model for the induction of oral cavity cancer in rodents by tobacco extracts, despite strong human data. There are probably cofactors that contribute to human oral cancer upon tobacco use, which are not reproduced in animal studies.

III. CARCINOGENS IN TOBACCO AND TOBACCO SMOKE

A second important goal of scientists in the field of tobacco carcinogenesis has been the identification of carcinogens in tobacco products. When these compounds are identified, studies can be designed to investigate the mechanisms by which they cause cancer, which in turn can provide important insights on the ways in which tobacco products cause cancer in humans.

When cigarette tobacco is burned, mainstream smoke and sidestream smoke are produced. Mainstream smoke is the material drawn from the mouth end of a cigarette during puffing. Sidestream smoke is the material released into the air from the burning tip of the cigarette plus that which diffuses through the paper.

The mainstream smoke emerging from the cigarette is an aerosol containing about 1×10^{10} particles/ml, ranging in diameter from 0.1 to 1.0 μm (mean diameter 0.2 μm). About 95% of the smoke is made up of gases— predominantly nitrogen, oxygen, and carbon dioxide. For chemical analysis, the smoke is arbitrarily separated into a vapor phase and a particulate phase, based on passage through a glass-fiber filter pad called a Cambridge filter. In addition to nitrogen, oxygen, and carbon dioxide, the gas phase contains substantial amounts of carbon monoxide, water, argon, hydrogen, ammonia, nitrogen oxides, hydrogen cyanide, hydrogen sulfide, methane, isoprene, butadiene, formaldehyde, acrolein, pyridine, and other compounds. The particulate phase contains more than 3500 compounds, and most of the carcinogens. Some major constituents of the particulate phase include nicotine and related alkaloids, hydrocarbons, phenol, catechol, solanesol, neophytadienes, fatty acids, and others. Many of the components are present in higher concentration in sidestream smoke than in mainstream smoke; this is especially true of nitrogen-containing compounds. However, a person's exposure to sidestream smoke is generally far less than to mainstream smoke because of dilution with room air.

There are over sixty carcinogens in cigarette smoke that have been evaluated by the International Agency for Research on Cancer and for which there is "sufficient evidence for carcinogenicity" in either laboratory animals or humans. The types of carcinogens, based on their chemical classes, are listed in Table I. Carcinogens specifically associated with lung cancer are listed in Table II. The 20 compounds included in this list have been found convincingly to induce lung tumors in at least one animal species and have been positively identified in cigarette smoke. Structures of the organic compounds are shown in Fig. 1. These compounds are most likely involved in lung cancer induction in people who smoke.

Polycyclic aromatic hydrocarbons are condensed ring aromatic compounds that are formed during all incomplete combustion reactions, such as those that occur in the burning cigarette. Among these, benzo[a]pyrene (BaP) is the most extensively studied compound. Its presence in cigarette smoke and ability to induce lung tumors upon local administration or inhalation are firmly established. It causes lung tumors in mice, but not in rats, when administered systemically. In studies of lung tumor induction by implantation in rats, BaP is more carcinogenic than several other polycyclic aromatic hydrocarbons in tobacco smoke.

Aza-arenes are nitrogen-containing analogs of polycyclic aromatic hydrocarbons. Two aza-arenes, dibenz[a,h]acridine and 7H-dibenzo[c,g]carbazole, are pulmonary tumorigens when tested by implantation in the rat lung and instillation in the hamster trachea, respectively. The carcinogenic activity of dibenz[a,h]acridine is less than that of BaP, whereas that of 7H-dibenzo[c,g]carbazole is greater than BaP. The levels of both compounds in cigarette smoke are relatively low.

N-Nitrosamines comprise a large group of potent carcinogens. Among these, N-nitrosodiethylamine is an effective pulmonary carcinogen in the hamster, but not the rat. Its levels in cigarette smoke are low compared to those of other carcinogens. 4-(Methylnitrosamino)-1-(3-pyridyl)-1-butanone (NNK) is a potent lung carcinogen in rats, mice, and hamsters. NNK is called a tobacco-specific N-nitrosamine because it is a chemical derivative of nicotine, and thus occurs only in tobacco products. It is the only compound in Table II that induces lung tumors systemically in all three commonly used rodent models. The specificity of NNK for tumor induction in the lung is remarkable; it induces lung tumors independent of the route of administration and in

TABLE I
Summary of Carcinogens in
Cigarette Smoke

Type	Number of compounds
Polycyclic aromatic hydrocarbons	10
Aza-arenes	3
N-Nitrosamines	10
Aromatic amines	4
Heterocyclic aromatic amines	8
Aldehydes	2
Miscellaneous organic compounds	18
Inorganic compounds	7
Total	62

TABLE II
Pulmonary Carcinogens in Cigarette Smoke

Carcinogen class	Compound	Amount in mainstream cigarette smoke (ng/cigarette)	Sidestream/mainstream smoke ratio	Representative lung tumorigenicity in species
Polycyclic aromatic hydrocarbons	Benzo[a]pyrene	20–40	2.5–3.5	Mouse, rat, hamster
	Benzo[b]fluoranthane	4–22		Rat
	Benzo[j]fluoranthane	6–21		Rat
	Benzo[k]fluoranthane	6–12		Rat
	Dibenzo[a,i]pyrene	1.7–3.2		Hamster
	Indeno[1,2,3-cd]pyrene	4–20		Rat
	Dibenz[a,h]anthracene	4		Mouse
	5-Methylchrysene	0.6		Mouse
Aza-arenes	Dibenz[a,h]acridine	0.1		Rat
	7H-Dibenzo[c,g]carbazole	0.7		Hamster
N-Nitrosamines	N-Nitrosodiethylamine	ND–2.8	<40	Hamster
	4-(Methylnitrosamino)-1-(3-pyridyl)-1-butanone	80–770	1–4	Mouse, rat, hamster
Miscellaneous organic compounds	1,3-Butadiene	$20–70 \times 10^3$		Mouse
	Ethyl carbamate	20–38		Mouse
Inorganic compounds	Nickel	0–510	13–30	Rat
	Chromium	0.2–500		Rat
	Cadmium	0–6670	7.2	Rat
	Polonium-210	0.03–1.0 pCi	1.0–4.0	Hamster
	Arsenic	0–1400		None
	Hydrazine	24–43		Mouse

both susceptible and resistant strains of mice. The systemic administration of NNK to rats is a reproducible and robust method for the induction of lung tumors. Cigarette smoke contains substantial amounts of NNK, and the total dose experienced by a smoker in a lifetime of smoking is remarkably close to the lowest total dose shown to induce lung tumors in rats. Levels of NNK and total polycyclic aromatic hydrocarbons in cigarette smoke are similar.

Lung is one of the multiple sites of tumorigenesis by 1,3-butadiene in mice, but is not a target in the rat. Ethyl carbamate is a well-established pulmonary carcinogen in mice but not in other species. Nickel, chromium, cadmium, and arsenic are all present in tobacco and a percentage of each is transferred to mainstream smoke; arsenic levels are substantially lower since discontinuation of its use as a pesticide in 1952. Metal carcinogenicity depends on the valence state and anion; these are poorly defined in many analytical studies of tobacco smoke. Thus, although some metals are effective pulmonary carcinogens, the role of metals in tobacco-induced lung cancer is un-

clear. Levels of polonium-210 in tobacco smoke are not believed to be great enough to appreciably impact lung cancer in smokers. Hydrazine is an effective lung carcinogen in mice and has been detected in cigarette smoke in limited studies.

Considerable data indicate that polycyclic aromatic hydrocarbons and NNK play very important roles as causes of lung cancer in people who smoke. The other compounds discussed earlier may also contribute, but probably to a lesser extent.

Polycyclic aromatic hydrocarbons and N-nitrosamines such as NNK and N'-nitrosonornicotine (NNN) are probably involved as causes of oral cavity cancer in smokers. N-Nitrosamines such as NNN and NDEA are likely causes of esophageal cancer in smokers. The risk of oral cavity cancer and esophageal cancer in smokers is markedly enhanced by the consumption of alcoholic beverages. NNK is also believed to play a prominent role in the induction of pancreatic cancer in smokers, whereas aromatic amines such as 4-aminobiphenyl and 2-naphthylamine are the most likely causes of bladder cancer.

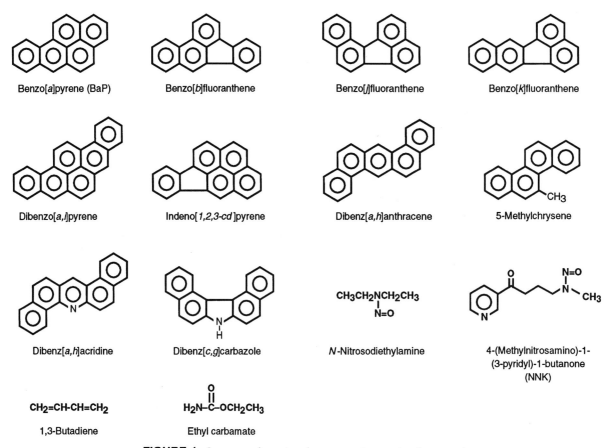

FIGURE 1   Structures of organic pulmonary carcinogens in tobacco smoke.

Cigarette smoke and CSC are tumor promoters, e.g., they enhance the carcinogenicity of tumor initiators when administered subsequent to the initiators. The majority of the tumor-promoting activity seems to be due to uncharacterized weakly acidic compounds. Substantial levels of cocarcinogens, which enhance the carcinogenicity of tumor initiators when applied together with the initiators, are present in cigarette smoke. Catechol is prominent among these. In addition, cigarette smoke contains high levels of acrolein, which is toxic to the pulmonary cilia, and other agents such as nitrogen oxides, acetaldehyde, and formaldehyde, which could contribute indirectly to pulmonary carcinogenicity through their toxic effects.

While cigarette smoke is extraordinarily complex, unburned tobacco is simpler. With respect to carcinogens, the tobacco-specific nitrosamines NNK and NNN are the most prevalent strong cancer-causing agents in unburned tobacco products. A mixture of

NNK and NNN induces oral tumors in rats, and consequently these compounds are considered to play an important role as causes of oral cavity cancer in people who use smokeless tobacco products.

IV. MECHANISMS OF TUMOR INDUCTION

The mechanisms by which tobacco causes cancer can best be illustrated by considering the relationship between cigarette smoking and lung cancer because it is here that the most information is available. The overall framework for discussing this information is illustrated in Fig. 2. Carcinogens form the link between nicotine addiction and cancer. Nicotine addiction is the reason that people continue to smoke. While nicotine itself is not considered to be carcinogenic, each cigarette contains a mixture of carcinogens.

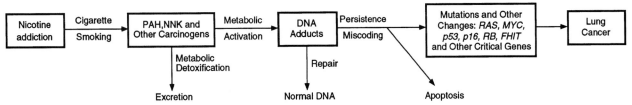

FIGURE 2 Scheme linking nicotine addiction and lung cancer via tobacco smoke carcinogens and their induction of multiple mutations in critical genes. PAH, polycyclic aromatic hydrocarbons; NNK, 4-(methylnitrosamino)-1-(3-pyridyl)-1-butane.

Thus, cigarettes are disastrous nicotine delivery devices. Most of the carcinogens in cigarette smoke require metabolic activation, i.e., they must be enzymatically transformed by the host into reactive intermediates in order to exert their carcinogenic effects. There are competing detoxification pathways, which result in harmless excretion of the carcinogens. The balance between metabolic activation and detoxification differs among individuals and will affect cancer risk.

A great deal is known about mechanisms of carcinogen metabolic activation and detoxification. The metabolic activation process leads to the formation of DNA adducts, which are carcinogen metabolites bound covalently to DNA, usually at guanine or adenine. There have been major advances in our understanding of DNA adduct structure and its consequences in the past two decades and there is now a large amount of mechanistic information available. If DNA adducts escape cellular repair mechanisms and persist, they can cause miscoding, resulting in a permanent mutation in DNA. This occurs when DNA polymerase enzymes read an adducted DNA base incorrectly, resulting in the insertion of the wrong base. Other errors can also occur due to the presence of DNA adducts. Cells that contain damaged DNA may be removed by apoptosis, or programmed cell death. If a permanent mutation occurs in a critical region of an oncogene or tumor suppressor gene, it can lead to activation of the oncogene or deactivation of the tumor suppressor gene. Oncogenes and tumor suppressor genes play critical roles in the normal regulation of cellular growth. Changes in multiple oncogenes or tumor suppressor genes result in the production of aberrant cells with loss of normal growth control. Ultimately, this leads to lung cancer. While the sequence of events has not been well defined, there can be lit-

tle doubt that these molecular changes are important. There is now a large amount of data on mutations in the human K-*ras* oncogene and *p53* tumor suppressor gene in lung tumors from smokers.

Blocking any of the horizontal steps in Fig. 2 may lead to decreased lung cancer, even in people who continue to smoke. The following discussion considers some of these steps in more detail.

Upon inhalation, cigarette smoke carcinogens are enzymatically transformed to a series of metabolites as the exposed organism attempts to convert them to forms that are more readily excreted. The initial steps are usually carried out by cytochrome P450 (P450) enzymes, which add oxygen to the substrate. These enzymes typically are responsible for the metabolism of drugs, other foreign compounds, and some endogenous substrates. Other enzymes, such as lipoxygenases, cyclooxygenases, myeloperoxidase, and monoamine oxidases, may also be involved, but less frequently. The oxygenated intermediates formed in these initial reactions may undergo further transformations by glutathione-*S*-transferases, uridine-5'-diphosphate-glucuronosyltransferases, sulfatases, and other enzymes, which are typically involved in detoxification. Some of the metabolites produced by P450s react with DNA or other macromolecules to form adducts. Metabolic pathways of BaP and NNK, representative pulmonary carcinogens in cigarette smoke, have been extensively defined through studies in rodent and human tissues. The major metabolic activation pathway of BaP is conversion to a reactive diol epoxide metabolite called BPDE; one of the four isomers produced is highly carcinogenic and reacts with DNA to form adducts with N^2- of deoxyguanosine. The major metabolic activation pathways of NNK and its main metabolite, 4-(methylnitrosamino)-1-(3-pyridyl)-1-butanol (NNAL), occur by hydroxylation of the carbons adjacent to the N-nitroso group (α-hydroxylation), which leads to the formation of two types of DNA adducts: methyl adducts, such as 7-methyguanine or O^6-methylguanine, and pyridyloxobutyl adducts.

Considerable information is available on pulmonary carcinogen metabolism *in vitro*, both in animal and in human tissues, but fewer studies have been carried out on uptake, metabolism, and adduct formation of cigarette smoke lung carcinogens in smokers. Various measures of cigarette smoke uptake in humans have been used, including exhaled carbon monoxide, carboxyhemoglobin, thiocyanate, and urinary mutagenicity. However, the most specific and widely used biochemical marker is the nicotine metabolite cotinine. While cotinine and other nicotine metabolites are excellent indicators of tobacco smoke constituent uptake by smokers, the NNK metabolites NNAL and its O-glucuronide (NNAL-Gluc) are excellent biomarkers of tobacco smoke lung carcinogen uptake.

BaP has been detected in human lung; no differences between smokers and nonsmokers were noted. 1-Hydroxypyrene and its glucuronide, urinary metabolites of the noncarcinogen pyrene, have been widely used as indicators of polycyclic aromatic hydrocarbon uptake. 1-Hydroxypyrene levels in smokers are generally higher than in nonsmokers. Overall, there is considerable evidence that pulmonary carcinogens in cigarette smoke are taken up and metabolized by smokers as well as by nonsmokers exposed to environmental tobacco smoke.

Less than 20% of smokers will get lung cancer. Susceptibility will depend in part on the balance between carcinogen metabolic activation and detoxification in smokers. This is an important area requiring further study. Most investigations have focused on the metabolic activation pathways by quantifying DNA or protein adducts. There is considerable data demonstrating the activation of BaP to DNA adducts in the lungs of smokers. Earlier investigations demonstrated that cigarette smoke induces aryl hydrocarbon hydroxylase (AHH) activity and proposed a relationship between AHH activity and lung cancer. AHH metabolizes BaP and is equivalent to P450 1A1. Cigarette smoking induces expression of this enzyme. Lung tissue from recent smokers with elevated AHH activity metabolically activated BaP to a greater extent than lung tissue from nonsmokers or ex-smokers. DNA adduct levels correlated with AHH activity in the same samples. Collectively, these results support the existence of a cigarette smoke-inducible pathway leading to BaP–DNA adducts in smokers' lungs (Fig. 2).

Several studies have detected 7-methylguanine in human lung. Levels were higher in smokers than in nonsmokers in two studies, suggesting that NNK may be one source of these adducts. While 7-methylguanine is not generally considered as an adduct that would lead to miscoding in DNA and the introduction of a permanent mutation, other methyl adducts that do have miscoding properties, such as O^6-methylguanine, are formed at the same time, but at lower levels. Pyridyloxobutylated DNA also has been detected in lung tissue from smokers, reflecting metabolic activation of NNK or NNN. The detection of methyl and pyridyloxobutyl adducts in DNA from smokers' lungs is consistent with the ability of human lung tissue to metabolically activate NNK, but the quantitative aspects of the relationship of metabolism to DNA adduct levels are unclear.

DNA repair processes are important in determining whether DNA adducts persist. Because smoking is a chronic habit, one would expect a steady-state DNA adduct level to be achieved by the opposing effects of damage and repair. Mechanisms of DNA repair include direct repair, base excision repair, and nucleotide excision repair. With respect to smoking and lung cancer, direct repair of O^6-methylguanine by O^6-methylguanine–DNA alkyltransferase and nucleotide excision repair of polycyclic aromatic hydrocarbon–DNA adducts would appear to be the most relevant processes.

As indicated in Fig. 2, the direct interaction of metabolically activated carcinogens with critical genes such as the p53 tumor suppressor gene and the K-*ras* oncogene is central to the hypothesis that specific carcinogens form the link between nicotine addiction and lung cancer. The p53 gene plays a critical role in the delicate balance of cellular proliferation and death. It is mutated in about half of all cancer types, including over 50% of lung cancers, leading to loss of its activity for cellular regulation. Point mutations at guanine (G) are common. In a sample of 550 p53 mutations in lung tumors, 33% were G $\rightarrow$ T transversions, whereas 26% were G $\rightarrow$ A transitions. (A purine $\rightarrow$ pyrimidine or pyrimidine $\rightarrow$ purine mutation is referred to as a transversion, whereas a purine $\rightarrow$ purine or pyrimidine $\rightarrow$ pyrimidine mutation is called a transition.) A positive relationship between lifetime cigarette consumption and the frequency of p53 mutations and of G → T transversions on the nontranscribed DNA strand also has been noted. These observations are generally consistent with the fact that most activated carcinogens react predominantly at G and that repair of the resulting adducts would be slower on the nontranscribed strand, thus supporting the hypothesis outlined in Fig. 2.

Mutations in codon 12 of the K-*ras* oncogene are found in 24–50% of human primary adenocarcinomas but are rarely seen in other lung tumor types. When K-*ras* is mutated, a complex series of cellular growth signals is initiated. Mutations in K-*ras* are more common in smokers and ex-smokers than in nonsmokers, which suggests that they may be induced by direct reaction of the gene with an activated tobacco smoke carcinogen. The most commonly observed mutation is GGT → TGT, which typically accounts for about 60% of the codon 12 mutations, followed by GGT → GAT (20%) and GGT → GTT (15%).

The p16^{INK4a} tumor suppressor gene is inactivated in more than 70% of human nonsmall cell lung cancers via homozygous deletion or in association with aberrant hypermethylation of the promoter region. In the rat, 94% of adenocarcinomas induced by NNK were hypermethylated at the p16 gene promoter. This change was frequently detected in hyperplastic lesions and adenomas, which are precursors to the adenocarcinomas induced by NNK. Similar results were found in human squamous cell carcinomas of the lung. The p16 gene was coordinately methylated in 75% of carcinoma *in situ* lesions adjacent to squamous cell carcinomas that had this change. Methylation of p16 was associated with loss of expression in tumors and precursor lesions, indicating functional inactivation of both alleles. Aberrant methylation of p16 has been suggested as an early marker for lung cancer. The expression of cell cycle proteins is related to the p16 and retinoblastoma tumor suppressor genes; NNK-induced mouse lung tumors appear to resemble human nonsmall cell lung cancer in the expression of cell cycle proteins. The estrogen receptor gene is also inactivated through promoter methylation. There was concordance between the incidence of promoter methylation in this gene in lung tumors from smokers and from NNK-treated rodents.

Loss of heterozygosity and exon deletions within the fragile histidine triad (FHIT) gene are associated with smoking habits in lung cancer patients and have been proposed as a target for tobacco smoke carcinogens. However, point mutations within the coding region of the FHIT gene were not found in primary lung tumors.

Collectively, evidence favoring the sequence of steps illustrated in Fig. 2 as an overall mechanism of tobacco-induced cancer is extremely strong, although there are important aspects of each step that require further study. These include carcinogen metabolism and DNA binding in human lung, the effects of cigarette smoke on DNA repair and adduct persistence, the relationship between specific carcinogens and mutations in critical genes, and the sequence of genetic changes leading to lung cancer.

Using a weight of the evidence approach, specific polycyclic aromatic hydrocarbons such as BaP and the tobacco-specific nitrosamine NNK can be identified as probable causes of lung cancer in smokers, but the contribution of other agents, such as those listed in Table II, cannot be excluded. The chronic exposure of smokers to the DNA-damaging intermediates formed from these carcinogens is consistent with our present understanding of cancer induction as a process that requires multiple genetic changes. Thus, it is completely plausible that the continual barrage of DNA damage produced by tobacco smoke carcinogens causes the multiple genetic changes that are associated with lung cancer. While each dose of carcinogen from a cigarette is extremely small, the cumulative damage produced in years of smoking is substantial.

V. SUMMARY

Although substantial progress has been accomplished in reducing the tobacco habit, worldwide use of tobacco products is still immense, due mainly to the addictive power of nicotine, arguably the single compound responsible indirectly for more cancer death than any other chemical. Tobacco products cause about 30% of all cancer death. Since the mid-1950s, studies in tobacco carcinogenesis have identified the major carcinogens in tobacco smoke and have elucidated the overall framework by which these carcinogens cause cancer in people. This series of steps, as illustrated in Fig. 2, is well established, although many details remain unclear. Blocking any of the horizontal steps in Fig. 2, even in people who continue to smoke, would result in decreased cancer mortality. Identification of individuals particularly susceptible to the carcinogenic properties of tobacco products would also be important. Rational approaches are now possible in this regard and, even if only partially successful, could have a major impact on cancer mortality because of the sheer magnitude of the epidemic of cancer death caused by tobacco products.

Acknowledgments

Our studies in tobacco carcinogenesis are supported by Grants CA-44377, CA-81301, and CA-85702 from the National Cancer Institute. The author is an American Cancer Society Research Professor, supported by Grant RP-00-138.

See Also the Following Articles

Bibliography

Blot, W. J., and Fraumeni, J. F., Jr. (1996). Cancers of the lung and pleura. *In* "Cancer Epidemiology and Prevention" (D. Schottenfeld and J. Fraumeni, eds.), pp. 637–665. Oxford Univ. Press, New York.

Doll, R. (1996). Cancers weakly related to smoking. *Brit. Med. J.* **52,** 35–49.

Guengerich, F. P., and Shimada, T. (1998). Activation of procarcinogens by human cytochrome P450 enzymes. *Mutat. Res.* **400,** 201–213.

Guerin, M. R., Jenkins, R. A., and Tomkins, B. A. (1992). "The Chemistry of Environmental Tobacco Smoke: Composition and Management." Lewis Publishers, Chelsea, MI.

Hecht, S. S. (1998). Biochemistry, biology, and carcinogenicity of tobacco-specific *N*-nitrosamines. *Chem. Res. Toxicol.* **11,** 559–603.

Hecht, S. S. (1999). Tobacco smoke carcinogens and lung cancer. *J. Natl. Cancer Inst.* **91,** 1194–1210.

Hoffmann, D., and Hecht, S. S. (1990). Advances in tobacco carcinogenesis. *In* "Handbook of Experimental Pharmacology" (C. S. Cooper and P. L. Grover, eds.), pp. 63–102. Springer-Verlag, Heidelberg.

Hoffmann, D., and Hoffmann, I. (1997). The changing cigarette, 1950–1995. *J. Toxicol. Environ. Health* **50,** 307–364.

International Agency for Research on Cancer (1985). Tobacco habits other than smoking: Betel quid and areca nut chewing and some related nitrosamines. *In* "Monographs on the Evaluation of the Carcinogenic Risk of Chemicals to Humans," Vol. 37. IARC, Lyon.

International Agency for Research on Cancer (1986). Tobacco smoking. *In* "Monographs on the Evaluation of the Carcinogenic Risk of Chemicals to Humans," Vol. 38. IARC, Lyon.

Sekido, Y., Fong, K. W., and Minna, J. D. (1998). Progress in understanding the molecular pathogenesis of human lung cancer. *Biochim. Biophys. Acta* **1378,** F21–F59.

Smith, T. J., Livingston, S. D., and Doolittle, O. J. (1997). An international literature survey of "IARC group I carcinogens" reported in mainstream cigarette smoke. *Food Chem. Toxicol.* **35,** 1107–1130.

World Health Organization (1997). "Tobacco or Health: A Global Status Report." World Health Organization, Geneva.

Total Body Irradiation

Brenda Shank

Doctors Medical Center, San Pablo, and
University of California, San Francisco

GLOSSARY

boosting Giving an additional dose of irradiation to a smaller volume within a large treatment volume so that the smaller volume reaches a higher total dose than the large volume; usually done so that the area at greatest risk of having a larger concentration of tumor cells receives a higher dose to eradicate those cells.

cell survival curve A graphic representation of the percentage of cells surviving after treatment with a chemical or physical agent on the y-axis versus the dose of the agent on the x-axis.

compensator A device usually constructed out of a metal or a metal alloy placed between the radiation beam and the patient to compensate for irregularities in the contour of the patient so that the dose actually delivered to a volume within the patient is as homogeneous as possible.

linear quadratic (LQ) model A formula to calculate cell survival as a function of the dose per fraction of irradiation and the number of fractions of irradiation.

T otal body irradiation (TBI) and other large field variations, such as total lymphoid irradiation (TLI) and total abdominal irradiation (TAI), play an important role in preparative cytoreductive regimens for bone marrow transplantation (BMT). There are three main purposes of TBI: immunosuppression (lymphocyte cell kill) to allow engraftment of donor marrow, eradication of malignant cells (leukemias, lymphomas, and some solid tumors), and eradication of cell populations with genetic disorders (Fanconi's anemia, thalassemia major, etc.).

I. INTRODUCTION

A. Advantages of TBI Compared with Chemotherapy

There are many theoretical advantages of TBI as a systemic agent when compared with chemotherapy: (1) there is no sparing of "sanctuary" sites such as the testes; (2) the dose delivered is fairly homogeneous and independent of blood supply; (3) there is no cross-resistance with other agents; (4) because no detoxification or excretion of a chemical agent is necessary, there is no alteration of dose if these mechanisms are impaired; and (5) the dose distribution within the body may be tailored by either blocking normal tissues that are more sensitive or "boosting" areas at greater risk of recurrence.

Because of the toxicity of the high TBI doses that would be required to immunosuppress adequately for consistent donor marrow engraftment and to eradicate malignancies sufficiently to obtain cures, TBI has been combined with chemotherapeutic agents.

B. Current Cytoreductive Therapy Usage

From data published by the International Bone Marrow Transplant Registry (IBMTR) in 1992, the majority of allogeneic marrow transplants (73%) are performed for leukemia. Other malignancies make up 10%, aplastic anemia, 8%, with the remainder being for genetic disorders and immune deficiencies. TBI has been a major component of most regimens for leukemia, although many centers have been investigating the use of alternative chemotherapy-only regimens with some success. TAI and TLI fields may be adequate when only immunosuppression is needed, as for aplastic anemia, or when only nodal areas need to be treated, as in refractory Hodgkin's disease without marrow involvement.

Many investigators have been looking at alternative regimens containing only chemotherapy for cytoreduction to avoid the toxicities attributed to TBI.

Several randomized studies have been done comparing busulfan and cyclophosphamide (Bu-Cy) to TBI-containing regimens. Although there may be some advantage of TBI-containing regimens in patients with acute myeloid leukemia (AML), no advantage has been seen with patients with chronic myeloid leukemia (CML) in the chronic phase, even with follow-up longer than 7 years, as demonstrated in Seattle data. However, for patients with later stages of CML studied in the Nordic Bone Marrow Transplant Group, there was a significant leukemia-free survival advantage and less transplant-related morbidity.

II. BIOLOGICAL PRINCIPLES

A. Normal Lymphocytes and Leukemic Cells

Immunosuppression, the clinical manifestation of reduced lymphocyte numbers or activity, is an important function of TBI. Cell culture studies, supported by studies of lymphocyte survival *in vivo*, demonstrate either no or a very small shoulder to the cell survival curve,

indicating minimal repair. Lymphocyte survival in patients undergoing TBI appears similar to *in vitro* data.

Leukemic cells also have either no shoulder or a minimal shoulder to the cell survival curve. Because many investigators have now studied survival in a variety of leukemic cells, sufficient data indicate the following: (1) the shoulder and slope of survival curves vary widely for different cell types and for different cell lines from the same type of leukemia, (2) some cell lines have no repair at all, whereas others exhibit definite repair, and (3) most human hematopoietic cell lines studied have survival curves that fit the linear quadratic (LQ) model of cell survival.

B. Animal Data

In marrow transplantation, the degree of immunosuppression is reflected clinically in the success of engraftment of donor marrow. In dogs, the rate of engraftment increases with increasing doses of irradiation, and single-dose irradiation is more immunosuppressive than fractionated irradiation for the same total dose. Other studies in mice, rats, and monkeys support this; with fractionated irradiation, higher total doses are necessary for engraftment when compared with single-dose irradiation. In mice, engraftment depends critically on the TBI dose; the required TBI dose increases with greater genetic disparity between donor and host.

One important question has been the issue of sequencing of TBI with Cy; traditionally, marrow transplantation regimens gave Cy prior to TBI, but in the last decade, many centers changed to delivering TBI up-front, with the advantage of better tolerance of the many fractions of TBI in fractionated regimens, especially when the patient was in the standing position. Radiobiological studies in animals and humans have shown that increasing the number of fractions, for a given total dose, contributes greatly to decreasing the incidence of interstitial pneumonitis (IP). As a corollary, increasing the number of fractions allows one to increase the total dose for the same biologic effect.

C. Schedule Optimization

Many investigators have attempted to use available data to model the effects of TBI and to optimize its schedule. Theoretical studies have generally suggested that fractionated regimens (daily or two to three fractions/day) have an advantage with regard to minimizing toxicity and allowing higher total doses to be given, thereby maximizing leukemic cell kill. Single-dose, low-dose rate TBI could potentially be radio-biologically equivalent to fractionated TBI, but this would require unduly long treatment times (about 24 h).

D. Interaction with Chemotherapy

The principal chemotherapeutic agents that have been used with TBI are Cy, VP-16, and AraC. With Cy, toxicities of greatest concern have been IP and hemorrhagic cystitis. VP-16 has been used increasingly in regimens for acute lymphoblastic leukemia (ALL). Major toxicities in combination with TBI have not appeared to be a problem. AraC, however, has been implicated in an increased risk for renal toxicity.

E. Physiologic Considerations

1. Orthostatic Hypotension

Occasionally, patients have experienced syncope during the course of TBI in the standing position; most often, this has been attributable to the administration of a phenothiazine, which can cause orthostatic hypotension. Use of nonphenothiazine antiemetics usually ameliorates this problem. Occasionally, especially in patients with aplastic anemia, syncope may be caused by brain hypoxia resulting from a combination of their anemia and hypotension in the standing position. Transfusion with packed red cells usually eliminates this problem.

2. Nausea and Vomiting

The most common acute side effects observed, regardless of regimen used, have been nausea and vomiting. These have been noted to be less intense with fractionated regimens compared with single-dose regimens, but they have persisted. Both ondansetron and granisetron have demonstrated effectiveness in decreasing the number of emetic episodes in randomized trials.

III. PHYSICAL PRINCIPLES

A. Reproducibility

To ensure reproducibility from one fraction to another and consistency throughout the course of one fraction, patient position and immobilization must be considered. In brief, patients today are treated either standing up with anterior and posterior fields or lying supine and/or prone with anterior and posterior fields, lateral fields, or a combination of both. When the patient is lying down, the patient is comfortable and motion during relatively short fractions (10–15 min) is minimal. When the patient is standing for that long, however, some form of immobilization is necessary. Many centers have developed some form of a TBI stand to help support and immobilize the patient. A stand developed at Memorial Sloan-Kettering Cancer Center (MSKCC) incorporates a bicycle seat and hand grips for greater patient security, as well as devices to control movement of the thorax region and support lung shields and port film holders. This stand was demonstrated to increase accuracy and reproducibility of lung shield placement.

B. Homogeneity

It is assumed, in patients with leukemia, that leukemic cells may be dispersed anywhere throughout the body, including within the skin. Most centers in the United States have used energies that range from that of Co-60 (1.25 MV) to 10 MV with a linear accelerator; these have a dose build-up region upon entering tissue, which could potentially result in underdosing the skin. To prevent this potential underdosage when energies greater than that of Co-60 are utilized, it is necessary to introduce a screen made of a tissue-equivalent material between the beam and the patient to maintain dose homogeneity.

At some institutions, compensators have also been used at the neck, feet, and other areas to increase homogeneity, especially when beams of $\geq$10 MV have been used. TBI dose variability within the patient of $\pm$5% is considered excellent, but $\pm$10% is considered acceptable.

C. Dose Rate

When TBI is given in a single dose to a total dose of 10 Gy, it is necessary to use a low-dose rate ($\leq$0.05 Gy/min) to decrease the probability of IP. With higher dose rates, the total dose given would have to be reduced, but this may contribute to a higher relapse rate. For fractionated TBI schedules with a small dose per fraction, dose rate becomes less important. When fraction sizes of $\leq$1.5 Gy are used, dose rates usually range from 0.05 to 0.18 Gy/min.

D. Blocking

Many centers use lung shields during TBI. Some institutions have attempted to shield the lungs with the patient's arms by treating the patient laterally. This is, however, difficult to both reproduce and assess the dosimetry and is not recommended.

One institution has used partial transmission liver shielding to decrease the incidence of veno-occlusive disease (VOD) and has also used renal shielding (70% transmission) to minimize renal dysfunction in the setting of cytoreduction, which included both AraC and Cy. Renal dysfunction at 18 months is significantly less with the use of these blocks, but long-term results with respect to relapse and survival are not available.

E. "Boosting"

When lung blocks were used, it was originally felt that it was necessary to supplement the dose by means of electrons to marrow-containing ribs in the area of the lung blocks ("boosting") to ensure that an adequate dose was given to all potential sites of leukemia. It has been calculated that blocking lungs is theoretically equivalent to merely lowering the total body dose by a small percentage. Because the Institut Gustave-Roussy did not add an electron boost to lungs and reported no difference in the relapse rate in their patients compared with other centers where lung boosts were given, many centers have eliminated this boost.

In the Seattle experience, 25% of the boys who survived >5 months after transplant developed primary testicular relapse. A 4-Gy testes boost with electrons was sufficient to prevent such relapse in the MSKCC experience.

Splenic irradiation prior to TBI is a logical boost treatment in patients with CML, especially when the spleen is enlarged because it frequently harbors a large leukemic cell burden. In a randomized European study, there appeared to be an advantage to such treatment in an intermediate risk CML group. If splenic irradiation is done, a liver/spleen radionuclide scan is very useful to carefully plan this treatment.

In some diseases, it is desirable to boost sites of residual gross disease or other areas at particular risk; e.g., boost treatments to total doses of 12 to 20 Gy have been added to TBI regimens in areas of gross residual lymphoma, such as the mediastinum.

IV. CLINICAL RESULTS

A. Immunosuppression

1. Engraftment

With conventional matched sibling allografts, nonengraftment is rare (1–2%); engraftment, as measured by a WBC >500/mm^3, occurs from 1.5 to 3 weeks from the day of BMT (median: 17 days). In HLA-nonidentical transplants from related nonsibling donors, graft failure was found to be a function of the degree of donor incompatibility.

When donor marrow has been T-cell depleted as a means of preventing graft-versus-host disease (GVHD), graft failures have been noted to be higher. Single dose TBI (7.5–10 Gy) has been shown to be more effective in preventing rejection than fractionated TBI to a relatively low total dose of 10 to 12 Gy. Many reports have indicated that either higher total doses of fractionated TBI or the addition of TLI to TBI may prevent graft rejection in a large proportion of patients receiving T-cell-depleted marrow.

2. Aplastic Anemia

TBI is used only to prevent rejection in severe aplastic anemia, as there are no malignant cells to eradicate. Because cyclophosphamide alone is insufficient to prevent rejection, cytoreductive regimens have usually included either TBI or TLI to enhance engraftment, either as a single dose or fractionated. The advantage of using TLI for immunosuppression is that normal tissues outside of the field can be spared, namely brain and eye, kidneys, lungs, and much of the small bowel.

Long-term survival in severe aplastic anemia is generally in the range of 65 to 75%, but GVHD has generally remained a problem. The most serious long-term complication encountered with anemias has been second malignancies.

B. Eradication of Malignancy

1. Relapse Rate

Leukemic relapse is a reflection of the efficacy of leukemic cell kill, which is dependent on many factors in addition to the cytoreductive transplant regimen; these factors include leukemic cell burden, pretransplant chemotherapy, drug resistance, and graft-versus-leukemia effect.

Three randomized studies from Seattle (described under the specific leukemias) showed that higher TBI doses, achieved with fractionation, decreased the relapse rate as might be expected radiobiologically, but the survival rate was not always improved. A nonrandomized study of 160 patients with various malignancies suggested that multiple fractions per day, or hyperfractionated TBI (HFTBI), at 14.85 Gy total dose were more efficacious than STBI (10 Gy) for both overall survival and cause-specific survival.

2. Acute Lymphoblastic Leukemia

Comparative studies between allogeneic BMT and maintenance chemotherapy for ALL have shown decreased relapse rates and improved disease-free survival in the BMT arm, although this is not always statistically significant. Success of transplant depends on the remission status.

The Seattle group compared two fractionated dose schedules in a nonrandomized study: 2.25 Gy daily for 7 days to 15.75 Gy total dose (26 patients), or 1.2 Gy t.i.d. for 4 days to 14.4 Gy total dose (23 patients). The group receiving the 15.75-Gy total dose had a lower relapse rate and better disease-free survival at 3 years, but these differences were not statistically significant.

3. Acute Myeloid Leukemia

In AML, a large number of studies have shown an improved disease-free survival with BMT compared with continued chemotherapy. Not much difference has been observed between allogeneic and autologous BMT, with disease-free survival for either being about 50%. Long-term leukemia-free survival from IBMTR data is 51% for patients in first remission, 31% in second remission, and 21% in relapse. Low relapse rates for children with AML treated at MSKCC were attributed to the high total TBI dose (13.2–14.4 Gy) used with their HFTBI regimen, the addition of a 4-Gy testes boost, and the sequencing of Cy after TBI.

Two randomized scheduling trials for AML in first remission have been done in Seattle. First, single dose TBI (10 Gy) was compared with daily fractionation to a higher total dose (six fractions of 2 Gy each for a total dose of 12 Gy). Event-free survival was significantly better with the daily fractionation scheme, primarily due to decreased early mortality. When this same fractionation scheme was compared with another daily fractionation scheme (seven fractions of 2.25 Gy each for a total dose of 15.75 Gy) in a second trial, there was no difference in relapse-free survival (both ~55% at 6 years). Although the relapse rate was less with the regimen with the higher total dose of 15.75 Gy, mortality was also greater.

4. Chronic Myeloid Leukemia

Many studies have shown that CML patients have a better survival when transplanted in first chronic phase (CP). Long-term disease-free survival for patients in first CP who have been transplanted with unmanipulated marrow from a matched sibling donor is about 60–70%. With T-cell depletion of donor marrow, there is an increased risk of relapse, resulting in a lower DFS. In either group, with or without T-cell depletion, patients who develop chronic GVHD have a lesser risk of relapse, demonstrating a graft-versus-leukemia effect as well.

In a Genoa nonrandomized study, patients who had received a higher mean TBI dose (>9.9 Gy) were more likely to remain in remission. In the Seattle randomized CML study, survival was initially lower in the fractionated high dose group due to an increased early mortality, but at 5 years, there was no statistically significant difference in survival.

5. Lymphomas

The first marrow transplants in patients with non-Hodgkin's lymphoma were done on patients in relapse; the surprising success in some of these otherwise hopeless patients encouraged others to perform BMT earlier in the course of intermediate or high grade non-Hodgkin's lymphoma. It was shown in an MSKCC study that aggressive cytoreduction (TBI-Cy) followed by ABMT as early treatment was highly successful in patients with the poor prognostic features of high serum lactic dehydrogenase and/or bulky mediastinal or abdominal disease. At 5 years, 79% of patients were alive free of disease in the group who underwent ABMT after induction chemotherapy compared with only 31% in the group of patients who elected to wait and undergo BMT only at failure of chemotherapy. With a more aggressive cytoreductive regimen (TBI/VP-16/Cy), even patients with relapsed and resistant disease may be successfully treated (57% DFS at a median follow-up of 42+ months).

Patients with refractory or relapsed Hodgkin's disease may be salvaged by marrow transplantation also. Patients who have received prior irradiation usually are not eligible for either a TLI- or a TBI-containing preparative regimen.

V. TOXICITY

A. Acute Side Effects

The most obvious acute side effects are nausea and vomiting, which tend to occur a few hours after the first fraction of fractionated irradiation, and have been noted to decrease with time over a course of hyperfractionated irradiation.

Other acute side effects frequently encountered include oral mucositis, diarrhea, and parotiditis. These, along with nausea and vomiting, have been shown to be less with HFTBI (b.i.d.) compared with single dose irradiation. Another study showed that no parotiditis occurred with fractionated TBI (12 Gy in six fractions) compared with a 40% incidence with single dose TBI (10 Gy).

TBI is probably the major factor responsible for the transient xerostomia associated with BMT. Some patients develop severe dental caries without fluoride prophylaxis; dental assessment and fluoride prophylaxis are recommended for all TBI patients. Prophylactic acyclovir, which is effective against herpes simplex virus (HSV), has been found to be very effective in decreasing the severity of mucositis. A fatigue syndrome has been observed in 49% of women and 28% of men receiving FTBI (6 × 2 Gy). Some patients develop skin erythema and, later, even hyperpigmentation.

B. Late Toxicities

1. Regimen-Related Toxicity

The term "regimen-related toxicity" refers to all toxicities related to the preparative (cytoreductive) regimen and should be distinguished from transplant-related morbidity, which can refer to other toxicities related to

transplantation, such as from prophylactic medications, pancytopenia, or GVHD. When all regimen-related toxicities were grouped together, the only major factor that increased risk in allogeneic transplant patients was a higher TBI dose when two regimens with daily fractionation were compared (12 Gy in six fractions of 2 Gy versus 15.75 Gy in seven fractions of 2.25 Gy).

2. Interstitial Pneumonitis

IP has been one of the major contributors to mortality following BMT, with a minimum incidence of about 20% even in patients who have not received TBI as part of their cytoreductive regimen. IP has usually been fatal in approximately two-thirds of patients who develop it, although there now may be somewhat fewer fatalities with the advent of a useful treatment, namely combined gancyclovir and immunoglobulin, for IP caused by one of the organisms most frequently responsible, cytomegalovirus (CMV).

Factors related to the transplant procedure that influence IP are the cytoreductive regimen, including Cy and TBI, and agents used after BMT for GVHD prophylaxis, such as methotrexate.

TBI techniques may be altered in various ways to minimize IP. There is a lower incidence of IP and fewer fatalities from IP when TBI is fractionated compared with single dose TBI, even when the total dose with the fractionated regimen is higher.

Lung shields can reduce the dose to a large percentage of the lung and, theoretically, reduce IP as a result. Some of the decrease in IP in fractionation studies may be attributable to the concomitant use of lung blocks when TBI was fractionated. In a study from the Institut Gustave-Roussy, however, lung shields were used in both single dose and fractionated TBI, and the beneficial effect of fractionation in reducing IP was still observed.

Reducing the total lung dose in a single dose (10 Gy) regimen does not appear to be the definitive answer to reducing IP. When this was attempted in a study that randomized patients between total lung doses of 6 and 8 Gy, IP was essentially the same (23% vs 28%, respectively), and relapse was significantly higher in the 6-Gy group.

Dose rate is important with single dose TBI, with very low dose rates (0.025 Gy/min) resulting in a low incidence of IP (10%) and fatal IP (5%), but treatment times are extremely lengthy to achieve this, i.e., up to 7 h. With fractionated TBI, the dose rate is of little importance, which is the expected result when the dose/fraction is within the shoulder of the cell survival curve for the tissue of interest.

3. Cataracts

With single dose TBI, it has been found that the incidence of cataract development is very high, 80 to 100%, when patients are followed long enough. As many as 50% of these patients required surgery for this condition. The incidence of cataract development is considerably less (5–30%) when TBI is fractionated, as has been shown in many studies, with only about 20% requiring surgery.

4. Hepatic Dysfunction

Many hepatic disorders may occur after BMT: GVHD, chronic hepatitis, infections (viral, fungal, bacterial), drug reactions, leukemic infiltrates, and, a potentially fatal complication, venoocclusive disease of the liver (VOD), which has risen in incidence as cytoreductive regimens have become more intense. Chemotherapy and TBI are considered to be the principal causes of VOD, but the etiology of the disease is undoubtedly multifactorial. With respect to TBI, higher total dose (>12 Gy compared to 12 Gy) has played a role. Results of fractionated (12–15 Gy) versus single dose (10 Gy) TBI have been variable. In single dose regimens, the dose rate has been important, with minimal VOD with dose rates of less than 0.07 Gy/min, compared with an incidence as high as 50% with dose rates of 0.18 to 1.20 Gy/min. However, a randomized study of dose rate with both single dose and fractionated TBI did not show a difference in VOD rates.

5. Renal Dysfunction

Renal dysfunction has been noted in some studies after BMT. Analyses have suggested various risk factors that contribute to this morbidity, such as the combination of AraC plus Cy, TBI, the use of cyclosporine for GVHD prophylaxis, and the use of the antifungal agent, amphotericin B.

6. Endocrine Dysfunction

Many abnormalities in endocrine function have been noted after BMT, manifested, for example, as hypothy-

roidism, growth deficits, impaired sexual development, and infertility. Decreased morbidity has generally been noted with fractionated TBI compared with single dose TBI. An excellent review of this subject has been published by Sanders and colleagues from Seattle.

Thyroid function has been shown to be altered more frequently with transplant regimens containing TBI. In several studies, a much higher incidence of compensated hypothyroidism, as well as overt hypothyroidism, was found in children who had received single dose TBI (10 Gy) compared to fractionated TBI (12–15.75 Gy over 4 to 7 days).

Gonadal function is depressed in the majority of patients who receive single dose TBI, but appears to be less frequently affected in patients who receive fractionated TBI. Although most women develop primary gonadal failure, a few have recovered and pregnancies have been reported from several institutions.

7. Growth Retardation

Two factors can contribute to growth retardation of children who receive TBI: depressed growth hormone and a direct radiation effect on bone growth. Growth hormone deficiency is found in about 40 to 55% of children who have received TBI, but if they have had prior cranial irradiation, this incidence climbs to as high as 90%. Less growth retardation occurs with fractionated TBI compared to single dose TBI.

8. Alteration in Cognitive Function

Few studies have looked at cognitive function after marrow transplantation. A study in children showed no significant changes in IQ or in an adaptive behavior scale.

One study of patients who received TBI demonstrated an increasing cognitive dysfunction with increasing TBI dose by both univariate and multivariate analysis. Long-term neurobehavioral toxicity was very low in 20 patients who received HFTBI to 14.4 Gy followed from 16 to 50 years in a German study; only one patient developed any problem (a peripheral movement disorder of unknown origin).

9. Secondary Malignancies

An association between irradiation for BMT and the development of secondary malignancies (SM) is controversial. In severe aplastic anemia and Fanconi's anemia patients who were transplanted, a report from

Paris implicated TAI in an unusually high incidence of SM at 8 years (22%) in contrast to only 1.4% at 10 years in Seattle when aplastic anemia patients were prepared with chemotherapy only. It should be noted that there is an association of squamous cell carcinoma with Fanconi's anemia, even without irradiation. Another analysis from Seattle with 2246 patients (320 with aplastic anemia and 1926 with hematologic malignances) cited a 1.4% incidence of SM and implicated TBI as well as ATG given for GVHD as risk factors. In contrast to the studies just given, others have suggested no association with irradiation.

See Also the Following Articles

BRACHYTHERAPY • DOSIMETRY AND TREATMENT PLANNING FOR THREE-DIMENSIONAL RADIATION THERAPY • LATE EFFECTS OF RADIATION THERAPY • PROTON BEAM RADIATION THERAPY • RADIATION RESISTANCE • RADIOBIOLOGY, PRINCIPLES OF

Bibliography

Bortin, M. M., Horowitz, M. M., and Rimm, A. A. (1992). Progress report from the international bone marrow transplant registry. *Bone Marrow Transpl.* **10**, 113–122.

Briot, E., Dutreix, A., and Bridier, A. (1990). Dosimetry for total body irradiation. *Radiother. Oncol.* **18** (Suppl. 1): 16–29.

Buckner, C. D., Doney, K., Sanders, J., *et al.* (1992). Marrow transplantation for patients with acute lymphoblastic leukemia: the Seattle experience. *Leukemia* **6**(Suppl. 2), 193–195.

Clift, R., Buckner, C. D., Bianco, J., *et al.* (1992). Marrow transplantation in patients with acute myeloid leukemia. *Leukemia* **6**(Suppl.2), 104–109.

Sanders, J. E., Long-term Follow-up Team (1991). Endocrine problems in children after bone marrow transplant for hematologic malignancies. *Bone Marrow Transpl.* **8** (Suppl. 1), 2–4.

Shank, B. (1983). Techniques of magna-field irradiation. *Int. J. Rad. Oncol. Biol. Phys.* **9**, 1925–1931.

Shank, B. (1998). Total body irradiation. *In* "Textbook of Radiation Oncology" (S. Leibel and T. Phillips, eds.), pp. 253–275. W. B. Saunders, Philadelphia.

Shank, B. (1998). Total body irradiation for marrow or stem-cell transplantation. *Ca Invest.* **16**, 397–404.

Thomas, E. D. (1990). Total body irradiation regimens for marrow grafting. *Int. J. Radiat. Oncol. Biol. Phys.* **19**, 1285–1288.

Van Dyk, J., Galvin, J. M., Glasgow, G. P., and Podgorsak, E. B. (1986). "The Physical Aspects of Total and Half Body Photon Irradiation (AAPM Report No. 17)." American Institute of Physics, New York.

TP53 Tumor Suppressor Gene: Structure and Function

D. Joseph Jerry

University of Massachusetts, Amherst

Michelle A. Ozbun

University of New Mexico School of Medicine, Albuquerque

GLOSSARY

apoptosis A specific mechanism by which cells die. This is an ATP-dependent mechanism as compared to necrosis, which is a passive process for cell death.

conformation The three-dimensional folding (tertiary structure) of a protein.

dominant negative A protein that is able to inactivate the function of its wild-type counterpart.

frameshift mutation Mutations in which deletion or insertion of nucleotides causes a shift in the reading frame, altering all the succeeding codons.

Li–Fraumeni-like syndrome A rare autosomal dominant syndrome characterized by a high incidence of multiple pri-

mary tumors. This is distinguished from Li–Fraumeni syndrome by the lack of requirement of a sarcoma in the founding ancestor in a pedigree.

Li–Fraumeni syndrome A rare autosomal-dominant syndrome characterized a wide spectrum of primary tumors and soft tissue sarcomas at an early age. A high percentage of families with this syndrome carry a germline mutation in one allele of the *TP53* gene.

missense mutation A change in a single amino acid of a protein as a result of a point mutation affecting a single codon.

nonsense mutation Mutations that result in a premature termination signal (stop codon), resulting in truncated proteins that may have altered functions or be unstable.

senscence Phenomenon observed where normal diploid cells exhibit a finite proliferative capacity *in vitro* and is believed to be a measure of cellular aging.

transactivation Activity whereby nuclear proteins bind to specific sequences within promoters of genes and activate the synthesis of the mRNA encoded by the gene (transcription).

tumor suppressor gene A gene encoding a protein that is involved in the negative growth regulation of cells and can

inhibit formation of tumors. These are commonly identified as genes that undergo selective allelic loss during tumor formation.
wild type The gene as it is found in normal diploid cells.

The *TP53* gene in humans (designated *Trp53* in the mouse) encodes a 53-kDa protein that has characteristics of a tumor suppressor gene. The *TP53* gene is either mutated or compromised functionally in the majority of human solid tumors exposing its critical role in tumor suppression. Disruption of the p53 protein is also critical for the transformation of cells by oncogenic viruses. These observations initiated detailed analysis of the biochemical activities of the p53 protein and its biological roles in cells. The majority of mutations identified in human tumors are found within the central domain of p53, causing a loss of its ability to transcriptionally activate target. The mutational spectrum found in tumors underscores the conformational sensitivity of the p53 protein. Mutant p53 proteins often form complexes with the wild-type p53 protein and act in a dominant-negative fashion to abrogate the function of p53 in cells retaining a wild-type allele of p53. These observations identified transcriptional activation as a central activity of the wild-type p53 protein. Although the role of p53 as a transcription factor is important for enforcement of cell cycle arrest and apoptosis, multiple overlapping biochemical activities appear to be essential for p53 to fulfill its role as "guardian of the genome." Investigations of the biochemical activities of p53 continue in an effort to exploit these pathways to treat and prevent a variety of human cancers.

I. INTRODUCTION

A. History

The p53 protein was first recognized in the late 1970s when it was found to be bound to the large tumor antigen (T-Ag) from simian virus 40 (SV40). The SV40 large T antigen was required for oncogenic transformation and immortalization of cells in culture. Quantities of the p53 protein were elevated 5- to 100-fold in many transformed and tumor cell lines, whereas the protein was virtually undetectable in normal cells. These characteristics suggested that p53 might be oncogenic. The p53 cDNA was cloned in the early 1980s and was shown to cooperate with an activated *ras* oncogene in the transformation of normal fibroblasts from rat embryos. These experiments appeared to confirm the identity of p53 as an oncogenic protein. However, the oncogenic properties of p53 were questioned when investigators found that one mouse p53 cDNA inhibited the transformation of cells by the activated *ras* oncogene. Subsequent experiments demonstrated that this clone was the bona fide wild-type p53 cDNA and that mutation of p53 was required to render the p53 protein oncogenic. Therefore, one role of SV40 large T antigen in cellular transformation was to inactivate wild-type p53 by direct binding. The absence of active p53 rendered cells susceptible to oncogenic transformation. Overexpression of the wild-type p53 protein not only failed to transform cells, but elicited growth suppression when introduced into tumor cells. Thus, the activity of p53 in the suppression of transformation of cells in culture was established.

B. Mutations in Human Cancers

The role of p53 as a tumor suppressor gene was firmly established when mutations were detected in human tumors. Screening human tumors for mutations dominated efforts during the late 1980s through the early 1990s and provided a rich harvest compared to previous efforts searching for activating mutations in protooncogenes. Mutations in the human p53 gene (*TP53*) have been reported for thousands of tumors representing nearly all tissue types. (Mutations and polymorphisms in *TP53* are compiled in a database and can be accessed at http://www.iarc.fr/p53/.) The prevalence of mutations in human cancers identified p53 as a critical regulator that had to be abrogated during the ontogeny of most tumors. Mutations were frequently detected in one allele of the tumors along with loss of the remaining wild-type allele termed loss of heterozygosity (LOH). Unlike oncogenes that had been shown to become constitutively activated when a critical codon was mutated, the mutations in *TP53* were distributed broadly throughout a large portion of the gene. The most frequent types of mutations involved changes of one nucleotide (point mutation), resulting in the replacement of a single amino acid residue (missense mutation). This differs from other tumor suppressor genes where mutations most often are frameshift mutations that result in the premature termination of translation and truncated proteins. The apparent selection of missense mutations of the *TP53* gene in human tumors may reflect the loss of tumor suppressor function by these mutations, as well as the dominant-negative activities (gain of function) possessed by many mutant p53 proteins.

The spectrum of mutations varies considerably among tumor types and has been used as a fingerprint implicating specific environmental mutagens as the sources of the mutations (Table I). Skin cancer provides the clearest example of carcinogen-specific mutations. Exposure to UV light increases the risk of basal cell and squamous cell carcinoma, as well as the melanoma. Tandem mutation of pyrimidines is characteristic of UV light exposure in experimental systems and occurs in ~25% of skin cancers, but is rare in other types of cancer. The mutagenic spectrum of other agents is less specific, but comparisons of mutagenic spectra among types of cancers can implicate specific mutagens. There is a prevalence of G → T transversions in lung cancer patients reporting a history of smoking that is not observed in lung cancers from nonsmokers or other types of cancers. Furthermore, there is a dose-dependent correlation between smoking history and the prevalence of G → T mutations. The pattern of mutations in smokers is consistent with the mutations induced by cigarette smoke in experimental systems. The pattern of mutations observed in lung cancers among coal miners has been

suggested to be related to chronic exposure to radon. Mutations in liver cancers also exhibit differences among groups. The most striking was the frequent mutation of codon 249 in liver cancers in the Quidong province of China (95%), whereas mutation of this codon is infrequent in liver cancers among Western populations. This selective mutation is consistent with the mutagenic spectrum of aflatoxin, which often contaminates grains in developing countries. Therefore, mutations in *TP53* can be used to provide molecular epidemiological evidence to discover the underlying causes of some cancers. Unfortunately, the majority of mutations involve GC→AT transversions, which can be induced by a variety of exogenous agents, as well as damage by reactive oxygen species (ROS), which are by-products of normal cellular metabolism. In tumors, mutation of one allele is commonly observed along with large-scale deletions, including the *TP53* gene on the second allele, resulting in "loss of heterozygosity" for markers surrounding the *TP53* locus. These features suggested that p53 is acting as a classical tumor suppressor gene in a "two-hit" mechanism proposed by Alfred Knudson.

The frequent mutation of the *TP53* gene in sporadic human tumors led to investigations of its possible role in heritable cancer syndromes. The Li–Fraumeni syndrome was originally characterized by the frequency of a number of different tumor types in affected families, with pediatric soft tissue sarcomas being a critical feature. As more stringent criteria for the clinical description were defined, it became evident that breast cancer was the most prevalent form of cancer in women affected by Li–Fraumeni syndrome (Fig. 1). In 1990, germline mutations were found in Li–Fraumeni syndrome

TABLE I
Molecular Epidemiology of Human Cancer and Mutation of *TP53*[a]

Tumor type	Mutations	Source of lesions
Skin cancer	CC→TT	UV light causes pyrimidine dimers
Lung cancer		
Smokers	G:C→T:A	Polycyclic aromatic hydrocarbons
Nonsmokers	G:C→A:T	Endogenous mutagens likely
Liver cancer		
United States	G:C→A:T at Ser[149] are rare	Endogenous mutagens likely
China	G:C→A:T at Ser[149] predominate	Aflatoxin B_1

[a]For details, see Bennett *et al.* (1999) and Greenblatt *et al.* (1994).

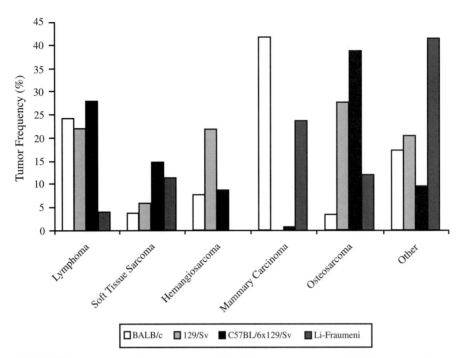

FIGURE 1 Comparison of tumor spectra of *Trp53* heterozygous mice and Li–Fraumeni syndrome in humans. Data for 129/Sv and C57BL/6 backcross mice were compiled from Donehower and coworkers. Tumor data for Li–Fraumeni syndrome are summaries of over 700 patients. Data were from both male and females; however, breast cancer was only observed in females.

probands. In these families, the multiple tumor susceptibility segregated as an autosomal dominant phenotype associated with heterozygosity for the mutant allele of *TP53*. Tumors showed loss of the wild-type allele (LOH). Although not all Li–Fraumeni families harbor mutations in *TP53*, they may harbor alterations in other genes that abrogate the function of p53, possibly through overexpression of cellular antagonists of p53.

C. Mutations in Mouse Models

Germline knockout alleles were created in mice and served to fortify the role of the p53 pathway in tumor susceptibility. Mice homozygous for p53 knockout alleles (*Trp53*^null^) developed normally, but exhibited multiple tumor types at young ages, confirming the significant role of *Trp53* in the susceptibility to tumors. The preponderance of tumors were lymphomas, suggesting the special importance of p53 in this tissue. Early death due to lymphoma precluded the analysis of other tumor types that may occur at later ages.

Therefore, transplantation was used to demonstrate the extreme tumor susceptibility exhibited by mammary epithelium devoid of p53.

Although *p53*-deficient mice exhibited increased tumor susceptibility, the tumor spectrum in mice that were heterozygous for the *Trp53*^null^ allele differed from that observed for Li–Fraumeni syndrome in humans (Fig. 1). The tumor spectrum varied when the *Trp53*^null^ allele was transferred to different strains of inbred mice. When the *Trp53*^null^ allele was transferred to the genetic background of Balb/c mice, mammary tumors became the most frequent tumor in females that were heterozygous for the *Trp53*^null^ allele, providing a valuable model of Li–Fraumeni syndrome in which breast cancer is the most common tumor. These results demonstrate the presence of genes that can influence the susceptibility and tumor spectrum of individuals bearing germline mutations in *TP53*. Identification of these genes may serve to not only predict tumor sensitivities in individuals, but may provide targets for therapy that can modulate the function of p53.

II. STRUCTURE AND FUNCTION

A. The Structural Gene and Protein Conformation

The gene encoding p53 in humans *(TP53)* resides on the short arm of chromosome 17 (17p13.1). The mouse genome contains both a functional gene that encodes the p53 protein *(Trp53)* on chromosome 11 and a processed pseudogene on chromosome 14. Structural homologues of the p53 gene are present in all vertebrates and are composed of 11 exons with near identical exonic borders (Fig. 2). In mammals, the p53 gene spans approximately 20 kb with a large intron (8–10 kb) separating the noncoding exon 1 from exon 2, which contains the translational start site. mRNA transcripts of p53 vary among species (ranging from 1.8 to 3.0 kb) due to differences in the lengths of the 3'-untranslated regions. In addition to p53, a family of p53-related proteins has been uncovered. Although the genes for p63 and p73 have similarities to p53 in both structure and biochemical activities, they have not been found to be mutated in human cancers. Therefore, they appear to be unable to mediate the broad genome guardian role ascribed to p53.

Alignments of the amino acid sequences of the p53 proteins from vertebrates provided the first insights into the structure of the p53 protein. Five regions of sequence conservation were identified by Soussi and co-workers. These regions coincided with clustering of mutations in human tumors (Fig. 3A) and, therefore, contained functional domains that were essential for the tumor suppressor function of p53. A transactivation motif lays in the extreme N terminus and contains conserved domain I. The "core domain" is essential for sequence-specific DNA binding, overlaps conserved domains II–V, and is mutated in the majority of human tumors. Zinc is bound by the core domain and stabilizes the tertiary structure of this region. The C terminus is less conserved, but contains the nuclear localization signal (NLS) that is required for proper subcellular localization of the p53 protein. The C-terminal domain serves a regulatory role by maintaining p53 in a "latent" form. Tetramerization is mediated by the C-terminal domain leading to DNA binding and transactivation of target genes by p53. The C terminus appears to mask the N terminus, as deletion of the C terminus leads to constitutive activation of p53.

The peculiar sensitivity of p53 to disruption of its function by point mutations over a relatively large region remained obscure until the three-dimensional crystal structure was solved. Although the evolutionarily conserved domains mediate specific activities of p53, the region from amino acid residues 112 to 290 appears important for stable folding of the core domain that is responsible for sequence-specific binding to DNA. Therefore, point mutations within this do-

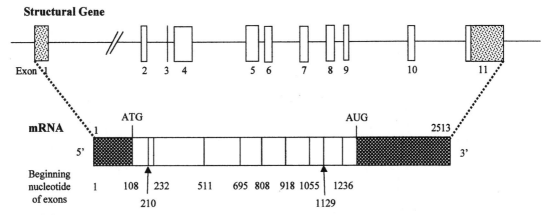

FIGURE 2 Structure of the human p53 gene *(TP53)*. The structural gene for human *TP53* is shown with mature mRNA. Sequences coding for the protein begin with exon 2 and end in exon 11. Stipled areas indicate noncoding regions (exon 1 and a portion of exon 11).

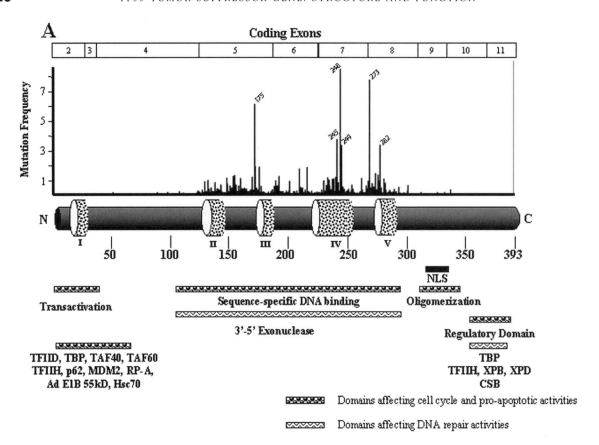

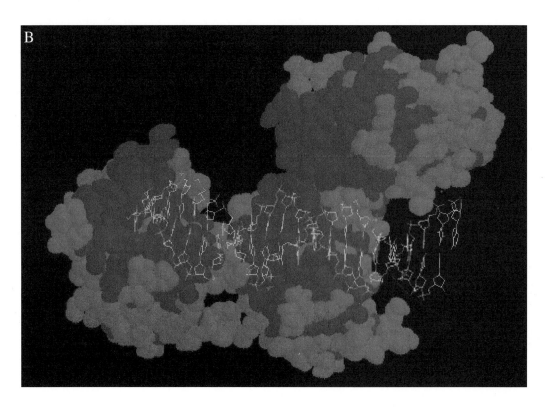

main can destabilize the three-dimensional conformation of the protein, rendering it inactive. The degree of conservation of the amino acid sequence among species ranging from amphibians to humans emphasizes the critical role of the core domain. In Fig. 3B, the three-dimensional structure of the core domain is shown bound to DNA. Amino acid residues that are identical among the 10 species compared dominate the surfaces contacting DNA. The degree of conservation of the core domain is 64%, whereas conservations of the N-terminal and C-terminal domains are 11 and 24%, respectively. The loop motifs that contact DNA have little regular secondary structure; therefore, mutations in these residues can disrupt folding of the core domain. A zinc atom coordinated by conserved amino acids provides additional stability, but like mutations, shifts in the redox status of the zinc can alter the activity of the p53 protein.

Conformational shifts in p53 protein can be detected using monoclonal antibodies (Table II). N and C termini of p53 protein form charged regions that are quite stable, whereas the central core region is hydrophobic and resistant to proteases when in an active conformation. Therefore, antibodies directed against the termini will react whether the protein adopts an active or denatured conformation. In contrast, antibodies directed against epitopes within the central region recognize the active conformation in which unique surfaces are exposed (PAb246 and PAb1620), whereas other epitopes are buried within the hydrophobic region (absence of reactivity with PAb240). However, when the p53 protein becomes denatured, the hydrophobic epitopes are exposed and the surface epitopes are lost. Most mutations destabilize the conformation of p53 protein, causing it to expose epitopes for PAb240 and lose reactivity with PAb1620 or PAb246 when analyzed by immunoprecipitation. Loss of the native conformation by mutation causes the p53 protein to be stabilized in cells,

leading to an accumulation of mutant p53 protein within the nucleus. Because levels of wild-type p53 protein are usually below the limit of detection by immunohistochemical procedures, accumulation of p53 protein is often an indicator of the presence of mutations. However, wild-type p53 has also been shown to accumulate within some tumor cells. In these instances, it is likely that p53 function may be compromised by the disruption of other players in the p53 pathway.

B. Biochemical Activities

Identification of conserved domains within p53 protein has been used to direct the search for functional domains (Fig. 3A). The diverse biochemical activities attributed to p53 protein reflect the breadth of cellular processes which are essential for the global role of p53 as "guardian of the genome." The role of p53 as a transcription factor has been characterized extensively and appears to be essential to induce cell cycle arrest and apoptosis in response to DNA damage. Although somatic mutations in tumors are most frequent in the central core region, mutations in N or C termini that disrupt transactivation also cause loss of the cell cycle arrest and proapoptotic activities of p53, along with loss of tumor suppression. Transactivation by p53 is optimal when it forms tetramers, which requires the oligimerization domain overlapping the NLS in the C terminus. A regulatory domain is also located within the extreme C terminus, which causes p53 to adopt a "latent" conformation. This allows p53 protein to be present in cells without eliciting an unwanted transcriptional activation of target genes and yet is available to mediate rapid responses to genotoxic stress. This domain prevents transcriptional activation by p53 tetramers. When cells suffer DNA damage, the C terminus undergoes posttranslational modifications, causing activation of the

---

FIGURE 3 Biochemical activities and structure of p53 protein. (A) The frequency of mutations and their location are shown relative to the coding exons (above) and the primary sequence of the p53 protein (below). Regions of sequence conservation among species (stippled areas, I–V) are shown on the protein. Major functional domains are shown below the diagram of the p53 protein. These are separated into domains controlling cell cycle and apoptosis and domains implicated in DNA repair. Adapted from Albrechtsen *et al.*, 1999. (B) The three-dimensional space-filling model of residues 94–289 is shown bound to DNA as determined by Cho and colleagues. The p53 structure is shaded according to the conservation of each residue among species ranging from *Xenopus* to human. Residues that are identical among all the sequences compared are colored dark gray. The remaining residues are colored light gray. Alignments and images were provided courtesy of Paul Stothard (University of Alberta).

TABLE II
Monoclonal Antibodies Frequently Used to Detect p53

Epitope location and name of monoclonal	Epitope sensitivity[a]
N-terminus	
DO1	Native and denatured
DO7	Native and denatured
PAb1801	Native and denatured
Central core region	
PAb240	Denatured conformation only
PAb246	Native conformation only (mouse p53 only)
PAb1620	Native conformation only
C-terminus	
PAb421	Native and denatured

[a]Antibodies that react with both native and denatured p53 protein are indicated. Those that are specific for the denatured conformation are diagnostic for inactive or mutant p53 protein. Those that react against the native conformation only indicate the presence of wild-type p53 protein that is biochemically active.

"latent" p53, which increases the transcriptional activation of target sequences by p53. Peptides have also been used to activate latent p53 and may be useful therapeutically.

The transactivation and oligomerization domains of p53 are not targets of somatic mutation, but do mediate important interactions with a broad range of proteins. Multiple components of the basal transcription machinery bind to the transactivation domain (TFIID, TBP, TAFs), allowing p53 to bind to an enhancer and then recruit these essential transcription factors to the gene. These regions are also targets of extensive posttranslational modification (Fig. 4). Histone acetyltransferases (PCAF and P300) can enhance sequence-specific transcriptional activation by acetylation of the C terminus of p53. Both N and C termini of p53 are subject to extensive phosphorylation of critical amino acid residues, which enhances the activity of p53 (transactivation and proapoptotic functions). Amino acid residues within the transactivation domain are substrates for several kinases (DNA-PK, CAK, ATM), which can inhibit the binding of p53 by MDM2, a negative regulator of p53 that causes the nuclear export and ubiquitin-dependent degradation of p53, leading to stabilization of the p53 protein within cells. Phosphorylation of the C termi-

nus also regulates interactions with 14-3-3σ, which is critical for G2 checkpoint function.

Additional biochemical activities of p53 have been identified that suggest a more direct participation of p53 in DNA repair pathways and have been reviewed in detail by Albrechtsen and colleagues. These include $3' \rightarrow 5'$ exonuclease activity localized within the central core domain. The C terminus of p53 can also bind to single-stranded and double-stranded DNA in a nonsequence-specific manner, which may be important in the "sensing" of damaged DNA. Direct interactions between p53 protein and several DNA repair proteins have also been reported (RPA, Rad51, Cockayne syndrome B protein, xeroderma pigmentosum B and D proteins, BRCA1, BRCA2). Cells that are deficient in p53 are defective in multiple pathways of DNA repair (nucleotide excision repair and double strand break repair). Similarly, p53 appears to be important for the suppression of homologous recombination. The ability of p53 to interact with helicases that are disrupted in Cockayne and Werner syndromes, which display premature aging as well as genetic instability, suggests more wide-ranging roles for p53 in these processes. These observations have led to the proposal that p53 in the uninduced or latent state may perform essential roles in DNA repair, suppression of recombination, and control of DNA replication. Upon activation by posttranslational modification, transcriptional activation becomes the dominant activity that leads to cell cycle arrest and apoptosis (Fig. 4). This model provides a means by which p53 may discriminate between its role in maintenance of the genome and its acute responses, which favor apoptosis.

III. REGULATION OF p53 FUNCTION: THE CELLULAR VIEW

A. Sensors Signaling to p53

The p53 pathway is activated in response to a broad range of cellular stresses (Fig. 5). Although the identities of the sensors of cellular stress remain elusive, it is clear that a variety of perturbations in the environment of a cell can lead to p53-dependent re-

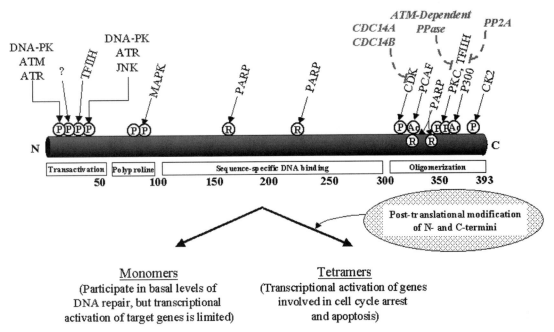

FIGURE 4 Cellular regulators of p53 function. The posttranslational modifications of p53 that have been shown to regulate major biochemical activities are summarized. Arrows designate the enzymes acting on these sites. Enzymes that are inhibitory are indicated by dotted lines. P, phosphorylation; Ac, acetylation; R, ribosylation.

sponses. Cells monitor their context and polarity through interactions with the extracellular matrix, which appears to involve appropriate signaling through integrins and E-cadherin, and can activate p53-dependent responses. Alterations in metabolic status, both in terms of nutrients and oxidative state, can activate p53. Inappropriate cellular proliferation also can cause p53-dependent senescence or apoptosis. Both activation of protooncogenes and infection with DNA tumor viruses that stimulate proliferation initiate p53-dependent apoptosis. Similarly, the integrity of genomic DNA is under surveillance by multiple mechanisms, which detect breaks and mismatched base pairs within the DNA, stalled replication, and disruption of microtubules, which can lead to the failure of proper segregation during mitosis. Therefore, p53-dependent responses can be initiated by receptor-mediated signaling at the membrane as well as by cytoplasmic and nuclear sensing mechanisms. All of these mechanisms represent potent blockades that must be overcome for cells to become tumors. The fact that all these mechanisms converge upon p53 for a portion of their effects on inhibition

of tumorigenesis underscores the central role of p53 in orchestrating primary defenses against unregulated growth or inappropriate survival of cells.

B. Mechanisms Regulating p53 Activity

Activation of p53 in response to genotoxic stress has been examined extensively, yielding a complicated network of genes, which can signal to p53 and engage the coordinated cellular responses of cell cycle arrest, DNA repair, or apoptosis. The radiosensitivity exhibited by patients with ataxia-telangiectasia provided an important clue to the cellular mechanisms for sensing and responding to double strand breaks. The *ATM* gene (ataxia-telangiectasia mutated) is a crucial participant in the response to double strand breaks. Its activity is to initiate a cascade of kinases, which cause two distinct effects: arrest of the cell cycle and assist repair of the double strand breaks. The ATM protein is a serine/threonine kinase that can phosphorylate Ser15 of human p53, leading to a stabilization of p53 protein. Therefore, ATM senses the DNA damage following ionizing radiation and then engages the p53

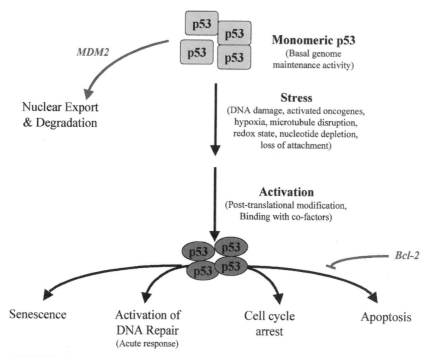

FIGURE 5 Pathways for regulation of p53 and responses. The p53 protein can exist in multiple states within cells. Under normal conditions, levels of p53 protein are very low due to rapid turnover. Stability is controlled, in part, by factors like MDM2. Activation of cellular stress pathways causes covalent modification and tetramerization of p53 that stabilize the protein, leading to accumulation within the nucleus. The cellular outcome depends on the balance of factors present in cells, which may antagonize one response (e.g., diminished apoptosis in cells with high levels of Bcl-2).

pathway, which is required for the cell cycle arrest and apoptosis. Other genes that participate in DNA repair include poly-ADP-ribose polymerase (PARP), DNA-dependent protein kinase (DNA-PK), and AT-related protein (ATR). These genes also cause post-translational modifications of p53 protein that enhance its stability and transcriptional activation of target genes. Therefore, p53 integrates the signals from pathways that are activated by different types of DNA damage (double strand breaks, bulky adducts, mismatches) by being a target for multiple posttranslational modifications. The transcriptional activation of p53-dependent genes has been shown to be essential for both cell cycle arrest and apoptotic responses induced by p53.

Other types of cell stress that participate in tumor development can also lead to activation of p53, but accomplish this through distinct mechanisms. Activation of proliferation of cells by expression of onco-

genes can initiate events leading to formation of tumors. However, cells recognize illegitimate proliferation and undergo p53-dependent apoptosis, providing a potent suppression of tumorigenesis. In this instance, ARF (alternative reading frame of the *INK4A* gene encoding the p14 protein in human and p19 protein in mouse) is induced in response to mitogenic stimulation, leading to stabilization of p53. Hypoxia can also signal the activation of p53, which further limits the growth of tumors by inhibiting angiogenesis and proliferation. Hypoxia results in the production of Hif1α, which enhances p53-dependent transcriptional activation by direct binding to p53 protein. In contrast, the extracellular matrix provides survival signals, causing cells to resist proapoptotic signals induced by DNA damage. Disruption of contacts between cells and the basement membrane can initiate p53-dependent apoptosis, a mechanism that appears important for preventing metastases. The mechanisms by which p53-dependent responses are activated in response to these varying stresses have not been characterized in great detail, but appear to activate p53 through multiple pathways that include increased transcription of the *TP53* gene, stabilization of the protein, and posttranslational modifications.

Given the dire consequences to a cell if p53 should be inappropriately activated, it is not surprising that antagonists are also present to enforce strict regulation of p53. The MDM2 protein is encoded by the *HDM2* gene (*mdm2* in mouse) and was discovered as an oncogene that antagonized the tumor suppressor function of p53 through direct interaction with p53 in a manner resembling that of SV40 large T antigen. However, MDM2 not only inhibits the transactivation function of p53 by binding to the extreme N terminus, but also has a nuclear export signal and E3 ubiquitin ligase activity. Therefore, MDM2 mediates the export of p53 from the nucleus to the cytoplasm where it is ubiquitinated and targeted for rapid degradation in the proteosomes. The importance of this pathway appears to be emphasized by the critical regulation of the p53–MDM2 complex at multiple levels. First, MDM2 was shown to be a target gene that is transcriptionally activated by p53. This would appear to be a valuable response so that cells can respond to stress by activation of p53, but a prolonged response could lead to apoptosis of the cell. Therefore, activation of p53 also induces MDM2, which would rapidly destroy p53, minimizing inappropriate apoptosis. The level of p53 response is further regulated by the reciprocal phosphorylation of both MDM2 and p53 by kinases involved in DNA repair pathways. Phosphorylation of the N terminus of p53 leads to increased activity and inhibits the interaction with MDM2. MDM2 is also phosphorylated by these kinases, leading to decreased interaction with p53 as well. The ARF tumor suppressor protein also binds to the p53–MDM2 complex and serves to stabilize p53, despite the presence of MDM2. These molecules provide redundant mechanisms to finely tune the levels of p53 activity that are appropriate for the situation faced by a cell.

The levels of p53 mRNA are also induced when cells become stressed, indicating transcriptional regulation of p53 activity. Despite this observation, the structure of the p53 promoter has not been examined extensively. Both positive and negative *cis*-acting regulatory elements have been identified within the p53 promoter. These elements appear to mediate transcriptional activation of p53 in response to specific types of cellular stress. NF-κB and AP-1-binding sites have been shown to be essential for mitogen-induced transcription of the p53 promoter. Elements that mediate transcription of the p53 gene following exposure to UV radiation also are essential for basal transcription. The p53 promoter lacks homology to motifs, which identify conventional basal promoters and initiation sites, and therefore appears to be a new class of eukaryotic promoter elements.

Although redundant mechanisms serve to enforce the proper function of p53, these mechanisms can also serve as targets for the disruption of p53 during oncogenic transformation. Posttranslational mechanisms provide a rapid means to invoke p53-dependent responses by both stabilization of p53 and increased activity of the protein. These mechanisms have been shown to be disrupted in tumors. Oncogenic viruses have evolved to inhibit p53 function by stimulating ubiquitin-dependent degradation (e.g., human papillomavirus), as well as inhibition via direct binding to the p53 protein (e.g., SV40 and adenovirus). Likewise, amplification of cellular antagonists of p53 (e.g., MDM2 and Bcl-2) has been observed in human cancers. Although infrequent, methylation of the p53 promoter can lead to transcriptional silencing of the gene in some instances. Therefore, p53 function can be compromised by multiple mechanism during tumorigenesis in addition to direct mutation of *TP53*.

IV. FUNCTION AND REGULATION OF p53 IN TISSUES

A. Embryonic Development

Considering the pivotal functions of p53 identified in cultured cells, it was anticipated that its function would be essential for the proper development of tissues. Patterns of expression suggested precise developmental regulation in the embryo. Nonetheless, mice deficient in p53 developed normally. Although tumors developed frequently in these mice, they were observed primarily in animals that have reached maturity. Therefore, the role of p53 in tissue development appeared to be more subtle.

Analysis of p53 in embryos revealed tissue-specific patterns of expression. However, high levels of mRNA were detected in tissues undergoing rapid proliferation as well as tissues that were composed largely of postmitotic cells (e.g., neural tissues). Similar patterns of protein expression were detected by immunohistochemical staining. The precise regulation of expression suggested that p53 may participate in the differentiation of tissues, rather than simply acting to determine whether the DNA was intact. Indeed, inappropriate expression of wild-type p53 transgenes in the developing lens or kidney of mice led not only to increased apoptosis, but failure of differentiation as well. Although embryonic development can occur in the absence of p53, embryonic mortality was increased in *p53*null mice due to failure of neural tube closure in female embryos. The important role of p53 in ensuring proper embryonic development is emphasized by the increased number of birth defects in p53-deficient neonatal mice that were subjected to sublethal doses of radiation *in utero*. Similarly, p53 deficiency has been used to partially rescue embryonic lethal phenotypes in genetically engineered mice. Therefore, p53 appears to play a "quality assurance" role in the developing embryo. This might be expected, as p53 has been shown to be activated in cells when they encounter inappropriate extrinsic signals from either the matrix or surrounding cells (Fig. 5).

B. Postnatal Development

Appropriate regulation of p53 is also important in tissues undergoing development postnatally. Early onset thymic lymphomas are the major tumor type observed in *p53*null mice. Impaired differentiation appears to be a significant factor, as lymphomas consist of primarily immature T cells (CD4$^+$CD8$^+$). In the prostate, apoptotic cell death following androgen ablation was reduced in *p53*null mice, resulting in delayed involution. The mammary epithelium also undergoes apoptosis following weaning of the neonates. Similar to the prostate, involution of the mammary gland was delayed in *p53*null mice. These data emphasize the physiological role of p53 in coordinating the remodeling of tissues undergoing normal developmental changes.

C. Regulation of p53 in Tissues and Relationship to Tumor Development

Although the consequences of loss of p53 have been documented in numerous human tumors, the levels and patterns of p53 expression vary among normal tissues. In some tissues, p53 is regulated at the level of gene transcription. However, in the majority of tissues, p53 mRNA is expressed constitutively and regulation is achieved by altering the stability of p53 protein in response to varying conditions. Therefore, the activity of the p53 pathway in response to genotoxic agents provides a more meaningful assessment of p53 function than measuring p53 protein or mRNA levels alone. Several investigators have used γ radiation as a means to introduce DNA damage to test the p53 pathway because responses to this type of agent are p53 dependent. Distinct patterns of responses to γ radiation in normal tissues have emerged from these experiments. First were tissues that had low basal levels of p53 protein, but responded to radiation with an accumulation of p53 protein within nuclei resulting in apoptosis. Tissues of this type included spleen, thymus, bone marrow, and intestinal crypts. Second were tissues in which the nuclear accumulation of p53 was observed following γ radiation, but failed to undergo apoptosis (e.g., salivary gland, myocardium, adrenal, lung parenchyma, and kidney). A third category was composed of tissues in which no responses to γ radiation were observed (e.g., skeletal muscle, brain, liver), suggesting a relative inactivity of p53 in these tissues. In most instances, tissues that failed to activate p53 following DNA damage showed no significant expression of p53. An example is quiescent mammary epithelium where responses to γ radiation were minimal. However, the refractory state of p53 was reversed following hormonal stimulation, resulting in potent induction of p53-dependent target genes and apoptosis suggesting that responsiveness of tissues may be related to the proliferative status. In intestinal epithelium, crypt cells show the strongest responses to γ radiation, whereas cells undergoing differentiation are relatively resistant.

The spectrum of responses to genotoxic stress among tissues offers examples of the complexity of p53 regulatory pathways. Classical paradigms suggest that p53 becomes activated in response to DNA damage and binds to promoters of target genes, causing increased transcription of both cell cycle arrest genes and proapoptotic genes. However, in the normal life of a cell, it would be advantageous for cells to discriminate between DNA damage that can be repaired and damage that is so profound that the cell should be eliminated by apoptosis. Indeed, selective activation of p53 responsive genes has been demonstrated for several tissues. Investigations of radiosensitive tissues (e.g., spleen, thymus, small intestine) showed a strong induction of genes involved in cell cycle regulation followed by the induction of proapoptotic genes at later times, whereas only a subset of genes was induced in radioresistant tissues (brain, heart, liver). These patterns of expression offer insights into how normal tissues may respond to cytotoxic therapies, especially radiation therapy.

The pattern of p53-dependent responses in normal tissues does not, however, predict whether loss of p53 is important for the evolution of tumors. For example, liver cancers frequently involve mutations in *TP53*, and yet p53 responses to γ radiation in the liver are negligible. Therefore, it would appear that different biochemical functions of p53 may be emphasized among tissues and among developmental states. In the quiescent liver and mammary epithelium, DNA repair activities may be unnecessary, as the cells are largely nonproliferative. However, p53 may become active in these tissues in response to proliferative stimuli causing apoptosis of rogue cells without needlessly compromising cells that are dutifully fulfilling their functions as part of the tissue.

V. CLINICAL USES OF p53

A. Prognostic Indicator

The mutational status of *TP53* in human tumors has led to its being proposed as a prognostic indicator. Mutation of *TP53* is found in larger tumors that are high grade and aneuploid. Although mutation of *TP53* is associated with poor prognosis, inclusion of p53 status has not provided an improvement in predicting responses to therapy or clinical outcomes when compared to routine histopathologic criteria. Furthermore, the p53 pathway can be disrupted by alterations at multiple levels, making it necessary to either directly assess the function of p53 in a tumor or determine the patterns of expression of molecules that regulate p53 function (e.g., MDM2, p14/ARF). However, in subsets of tumors in which the clinical outcome is difficult to predict, p53 status is becoming a valuable aid in therapeutic decisions. In bladder cancer patients who lack detectable p53 (suggesting that wild-type p53 is preserved) and the cancer is confined to the bladder, survival was dramatically better following therapy. Similarly, p53 is a useful independent prognostic indicator in stage II breast cancer, but not stage III.

B. Strategies for p53-Targeted Therapies

Classic cancer therapies depend on delivering a severe cytotoxic insult to tumor cells, resulting in their destruction. Restoring p53 function in tumor cells would increase sensitivity to many chemotherapeutic agents. Therefore, replacement of p53 in tumor cells has been explored because mutation of p53 is the most common mechanism for the disruption of p53 in human cancers. This approach requires the efficient delivery of the wild-type p53 gene to the overwhelming majority of tumor cells in an effort to activate apoptosis in the tumor cells, while infection of normal cells must be minimized because expression of high levels of wild-type p53 is toxic. Viral vectors provide a vehicle for the efficient delivery of genes with adenoviral vectors being preferred. However, adenoviral proteins cause vigorous immune responses, rendering subsequent treatments ineffective. Preferential infection of tumor cells, but not normal cells, also remains a challenge. The Onyx-015 adenovirus was designed so that it could replicate only in cells lacking p53 and, therefore, effectively targets only tumor cells. Although clinical results show promise, the immune responses initiated by this adenovirus remain a limitation to its use in clinical settings.

Small molecules have also been shown to have potential for activating the function of both wild-type and mutant p53 proteins in cancer cells. These drugs take advantage of the conformational flexibility of p53 and appear to stabilize the "active" conformation of wild-type p53, increasing its DNA binding and transactivation functions. Initial work demonstrated the ability of peptides to bind to the C terminus of latent p53 and activate it. In tumors where wild-type p53 is sequestered in the cytoplasm, C-terminal peptides were shown to stimulate p53 function by translocating p53 to the nucleus. Some peptides were able to activate the function of both wild-type and mutant p53 proteins. Screens of drug libraries identified additional molecules that can restore p53 function by stabilizing the "active" conformation of mutant and wild-type p53 proteins. Conversely, p53 function can be transiently inhibited by drugs and were shown to limit hair loss in mice following γ radiation. Alternative therapies may take advantage of the interactions of p53 with other proteins. Peptides have been designed that competitively inhibit the interaction of MDM2 and p53 proteins and restore the function of p53 in cases where MDM2 has been overexpressed.

VI. SUMMARY

Although discovered in the 1980s, p53 remains unique among tumor suppressor genes in its range of functions and widespread importance in tumor suppression. The p53 protein is inactivated by several oncogenic viruses and is the most common genetic lesion in human tumors. These features reflect the central role of p53 in human cancer. It is distinguished from other tumor suppressor genes by its sensitivity to a variety of point mutations that render it nonfunctional. The protein can perform multiple biochemical functions mediating both cell cycle arrest and apoptosis, as well as participating in DNA repair pathways. Therefore, it is uniquely poised to serve as the arbiter of whether cells should live or die by integrating diverse signals from the cell. These pathways provide a quality-assurance function, ensuring the proper development of tissues as well as the elimination of oncogenic cells. Although the complexities of the regulation of p53 have hindered its use as a diagnostic tool, it is becoming valuable as a prognostic indicator for tumors that are presently difficult to diagnose accurately. The challenge that awaits us now is to develop therapies that can selectively exploit the various activities of p53 for the treatment of human cancers.

See Also the Following Articles

Bibliography

Albrechtsen, N., Dornreiter, I., Grosse, F., Kim, E., Wiesmuller, L., and Deppert, W. (1999). Maintenance of genomic integrity by p53: Complementary roles for activated and non-activated p53. *Oncogene* **18,** 7706–7717.

An, W. G., Kanekal, M., Simon, M. C., Maltepe, E., Blagosklonny, M. V., and Neckers, L. M. (1998). Stabilization of wild-type p53 by hypoxia-inducible factor 1alpha. *Nature* **392,** 405–408.

Armstrong, J. F., Kaufman, M. H., Harrison, D. J., and Clarke, A. R. (1995). High-frequency developmental abnormalities in p53-deficient mice. *Curr. Biol.* **5,** 931–936.

Bennett, W. P., Hussain, S. P., Vahakangas, K. H., Khan, M. A., Shields, P. G., and Harris, C. C. (1999). Molecular epidemiology of human cancer risk: Gene-environment interactions and p53 mutation spectrum in human lung cancer. *J. Pathol.* **187,** 8–18.

Bhatavdekar, J. M., Patel, D. D., Shah, N. G., Vora, H. H., Suthar, T. P., Chikhlikar, P. R., Ghosh, N., and Trivedi, T. I. (2000). Prognostic significance of immunohistochemically localized biomarkers in stage II and stage III breast cancer: A multivariate analysis. *Ann. Surg. Oncol.* **7,** 305–311.

Birch, J. M., Blair, V., Kelsey, A. M., Evans, D. G., Harris, M., Tricker, K. J., and Varley, J. M. (1998). Cancer phenotype correlates with constitutional TP53 genotype in families with the Li-Fraumeni syndrome. *Oncogene* **17,** 1061–1068.

Bischoff, J. R., Kirn, D. H., Williams, A., Heise, C., Horn, S., Muna, M., Ng, L., Nye, J. A., Sampson-Johannes, A., Fattaey, A., and McCormick, F. (1996). An adenovirus mutant that replicates selectively in p53-deficient human tumor cells. *Science* **274,** 373–376.

Bottger, V., Bottger, A., Howard, S. F., Picksley, S. M., Chene, P., Garcia-Echeverria, C., Hochkeppel, H.-K., and Lane, D. P. (1996). Identification of novel mdm2 binding peptides by phage display. *Oncogene* **13,** 2141–2147.

Bouvard, V., Zaitchouk, T., Vacher, M., Duthu, A., Canivet, M., Choisy-Rossi, C., Nieruchalski, M., and May, E. (2000). Tissue and cell-specific expression of the p53-target genes: bax, fas, mdm2 and waf1/p21, before and following ionising irradiation in mice. *Oncogene* **19,** 649–660

Bullock, A. N., Henckel, J., and Fersht, A. R. (2000). Quantitative analysis of residual folding and DNA binding in mutant p53 core domain: definition of mutant states for rescue in cancer therapy. *Oncogene* **19,** 1245–1256.

Cai, W. B., Roberts, S. A., Bowley, E., Hendry, J. H., and Potten, C. S. (1997). Differential survival of murine small and large intestinal crypts following ionizing radiation. *Int. J. Radiat. Biol.* **71,** 145–155.

Carmeliet, P., Dor, Y., Herbert, J. M., Fukumura, D., Brusselmans, K., Dewerchin, M., Neeman, M., Bono, F., Abramovitch, R., Maxwell, P., Koch, C. J., Ratcliffe, P.,

Moons, L., Jain, R. K., Collen, D., Keshert, E., and Keshet, E. (1998). Role of HIF-1alpha in hypoxia-mediated apoptosis, cell proliferation and tumour angiogenesis [published erratum appears in *Nature* 1, 395(6701).525(1998)]. *Nature* **394,** 485–490.

Cho, Y., Gorina, S., Jeffrey, P. D., and Pavletich, N. P. (1994). Crystal structure of a tumor suppressor-DNA complex: Understanding tumorigenic mutations. *Science* **265,** 346–355.

Colombel, M., Radvanyi, F., Blanche, M., Abbou, C., Buttyan, R., Donehower, L. A., Chopin, D., and Thiery, J. P. (1994). Androgen suppressed apoptosis is modified in p53 deficient mice. *Oncogene* **10,** 1269–1274.

Debbas, M., and White, E. (1993). Wild-type p53 mediates apoptosis by E1A, which is inhibited by E1B. *Genes Dev.* **7,** 546–554.

de Stanchina, E., McCurrach, M. E., Zindy, F., Shieh, S. Y., Ferbeyre, G., Samuelson, A. V., Prives, C., Roussel, M. F., Sherr, C. J., and Lowe, S. W. (1998). E1A signaling to p53 involves the p19(ARF) tumor suppressor. *Genes Dev.* **12,** 2434–2442.

Donehower, L. A., Godley, L. A., Aldaz, C. M., Pyle, R., Shi, Y.-P., Pinkel, D., Gray, J., Bradley, A., Medina, D., and Varmus, H. E. (1995). Deficiency of *p53* accelerates mammary tumorigenesis in *Wnt-1* transgenic mice and promotes chromosomal instability. *Genes Dev.* **9,** 882–895.

Donehower, L. A., Harvey, M., Slagle, B. L., McArthur, M. J., Montgomery, C. A., Butel, J. S., and Bradley, A. (1992). Mice deficient for p53 are developmentally normal but susceptible to spontaneous tumors. *Nature* **356,** 215–221.

Dudenhöffer, C., Kurth, M., Janus, F., Deppert, W., and Wiesmüller, L. (1999). Dissociation of the recombination control and the sequence-specific transactivation function of P53. *Oncogene* **18,** 5773–5784.

Foster, B. A., Coffey, H. A., Morin, M. J., and Rastinejad, F. (1999). Pharmacological rescue of mutant p53 conformation and function. *Science* **286,** 2507–2510.

Godley, L. A., Kopp, J. B., Eckhaus, M., Paglino, J. J., Owens, J., and Varmus, H. E. (1996). Wild-type p53 transgenic mice exhibit altered differentiation of the uretic bud and possess small kidneys. *Genes Dev.* **10,** 836–850.

Greenblatt, M. S., Bennett, W. P., Hollstein, M., and Harris, C. C. (1994). Mutations in the p53 tumor suppressor gene: Clues to cancer etiology and molecular pathogenesis. *Cancer Res.* **54,** 4855–4878.

Hainaut, P., Soussi, T., Shomer, B., Hollstein, M., Greenblatt, M., Hovig, E., Harris, C. C., and Montesano, R. (1997). Database of p53 gene somatic mutations in human tumors and cell lines: Updated compilation and future prospects. *Nucl. Acids Res.* **25,** 151–157.

Herr, H. W., Bajorin, D. F., Scher, H. I., Cordon-Cardo, C., and Reuter, V. E. (1999). Can p53 help select patients with invasive bladder cancer for bladder preservation? *J. Urol.* **161,** 20–22.

Hupp, T. R., Sparks, A., and Lane, D. P. (1995). Small peptides activate the latent sequence-specific DNA binding function of p53. *Cell* **83,** 237–245.

Jacks, T., Remington, L., Williams, B. O., Schmitt, E. M., Halachmi, S., Bronson, R. T., and Weinberg, R. A. (1994). Tumor spectrum analysis in p53-mutant mice. *Curr. Biol.* **4,** 1–7.

Jeffrey, P. D., Gorina, S., and Pavletich, N. P. (1995). Crystal structure of the tetramerization domain of the p53 tumor suppressor at 1.7 angstroms. *Science* **267,** 1498–1502.

Jerry, D. J., Kittrell, F. S., Kuperwasser, C., Laucirica, R., Dickinson, E. S., Bonilla, P. J., Butel, J. S., and Medina, D. (2000). A mammary-specific model demonstrates the role of the p53 tumor suppressor gene in tumor development. *Oncogene* **19,** 1052–1058.

Jerry, D. J., Kuperwasser, C., Downing, S. R., Pinkas, J., He, C., Dickinson, E. S., Marconi, S., and Naber, S. P. (1998). Delayed involution of the mammary epithelium in BALB/c-p53null mice. *Oncogene* **17,** 2305–2312.

Khuri, F. R., Nemunaitis, J., Ganly, I., Arseneau, J., Tannock, I. F., Romel, L., Gore, M., Ironside, J., MacDougall, R. H., Heise, C., Randlev, B., Gillenwater, A. M., Bruso, P., Kaye, S. B., Hong, W. K., and Kirn, D. H. (2000). A controlled trial of intratumoral ONYX-015, a selectively-replicating adenovirus, in combination with cisplatin and 5-fluorouracil in patients with recurrent head and neck cancer. *Nature Med.* **6,** 879–885.

Kirch, H.-C., Flaswinkel, S., Rumpl, H., Brockmann, D., and Esche, H. (1999). Expression of human *p53* requires synergistic activation of transcription from the *p53* promoter by AP-1, NF-κB and Myc/Max. *Oncogene* **18,** 2728–2738.

Kleihues, P., Schauble, B., zur, H. A., Esteve, J., and Ohgaki, H. (1997). Tumors associated with p53 germline mutations: A synopsis of 91 families. *Am. J. Pathol.* **150,** 1–13.

Komarov, P. G., Komarova, E. A., Kondratov, R. V., Christov-Tselkov, K., Coon, J. S., Chernov, M. V., and Gudkov, A. V. (1999). A chemical inhibitor of p53 that protects mice from the side effects of cancer therapy. *Science* **285,** 1733–1737.

Komarova, E. A., Christov, K., Faerman, A. I., and Gudkov, A. V. (2000). Different impact of p53 and p21 on the radiation response of mouse tissues. *Oncogene* **19,** 3791–3798.

Kuerbitz, S. J., Plunkett, B. S., Walsh, W. V., and Kastan, M. B. (1992). Wild-type p53 is a cell cycle checkpoint determinant following irradiation. *Proc. Natl. Acad. Sci. USA* **89,** 7491–7495.

Kuperwasser, C., Hurlbut, G. D., Kittrell, F., Medina, D., Naber, S. P., and Jerry, D. J. (2000). Development of mammary tumors in Balb/c *p53*-heterozygous mice: A model for Li-Fraumeni syndrome. *Am. J. Pathol.*

Kuperwasser, C., Pinkas, J., Hurlbut, G. D., Naber, S. P., and Jerry, D. J. (2000). Cytoplasmic sequestration and functional repression of p53 in the mammary epithelium is reversed by hormonal treatment. *Cancer Res.* **60,** 2723–2729.

Ljungman, M. (2000). Dial 9-1-1 for p53: Mechanisms of p53 activation by cellular stress. *Neoplasia* **2,** 208–225.

Lowe, S. W., Jacks, T., Housman, D. E., and Ruley, H. E. (1994). Abrogation of oncogene-associated apoptosis allows transformation of p53-deficient cells. *Proc. Natl. Acad. Sci. USA* **91,** 2026–2030.

Ludwig, T., Chapman, D. L., Papaioannou, V. E., and Efstratiadis, A. (1997). Targeted mutations of breast cancer susceptibility gene homologs in mice: Lethal phenotypes of Brca1, Brca2, Brca1/Brca2, Brca1/p53, and Brca2/p53 nullizygous embryos. *Genes Dev.* **11,** 1226–1241.

MacCallum, D. E., Hupp, T. R., Midgley, C. A., Stuart, D., Campbell, S. J., Harper, A., Walsh, F. S., Wright, E. G., Balmain, A., Lane, D. P., and Hall, P. A. (1996). The p53 response to ionising radiation in adult and developing murine tissues. *Oncogene* **13,** 2575–2587.

Malkin, D., Li, F. P., Strong, L. C., Fraumeni, J. F., Nelson, C., Kim, D. J., Kassel, J., Gryka, M. A., Bischoff, F. Z., Tainsky, M. A., and Friend, S. H. (1990). Germ line p53 mutations in a familial syndrome of breast cancer, sarcomas and other neoplasms. *Science* **250,** 1233–1238.

Meek, D. W. (1999). Mechanisms of switching on p53: A role for covalent modification? *Oncogene* **18,** 7666–7675.

Merritt, A. J., Potten, C. S., Kemp, C. J., Hickman, J. A., Balmain, A., Lane, D. P., and Hall, P. A. (1994). The role of p53 in spontaneous and radiation-induced apoptosis in the gastrointestinal tract of normal and p53-deficient mice. *Cancer Res.* **54,** 614–617.

Mummenbrauer, T., Janus, F., Muller, B., Wiesmuller, L., Deppert, W., and Grosse, F. (1996). p53 protein exhibits 3′-to-5′ exonuclease activity. *Cell* **85,** 1089–1099.

Nakamura, T., Pichel, J. G., Williams, S. L., and Westphal, H. (1995). An apoptotic defect in lens differentiation caused by human p53 is rescued by a mutant allele. *Proc. Natl. Acad. Sci. USA* **92,** 6142–6146.

Noda, A., Toma-Aiba, Y., and Fujiwara, Y. (2000). A unique, short sequence determines p53 gene basal and UV-inducible expression in normal human cells. *Oncogene* **19,** 21–31.

Nomoto, S., Ootsuyama, A., Shioyama, Y., Katsuki, M., Kondo, S., and Norimura, T. (1998). The high susceptibility of heterozygous p53(+/−) mice to malformation after foetal irradiation is related to sub-competent apoptosis. *Int. J. Radiat. Biol.* **74,** 419–429.

Norimura, T., Nomoto, S., Katsuki, M., Gondo, Y., and Kondo, S. (1996). p53-dependent apoptosis suppresses radiation-induced teratogenesis. *Nature Med.* **2,** 577–580.

Ostermeyer, A. G., Runko, E., Winkfield, B., Ahn, B., and Moll, U. M. (1996). Cytoplasmically sequestered wild-type p53 protein in neuroblastoma is relocated to the nucleus by a C-terminal peptide. *Proc. Natl. Acad. Sci. USA* **93,** 15190–15194.

Pavletich, N. P., Chambers, K. A., and Pabo, C. O. (1993). The DNA-binding domain of p53 contains the four conserved regions and the major mutation hot spots. *Genes Dev.* **7,** 2556–2564.

Picksley, S. M., Spicer, J. F., Barnes, D. M., and Lane, D. P. (1996). The p53-MDM2 interaction in cancer-prone family, and the identification of a novel therapeutic target. *Acta Oncol.* **35,** 429–434.

Ravi, R., Mookerjee, B., Bhujwalla, Z. M., Sutter, C. H., Artemov, D., Zeng, Q., Dillehay, L. E., Madan, A., Semenza, G. L., and Bedi, A. (2000). Regulation of tumor angiogenesis by p53-induced degradation of hypoxia-inducible factor 1alpha. *Genes Dev.* **14,** 34–44.

Reinke, V., and Lozano, G. (1997). The p53 targets mdm2 and Fas are not required as mediators of apoptosis in vivo. *Oncogene* **15,** 1527–1534.

Reisman, D., and Loging, W. T. (1998). Transcriptional regulation of the p53 tumor suppressor gene. *Semin. Cancer Biol.* **8,** 317–324.

Rotman, G., and Shiloh, Y. (1999). ATM: A mediator of multiple responses to genotoxic stress. *Oncogene* **18,** 6135–6144.

Sah, V. P., Attardi, L. D., Mulligan, G. J., Williams, B. O., Bronson, R. T., and Jacks, T. (1995). A subset of p53-deficient embryos exhibit exencephaly. *Nature Genet.* **10,** 175–180.

Schmid, P., Lorenz, A., Hameister, H., and Montenarh, M. (1991). Expresion of p53 during mouse embryogenesis. *Development* **113,** 857–865.

Selivanova, G., Iotsova, V., Okan, I., Fritsche, M., Strom, M., Groner, B., Grafstrom, R. C., and Wiman, K. G. (1997). Restoration of the growth suppression function of mutant p53 by a synthetic peptide derived from the p53 C-terminal domain. *Nature Med.* **3,** 632–638.

Selivanova, G., Ryabchenko, L., Jansson, E., Iotsova, V., and Wiman, K. G. (1999). Reactivation of mutant p53 through interaction of a C-terminal peptide with the core domain. *Mol. Cell Biol.* **19,** 3395–3402.

Serrano, M., Lin, A. W., McCurrach, M. E., Beach, D., and Lowe, S. W. (1997). Oncogenic *ras* provokes premature cell senescence associated with accumulation of p53 and p16$^{\text{INK4a}}$. *Cell* **88,** 593–602.

Sionov, R. V., and Haupt, Y. (1999). The cellular response to p53: The decision between life and death. *Oncogene* **18,** 6145–6157.

Soengas, M. S., Alarcon, R. M., Yoshida, H., Giaccia, A. J., Hakem, R., Mak, T. W., and Lowe, S. W. (1999). Apaf-1 and caspase-9 in p53-dependent apoptosis and tumor inhibition. *Science* **284,** 156–159.

Soussi, T., Caron, D. F., and May, P. (1990). Structural aspects of the p53 protein in relation to gene evolution. *Oncogene* **5,** 945–952.

Tang, W., Willers, H., and Powell, S. N. (1999). p53 directly enhances rejoining of DNA double-strand breaks with cohesive ends in gamma-irradiated mouse fibroblasts. *Cancer Res.* **59,** 2562–2565.

Turner, B. C., Gumbs, A. A., Carbone, C. J., Carter, D., Glazer, P. M., and Haffty, B. G. (2000). Mutant p53 protein overexpression in women with ipsilateral breast tumor recurrence following lumpectomy and radiation therapy. *Cancer* **88,** 1091–1098.

Vahakangas, K. H., Samet, J. M., Metcalf, R. A., Welsh, J. A., Bennett, W. P., Lane, D. P., and Harris, C. C. (1992). Mutations of p53 and ras genes in radon-associated lung cancer from uranium miners. *Lancet* **339,** 576–580.

Varley, J. M., Evans, D. G., and Birch, J. M. (1997). Li-Fraumeni syndrome: A molecular and clinical review. *Br. J. Cancer* **76,** 1–14.

Varley, J. M., McGown, G., Thorncroft, M., Santibanez-Koref, M. F., Kelsey, A. M., Tricker, K. J., Evans, D. G., and Birch, J. M. (1997). Germ-line mutations of TP53 in Li-Fraumeni families: An extended study of 39 families. *Cancer Res.* **57,** 3245–3252.

Vineis, P., Malats, N., Porta, M., and Real, F. X. (1999). Human cancer, carcinogenic exposures and mutation spectra. *Mutat. Res.* **436,** 185–194.

Willers, H., McCarthy, E. E., Wu, B., Wunsch, H., Tang, W., Taghian, D. G., Xia, F., and Powell, S. N. (2000). Dissociation of p53-mediated suppression of homologous recombination from G1/S cell cycle checkpoint control. *Oncogene* **19,** 632–639.

Wilson, J. W., Pritchard, D. M., Hickman, J. A., and Potten, C. S. (1998). Radiation-induced p53 and p21WAF-1/CIP1 expression in the murine intestinal epithelium: Apoptosis and cell cycle arrest. *Am. J. Pathol* **153,** 899–909.

Transfer of Drug Resistance Genes to Hematopoietic Precursors

Thomas Moritz

University of Essen Medical School, Essen, Germany

David A. Williams

Herman B. Wells Center for Pediatric Research

GLOSSARY

chemotherapy resistance genes (CTX-R genes) Genes whose expression protects cells from the cytotoxic effects of chemotherapy drugs.

DNA glycosylases A class of enzymes that initiate the excision repair process of alkylation-damaged DNA.

DNA methyltransferases A class of proteins that repair alkylation-damaged DNA by the transfer of methyl groups.

hematopoietic progenitor cells Cells in the hematopoietic differentiation pathway that give rise to colonies *in vitro* with a restricted subset of mature hematopoietic cells [burst-forming unit-erythroid (BFU-E), colony-forming unit-granulocyte–macrophage (CFU-GM), mixed colony-forming unit (CFU-MIX), burst-forming unit-megakaryocyte (BFU-Mk), colony-forming unit-megakaryocyte (CFU-Mk)].

hematopoietic stem cells Primitive cells in the hematopoietic differentiation pathway that can give rise to all forms of hematopoietic cells and that have self-renewal capacity.

high-dose chemotherapy Dose-intensified form of chemotherapy, in which 3- to 10-fold increased doses are used and the hematopoietic system is supported by autologous stem cell transfusions and hematopoietic growth factor application.

multidrug resistance A mechanism that confers increased resistance to multiple chemotherapeutic agents to individual cells.

recombinant retrovirus vectors Engineered viral particles consisting of a retroviral backbone but lacking most of the retrovirus genome and carrying heterologous DNA sequences used for the purpose of gene transfer.

somatic gene therapy The introduction and expression of foreign genes in the somatic cells of a person for therapeutic purposes.

Since the early 1980s, somatic gene therapy has emerged as a potential new treatment modality. The lymphohematopoietic system, with its extensive proliferative and self-renewal capacities, has been considered one of the optimal targets for genetic manipulation. One approach to the clinical use of gene transfer technology is the introduction of chemotherapy resistance (CTX-R) genes into hematopoietic stem and progenitor cells. A number of CTX-R genes that confer resistance to some of the most frequently used chemotherapeutic agents have been defined and cloned. Stable introduction and expression of these genes in long-lived hematopoietic cells may result in protection from dose-limiting hematologic side effects of cancer chemotherapy and may allow dose intensification of current chemotherapy regimens.

I. INTRODUCTION

Severe and often dose-limiting side effects of anticancer chemotherapy include toxicity to the hematopoietic system, leading to neutropenia and thrombocytopenia. Reducing or eliminating these side effects is a major aim of current hematological research. Reducing such side effects would be expected to lower morbidity and mortality of current chemotherapy protocols. Subsequently, further dose intensification may improve survival rates. Currently, transfusions of red cells, platelets, and autologous hematopoietic progenitor and stem cells, as well as administration of recombinant hematopoietic growth factors, are used toward this aim. While these approaches provide some degree of protection to the hematopoietic system after chemotherapy, a 10- to 20-day period of severe myelosuppression significantly contributing to the morbidity and mortality of dose intensified chemotherapy regimens usually cannot be avoided. In this situation, the transfer of chemotherapy resistance genes into autologous hematopoietic cells prior to retransfusion is being investigated as a strategy to further reduce the hematological side effects of chemotherapy and/or to increase the dose intensity of treatment. CTX-R genes code for proteins, which protect cells from the toxic effects of chemotherapeutic drugs. A number of such genes have been identified and cloned (Table I). According to their function and subcellular localization, the products of CTX-R genes can roughly be subclassified into three groups: (i) membrane-bound proteins, which function as efflux pumps for cytotoxic drugs, such as the multidrug drug resistance protein 1 (MDR-1) or the multidrug resistance related protein (MRP); (ii) cytoplasmic proteins, which are involved in the metabolism of cytotoxic drugs or interfere with their mode of action, such as aldehyde dehydrogenase (ALDH), mutant forms of dihydrofolate reductase (ΔDHFR), glutathione S-transferase (GST), or cytidine deaminase (CDD); and (iii) nuclear proteins with DNA repair capacities, such as apurinic/apyrimidinic endonucleases (APE), methylpurine DNA glycosylases (MPG), or O^6-methylguanine DNA methyltransferases (MGMT).

The hematopoietic system is composed of several functional cell compartments (Fig. 1). Cells within these compartments differ significantly with respect to the capacity to proliferate and differentiate. The most primitive cells, pluripotent hematopoietic stem cells, have the capacity to generate additional stem cells (self-renewal) and to give rise to cells of all hematopoietic lineages (pluripotency). Functionally, the stem cell compartment has the capacity to reconstitute the hematopoietic system when used as a donor source for bone marrow transplantation (long-term reconstitution). To generate terminally differentiated and mature cells, pluripotent stem cells produce clonally derived progeny cells through a process termed commitment. During commitment, cells differentiate and simultaneously lose self-renewal capacity while becoming progressively restricted to a single blood cell lineage. Extensive cell proliferation is seen during commitment, allowing relatively few stem cells to generate the large cell numbers required daily for the normal functioning of the hematopoietic system.

Pluripotent hematopoietic stem cells maintain self-renewal capacity and therefore may allow long-lived

TABLE I
Candidate Chemotherapy Resistance Genes

Gene	Causes resistance to	Resistance mechanism
Plasma membrane		
Multidrug resistance 1	Vinca alkaloids, etoposide, taxol, anthracyclines, colchicine	Transmembrane drug efflux pump
Multidrug resistance-related protein	Vinca alkaloids, etoposide, anthracyclines	Transmembrane drug efflux pump
Cytoplasmic		
Dihydrofolate reductase	Methotrexate, trimetrexate	Mutant form is not inhibited by drug
Aldehyde dehydrogenase	Cyclophosphamide	Intracellular detoxification
Glutathione *S*-transferase	Cyclophosphamide	Intracellular detoxification
Thymidylate synthase	5-Fluorodeoxyuridine	Mutant form is not inhibited by drug
Ribonucleotide reductase	Hydroxyurea	Mutant form is not inhibited by drug
Tubulin	Vinca alkaloids and taxol	Mutant form is not inhibited by drug
Nuclear		
Methyltransferase	Alkylating agents	Repairs O^6 adduct
ada (encodes bacterial methyltransferase)	Alkylating agents	Repairs O^6 adduct
AP-endonuclease	Alkylating agents, etoposide, anthracyclines	Repairs AP sites after alkylation and oxidative DNA damage
APN-1 (encodes bacterial AP-endonuclease)	Alkylating agents, etoposide, anthracyclines	Repairs AP sites after alkylation and oxidative DNA damage
Methylpurine glycosylase	Alkylating agents	Removes alkylated bases
Superoxide dismutase	Anthracyclines and paraquat	Protects against oxidative damage
Topoisomerase I	Camptothecin	Role in DNA repair
Topoisomerase II	Anthracyclines and etoposide	Role in DNA repair

gene expression of heterologous DNA sequences in the hematopoietic system. Also, committed progenitors, such as CFU-E, CFU-GM, and CFU-Mix (see Fig. 1), have extensive proliferative capacities. Together with the relatively long-lived nature of progeny from these cells, committed progenitors may also prove useful targets for gene transfer. Transduction of relatively few primitive cells would be expected to generate large numbers of gene-modified mature progeny cells *in vivo*. Therefore, the design of clinical gene transfer protocols utilizing chemotherapy resistance genes should take into consideration both pluripotent stem cells and committed progenitor cells as potential targets.

Most current research focuses on the transduction of pluripotent stem cells. Although gene transfer into these cells has been achieved in murine systems by a number of research groups, the transfer of this technology to large outbred species, such as canines or primates and certainly humans, is still problematic, although considerable progress has been achieved in this area over the last few years. Gene transfer into committed progenitor cells, however, is a well-established procedure, but these target cells have not been extensively investigated for clinical applications. Although this approach does not seem suitable for repair of genetic defects requiring a life-long replacement of a missing gene product, it should allow the generation of chemotherapy-resistant hematopoietic cells *in vivo* for several weeks.

II. BACKGROUND: TRANSFER OF GENES INTO HEMATOPOIETIC CELLS

A. Methods of Gene Transfer

Due to the rapid progress in recombinant DNA technology, a variety of methods that allow introduction and expression of foreign genes in mammalian cells is available. Microinjection of DNA, calcium phosphate or diethylaminoethyl dextran (DEAE) precipitation, liposome-mediated transfection, electroporation, and a variety of biological gene transfer systems based on

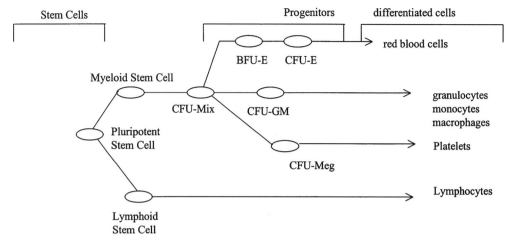

FIGURE 1 Model of hematopoietic stem cell differentiation illustrating progenitor cells of increasingly restricted potential that give rise to the maturing cells. CFU, colony-forming unit; Mix, granulocyte–erythrocyte–monocyte (or macrophage)–megakaryocyte; BFU, burst-forming unit; E, erythroid; GM, granulocyte–monocyte (or macrophage); Meg, megakaryocyte.

viral agents [herpesvirus, adenovirus, adeno-associated virus (AAV), and retroviruses, including lentiviruses and foamy viruses] are currently under investigation. Physical and chemical methods, which transduce DNA relatively inefficiently, are not considered clinically useful for gene transfer into hematopoietic cells. Because of the high efficiency of gene transduction, retrovirus-based vectors are the most commonly used vehicles for gene transfer into hematopoietic cells. Other virus-based systems have been hampered by safety problems and poor transduction efficiencies, although several have potential advantages over recombinant retroviral vectors. For instance, herpesvirus- and adenovirus-based systems allow transfer of large DNA sequences; AAV-, foamy virus-, and lentivirus-based vectors may allow the transduction of noncycling cells; and AAV-based systems also appear to lead to site-specific gene integration. Therefore, adenovirus-based systems (capable of mediating high-level gene expression for several weeks) may be a future alternative for gene transfer into committed progenitor cells, and with improvements, AAV-based vectors (the only vectors apart from retroviral vector that lead to stable integration of the gene) may offer new options for gene therapy utilizing both hematopoietic stem and progenitor cells. The most interesting alternative to retrovirus vectors, however, at present are lentiviral vectors, which are based on

the genome of HIV-1 or HIV-2. While initial constructs were restricted in their tropism to CD4-positive cells, envelope protein modification has extended the host range of modern lentiviral vectors substantially, and transduction rates of up to 90% have been reported for primary hematopoietic cells using these vectors. Studies on the transduction efficiency for long-lived stem cells are currently being performed. The outcome of these studies (in particular gene transfer efficiency in comparison to retroviral transduction) will determine the future role of lentivirus vectors in hematopoietic gene therapy, if safety problems associated with these HIV-1-related vectors can be resolved.

B. Retrovirus-Mediated Gene Transfer into Hematopoietic Cells

The first successful gene transfer into hematopoietic cells was described in 1983, when the dominant selectable marker gene for neomycin phosphotransferase (NEO) was introduced into a small proportion of murine CFU-GM via a retroviral vector. This was followed, in 1984, by gene transfer into murine colony-forming unit-spleen (CFU-S) cells, a transplantable, multilineage stem cell with limited self-renewal capacity. In 1985 the feasibility of successful gene transfer into pluripotent stem cells capable of long-term and multilineage reconstitution was further verified by retroviral integration pattern analysis showing clonally derived NEO-containing cells in murine bone marrow, thymus, and spleen after reconstitution following bone marrow transplant (BMT) of transduced hematopoietic stem cells. Since these early reports, a wide variety of different genes has been introduced *in vitro* into bone marrow cells from mice, humans, primates, and other animals. In contrast, efficient transduction of long-term repopulating cells in large animal models and in the clinical setting has been problematic. Although the initial gene marking trials in children with leukemia and neuroblastoma achieved long-term marker gene expression in up to 15% of peripheral blood progeny of transduced stem cells, until very recently the experience of other investigators has been disappointing.

Over the last several years the difficulties that must be overcome to establish gene transfer into hematopoietic cells as a feasible therapeutic option have become clearer. For instance, it is now well established that it is impossible to predict the efficiency of infection and expression of transferred sequences in primary hematopoietic cells of any specific vector based on *in vitro* testing. For instance, recombinant vectors selected on the basis of expression in primary fibroblast or permanent hematopoietic cell lines do not necessarily function well in primary hematopoietic cells. In addition, some promoters that do not function well in murine hematopoietic cells lead to high-level expression in human cells. Vectors specifically suited to express heterologous genetic sequences in primitive hematopoietic cells have been designed. In addition, in other areas of retrovirus gene transfer technology, substantial progress has been achieved. This includes the use of retrovirus particles with altered receptor specificity and incorporation of novel growth factors into the transduction protocols for hematopoietic cells, as well as the use of fibronectin fragments to facilitate the initial target cell/retrovirus interaction. Due to these improvements, gene transfer and transgene expression in 10–20% of mature blood cells has been described in large outbred animal models as well as in some clinical studies.

Until the early 1990s, adult bone marrow has been the main source of hematopoietic cells in gene transfer studies. Currently, two other sources of human hematopoietic progenitor and stem cells are also available: peripheral blood and umbilical vein cord blood. Mobilized peripheral blood stem and progenitor cells appear very useful in the context of hematoprotective gene therapy. Numerous studies have demonstrated that large numbers of committed progenitor and stem cells can be harvested by apheresis from adult patients after chemotherapy and growth factor treatment. As few as one or two apheresis procedures can yield sufficient cells for use in autologous bone marrow rescue after otherwise lethal chemotherapy. Meanwhile, studies by several groups have demonstrated convincingly gene transfer into peripheral blood-derived hematopoietic progenitor and stem cells *in vitro* as well as in *in vivo* animal studies. To date, some of the most successful clinical studies evaluating hematopoietic cell gene therapy were performed with leukapheresed peripheral blood cells, making chemotherapy and/or cytokine-activated peripheral blood hematopoietic cells a suitable and readily available target source for gene therapy. However, umbilical cord blood-derived cells, although a promising target for gene therapy in pediatric patients suffering from inherited disorders, are an unlikely target for use in hematoprotection after chemotherapy. Problems with the use of cord blood include the relatively small aliquot of CD34-positive cells in single cord blood harvests and a somewhat high rate of graft failure when such cells are used as donor stem cells in allogeneic transplants.

III. TRANSFER OF CHEMOTHERAPY RESISTANCE GENE: GENERAL CONSIDERATIONS

Hematoprotection after chemotherapy appears to be the most interesting and most readily achievable clinical application of chemotherapy resistance gene transfer into hematopoietic cells. In addition to the problems of transfer efficiency and expression of genes in target cells, two other prerequisites related to hematoprotective gene therapy have to be met to improve therapeutic results by this technology: (1) hematologic side effects need to be dose-limiting for the clinical use of the drug(s) the gene protects against and (2) dose intensification of the drug(s) within chemotherapeutic regimens should improve the antitumor efficacy of these regimens.

The first point has been established for several drugs for which CTX-R genes have been identified and cloned, such as nitrosoureas, endoxan, etoposide, and anthracyclines, while it is less clear for other drugs, such as methotrexate. However, many drugs with predominantly hematopoietic side effects at conventional doses have other organ toxicities that become critical with high-dose chemotherapy protocols. Examples include cardiac toxicity for anthracyclines, gut toxicity for etoposides, lung and liver toxicity for nitrosoureas, or neurotoxicity for taxanes. Using these drugs, further dose escalation may be problematic unless strategies can be developed that also can avoid or overcome these additional toxicities in other organs. One approach to circumvent this problem may be the simultaneous transfer of multiple CTX-R genes, a strategy for which suitable retroviral constructs are already available. This should allow for the rational design of chemotherapy protocols, which reduce individual organ toxicity by combining different CTX-R associated drugs.

The second point is more controversial. Numerous clinical studies have shown that a direct relationship exists between the dose intensity of chemotherapy administered to a patient and the antitumor response observed. These observations have been made from randomized studies comparing regimens of different dose intensity between matched patient populations, as well as studies within one population reporting inferior therapeutic results in those patients who received less dose intensive therapy (usually due to side effects). However, nearly all of these studies investigated dose intensities only up to the point that was defined as dose limiting in the context of conventional chemotherapy (usually due to hematological side effects). It has not been proven universally that the same dose–response relationship exists when the dose intensities of standard chemotherapy are exceeded. While numerous studies have investigated high-dose chemotherapy regimens using hematopoietic growth factor and/or autologous stem cell support, data supporting the efficiency of this type of therapy are limited to a small number of diseases. Significantly better cure rates and/or overall survival following high-dose chemotherapy in prospectively randomized studies have been demonstrated only for patients suffering from mul-

tiple myeloma (stage II or III disease according to Salmon–Durie) or relapsed high-grade non-Hodgkin's lymphomas and are likely in primary progressive or relapsed Hodgkin's disease and high-risk germ cell tumors. For other disease entities, in particular breast and ovarian cancer, however, the benefit of high-dose chemotherapy is still controversial.

A specific therapeutic dilemma in which CTX-R gene transfer might be helpful is the treatment of recurrent disease after initial high-dose chemotherapy. Although the tumor often is responsive to chemotherapeutic treatment in this situation, therapeutic options may be hampered by a compromised hematopoietic system. In this situation, myelosuppression frequently represents the dose-limiting toxicity. Transfer of CTX-R genes into the autologous hematopoietic cells used for hematopoietic support during high-dose chemotherapy might be a way to secure further chemotherapeutic treatment options for patients who carry a high risk of recurrent disease.

Another possible application of CTX-R genes in gene therapy is their use as dominant selectable markers within vectors that are primarily designed to express another therapeutic gene. This strategy appears to be particularly suited for the genetic therapy of monogenic diseases affecting the hematopoietic system in which the introduced therapeutic gene does not confer a selective growth advantage to the transduced self-renewing stem cell population. This applies to diseases in which the genetic defect primarily affects the function of mature hematopoietic cells but is not associated with a defective stem cell. Strategies aiming at permanent cure of genetic diseases will require the transduction of primitive long-lived hematopoietic stem cells. However, given the limitations of current gene transfer technology, the percentage of initially transduced stem cells will probably be low and may not be sufficient for phenotypic correction and cure. Therefore, expression of the transferred gene in a therapeutically relevant number of effector cells will probably necessitate selection procedures. A major impediment to the use of CTX-R genes in this context is the considerable mutagenic potential of most of the associated chemotherapeutic drugs. Mutagenic side effects have not been described, however, following treatment with the folate antagonists methotrexate (MTX) and trimetrexate (TMTX). Transfer of mutant forms of DHFR in combination with MTX or TMTX application is currently under intensive investigation to enrich for genetically corrected cells in diseases such as chronic granulomatous disease or Gaucher's disease.

While transduction of long-term repopulating cells will be required for strategies aiming at the life-long cure of monogenic diseases affecting the hematopoietic system, transduction of more committed populations, such as clonogenic progenitor cells, may be sufficient for protection of the hematopoietic system from cytotoxic chemotherapy-induced myelosuppression. Clonogenic progenitors with granulocyte–macrophage (CFU-GM), erythroid (BFU-E), and multiple lineage (CFU-MIX) differentiation potential still possess high proliferative capacities and may generate large numbers of functional mature cells after adequate growth factor stimulation. In contrast to human stem cells, gene transfer into human clonogenic progenitor cells is a well-established and highly efficient procedure. In addition, clonogenic assays allow reliable quantification of human progenitor cells, the cells are well defined by their CD34$^+$ surface phenotype, and efficient enrichment using clinically applicable procedures is well established.

The choice of target cells for CTX-R gene transfer strategies will depend, at least to a certain degree, on the individual chemotherapeutic agent, as considerable differences in the relative toxicity for stem cells, progenitor cells, and more committed cells have been described for different agents. Progenitor cell gene transfer is most likely to be of clinical benefit in the context of agents with predominant toxicity at the level of clonogenic or more committed cells, such as methotrexate or cyclophosphamide, whereas efficient marrow protection from agents with predominant stem cell toxicity, such as nitrosoureas or busulfan, will presumably require CTX-R gene transfer into stem cells. Another point to be considered (especially in the context of high-dose chemotherapy) is the significant and long-lasting suppression of the lymphoid compartment associated with therapy. Gene transfer strategies targeting primarily primitive stem cells have been shown in some cases to confer some degree of protection to the lymphoid compartment.

Chemotherapy resistance gene transfer to committed progenitor cells as envisioned here would require more intensive manipulation to achieve hematoprotection than infection of stem cells, as this approach would need repeated infusions of transduced cells with each chemotherapy cycle. However, some evidence suggests that dose intensification during the first two to four cycles of chemotherapy is critical to improving therapeutic results. Intensification protocols utilizing gene transfer methods might target these early cycles in chemotherapy regimens.

A more theoretical problem with targeting committed progenitors for use in chemotherapy protocols is the subsequent risk of stem cell depletion. As reviewed earlier, current technology allows only a few primitive stem cells to be transduced. Although infection of committed progenitors may protect patients from the acute hematotoxicity of intensified chemotherapy, the lack of protection at the stem cell level may lead to bone marrow failure after the transduced progenitor cells have differentiated. Optimal candidate genes for use in such protocols might be expected to be those encoding resistance to cytotoxic agents that tend to spare more primitive cell populations.

IV. CANDIDATE CHEMOTHERAPY RESISTANCE GENES

A. Mutant Dihydrofolate Reductase

Dihydrofolate reductase is a key enzyme in folate metabolism catalyzing the reduction from dihydrofolate to the metabolically active tetrahydrofolate. The cytotoxic drug methotrexate, a folate analog that acts as a competitive inhibitor of DHFR, leads to depletion of tetrahydrofolate and accumulation of toxic amounts of dihydrofolates and related metabolic products, leading to cell death. Several mutant forms of DHFR have been cloned that catalyze the physiological reaction of the enzyme but are no longer inhibited by methotrexate. In a variety of cell systems, expression of ΔDHFR proteins confers resistance against MTX.

A mutant DHFR cDNA was the first CTX-R sequence successfully introduced into hematopoietic cells. Expression of ΔDHFR in committed progenitors (murine, canine, and human) was reported in 1986. In addition, two studies have demonstrated stable introduction of ΔDHFR into murine hematopoietic stem cells in bone marrow transplant models. In both studies, generation of MTX-resistant bone marrow following gene transduction was associated with improved hematologic recovery and survival when MTX was administered in the immediate posttransplant period. During this posttransplant period, bone marrow appears to have increased sensitivity to MTX, and hematologic side effects of MTX are dose-limiting in the mouse. These studies also demonstrated the presence of MTX-resistant committed progenitor cells in primary and secondary recipients of bone marrow transduced with the ΔDHFR vector 8 to 10 weeks after transplantation. Protection from MTX toxicity after ΔDHFR gene transfer, at least *in vitro*, has also been demonstrated for primary human hematopoietic cells from peripheral blood and cord blood, although data for ΔDHFR gene transfer into the human hematopoietic system are scarce. These initial studies were performed with DHFR mutants characterized by single amino acid changes at positions 22 or 31 such as arg22, tyr22, or ser31. Subsequent studies utilizing double mutants such as tyr22-ser31, tyr22-gly31, or tyr22-arg31 demonstrated even higher resistance to folate antagonists in hematopoietic cell lines and primary murine hematopoietic cells *in vitro*, and these mutants are presently being evaluated in a number of *in vivo* animal studies.

One drawback to the clinical application of ΔDHFR vectors is the fact that hematologic toxicity is often not a dose-limiting factor in MTX therapy. One possible exception, as noted earlier, is the immediate posttransplant period. In mice following BMT, hematologic side effects clearly limit the dose of MTX that can be administered. Administration of MTX to humans undergoing allogeneic bone marrow transplantation, where it is frequently used to prevent graft-versus-host disease, has also been noted to cause severe myelosuppressive episodes. Transfer of ΔDHFR genes into hematopoietic cells might be explored in this setting in the future. Outside the posttransplantation setting, ΔDHFR gene transfer for marrow protection will probably be most helpful in combinations with other CTX-R genes.

An attractive clinical application for the ΔDHFR/MTX or ΔDHFR/TMTX system may be *in vivo* selection, as MTX and TMTX differ from other CTX-R-associated drugs in their lack of mutagenic potential. *In vivo* selection strategies are most likely to be of benefit in the treatment of monogenic diseases, but have also been evaluated in the context of

bcr/abl antisense gene transfer for the treatment of CML. However, several studies suggest that the main toxicity of folate antagonists within the hematopoietic system is on a postclonogenic precursor cell population, whereas more primitive hematopoietic cells, such as clonogenic progenitors or stem cells, are relatively resistant to these drugs. This concept is supported by the fact that although several studies have shown marrow protection from MTX toxicity *in vivo*, convincing evidence for the selection of ΔDHFR-transduced cells has been lacking. The relative resistance of primitive hematopoietic cells to folate antagonists has been attributed to the ability of these cells to overcome some degree of MTX or TMTX toxicity by uptake and utilization of preformed nucleotide precursors present in the serum. It has been shown that the addition of thymidine and hypoxanthine to semisolid cultures of BM cells reduces the toxicity of MTX, and the protective effects of ΔDHFR gene transfer *in vitro* are best demonstrated in dialyzed or thymidine phosphorylase-pretreated (and thus thymidine-depleted) serum. Similarly, *in vitro* selection of ΔDHFR expressing cells also seems to require thymidine depletion of serum.

One way to circumvent this problem is the administration of inhibitors of thymidine uptake in combination with MTX or TMTX. Nucleosides enter cells via carrier proteins and these transporters can specifically be blocked by substances such as dipyridamole, draflazine, or nitrobenzylmercaptopurine-riboside (NBMPR). When TMTX treatment was combined with inhibitors of cellular nucleoside uptake, significantly increased toxicity for both myeloid progenitor cells and repopulating stem cells was observed. In subsequent studies the same group of investigators demonstrated in a murine bone marrow transplant/gene transfer model *in vivo* selection of ΔDHFR-transduced stem cells after combined treatment with TMTX and NBMPR.

B. Multidrug Resistance Caused by P-Glycoprotein and Other Detoxifying Transmembrane Pump Proteins

Resistance to a wide variety of chemotherapeutic drugs, including anthracyclines, vinca alkaloids, etoposide, and taxol, has been shown to be associated with expression of a 170-kDa glycoprotein (P-glycoprotein) on the cell surface. P-glycoprotein acts as an ATP-dependent transmembrane efflux pump for a variety of molecules, including the chemotherapeutic drugs mentioned. Although other membrane proteins with similar function have been reported in association with multidrug resistance, P-glycoprotein is by far the best characterized and probably most important of these transport systems. The gene for the P-glycoprotein (MDR-1) has been identified, and a cDNA was cloned in 1986. Transfection studies introducing the MDR-1 cDNA into a variety of cell lines, including hematopoietic lines, have shown a 20- to 30-fold increase in resistance of these cells to MDR-1-associated drugs. Additional studies using transgenic mice expressing human MDR-1 gene sequences have shown protection of the mice from the hematotoxicity of MDR-1 associated drugs *in vivo*. These results make MDR-1 an attractive candidate gene for gene transfer into hematopoietic cells for the purpose of bone marrow protection.

MDR-1 has been successfully introduced and expressed in murine and human hematopoietic progenitor cells via recombinant retroviral vectors. Expression of the introduced MDR-1 cDNA increased resistance to MDR-1-associated drugs in these cells. Transduction of MDR-1 has been demonstrated in unfractionated and CD34$^+$ human bone marrow cells. Several studies have also demonstrated successful transduction of long-term reconstituting stem cells with MDR-1 in murine BMT models. In these studies, significant *in vivo* selection for transduced cells was observed after repeated challenges of the transduced animals with taxol.

Based on these encouraging preclinical results, several groups have translated the concept of MDR-1 gene transfer to the clinic and applied it to the treatment of lymphomas or solid malignancies. Peripheral blood, as well as bone marrow-derived autologous hematopoietic cells, that were administered as supportive treatment in the context of high-dose chemotherapy were transduced with different MDR-1 expressing retrovirus vectors. Results of these early studies, however, have been disappointing, and gene transfer efficiency for stem cells, as well as long-term expression of the transgene in the hematopoietic system, was well below 1% of to-

tal hematopoietic cells. Significantly better gene transfer efficiency, as measured by proviral integration of the MDR-1 expressing vector construct, has only been reported from a recent study in patients with testicular cancer. In this study, however, retrovirus expression of MDR-1 sequences was deficient due to mRNA splicing.

Other investigators have also reported problems with expression of the MDR-1-encoded P-glycoprotein even in successfully transduced cells. At least in part these problems appear to be related to the relatively large size of the MDR-1 cDNA (4.2 kb) and the presence of a number of cryptic splice donor and splice acceptor sites within the gene. While it appears that the generation of more efficient vectors for MDR-1 expression and modifications in the MDR-1 cDNA will eventually solve these problems, a more serious potential issue has been raised by studies reporting a significant rate of myeloproliferative syndrome when mice were transplanted with MDR-1 transduced and *in vitro*-expanded donor cells. So far, other groups using different retroviral vectors have not reproduced these data, and it has been speculated that the myeloproliferative syndrome is related to sequences specific to the Harvey sarcoma virus backbone of the vector utilized in the original studies. At present, caution is being exercised in planning and conducting further clinical studies investigating MDR-1 gene transfer.

Similar to the ΔDHFR system, MDR-1 gene transfer to stem cells might also be utilized to select for transduced cells, and selection of MDR-1 expressing cells has been demonstrated *in vitro* for clonogenic human hematopoietic cells, as well as *in vivo* in mice. While *in vivo* application of this system in the context of gene therapy for monogenic diseases may be questionable due to the mutagenic side effects of MDR-1-related drugs, *in vivo* selection of MDR-1-transduced cells could be of relevance for strategies aiming at marrow protection. In this situation, repetitive application of MDR-1-associated drugs after MDR-1 gene transfer could generate widespread MDR-1-related drug resistance in the hematopoietic system, despite relatively low initial transduction rates. Whether selection at the stem cell level can be achieved in the clinical setting remains to be seen, as high endogenous expression of MDR-1, corresponding to a "rhodamine dull phenotype" previously utilized as a marker of stem cells in murine studies, has been reported for primitive human cells, including human cells, capable of repopulating immune-deficient mice.

In addition to MDR-1, a whole family of detoxifying membrane transport proteins containing the ATP binding cassette exists. The multidrug resistance associated protein (MRP) is another member of this family. MRP was originally cloned from a multidrug-resistant small cell lung cancer cell line (H69/AR) and confers resistance against vinca alkaloids, etoposide, and certain anthracyclines. Overexpression of the MRP-cDNA was demonstrated to confer an MRP-type multidrug resistance phenotype to fibroblasts, as well as several human cancer cell lines. Gene transfer of MRP into hematopoietic cells was investigated in a murine gene transfer/bone marrow transplant model. In these studies, retrovirus expression of MRP in transplanted cells reduced doxorubicin-induced myelosuppression and mortality substantially. In addition, *in vivo* selection of transgenic MRP-expressing cells was demonstrated.

C. O⁶-Methylguanine DNA Methyltransferase and Other DNA Repair Proteins

Highly conserved DNA repair mechanisms exist among such distantly related organisms as bacteria, yeast, insects, fishes, and mammals. These repair mechanisms protect cells from toxic effects of many alkylating agents. Modifications in all four major pathways, base excision repair (BER), nucleotide excision repair (NER), mismatch repair (MMR), and the direct reversal of mutations by O^6-methylguanine DNA methyltransferase (MGMT) have been demonstrated to be associated with alteration in cellular sensitivity to mono- and bifunctional alkylating agents. While in some cases increased activity of DNA repair pathways is associated with cellular resistance, with MMR the opposite phenotype has been reported, i.e., increased resistance with impairment of the pathway. Additionally, experiments with "knockout" mice have revealed that the relative activity of different pathways in primary hematopoietic cells is of importance. While the hematopoietic cells of MGMT-deficient knockout animals are significantly more sensitive to alkylating agents than cells from their wild-type lit-termates, additional loss of the mismatch repair pathway (MGMT $^{-/-}$; MLH1$^{-/-}$) restores the animals to the more resistant phenotype of the wild-type litter-mates. So far, very little is known concerning the expression of DNA repair enzymes in hematopoietic cells. Even less is known about the role of individual repair enzymes or repair pathways in the hematotoxicity induced by specific chemotherapeutic agents. This lack of information still significantly hampers the use of DNA repair genes in gene transfer strategies aiming at hematoprotection.

An exception is the DNA repair process performed by O^6-methylguanine DNA methyltransferases. These proteins repair O^6-guanine alkyl adducts, which are induced by cytotoxic drugs of the chloroethylnitrosourea (CENU) variety, such as ACNU, BCNU, and CCNU, or by triazene derivatives, such as dacarbazine and temozolomide. Among the various DNA lesions induced by these substances, O^6-guanine alkyl adducts are particularly cytotoxic, as they ultimately induce irreversible interstrand cross-links in the DNA. These cross-links can be prevented by early repair of the O^6-alkyl lesions. DNA methyltransferases perform this repair function by transfer of the damaging alkyl group to a cysteine in the acceptor pocket of the protein. It has been demonstrated that *in vitro* sensitivity to CENUs correlates inversely with cellular MGMT levels, and inhibition of MGMT by the specific pharmacologic inhibitor O^6-benzylguanine (6-BG) increases the toxicity of CENUs. Although MGMT is present in a variety of mammalian cells, bone marrow cells express the protein at low levels. In the clinical setting, a severe and delayed myelosuppression is the dose-limiting toxicity of CENU treatment. This clinical hematotoxicity of the nitrosoureas differs from the toxicity seen with most other cytotoxic drugs in that it is delayed, with the nadirs for white blood cells and platelets occurring 4–5 and 5–6 weeks, respectively, after drug administration. With repeated doses, this nadir becomes more severe and prolonged, and hematotoxicity can be fatal. In mouse models, CENU administration has been demonstrated to cause extensive damage to the stem cell compartment. Therefore, it seems likely that approaches aimed at the reduction of nitrosourea-induced hematotoxicity will require the successful transduction of hematopoietic stem cells. Other major side effects of CENUs are renal and pulmonary, but with the exception of BCNU, where pulmonary toxicity most likely will prohibit major dose escalation, dose intensification may be possible if gene transfer into hematopoietic stem cells successfully reduces bone marrow toxicity.

Several investigators have shown the feasibility of this approach *in vitro*. In addition, more recent studies in mice have demonstrated increased tolerance to nitrosourea chemotherapy following gene transfer of MGMT into transplanted repopulating stem cells. Also, selection of MGMT-modified cells in the myeloid and lymphoid compartment of these mice after nitrosourea treatment was detected. However, on a cellular level, the increase in MGMT resistance was only modest. This is particularly noteworthy, as some tumors have been demonstrated to increase expression of MGMT, and such expression may cause tumor chemoresistance. Thus, efforts are underway to manipulate MGMT activity in tumors through the systemic administration of inhibitors, such as 6-BG.

Potentially useful to this approach, mutant forms of MGMT (ΔMGMT) that are resistant to inhibition by 6-BG offer a chance to increase the level of protection of bone marrow-derived cells. 6-BG is a guanine analog that causes irreversible inactivation of the MGMT protein. *In vitro* studies with tumor cell lines and xenograft studies in tumor-bearing animals have demonstrated the potential of 6-BG to augment the tumor cytotoxic activity of nitrosoureas and other O^6-alkylating agents. This observation also has been verified in clinical phase I studies. In the clinical studies, as well as in preclinical toxicity analysis in murine models, severe myelosuppression was determined to be the dose-limiting toxicity of combined 6-BG and nitrosourea treatment. This finding was not unexpected given the low endogenous level of MGMT expression in bone marrow. Therefore, combined 6-BG/nitrosourea treatment supported by expression of ΔMGMT in the hematopoietic system may be a strategy to improve the treatment options for nitrosourea-resistant tumors.

Initial experiments with 6-BG-resistant forms of MGMT were performed with the bacterial ada methyltransferase gene. While expression of ada in primary murine hematopoietic progenitor cells *in vitro*

resulted in significantly increased resistance to combined 6-BG plus nitrosourea treatment, marrow protection in a murine bone marrow transplant/gene transfer model was only modest. Due to these results, which have been attributed to deficient nuclear distribution of the bacterial protein, and to concerns about possible immunologic responses to the expression of bacterial proteins in human cells, additional studies have been performed with human ΔMGMT. A greater than 8-fold increased resistance to combined 6-BG/nitrosourea treatment was demonstrated in human clonogenic progenitor cells after gene transfer of a human Gly→Ala mutant (G156A) of MGMT *in vitro*, and similar results were observed for the more primitive long-term culture initiating cells. In a murine bone marrow transplantation/gene transfer model, expression of G156A also allowed protection of the bone marrow from the combined toxicity of 6-BG/nitrosourea and enrichment for transduced hematopoietic cells. In comparison to gene transfer of wild-type MGMT, the selection advantage of ΔMGMT was more pronounced and ΔMGMT proviral sequences increased from 67% of CFU before treatment to nearly 100% after one cycle of chemotherapy treatment. Up to a 10-fold increased resistance to 6-BG/nitrosourea treatments was detected in committed progenitor cells harvested 13 to 23 weeks after transplantation. A selective advantage for ΔMGMT-transduced hematopoietic cells has also been demonstrated in nonmyeloablated mice. In this study, while there was no evidence of ΔMGMT proviral sequences in the bone marrow of mice injected with 5×10^4 to 1×10^6 BM cells and left untreated, mice receiving 6-BG/nitrosourea treatment following transplantation demonstrated ΔMGMT proviral sequences in 15 to 97% of bone marrow-derived CFU 24 to 30 weeks after transplantation. Meanwhile, other mutants of MGMT, which are more highly resistant to 6-BG, are being investigated and initial data using these mutants look promising.

The concept of treating MGMT-overexpressing malignancies with 6-BG plus nitrosoureas while protecting the hematopoietic system by ΔMGMT gene transfer has already been tested in a xenograft tumor model. Nude mice were transplanted with isogeneic ΔMGMT-expressing bone marrow and inoculated with SW480 human colon carcinoma cells (which are highly resistant to nitrosoureas due to high wild-type MGMT expression). Thereafter the mice are treated with a combined 6-BG/nitrosourea therapy. In comparison to control littermates transplanted with mock-transduced bone marrow, mice receiving ΔMGMT-transduced transplants tolerated higher dose intensities of treatment, resulting in a significant delay in tumor growth. These data clearly support the potential clinical relevance of marrow protection by ΔMGMT in the context of MGMT-overexpressing malignancies, and currently several groups are trying to evaluate this concept on a clinical level. Such phase I studies are examining toxicity of expression of wild-type MGMT cDNA in bone marrow cells. Based on preclinical data, the next trials in humans may involve 6-BG-resistant MGMT mutants.

A number of eukaryotic DNA glycosylase genes have been cloned from *Saccharomyces cerevisiae* (MAG), human (AAG), and murine (MAAG) cells. It seems likely that some of these enzymes recognize and repair base adducts produced by nitrosoureas, as has been shown for *Escherichia coli*-derived 3-methyladenine DNA glycosylase (3MeA). Overexpression of the human AAG gene does protect glycosylase-deficient *E. coli* strains substantially against nitrosoureas, but data for eukaryotic cells (in particular in mammalian cells) are still lacking. Glycosylase enzymes appear to be interesting candidates to protect against nitrosourea-induced hematotoxicity. However, other candidate genes in the BER pathway, particularly apurinic/apyrimidinic endonuclease (APE) and the yeast endonuclease, APN-1, appear to protect cells from some other agents, such as bleomycin. In addition, the *E. coli* gene, fpg, which repairs ring-open DNA lesions, appears useful in mediating cellular resistance to another commonly used alkylating agent, thiotepa.

D. Aldehyde Dehydrogenase, Glutathione S-Transferase, and Cyclophosphamide-Induced Toxicity

Cyclophosphamide is one of the most commonly used alkylating agents in the treatment of cancer and is also included in a dose-intensified protocol. Myelosuppression, which is relatively confined to progenitor and precursor cells and spares the stem cell compartment, is the dose-limiting toxicity of the drug. As intracellular detoxification of drugs appears to be an important mechanism to prevent alkylating agent-induced cross-linking of DNA, the relative resistance of stem cells to cyclophosphamide has been attributed to high expression of the detoxifying enzyme cytosolic aldehyde dehydrogenase (ALDH). In contrast, ALDH expression in hematopoietic progenitor or precursor cells is relatively low. This high ALDH expression also has allowed the use of 4-hydroperoxy-cyclophosphamide (4-HC), a metabolic product of cyclophosphamide, as a stem cell sparing agent for *in vitro* bone marrow purging prior to autologous bone marrow transplantation. ALDH is a cytosolic enzyme, which catalyzes the oxidative metabolism of aldophosphamide—the metabolic product of cyclophosphamide—to the nontoxic carboxyphosphamide. This conversion competes with the nonenzymatic breakdown of aldophosphamide to acrolein and phosphamide mustard, substances that are directly responsible for cyclophosphamide-induced DNA cross-linking.

Augmenting the expression of ALDH via gene transfer appears as an attractive strategy to improve cyclophosphamide resistance in the hematopoietic system, in particular in progenitor or precursor cells. A retroviral vector containing the human ALDH cDNA sequence was reported to increase the level of ALDH expression in both murine leukemia and human hematopoietic cell lines *in vitro*, conferring a significant increase in cyclophosphamide resistance—4-fold in the murine system and 1.5-fold more in the human system—to these cells. Increased resistance to 4-HC after retroviral transduction with ALDH was also reported in primary human clonogenic progenitor cells. At the moment it remains unclear as to whether ALDH gene transfer can also protect from cyclophosphamide hematotoxicity *in vivo*. Given the relative low level of protection conferred to human hematopoietic cells *in vitro*, ALDH gene transfer alone may not suffice for this purpose and a combination with another cyclophosphamide resistance conferring gene may be required.

Such a combination may utilize glutathione S-transferase. The polypeptide glutathione is a critical component in cellular defense against oxidative and radical-induced damage, including damage caused by alkylating agents, such as cyclophosphamide, cisplatinum, or anthracyclines. Depletion of glutathione sensitizes cells to these drugs, whereas increased glutathione levels in cell lines and primary tumor tissue have been associated with chemotherapy resistance. Glutathione is believed to exert its effects mainly by maintaining a reductive microenvironment within the cell. A variety of enzymes have been identified that interact with glutathione and/or regulate glutathione levels, such as GSTs, glutathione peroxidase, glutathione reductase, and γ-glutamyl transpeptidase (GGT). While all of these proteins theoretically might be used as targets in gene therapy approaches, the majority of work so far has been done with GSTs.

GSTs are a family of structurally diverse proteins that catalyze the formation of conjugates between toxic agents (including cytotoxic drugs) and glutathione. In mammals, these enzymes have been classified on the basis of sequence similarity into five classes: the cytosolic forms α, μ, π, φ, and a microsomal form. Transfection of GST cDNAs has been shown to confer resistance to alkylating drugs in several cell lines, and population studies have associated null mutants of GST genes with an increased susceptibility to cancers of the skin, lung, and cervix. In the context of cyclophosphamide, detoxification of aldophosphamide by conjugation with GSH to a nontoxic intermediate seems to be the most relevant reaction, but GST can also participate in the detoxification of acrolein and phosphamide mustard. The Yc isoform of GST, a member of the α family, which is not constitutively expressed in rat or human bone marrow cells, has been studied particularly in this respect.

In vitro studies of GST gene transfer in cell lines have reported modest increases (1.5- to 3-fold) in the relative resistance to a number of cytotoxic drugs, including alkylating agents. One study has also demonstrated significantly increased 4-HC resistance in CFU-GM progenitor cells after transfection of a GST expression vector into human CD34$^+$ peripheral blood cells. Although in principle, targeting the glutathione system offers the opportunity to confer resistance to many frequently used cytotoxic drugs, the combination with ALDH gene transfer to augment cyclophosphamide resistance from the level achievable with either gene alone would appear more promising. Retroviral vectors allowing simultaneous expression of both genes from one viral backbone are well within the scope of present retrovirus technology.

E. Cytidine Deaminase

Cytidine analogs such as cytosine arabinoside (Ara-C), 2′,2′-difluorodeoxycytidine (gemcitabine), or 5-aza-2′-deoxycytidine (deoxycoformycin) represent a class of potent chemotherapeutic agents with widespread applications in the treatment of hematological and, in the case of gemcitabine, also solid malignancies. The dose-limiting toxicity of these drugs is myelosuppression. Ara-C resistance has been observed in leukemic cell lines and primary human myeloblasts overexpressing cytidine deaminase (CDD). This enzyme catalyzes the deamination of cytosine nucleotides and analogs such as Ara-C and thus prevents the intracellular accumulation of Ara-CTP, the active metabolite of Ara-C. While CDD expression is relatively high in gut, liver, and differentiated myeloid cells (in particular granulocytes), primitive human CD34$^+$ hematopoietic cells express CDD at very low levels, which may explain the high hematotoxicity of Ara-C. CDD expression in primary "nonmalignant" CD34$^+$ cells is also lower than expression in AML myeloblasts. The cDNA of human CDD has been cloned, and several groups have reported increased resistance to Ara-C in murine fibroblasts expressing human CDD. In subsequent studies, induction of Ara-C resistance by CDD gene transfer was also demonstrated for hematopoietic cell lines and primary murine clonogenic progenitor cells *in vitro*. However, the level of protection conferred by CDD overexpression in individual studies varied considerably, ranging from 2.5- to 20-fold for cell lines and 2- to 10-fold for primary cells. CDD gene transfer has also been investigated in a murine bone marrow transplantation/gene transfer model in which after engraftment of CDD-transduced cells, recipient animals were exposed to three cycles of Ara-C treatment. In this model, despite successful gene transfer, only modestly increased Ara-C resistance in clonogenic progenitor cells harvested from recipient animals 1 year after transplantation was detected, and no convincing evidence of bone marrow protection from Ara-C toxicity or selection of transduced cells was seen.

Thus, at present, a myeloprotective effect of CDD gene transfer has not convincingly been demonstrated *in vivo*, nor are data available for primary human hematopoietic cells. However, in comparison to other CTX-R genes, studies on CDD overexpression in hematopoietic cells have just begun to emerge. If successful, this technology may have significant potential in the treatment of leukemic malignancies, especially AML. Here Ara-C is the most effective single chemotherapeutic agent, and its use in primary as well as relapsed disease is associated with severe and long-lasting myelosuppression.

V. SUMMARY AND FUTURE PERSPECTIVES

A number of CTX-R genes with relevance to the hematopoietic system have been identified since the 1980s and retrovirus vectors encoding a number of these genes have been developed. The effect of overexpression of such gene sequences has been studied *in vitro* in hematopoietic cell lines and primary hematopoietic cells, as well as *in vivo* in animal models. For MDR-1 and MGMT, the first clinical studies have also been performed, and for several other genes, clinical trials are planned. While clinical studies so far have been hampered by inefficient gene transfer or suboptimal transgene expression, advances in gene transfer technology should allow for significantly improved results in the future. Future studies should define the possible role of CTX-R gene transfer in the context of chemotherapeutic treatment with CTX-R-associated agents. In particular, it will be necessary to determine whether this technology reduces hematologic side effects sufficiently to allow dose intensification of current chemotherapy protocols.

Acknowledgments

This work is supported by National Cancer Institute Grant P01 CA75426 (DAW) and by a grant from Deutsche Forschungsgemeinschaft, Forschergruppe: "Tumorselektive Therapie und Therapieresistenz" (TM).

See Also the Following Articles

Cytokine Gene Therapy • Cytokines: Hematopoietic Growth Factors • DNA Methylation and Cancer • Genetic Basis for Quantitative and Qualitative Changes in Drug Targets • Multidrug Resistance I: P-Glycoprotein • Multidrug Resistance II: MRP and Related Proteins • Resistance to DNA-Damaging Agents • Retroviral Vectors • Stem Cell Transplantation

Bibliography

Allay, J. A., Persons, D. A., Galipeau, J., Riberdy, J. M., Ashmun, R. A., Blakley, R. L., and Sorrentino, B. P. (1998). *In vivo* selection of retrovirally transduced hematopoietic stem cells. *Nature Med.* **4**, 1136–1143.

Bank, A., Ward, M., and Hesdorffer, C. (1999). Transfer of the MDR-1 gene into hematopoietic cells. *In* "Marrow Protection" (J. R. Bertino, ed.), *Prog. Exp. Tumor Res.*, Vol. 36, pp. 50–64, Karger, Basel.

Beauséjour, C. M., Oanh Le, N. L., Létourneau, S., Cournoyer, D., and Momparler, R. L. (1998). Coexpression of cytidine deaminase and mutant dihydrofolate reductase by a bicistronic retroviral vector confers resistance to cytosine arabinoside and methotrexate. *Hum. Gene Ther.* **9**, 2537–2544.

Bertino, J. R., Zhao, S. C., Mineishi, S., Ercikan-Abali, E. A., and Banerjee, D. (1999). Use of variants of dihydrofolate reductase in gene transfer to produce resistance to methotrexate and trimetrexate. *In* "Marrow Protection" (J. R. Bertino, ed.), *Prog. Exp. Tumor Res.*, Vol. 36, pp. 82–94, Karger, Basel.

Bunting, K. D., Galipeau, J., Topham, D., Benaim, E., and Sorrentino, B. P. (1999). Effects of retroviral-mediated MDR1 expression on hematopoietic stem cell self-renewal and differentiation in culture. *Ann. N. Y. Acad. Sci.* **872**, 125–140.

Davis, B. M., Koc, O. N., Reese, J. S., and Gerson, S. L. (1999). O^6-benzylguanine-resistant mutant MGMT genes improve hematopoietic cell tolerance to alkylating agents. *In* "Marrow Protection" (J. R. Bertino, ed.), *Prog. Exp. Tumor Res.*, Vol. 36, pp. 65–81, Karger, Basel.

Eliopoulos, N., Beausjour, C., and Momparler, R. L. (1999). Chemoprotection against cytosine nucleoside analogs using the human cytidine deaminase gene. *In* "Marrow Protection" (J. R. Bertino, ed.), *Prog. Exp. Tumor Res.*, Vol. 36, pp. 124–142, Karger, Basel.

Flasshove, M., Banerjee, D., Mineishi, S., Li, M. X., Bertino, R., and Moore, M. A. S. (1995). *Ex vivo* expansion and selection of human CD34-positive peripheral blood progenitor cells after introduction of a mutated dihydrofolate reductase cDNA via retroviral gene transfer. *Blood* **85**, 566–574.

Harris, A. L., and Hochhauser, D. (1992). Mechanisms of multidrug resistance in cancer treatment. *Acta Oncol.* **31**, 205–213.

Jelinek, J., Fairbairn, L. J., Dexter, T. M., Rafferty, J. A., Stocking, C., Ostertag, W., and Margison, G. P. (1996). Long-term protection of hematopoiesis against the cytotoxic effects of multiple doses of nitrosourea by retrovirus-mediated expression of human O^6-alkylguanine-DNA-alkyltransferase. *Blood* **87**, 1957–1961.

Machiels, J.-P., Govaerts, A.-S., Guillaume, T., Bayat, B., Feyens, A.-M., Lenoir, E., Goeminne, J.-C., Cole, S., Deeley, R., Caruso, M., Bank, A., Symann, M., and D'Hondt, V. (1999). Retrovirus-mediated gene transfer of the human multidrug resistance-associated protein into hematopoietic cells protects mice from chemotherapy-induced leukopenia. *Hum. Gene Ther.* **10,** 801–811.

Magni, M., Shammah, S, Schiro, R., Mellado, W., Dalla-Favera, R., and Gianni, A. M. (1996). Induction of cyclophosphamide-resistance by aldehyde-dehydrogenase gene transfer. *Blood* **87,** 1097–1103.

Maze, R., Carney, J. P., Kelley, M. R., Glassner, B. J., Williams, D. A., and Samson, L. (1996). Increasing DNA repair methyltransferase levels via bone marrow stem cell transduction rescues mice from the toxic effects of 1,3-bis(2-chloroethyl)-1-nitrosourea, a chemotherapeutic alkylating agent. *Proc. Natl. Acad. Sci. USA* **93,** 206–210.

Maze, R., Kapur, R., Kelley, M. R., Hansen, W. K., Oh, S. Y., and Williams, D. A. (1997). Reversal of 1,3-bis(2-chloroethyl)-1-nitrosourea-induced severe immunodeficiency by transduction of murine long-lived hemopoietic progenitor cells using O^6-methylguanine DNA methyltransferase complementary DNA. *J. Immunol.* **158,** 1006–1013.

Moritz, T., Mackay, W. Glassner, B. J., Williams, D. A., and Samson, L. (1999). Retrovirus-mediated expression of a DNA repair protein in bone marrow protects hematopoietic cells from nitrosourea-induced toxicity *in vitro* and *in vivo.* *Cancer Res.* **55,** 2608–2614.

Moritz, T., and Williams, D. A. (1999). Methods for gene transfer: Genetic manipulation of hematopoietic stem cells. *In* "Hematopoietic Cell Transplantation" (E. D. Thomas, K. G. Blume, and S. J. Forman, eds.), 2nd ed., pp. 79–86. Blackwell Science, Malden, MA.

Reese, J. S., Koc, O. N., Lee, K. M., Liu, L., Allay, J. A., Phillips, W. P., Jr., and Gerson, S. L. (1996). Retroviral transduction of a mutant methylguanine DNA methyltransferase gene into human CD34 cells confers resistance to O6-benzylguanine plus 1,3-bis(2-chloroethyl)-1-nitrosourea. *Proc. Natl. Acad. Sci. USA* **93,** 14088–14093.

Samson, L. D. (1992). The repair of DNA alkylation damage by methyltransferases and glycosylases. *Essays Biochem.* 27, 69-78.

Sauerbrey, A., McPherson, J. P., Zhao, S.-C., Banerjee, D., and Bertino J. R. (1999). Expression of a novel double-mutant dihydrofolate reductase-cytidine deaminase fusion gene confers resistance to both methotrexate and cytosine arabinoside. *Hum. Gene Ther.* **10,** 2495–2504.

Schiedlmeier, B., Kühlcke, K., Eckert, H. G., Baum, C., Zeller, W. J., and Fruehauf, S. (2000). Quantitative assessment of retroviral transfer of the human multidrug resistance 1 gene to human mobilized peripheral blood progenitor cells engrafted in nonobese diabetic/severe combined immunodeficient mice. *Blood* **95,** 1237–1248.

Sorrentino, B. P., Allay, J. A., and Blakley, R. L. (1999). *In vivo* selection of hematopoietic stem cells transduced with DHFR-expressing retroviral vectors. *In* "Marrow Protection" (J. R. Bertino, ed.), *Prog. Exp. Tumor Res.,* Vol. 36, pp.143–161, Karger, Basel.

Sorrentino, B. P., Brandt, S. J., Bodine, D., Gottesman, M., Pastan, R., Cline, A., and Nienhuis, A. W. (1992). Selection of drug-resistant bone marrow cells *in vivo* after retroviral transfer of human MDR1. *Science* **257,** 99–103.

Williams, D. A., Hsieh, K., DeSilva, A., and Mulligan, R. C. (1987). Protection of bone marrow transplant recipients from lethal doses of methotrexate by the generation of methotrexate-resistant bone marrow. *J. Exp. Med.* **166,** 210–218.

Transgenic Mice in Cancer Research

Udayan Guha
James Hulit
Richard G. Pestell
Albert Einstein College of Medicine, New York, New York

GLOSSARY

gene targeting The introduction of a specific mutation or deletion into an endogenous gene.

heterozygous Having one allele or wild-type gene copy and one mutated allele.

homozygous Having two alleles of a gene.

oncogene A gene product, the activity of which induces tumorigenesis.

transgene A gene that has been introduced into an animal in a manner that leads to its propagation through subsequent offspring.

tumor suppressor A gene product, the inactivation of which results in tumorigenesis.

I. INTRODUCTION

The term "transgenic" refers to animals that have incorporated foreign DNA into their genome and includes a variety of species such as fish, poultry, rabbits, pigs, sheep, goats, cattle, and mice. Linear fragments of DNA can be integrated into the genome in a random fashion. If the gene-modified chromosome enters the germline cells, it can be passed onto the progeny, which thereby contain permanently altered genomes and are then said to be transgenic. DNA can be transferred into mice by retroviral infection, embryonic stem cell transfer, or cell/embryo aggregation, although direct microinjection of purified DNA into the male pronucleus is the most widely used.

The wide use of transgenic mice as a preferred biological system is a consequence of the finding that rodent genes can complement their human counterpart and that many rodent and human genes are highly homologous. The frequent similarities among the genetics, metabolism, and physiology of mice and humans, together with the fecundity, large numbers of progeny, and ease of maintenance, provide further practical reasons for investigating mouse transgenic models. The transgenic mouse has become an important ally for cancer biologists because the function of DNA fragments implicated as tumor suppressors or oncogenes through *in vitro* analysis can be more rigorously assessed in the presence of appropriate tissue-specific and local three-dimensional inputs provided by the transgenic context.

II. GENERATION OF TRANSGENIC MICE

The generation of transgenic mice is predicated upon several fundamental technological breakthroughs. First, the finding that foreign DNA, injected into the pronucleus of a fertilized mouse egg, would become a permanent component of the genetic makeup of the mouse (Fig. 1). Second, the finding that normal pluripotent embryonic stem (ES) cells, derived from the inner cell mass, when cultured and reintroduced into another blastocyst, colonized the host embryo and thereby contributed to cell lineages, including the germ cells, giving rise to chimeric animals (Fig. 2). Third, the finding that DNA introduced into mammalian cells can recombine into the genome via homologous recombination with a frequency as high as 1 in 100 to 1 in 500 (Fig. 3). Thus, cultured stem cells provided the opportunity to alter specific genes by homologous recombination and, after selection of the desired genotype, the reintroduction of the mutant stem cells could be used to make mice with a desired genotype.

The 129 mice strain has been useful for the derivation of ES cell lines; however, more than 17,000 substrains have been derived and their important differences have been catalogued. ES cells are maintained on a feeder layer consisting of mitotically inactivated STO fibroblasts or primary mouse embryo fibroblasts (MEFs). At the Albert Einstein College of Medicine, ES cells are maintained on STO/Neo cells, which are

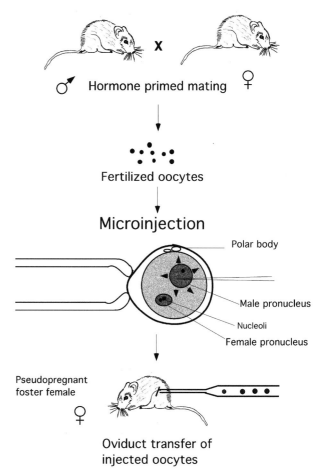

FIGURE 1 Generation of transgenic mice by the microinjection technique. Fertilized eggs are harvested from females after hormone primed mating and highly purified DNA is injected into the more prominent pronucleus (generally the male pronucleus). The injected eggs are implanted back to the oviduct of pseudopregnant foster mouse and the embryo allowed to proceed until term.

stable fibroblast lines integrating Neo[R] and leukemia inhibitory factor (LIF) (Collaborative Research). ES cells will behave like normal embryonic cells if implanted in the embryonic environment by injection into a host blastocyst or through aggregation with blastomere stage embryos. Such ES cells maintain a wide developmental potential.

Targeted mutagenesis in mice is a powerful tool for the analysis of gene function and investigation of human disease. Hundreds of new strains have been developed and thousands are expected to become available in the future (Table I). The successful targeting of a transgene to specific tissues requires the appropriate

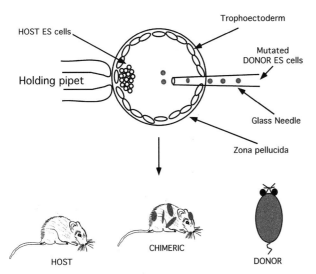

FIGURE 2 Generation of chimeric mice with mutant ES cells. The blastocyst is held by a suction pipette. Mutant ES cells are injected into the blastocyst from the opposite side. The blastocyst is then implanted into the uterus of a host pseudopregnant female mouse. The resulting chimeric pups contain cells from both the host and the donor injected ES cells.

promoter, regulatory sequences for RNA splicing and polyadenylation, and additional modifiers, such as silencer elements. The choice of promoter contributes to the level, timing, and site of transgene expression. Strong viral promoters [cytomegalovirus (CMV), simian virus 40 (SV40)] or ubiquitous cellular gene promoters (β-actin) and tissue-specific promoters (Table II) have been assessed and subsequently modified substantially by investigators over the last few decades. Because these modifications may alter tissue specificity substantially, one must examine closely the history of any given promoter construction.

Because the presence of prokaryotic sequences is inhibitory to the appropriate expression of certain genes (β-globin, α-actin, α-fetoprotein), most investigators remove prokaryotic sequences prior to microinjection of a construction. The expression level of the transgene may be influenced by the site of chromosomal integration, likely dependent on the presence of tissue-specific transactivators, nuclear matrix-binding sites, and other elements. Tissue-specific expression is influenced by enhancer–promoter-specific interactions. Furthermore, intrinsic sequences may determine the level of transcription in transgenic mice, although not observed in culture. The ability to modulate transgene expression *in*

vivo by external stimuli may be a key element in transgenic analysis. Inducible promoters include metallothionein promoters, which are induced by heavy metals; the *hsp68/lacZ*, which is induced by heat shock; the lac operator–promoter, which is coexpressed with the lac repressor and induced by the addition of isopropyl β-D-1-thiogalactopyvanoside (IPTG); the *tet* operon promoter; hormone inducible promoters such as MMTV (mouse mammory tumor virus) and WAP (whey acidic protein); the transferrin gene, the H-2E$_\alpha$ gene; and others (discussed in Section VI).

Appropriately purified transgene plasmid DNA is injected into one cell mouse embryos. The embryo is held in place by a pipette, and one of the two pronuclei is injected through a fine needle (Fig. 1). The embryos are implanted into pseudopregnant female mice, i.e., animals hormonally treated to mimic pregnancy. The injected embryos will implant into the uterus and develop to term. Gene transfer into pluripotent stem cells is performed by either electroporation or microinjection. Stably transfected ES cells are injected into the blastocyst cavity, whereupon

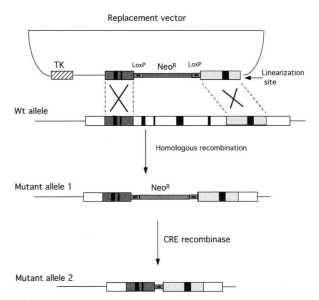

FIGURE 3 Replacement gene-targeting vector strategy. The replacement vector contains the Neo^R expression cassette, flanked by LOXp sites, for positive selection, and herpes simplex virus thymidine kinase gene expression cassette (TK) for negative selection. A region of chromosomal homology to the wild-type allele of approximately 5–8 kb, flanking the protein-coding exons and adjacent sequences to be deleted, is shown in gray. Mutant allele 1 is the result of homologous recombination. Mutant allele 2 is the result of removal of the Neo^R expression cassette by the addition of CRE recombinase.

TABLE I
Transgenics in Cancer Research Web Sites[a]

Index of biology servers

Biologist's Control Panel	http://gc.bcm.tmc.edu:8088/bio/
Search in the biology Web severs (Pasteur Institute)	http://www.pasteur.fr/recherche/BNB/bnb-en.html
GDB (The Genome Database)	http://gdbwww.gdb.org

Transgenics: nonmurine

The genome database (human)	http://gdbwww.gdb.org/
Flybase (Drosophila)	http://flybase.bio.indiana.edu:82
Whitehead Institute for Biomedical Research/MIT Center for Genome Research	http://www-genome.wi.mit.edu/
1. Maps of the Mouse Genome (MIT)	http://www-genome.wi.mit.edu/cgi-bin/mouse/index"
The Fish Net (zebrafish)	http://zfish.uoregon.edu
Worm web (C. elegans)	http://wormsrv1.sanger.ac.uk/cgi-bin/ace/simple/worm
Saccharomyces Genome Database	http://genome-www.stanford.edu/saccharomyces/
Japan Animal Genome Database	http://ws4.niai.affrc.go.jp/

Transgenics: murine

The Jackson laboratory (mouse)	http://www.jax.org/
1. MGD (The Mouse Genome Database)	http://www.informatics.jax.org/
2. The Encyclopedia of the Mouse Genome	http://www.informatics.jax.org/encyclo.html
3. GXD (Gene eXpression Database)	http://www.informatics.jax.org/exptools.html
4. Induced Mutant Resources	http://lena.jax.org/resources/documents/imr
5. TBASE (The Transgenic/Targeted Mutation Database)	http://www.jax.org/tbase/
6. Interspecific Backcross (JLBI) Mapping Panel	http://www.informatics.jax.org/mgd.html
The Mouse Atlas Project	http://genex.hgu.mrc.ac.uk/
The Portable Dictionary of the Mouse Genome	http://mickey.utmem.edu/front.html
Whole Mouse Catalog	http://www.rodentia.com/wmc/
Cybermouse Project	http://bitmed.ucsd.edu/cybermouse.html

Transgenic and knockout web sites

Database of Gene Knockouts	http://www.bioscience.org/knockout/knochome.htm
BioMedNet Mouse Knockout Database	http://biomednet.com/db/mkmd
UCD Medpath Transgenic Mouse Searcher 2.0	http://www-mp.ucdavis.edu/personaltgmouse1.html
Nagy Laboratory: Cre Transgenic and Floxed Gene Databases	http://www.mshri.on.ca/nagy/cre.htm
Gene Trap Insertions	http://socrates.berkeley.edu/~skarnes/resource.html
Transgenic Systems for Mutation Analysis—BigBlue and MutaMouse	http://eden.ceh.uvic.ca/bigblue.htm

Crossing organisms/phenotype analysis

TIGR Human Gene Index	http://tigr.org/tdb/hgi/hgi.html
National Center for Biotechnology Information	http://www.ncbi.nlm.nih.gov/index.html
1. Genbank	http://www2.ncbi.nlm.nih.gov/dbEST/index.html
2. Cross-referencing Model organisms with Mammalian phenotypes	http://www.ncbi.nlm.nih.gov/XREFdb/
3. OMIM (Online Mendelian Inheritance in Man)	http://www3.ncbi.nlm.nih.gov/omim
4. Unique Human Gene Sequence Collection	http://www.ncbi.nlm.nih.gov/Schuler/UniGene/
5. Human/Mouse Homology Relationships	http://www3.ncbi.nlm.nih.gov/Homology/
6. Biology of the Mammary Gland	http://mammary.nih.gov/
7. The Mammary Transgene Database	http://mbcr.bcm.tmc.edu:80/BEP/ERMB/mtdb.html
Dysmorphic Human–Mouse Homology Database	http://www.hgmp.mrc.ac.uk/DHMHD/dysmorph.html

Mapping/resource centers

UK MEC Human Genome Mapping Project Resource Center	http://www.hgmp.mrc.ac.uk/homepage.html
Resource Center of the German Human Genome Project	http://www.rzpd.de/
National Center for Genome Resources (nonprofit bioinformatics company)	http://www.ncgr.org
Web Resources of Genetic Linkage Analysis (Rockefeller University)	http://linkage.rockefeller.edu/
Stanford Human Genome Center	http://shgc-www.stanford.edu/

Mapping, sequencing, radiation hybrid mapping

The Cooperative Human Linkage Center (CHLC)	http://www.chlc.org/
Genethon Human Genome Research Center	http://www.genethon.fr/genethon en.html
Research Genetics (private company)	http://www.resgen.com/
The European Collaborative Interspecific Backcross EUCIB Mapping Panel	http://www.mgc.har.mrc.ac.uk/about-mgc.html
Frederick Interspecific Backcross Mapping Panel; Neal Copeland:	copeland@ncifcrf.gov
Nancy Jenkins:	jenkins@ncifcrf.gov
NIH interspecific Backcross Mapping Panel; Christine Kozak:	ckozak@nih.gov
Seldin interspecific Backcross Mapping Panel; Mike Seldin:	mfseldin@ucdavis.edu

[a]From http://www.aecom.yu.edu/pestell.

TABLE II
Tissue-Specific Promoters for Transgenic Mouse Models[a]

Breast
MMTV, WAP

Prostate
Probasin, C3(1), MMTV, SV40 T antigen, Cryptidin-2 (CR2), Fetal γ globin, gp91-phox

Hematopoietic system
B cells—immunoglobulin heavy chain enhancer (Eμ)
Erythroid cells—β-globin
T cells—T cell receptor
Macrophages—M- MuLV LTR

Nervous system
Brain—NSE, MBP, *Thy-1*, NFP, GRH, VP

Cardiovascular system
Mouse cardiac myosin heavy chain (MHC)

Gastrointestinal system
Pancreas—insulin, eastase
Kidney—Ren-2
Liver—albumin, AGP-A, CRP, α2U-G, AAT, HBV
Spermatids—protamine

Muscle
Muscle-α-actin, myosin light chain

---

[a]AAT, α1 antitrypsin; AGP-A, α1-acid glycoprotein; Alb, albumin; α2U, globulin; CRP, C reactive protein; HBV, hepatitis B virus; HLA, histocompatability antigen class; NSE, neurone specific enolase; MBP, myelin basic protein; MMTV, mouse mammary tumor virus (N.B. several different MMTV promoters are used); MSV, murine sarcoma virus; NSE, neurone specific enolase; NFP, neurofilament protein; GRH, gonadotropin releasing hormone; VP, vasopressin; WAP, whey acidic protein.

they colonize the embryo and contribute in part to the somatic and germline cells of the developing mouse.

Originally, standard transgenic technology was limited in the size of the fragments that could be introduced to approximately 40–50 kb. Subsequently, cloning vectors with a large DNA capacity such as P1s, bacterial artificial chromosomes (BACs), and yeast artificial chromosome (YAC) cloning vectors with a DNA capacity of over 2 Mb were developed to enhance analyses of more complex murine genomic regions. YACs have been introduced into the mouse germline through spheroplast fusion of yeast containing a YAC with totipotent mouse ES cells, lipofection of purified YAC DNA into ES cells, and microinjection of purified YAC DNA into single cell mouse embryos. This type of technology has been highly valuable in cancer genetic analysis.

III. UTILITY OF TRANSGENIC REPORTER MICE

The transgenic mouse has been used for fate mapping, to assess cell ancestry, location, and commitment, and more recently for studies of tumorigenesis. Several different approaches have been used. In one approach, a reporter gene, such as green fluorescent protein (GFP), is knocked into a locus to thereby enable an endogenous promoter to drive reporter gene expression. Alternatively, endogenous promoter gene function can be followed through ablation studies in which toxic genes such as diptheria toxin are driven by the specific promoter. In this strategy, expression of the diptheria toxin under control of the particular promoter leads to ablation of the cell lineage in which the promoter is expressed. Transgenic mice that contain specific DNA enhancer sequences (NFκB, AP-1) linked to a reporter gene have also been used to dissect the molecular pathogenesis and signaling pathways involved in tumorigenesis. These reporter genes included the β-galactosidase, or luciferase reporter genes. DNA enhancer reporter mice have been used to follow the role of nuclear transcription factors during development and tumorigenesis. Through analysis of reporter gene activity, the role of candidate transcription factors in the onset and progression of tumorigenesis can be assessed.

Advances in this field have been the generation of reporter mice to study somatic excision using CRE recombinase (i.e., ZAP or ROSA26 lines). Transgenic mice in which the gene of interest is flanked by LOXp sites (i.e., bacterial recombinase recognition sequence) can be crossed with the CRE reporter mouse to follow the efficiency of somatic excision. In ZAP transgenic line (β-galactosidase/alkaline phosphatase) reporter mice, LacZ expression is driven relatively ubiquitously by the pCAGG (chicken β-actin hybrid gene promoter). In this transgenic line the LOXp site flanks the β-galactosidase gene. Upon excision with CRE recombinase, an open reading frame for alkaline phosphatase is introduced, the expression of which can be assessed by the resulting brown staining of the tissue. Colorimetric or immunohistochemical analysis can then be used to follow cells in which excision by CRE has taken place.

IV. TARGETED TISSUE-SPECIFIC ONCOGENES AND TUMOR SUPPRESSORS

Tumorigenesis involves a multistep process progressing from preneoplastic lesions. Retroviral oncogenes were found to have cellular counterparts or protooncogenes. As normal cellular genes they control growth and metabolism by encoding growth factors, cell surface receptors, membrane-associated proteins, cytoplasmic protein kinases, nuclear transcription factors and cell cycle regulatory proteins. Dominant oncogenes cause cancer when they are expressed in altered form or amount. Recessive oncogenes predispose to cancer when their expression is eliminated, e.g., by mutation. The sequential acquisition of aberrantly functioning cellular protooncogenes or viral transforming genes contributes to the stepwise progression of the tumorigenic phenotype. In addition, immortalization, cellular senescence, and telomerase activity contribute in a dynamic oncogene-specific manner to the process of tumor progression and metastasis.

The transgenic mouse has served an important function in dissecting this dynamic interplay. Initially, transgenic mice were generated in which candidate oncogenes were targeted and overexpressed in specific tissues to examine their contribution to the malignant phenotype. A very large number of oncogenes were introduced into mice. Cross-breeding of oncogenic mouse models often resulted in accelerated rates of tumorigenesis. These tumors often arose stochastically and clonally, indicating that activation of more than one oncogene may be necessary for the development of tumors. One important advance in the understanding of mouse cancer models has been the introduction of accurate and unified pathologic descriptors. The availability of these descriptions on the web has also enhanced collaborative interactions between investigators (Table I). Although a variety of mouse tumor models have been developed, herein transgenic approaches to the analysis of breast and prostate cancer are outlined, with an emphasis on comparative database sources.

A. Transgenic Models of Breast Cancer

A variety of oncogenes, implicated in human breast cancer, induce tumor formation when overexpressed in the mammary gland of transgenic mice (Table III). These mammary oncogenes include activating mutations of membrane receptors [Erb-B2 (Neu)], nonreceptor tyrosine kinase proteins (pp60Src), and cytoplasmic (p21Ras) and nuclear (c-Myc) oncogenes (Table III). The analysis of transgenic mice engineered to understand mammary gland biology and cancer is now in its second decade, and with almost 100 transgenes, targeted mutations, and combinations of transgenics to hand, consensus reports have been issued to simplify morphologic nomenclature. Nomenclature developed at the NIH-sponsored Annapolis meeting proposed the use of morphological descriptors, criteria for malignancy, grading, properties, topology, etiology, "signature" features (morphological changes within the tumor that commonly correlate with a specific oncogenic initiator), and metastasis. To enhance uniformity in pathological interpretation, a web-based interactive histology atlas was developed (http://histology.nih.gov).

B. Transgenic Models of Prostate Cancer

Prostate cancer models have included models in the dog, the rat, heterotopic transplantation of cell lines into immune-deficient mice, and the use of the transgenic mouse. The mouse has limitations for modeling prostate cancer because of structural differences between the human and the murine prostate and the lack of spontaneous prostate cancer in the mouse. Nonetheless, prostatic hyperplasia has been observed in mice homozygously deleted of candidate tumor suppressor genes (*Mxi1, estrogen receptor* β, *pten, p27^{Kip1}, nkx3.1*), and a number of genetically engineered strains of murine prostate cancer have been generated (Table IV). Promoters used to induce prostate-directed expression include the probasin promoter (either a minimal 454-bp or 1.5-kb 5' flanking sequence), the C3(1) promoter, the MMTV LTR, Cryptidin-2 (CR2), fetal γ globin, and gp91-phox.

V. EVOLUTION OF KNOCKOUT TECHNOLOGY

The analysis of transgenic mice inactivated or deleted of specific genes, in conjunction with mice expressing

TABLE III
Transgenic Mouse Models of Mammary Cancer[a]

Models	Transgene	Bi-transgene	Promotors
Differentiation			
	Wnt 1		MMTV-LTR
	Wnt10b		MMTV-LTR
	Notch (INT3)	TGFβ	MMTV-LTR, WAP
Oncogenes cell-cycle			
	pp60Src		MMTV-LTR
	PyV-mT		MMTV-LTR
	Ras		MMTV-LTR
	Cyclin D1		MMTV-LTR
	Myc	Bcl-2	MMTV-LTR, WAP
	p53-172H,	p53	WAP, Null
	SV40 T Ag	Bcl-2	WAP, C(3)1
	β-catenin Y33		MMTV-LTR
Receptors			
	TGF-β MMTV-infected		WAP
	TGFβ DNIIR		MMTV-LTR
	Erb-B2 (neu) p53-172H		MMTV-LTR
	Ret-1		MMTV-LTR
	Tpr-MET		MMTV-LTR
	CDC37		MMTV-LTR
	Aromatase		MMTV-int-5/aromatase
Growth fractors			
	FGF3 (INT2)	Wnt1	MMTV-LTR
	FGF7 ((KGF)		MMTV-LTR
	Heregulin (NDF)	Myc	MMTV-LTR
	HGF		MT
	IGFII		BGL, H19
	TGFα	p53-172H, myc	WAP, MMTV-LTR

[a]From Zafonte et al. (2000).

TABLE IV
Transgenic Mouse Models of Prostate Cancer[a]

Promoter	Transgene	Pathology
Probasin (-454)	SV40 T antigen	Metastatic adenocarcinoma
Probasin (-454)	Ras	Epithelial and stromal hyperplasia
Large probasin	SV40 T antigen	Invasive adenocarcinoma
C3(1)	SV40 T antigen	Invasive adenocarcinoma, rare metastasis
C3(1)	Polyoma middle T	Invasive adenocarcinoma
C3(1)	bcl-2	Epithelial and stromal hyperplasia
MMTV	SV40 T antigen	Prostate and/or seminal vesicle adenocarcinoma
MMTV	int-2	Hyperplasia of urogenital organ epithelium
MMTV	kgf	Hyperplasia of urogenital organ epithelium
Cryptdin	SV40 T antigen	Androgen-independent metastatic prostate adenocarcinoma
Fetal gamma globin	SV40 T antigen	Androgen-independent metastatic prostate adenocarcinoma
gp91-phox	SV40 T antigen	Neuroblastoma of neuroectodermal origin

[a]From Amanatullah et al. (2000).

specific oncogenes or growth factors, has dramatically enhanced our understanding of oncogenic signaling pathways, previously only assessed in cultured cells. As noted earlier, advances in the analysis of a specific gene product in the mouse were propelled by technological breakthroughs in ES cell technology and recombinant vector design. Exogenous DNA introduced into mammalian cells recombines into the genome via homologous recombination with a frequency of 1 in 100 to 1 in 500. One approach to targeted gene disruption involves the introduction of a promoterless Neo^R gene fused to exons of the target gene just downstream of the promoter to disrupt the coding region of the target gene. The Neo^R gene functions as a selectable marker of homologous recombination. The Neo^R cassette, however, can affect the transcription of nearby genes and/or result in hypomorphs of the target gene and is therefore typically deleted in current strategies.

Screening approaches to identify recombinant clones require selection markers within the transgenic knockout cassette. Double selection, which enhances the rate of screening, uses "positive" (a drug conferring resistance to neomycin, G418, Neo^R) and "negative" (herpes simplex virus thymidine kinase, HSV-TK) selection (Fig. 3). The HSV-TK gene is lethal to cells grown in the presence of a nucleotide analog such as gancyclovir. Integration of DNA by homologous recombination usually retains homologous sequences but eliminates nonhomologous sequences that flank the homologous sequences. A typical targeting cassette therefore contains the Neo^R gene within the target gene sequences, whereas the HSV-TK gene usually flanks the homologous gene sequences. In this manner, cells expressing the HSV-TK gene can be eliminated by the addition of gancyclovir and those that express Neo^R will be resistant to G418. Cells that have undergone homologous recombination will have excluded the HSV-TK and will retain the Neo^R, allowing double selection for recombinant clones.

Once appropriate ES cells bearing the targeted mutation have been identified, they are injected into mouse embryos at the blastocyst stage (Fig. 2), the same embryonic stage from which the ES cells were isolated. ES cells derived for homologous recombination are isolated from white or agouti mice and are in-

jected into blastocysts from black mice to allow selection by coat color. The injected ES cells adhere to the embryonic cells of the blastocyst and the embryos are implanted into pseudopregant female mice. Chimeric mice born from these injected blastocysts have patches of white or agouti fur and patches of black fur. The subsequent generation will be either completely black (nonmutant) or completely white or agouti (mutant). The mutant mice are heterozygous, as homologous recombination occurs on only one chromosome and thus these mice must be bred to homozygosity.

Gene targeting has been used to generate mice that lack candidate tumor suppressor genes (p53, pRB, p16Ink4a/ARF, p27^Kip1, telomerase, BRCA1) or oncogenes (Wnt-1 and the pp60src protooncogene). General themes deduced from these studies suggest that tumor suppressors have tissue- and oncogene-specific interactions. Mice with targeted deletion of the p53 gene, for example, develop tumors in a wide variety of tissues, whereas p16Ink4/ARF-deleted mice develop a preponderance of lymphomas and sarcomas. These studies have also shown that the loss of candidate tumor suppressors results in different tumor tissue types in humans compared with mice. For example, loss of the pRB gene is associated with retinal tumors in humans. Deletion of the pRB gene in mice, however, is embryonic lethal, and mice heterozygote for pRB develop intermediate lobe pituitary tumors in an E2F-1-dependent manner.

VI. TEMPORAL REGULATION OF TRANSGENE EXPRESSION

The generation of murine models that accurately represent human disease requires a recapitulation of temporal and spatial expression in the mouse that more closely reflects the predicted dynamics in the human counterpart. The ability to regulate target genes in transgenic mice with both temporal and spatial specificity facilitates the analysis of gene function, particularly for genes required for development that have been implicated in tumorigenesis.

The ability to modulate gene expression *in vitro* and *in vivo* has become a powerful tool in understanding the role(s) of specific gene products in the normal growth and development of cells, tissues, and through transgenesis in the whole animal. The utility of tissue-specific transgenic models to examine the function of a target gene is limited by several practical limitations. Characteristics inherent to an ideal inducible transgenic system include low basal level expression, high inducibility, tissue-specific targeting, and sustained induction. The fidelity of these characteristics is particularly important in the delivery of toxic or lethal genes and for the delivery of CRE recombinase to allow efficient somatic excision. Binary systems, in which one mouse line contains an activator of expression and the second mouse line contains the silenced gene of interest, have been developed to examine the expression of potentially lethal or hypomorphic genes. Furthermore, as the acquisition of somatic mutations in the adult contributes to the onset and progression of tumorigenesis, genetic manipulation postnatally in a defined tissue is likely to recapitulate oncogenic mechanisms more faithfully and therefore provide a more informative model for the study of disease.

Transgenic approaches to controlled inducible target gene expression have utilized a transactivator such as the VP16 and Gal4/UAS activation system driven by tissue-specific promoters. The tetracycline-regulated system provides temporal and spatial control of gene expression. In the presence of the ligand, the transactivator, tTA, is bound to the tetO promoter and gene activity is silent until the ligand is removed. Transcriptional activity is induced by the addition of ligand in the reverse tTA system. Successful application of this system to transgenics has been balanced by reports of mosaic induction, background leakiness, and poor expression of the transactivator, perhaps related in part to the inefficient processing of the *tetR* gene in mammalian cells. Steroid hormone-inducible systems have centered on the expression of chimeric receptors that bind nontoxic hormone ligands. Estrogen receptor chimeric transgenics induced by tamoxifen show promise; however, evidence of mosaic transgene expression in target tissues and the need to use toxic and teratogenic doses for robust expression suggest that components of this system require further modifications.

The molting hormone, 20 OH-ecdysone, ponasterone A, and muristerone serve as ligands for the ecdysone system. These ligands bind a heterodimer of the *Drosophila* ecdysone receptor (EcR) and the product of the ultraspiracle gene (USP) in the context of a specific DNA-binding site. Ecdysteroids are neither teratogenic nor known to affect mammalian physiology. Pioneering studies by the laboratory of Dr. R. Evans led to the development of a chimeric receptor, consisting of the VP16 transactivation domain fused to an N-terminal truncation of the modified EcR (VgEcR), which conveyed low basal level activity and high ligand-induced activity in mammalian cells. Subsequent studies have verified its utility in transgenic mice, providing sustained *in vivo* expression.

VII. APPLICATION OF THE TRANSGENIC MOUSE IN RATIONAL THERAPEUTICS

Considerable progress has been made in correlating genetic alterations in specific tumors with patterns of chemotherapeutic drug sensitivity *in vitro*. Increasing evidence suggests that the local tumoral context directly affects tumor growth and survival, which is likely mediated through stromal, vascular, and paracrine interactions. Because *in vitro* chemosensitivity studies may not correlate with findings *in vivo*, there has been an increasing tendency to analyze therapeutic interactions using transgenic mice engineered to develop specific tumors. Transgenic mice engineered to express activated v-Ha-Ras or c-Myc oncogenes in the mammary gland, together with deficiencies in p53, were analyzed for chemotherapeutic responses to doxorubicin or paclitaxel. The p53 status determined the doxorubicin response but not the paclitaxil response in the MMTV-Ras mammary tumors. Transgenic mice harboring activated oncogenes and/or inactivated tumor suppressors provide intuitively useful model systems to analyze novel therapeutics and combination therapies with the long-term vision of providing therapies tailored to a patient's tumor genotype.

Acknowledgments

This work was supported in part by NIH grants (RO1CA75503, RO1CA86072, RO1 CA70896) and awards (to R.G.P.) (Irma

T. Hirschl and Weil-Caulier Charitable Trust, Susan G. Komen Breast Cancer Foundation, Breast Cancer Alliance Inc). We apologize for the citations that were omitted due to publication restrictions. Work conducted at the Albert Einstein College of Medicine was supported by Cancer Center Core National Institute of Health Grant 5-P30-CA13330-26.

See Also the Following Articles

BREAST CANCER • PROSTATE CANCER • STEM CELL TRANSPLANTATION • TARGETED VECTORS FOR CANCER GENE THERAPY • TUMOR SUPPRESSOR GENES: SPECIFIC CLASSES

Bibliography

Albanese, C., Reutens, A., D'Amico, M., Boumediene, B., Fu, M., Link, T., Nicholson, R., Depinho, R. A., and Pestell, R. G. (2000). Sustained mammary gland directed Ponasterone A-inducible expression in transgenic mice. *FASEB J.* **14,** 877–884.

Amanatullah, D. F., Reutens, B., Zafonte, B., Fu, M., Mani, S., and Pestell, R. G. (2000). Cell-cycle dysregulation in prostate cancer. *Front. Biosci.* **15,** 372–390.

Artandi, S. E., and DePinho, R. A. (2000). A critical role for telomeres in suppressing and facilitating carcinogenesis. *Curr. Opin. Genet. Dev.* **10,** 39–46.

Cardiff, R. D., Anver, M. R., Gusterson, B. A., Hennighausen, L., Jensen, R. A., Merino, M. J., Rehm, S., Russo, J., Tavassoli, F. A., Wakefield, L. M., Ward, J. M., and Green, J. E. (1999). The mammary pathology of genetically engineered mice: The consensus report and recommendations from the Annapolis meeting. *Oncogene* **19,** 968–988.

Furth, P. A., Onge, L. S., Boger, H., Gruss, P., Gossen, M., Kistner, A., Bujard, H., and Hennighausen, L. (1994). Temporal control of gene expression in transgenic mice by a tetracycline-responsive promoter. *Proc. Natl. Acad. Sci. USA* **91,** 9302–9306.

Gossen, M., Freunlieb, S., Bender, G., Muller, G., Hillen, W., and Bujard, H. (1995). Transcriptional activation of tetracycline in mammalian cells. *Science* **268,** 1766–1769.

Jaenisch, R. (1988). Transgenic animals. *Science* **240,** 1468–1474.

Moroy, T., Alt, F. W., and DePinho, R. (1991). Use of transgenic mice to study normal and abnormal mammalian development. *In* "Molecular Foundations of Oncology" (S. Broder, ed.), pp. 455–487. Williams and Wilkins, Baltimore, MD.

No, D., Yao, T.-P., and Evans, R. M. (1996). Ecdysone-inducible gene expression in mammalian cells and transgenic mice. *Proc. Natl. Acad. Sci. USA* **93,** 3346–3351.

Peterson, K. R., Clegg, C. H., Li, Q., and Stamatoyannopoulos, G. (1997). Production of transgenic mice with yeast artificial chromosomes. *Trends Genet.* **13,** 61–66.

Richa, J. (2000). Production of transgenic mice. *In* "Methods in Molecular Biology" (R. S. Tuan and C. W. Lo, ed.), Vol. 136, pp. 427–434. Humana Press, Totowa, NJ.

Rossant, J., and McMahon, A. (1999). "Cre"-ating mouse mutants: A meeting review on conditional mouse genetics. *Genes Dev.* **13,** 142–145.

Simpson, E. A., Linder, C. C., Sargent, E. E., Davisson, M. T., Mobraaten, L. E., and Sharp, J. J. (1997). Genetic variation among 129 substrains and its importance for targeted mutagenesis in mice. *Nature Genet.* **16,** 19–27.

Waldman, T., Zhang, Y., Dillehay, L., Yu, J., Kinzler, K., Vogelstein, B., and Williams, J. (1997). Cell-cycle arrest versus cell death in cancer therapy. *Nature Med.* **3,** 1034–1036.

Weinstein, J. N., Myers, T. G., O'Connor, P. M., Friend, S. H., Fornace, A. J. J., Kohn, K. W., Fojo, T., Bates, S. E., Rubinstein, L. V., Anderson, N. L., Buolamwini, J. K., van Osdol, W. W., Monks, A. P., Scudiero, D. A., Sausville, E. A., Zaharevitz, D. W., Bunow, B., Viswanadhan, V. N., Johnson, G. S., Wittes, R. E., and Paull, K. D. (1997). An information-intensive approach to the molecular pharmacology of cancer. *Science* **275,** 343–349.

Zafonte, B., Albanese, C., Reutens, A., Amanatullah, D., Hulit, J., Wang, C., Sparano, A., Lisanti, M., and Pestell, R. (2000). Cell-cycle dysregulation in breast cancer. *Front. Biosci.* **5,** 938–961.

Tumor Antigens

Karl Erik Hellström
Ingegerd Hellström
Pacific Northwest Research Institute, Seattle, Washington

GLOSSARY

costimulation The need for signaling by antigen via the T-cell receptor to be combined with a second signal(s) (e.g., via CD80) for an effective immune response to occur.

immunoconjugate An antibody that is chemically coupled with an anticancer agent, such as a chemotherapeutic drug.

immunotoxin A fusion protein commonly prepared between a single chain (sFv) antibody fragment and a toxin, such as *Pseudomonas* exotoxin PE40.

major histocompatibility complex (MHC) A cluster of genes whose products determine tissue compatibility. After processing, antigens are presented as peptides by MHC molecules (class I to be recognized by $CD8^+$ cytolytic T cells, CTL, and class II to be recognized by $CD4^+$ T helper cells).

T-cell immunity An immune response mediated by thymus-processed lymphocytes.

tumor antigenicity The expression of tumor-specific or tumor-associated antigens, which may be able to induce an immune response in the tumor host.

tumor immunogenicity The ability of a tumor to induce an immune response against itself in its host.

tumor vaccines Immunogens prepared to induce an active immune response to tumor antigens, used therapeutically in individuals with cancer or prophylactically against tumors associated with a viral etiology.

T he idea that tumors express antigens that can serve as targets for cancer treatment has been around since the late 1800s when Ehrlich postulated that immune mechanisms could provide "magic bullets" and Coley demonstrated tumor regression in some patients who had received immunostimulatory bacterial toxins. Since then there have been many hopes and many disappointments. We now know that cancer cells do, indeed, express a multitude of antigens, some of which can serve as therapeutic targets, and certain tumor antigens provide diagnostic markers.

I. MOUSE TUMORS ARE IMMUNOGENIC

Most of what has been learned about tumor immunogenicity comes from studies in mice. It was shown in the 1950s and 1960s that tumors experimentally induced by large doses of chemical carcinogens or by oncogenic viruses often are immunogenic. That is, they possess antigens that can both induce and serve as targets for an immune response leading to the rejection of tumor cells transplanted to a genetically identical animal that has been immunized with, e.g., X-irradiated tumor cells. The rejection antigens of chemically induced tumors were found to be unique for each neoplasm, whereas tumors induced by the same virus have shared antigens. The rejection antigens of virus-induced cancers, such as the polyoma T antigen, are viral products that are often intimately associated with the neoplastic state and are not likely to be lost during tumor progression.

Spontaneously occurring tumors were not rejected when tested under conditions used to immunize against chemically or virally induced tumors, and neither did tumors induced by low (more realistic) doses of chemical carcinogens. That led many to believe that human tumors (which after all are spontaneous) cannot be immunogenic. It was later shown that also spontaneous tumors do, indeed, have antigenic targets for a rejection response. However, to detect rejection antigens in such tumors or in tumors induced by lower doses of chemical carcinogens than those originally studied, one needs to immunize with tumor cells that have been modified in certain ways. Successful modifications include treating the immunizing cells with chemical mutagens, infecting them with certain viruses, transfecting a gene that encodes a lymphokine such as GMCSF, or transfecting a gene that encodes a costimulatory molecule (see later).

The same tumor cell can express several different antigens that can serve as a target for rejection. For example, tumors induced by a large dose of a chemical carcinogen not only express "strong" rejection antigens that are unique to each tumor, but also shared antigens against which a weak immune response is formed. Except for virally encoded antigens, most antigens shared by tumors are not tumor specific. Most of them are oncofetal and are, in addition to being present in tumor cells, also expressed in some fetal cells and, at a lower level, in some cells from the adult host. Several have sufficient selectivity for neoplastic cells to provide therapeutic targets.

II. IMMUNE RESPONSES TO TUMOR ANTIGENS

Tumor rejection is primarily mediated by T lymphocytes, although antibodies can also be involved and cause antibody-dependent cellular cytotoxicity (ADCC) or complement-mediated cytotoxicity (CDC). In addition, antibodies to growth factors or their receptors can have antitumor activity by interfering with growth-controlling mechanisms. While most antitumor antibodies bind to cell surface antigens, T lymphocytes recognize intracellular antigens presented as peptide epitopes by MHC molecules.

Both CD8$^+$ and CD4$^+$ T lymphocytes play roles in cell-mediated anti-tumor responses. CD8$^+$ lymphocytes can directly and specifically lyse antigen-positive neoplastic cells, whereas CD4$^+$ cells produce lymphokines that expand cytolytic T cells (CTL) and activate macrophages and natural killer (NK) cells with antitumor activity. Tumor destruction is primarily mediated by a Th1 type response, involving CTL and lymphokines, such as interferon γ, and it may be inhibited by Th2 type lymphokines (e.g., IL-10). The immune responses that can be induced to different tumor antigens may vary between those that cause tumor rejection and those that can suppress it. Circulating tumor antigen and immune complexes are often found in sera from tumor-bearing mice and humans and can interfere with the generation of an effective response as demonstrated in rodent models a long time ago.

III. HUMAN TUMOR ANTIGENS

Studies performed in the late 1960s showed that lymphocytes and sera from cancer patients often recognize antigens expressed on autologous and sometimes also on allogeneic tumor cells. Although the antigenic targets were not known, at least some of them were reported to be oncofetal. Much has since been learned, both about the tumor antigens and the immunological responses to them, as a result of advances in basic immunology, molecular biology, and biochemistry. Many cell surface antigens in human tumor cells have been identified using monoclonal antibodies (mAbs) of mouse and human origin and by recently developed SEREX technology. Many others have been identified because they are CTL targets (Table I). Genes encoding large numbers of human tumor antigens have been cloned and sequenced.

Many of the antigens identified by mAbs are also expressed in some fetal cells. Most of them are detectable in some adult tissues as well; e.g., Le^y is expressed at relatively high levels in epithelial cells of the stomach. Examples of antigens to which mAbs have been made include carcinoembryonic antigen

(CEA), α-fetoprotein (AFP), CA 125 and PSA, various mucin antigens (particularly MUC-1), an antigen identified by mAb 17.1A, and the transferrin-like glycoprotein p97, as well as Le^x- and Le^y-related antigens. Many of these antigens are overexpressed in carcinomas arising from different tissues, whereas CA125 is most frequently detected in ovarian carcinomas, and PSA is expressed in both normal and neoplastic prostate.

Antigens with absolute tumor specificity are of particular interest. They include unique antigens identified by antibodies or tumor-reactive T lymphocytes in certain tumors, e.g., some melanomas. Idiotypic determinants in B- or T-cell lymphomas serve the same purpose, as the only normal cells expressing the same determinants are those belonging to the clone from which the particular lymphoma originated. It is of

TABLE I

Examples of Antigens Identified in Human Tumors[a]

Type of antigen	Name	Tumors of greatest expression
Cell surface antigen recognized by antibodies[b]	CEA	Colon cancer
	AFP	Hepatoma
	PSA	Prostatic cancer[c]
	CA125	Ovarian cancer
	MUC-1	Various (breast, etc.) cancers
	GA 733 (mAb 17.1A defined)	Various cancers
	Antigen defined by mAb 72.3	Various cancers
	Le^y	Various (breast, etc.) cancers
	Le^x	Various cancers
	GD3	Melanoma
	GD2	Melanoma
	GM2	Melanoma
	Proteoglycan	Melanoma
	S100	Melanoma
	HER2	Breast cancer
	p97	Melanoma; some cancers
	CD20	B lymphoma[c]
	Mesothelin	Mesothelioma, ovarian cancer
Intracellular antigen recognized by T cells	HPV 16 encoded (E6;E7)	Cervical cancer
	EBNA	African Burkitt lymphoma
	Idiotypic determinants	B lymphoma; T lymphoma
	Encoded by mutated genes	e.g., mutated p53 in various tumors
	MAGE family members	Melanoma, cancer (varies)
	MART	Melanoma
	Tyrosinase	Melanoma

[a] A larger proportion of melanoma antigen is listed to demonstrate that the same tumor type often expresses many antigens as targets for both antibodies and CTL.

[b] Some antigens recognized by antibodies (e.g., CEA, HER2, MUC-2, and GA 733) can also be recognized as CTL targets following processing and presentation by MHC class I.

[c] Also expressed at high levels in normal prostate.

[d] Also expressed at high levels in normal B lymphocytes, but not in their precursors.

interest that the strongest rejection antigens in chemically induced mouse tumors are those that are unique to each neoplasm. Other tumor-specific antigens are encoded by the E6 and E7 genes of human papillomavirus type 16 (HPV-16), which plays a key role in the etiology of human cervical carcinoma. Because both E6 and E7 encode rejection antigens (as demonstrated in mouse models), there is a strong rationale for the construction of prophylactic and therapeutic vaccines against them. EBNA, detected in African Burkitt lymphoma, is another tumor-specific, virally encoded antigen. Mutated cellular oncogenes, e.g., ras p21 and mutated p53, can also encode tumor rejection antigens, as demonstrated in mouse models, and CTL responses to epitopes encoded by such genes have been identified, as has a CTL response to a mutated cyclin CDK4 that is expressed in some melanomas. Additional tumor-specific antigens are likely to be identified as more is learned about genetic differences between neoplastic and normal cells.

Most antigens in human cancers are tumor selective rather than tumor specific, although some of them have sufficient cancer selectivity to be therapeutic targets. These include many antigens (e.g., members of the MAGE family) that are expressed by tumors as well as by germ cells in testis. Antigen expression in testis is unlikely to complicate immunotherapy as the testis cells do not express MHC class I. Because the expression of many tumor antigens is heterogeneous within the same neoplasm, combination of antigens may be needed as a therapeutic target.

Several of the tumor-selective antigens are growth factor receptors. They are of great interest, as antibodies to them can interfere with the receptor function and sensitize tumor cells to apoptosis, particularly when used in combination with cytotoxic drugs. HER2, as well as receptors for EGF and the insulin-like growth factor, belong to this family. Antibodies to antigens that are growth factor receptors (given passively or induced by vaccination) can have an advantage over immune cells in that they often have low toxicity to antigen-positive normal cells.

A tumor can also share differentiation antigens with normal somatic cells in the adult individual. Such antigens can provide excellent therapeutic targets when the normal tissue is dispensable (e.g., prostate in patients with prostatic carcinoma).

IV. TUMOR ANTIGENS AS DIAGNOSTIC MARKERS

Anti-tumor mAbs can aid diagnosis in several ways. Immunohistological studies of tumor biopsies facilitate the identification of the tissue of origin, as well as the expression of markers known to influence prognosis (such as p53 and certain oncogenes). It can also help the selection of therapy, e.g., by learning whether a breast carcinoma expresses HER2 that can serve as a target for HER2-related therapy.

Detection of a tumor antigen in serum can be clinically informative. For example, CEA is elevated in sera from most patients with cancer of the colon as are CA125 and PSA in sera from patients with cancer of the ovary and prostate, respectively. In addition to aiding the primary diagnosis, these assays provide useful markers when assessing responses to therapy. Unfortunately, their sensitivity vs selectivity is not generally sufficient to screen large groups of healthy (or high risk) individuals to detect cancer at a very early stage. Nevertheless, AFP has been used in China with some success in screening for hepatomas. Searches are ongoing for additional tumor markers and antibodies in sera to be used alone or in combination with existent assays for diagnostic purposes. For example, LPA, a lysophospholipid growth factor, seems to be a potentially good marker for ovarian carcinoma, and molecules within the mesothelin family may provide additional such markers.

Substantial effort has gone into using radiolabeled mAbs for diagnostic "imaging" of tumors, and some promising findings have been obtained. However, in most situations this approach has not competed favorably with alternative diagnostic methods.

V. ANTIBODY-MEDIATED CANCER THERAPY

Unmodified mAbs have been given to thousands of patients with cancer, and clinical benefits have been shown, particularly with two products that have been approved for clinical use in the United States: a chimeric mAb ("Rituxan") to the CD20 molecule for the treatment of B-cell lymphomas and a chimeric mAb ("Herceptin") to HER2 for the treatment of HER2-positive breast carcinomas, the effect with Herceptin is dramatically increased when combined with chemotherapy. Furthermore, repeated infusions of mAb17.1A increased the time period of metastases-free survival, as compared to a parallel control group, in a randomized study with patients who had undergone surgery for Duke's stage C colon carcinoma.

The use of some "warhead" to make antitumor mAbs more effective has attracted much attention. Most effort has been given to three types of warheads: radioisotopes, chemotherapeutic drugs, and toxins. Provocative findings have been published using ^{131}I-labeled mAb to CD20 for treatment of patients with B lymphoma where long-lasting, complete remissions have been obtained. Other encouraging findings have been obtained in patients with ovarian carcinoma who received an yttrium-labeled mAb to MUC-1 subsequent to conventional therapy that debulked the tumor. Delivery of radioisotopes seems to be most effective using mAbs to tumor antigens, such as CD20, that do not internalize.

Work with a mAb (BR96)–doxorubicin (DOX) immunoconjugate (BR96-DOX) illustrates the possibilities as well as the challenges of drug–antibody conjugates. The target for BR96 is a fucosylated Le^y antigen that is abundantly expressed (>200,000 molecules/cell) on the surface of >75% of cells from >75% of carcinomas of the lung, breast, colon, ovary, and prostate. The mAb, which is of murine origin but has been chimerized (mouse–human), quickly internalizes once it has bound to the target cells. The immunoconjugate is stable at the pH of plasma but releases free DOX once it is internalized. It has been shown to be curative to nude mice carrying well-established transplants of human carcinoma of lung, colon, or breast. The Le^y antigen is not expressed in normal mouse tissues, but is present in gastrointestinal tissues not only of humans (constituting a problem for therapeutic use) but also in certain animals, including rats. It is, therefore, encouraging that BR96-DOX cured nude rats transplanted with human carcinoma as well as immunocompetent rats with a Le^y antigen-positive rat colon carcinoma growing either subcutaneously or in the liver. Free DOX had no effect in these systems, and neither did free mAb BR96 or a mixture of mAb and drug. On the basis of these findings, BR96-DOX was tested in the clinic. Although some partial tumor regressions were observed,

they were too infrequent to warrant continued studies on BR96-DOX for single agent therapy. This failure was attributed to gastrointestinal toxicity of the mAb protein that prevented the administration of more than a tenth of the dose needed for responses in rodents. Additional preclinical studies were then performed. They showed that a combination of BR96-DOX with Paclitaxel causes tumor regressions also at a dose expected to be tolerated in man, and the conjugate is now evaluated clinically in combination with cytotoxics.

A different approach is to use a protein toxin as the warhead, generally in the form of a recombinant immunotoxin. Complete tumor regressions and cures have been obtained in preclinical models. Clinical responses have been reported in human patients treated with an anti-Le^y fusion protein that consists of the scFv single-chain fragment part of a mAb joined with the PE40 part of *Pseudomonas* exotoxin PE40. Specificity of antibody binding seems to be most critical with this approach because of the potency of the toxin molecule. Immunotoxin therapy is also limited by the immunogenicity of the toxin, which leads to the rapid production of neutralizing antibodies.

VI. ACTIVE IMMUNOTHERAPY

Although spontaneous regression of human cancer is exceedingly rare, it does occur, particularly in neuroblastoma. Mechanisms involving tumor-reactive T cells are likely to play a role, as they are responsible for the spontaneous regression of some experimentally induced tumors, such as Moloney virus-induced sarcomas in mice. In addition to the high tumor specificity of some epitopes recognized by T cells, T-cell therapy has the advantage that it can provide immunological memory.

T cells can localize selectively into tumors to which they are immune, and adoptive transfer of immune lymphocytes can induce the regression of tumors in mouse models. Studies have been performed at the National Institutes of Health, in particular, in which large numbers of *in vitro*-expanded tumor-reactive lymphocytes were transferred to cancer patients. Long-term remissions were seen, but their frequency is low, and the infused lymphocytes often have a short life span. That problem may be circumvented by making the lymphocytes less likely to undergo apoptosis, e.g., by costimulation via CD28.

Why can antigenic tumors form in an immuno-competent host? An appealing explanation for this is that most tumors do not express certain costimulatory molecules that are needed to provide a second signal as tumor epitopes are presented to the T-cell receptor. Molecules of the B7 family (B7-1 or B7-2, also called CD80 and CD86) that are the natural ligands for CD28 on T cells provide the most important second signals. Unless CD28 is "triggered" via B7, antigen presentation not only fails to induce an immune response (immunological ignorance), but can even cause anergy.

There are two ways for a B7-negative tumor cell to induce a T-cell-mediated immune response leading to its destruction. First, a neighboring B7-positive antigen-presenting cell (APC), such as a dendritic cell, can provide "transcostimulation." Second, antigen released from the tumor cell can be taken up and presented by APC that express B7 as well as other costimulatory molecules. The latter mechanism, which occurs in regional lymph modes (draining the tumor) plays the major role.

Transfection of the CD80 (or the CD86) gene into a mouse tumor that is immunogenic according to the "old" criteria (rejection of "wild type" cells following immunization with X-irradiated tumor cells) increases its immunogenicity so it gets rejected after a short period of growth, and subsequently transplanted "wild-type" tumor cells are also rejected. Tumors that are nonimmunogenic according to the same criteria remain so even after transfection of a B7 gene. If, however, either CD48 (the mouse ligand for CD2) or the 4-1BB ligand is transfected in combination with B7 into such tumors, they will successfully immunize against wild-type cells. Furthermore, treatment of mice carrying "classically" nonimmunogenic tumors with an anti-4-1BB mAb will often induce the regression of large tumor nodules.

Several mechanisms may limit the extent to which an immune response can destroy tumors *in vivo*. Failure of tumor cells to present peptide epitopes via the class I molecules of the major histocompatibility complex has attracted much attention in view of the importance of CTL responses in tumor rejection. This is because studies with immunohistological techniques have demonstrated that the expression of MHC class I often decreases during tumor progression, sometimes leading to a complete loss, and damage to the antigen processing/transport mechanism has also been detected. It is important to emphasize, however, that losses detected by immunohistology may be quantitative rather than qualitative. A quantitative loss can prevent a tumor cell from inducing an immune response, but it may not prevent a tumor from destruction by CTL because much lower levels of presentation of peptide epitopes are then needed. It is noteworthy that at least two types of experiments, both performed in mice a long time ago, indicate that complete class I losses are rare. First, extensive transplantation studies on mouse tumors of homozygous or F_1 hybrid origin failed to demonstrate a single example of complete class I (then called H-2) loss, whereas partial losses were frequently seen. Second, polyoma virus-induced sarcomas in mice were found to retain their virus-encoded (polyoma T) rejection antigen (including their ability to present it via class I) even after intense selection for antigen-negative cells in polyoma-immune, syngeneic mice.

T-cell-mediated immune reactions to tumor antigens are often ineffective against large tumors. A likely reason for that is that there are various mechanisms that can downregulate these reactions, particularly at the tumor site. This is reflected by a low expression of several signal transduction molecules in T cells from tumor-bearing animals and human patients. Production by many tumors, and also by the host, of immunosuppressive molecules forms an important part of this downregulation. These include members of the transforming growth factor (TGF)-β family, which are produced by many tumors (gliomas in particular) and also by the tumor-bearing host, as well as NO and prostaglandins produced by macrophages. A high concentration of antigen released from the tumor may also play a part in a tumor's escape from destruction, most likely by deviating a Th1 response to a Th2 response. Furthermore, tumor-reactive T lymphocytes can be eliminated by apoptosis induced by Fas/Fas ligand interaction between the lymphocytes themselves and between the lymphocytes and tumor cells.

Various immunogens (cancer vaccines) can be used

to induce an active immune response to tumor antigens. They should preferably generate not only CTL but also T helper cells to provide lymphokines that not only expand CTL populations but also activate macrophages and NK cells to kill tumor cells via mechanisms that are not dependent on antigen presentation by MHC class I. Tumor cells that have been genetically modified to either express certain lymphokines (such as GMCSF) or costimulatory molecules (such as CD80 and/or 4-1BB ligand) can be used as immunogens. However, DNA vaccines, recombinant viruses, protein antigens that target dendritic cells, and peptide-pulsed dendritic cells have the advantage that the immune response is directed to defined tumor epitopes. This decreases the risk of autoimmunity to normal tissue antigens. However, some autoimmune damage to normal cells may be acceptable in a patient with metastatic cancer, and vaccines based on genetically modified tumor cells or dendritic cells pulsed with tumor homogenates have one advantage in that they provide a multitude of antigens expressed by the given patient's tumor. Promising findings have been obtained in melanoma patients given dendritic cells that have been pulsed with tumor-selective peptides. Furthermore, a randomized study with a carbohydrate (GM2) vaccine in stage II and III melanoma patients has demonstrated prolonged, tumor-free survival that correlated with the presence of anti-GM2 antibodies.

VII. CONCLUSIONS

The presence of a large variety of tumor antigens in most (probably all) neoplasms provides opportunities for therapy via passively transferred antibodies or immune lymphocytes, as well as by immunization with tumor vaccines, and several tumor antigens are being routinely used as diagnostic markers. mAbs have demonstrated success in the treatment of B-cell lymphomas and HER2-positive breast cancers, and clinical benefit of at least one cancer vaccine has been reported from a randomized study. Nevertheless, more needs to be learned before an immunological approach will contribute to the treatment of the majority of human cancers.

See Also the Following Articles

ANTIBODIES IN THE GENE THERAPY OF CANCER • ANTI-IDIOTYPIC ANTIBODY VACCINE • CELL-MEDIATED IMMUNITY TO CANCER • MOLECULAR BASIS FOR TUMOR IMMUNITY • T CELLS AGAINST TUMORS • T CELLS AND THEIR EFFECTOR FUNCTIONS

Bibliography

Baselga, J., Norton, L., Albanell, J., Kim, Y. M., and Mendelsohn, J. (1998). Recombinant humanized anti-HER2 antibody (Herceptin) enhances the antitumor activity of paclitaxel and doxorubicin against HER2/neu overexpressing human breast cancer xenografts. *Cancer Res.* **58,** 2825–2831.

Bast, R. C., Jr., Xu, F. J., Yu, Y. H., Barnhill, S., Zhang, Z., and Mills, G. B. (1998). CA 125: The past and the future. *Int. J. Biol. Mark.* **13,** 179–187.

Boon, T., Coulie, P. G., and Van den Eynde, B. (1997). Tumor antigens recognized by T cells. *Immunol. Today* **18,** 267–268.

Castelli, C., Rivoltini, L., Andreola, G., Carrabba, M., Renkvist, N., and Parmiani, G. (2000). T-cell recognition of melanoma-associated antigens. *J. Cell Physiol.* **182,** 323–331.

Coggin, J. H., Jr., Barsoum, A,L., and Roher, J. W. (1998). Tumors express both unique TSTA and crossprotective 44kDa oncofetal antigen. *Immunol. Today* **19,** 405–408.

Gopal, A. K., and Press, O. W. (1999). Clinical applications of anti-CD20 antibodies. *J. Lab. Clin. Med.* **134,** 445–450.

Hellstrom, I., Hellstrom, K. E., and Senter, P. D. (2000). Development and activities of the BR96-doxorubicin immunoconjugate. *In* "Methods in Molecular Biology: Immunotoxin Methods and Protocols" (W. A. Hall, ed.), Vol. 166, pp. 3–16.

Hellstrom, K. E., and Hellstrom, I. (1999). Cancer vaccines. *In* "Handbook of Experimental Pharmacology" (P. Perlmann and H. Wigzell, eds.), Springer, Heidelberg.

Herlyn, D., and Bircbent, B. (1999). Advances in cancer vaccine development. *Ann. Med.* **31,** 66–78.

Kaminski, M. S., Zasadny, K. R., Francis, I. R., Milik, A. W., Ross. C. W., Moon, S. D., Crawford, S. M., Burgess, J. M., Petry, N. A., Butchko, G. M., *et al.* (1993). Radioimmunotherapy of B-cell lymphoma with [131I]anti-B1 (anti-CD20) antibody. *N. Engl. J. Med.* **329,** 459–465.

Kochman, S., and Bernard, J. (1999). Antitumour immune response and cancer vaccination: The critical role of dendritic cells. *Curr. Med. Res. Opin.* **15,** 321–326.

Liebowitz, D. N., Lee, K. P., and June, C. H. (1998). Costimulatory approaches to adoptive immunotherapy. *Curr. Opin. Oncol.* **10,** 533–541.

Linsley, P. S., and Ledbetter, J. A. (1993). The role of the CD28 receptor during T cell responses to antigen. *Annu. Rev. Immunol.* **11,** 191–212.

Livingston, P. O., Wong, G. Y., Adluri, S., Tao, Y., Padavan, M., Parente, R., Hanlon, C., Calves, M. J., Helling, F., Ritter, G., *et al.* (1994). Improved survival in stage III melanoma patients with GM2 antibodies: A randomized trial of adjuvant vaccination with GM2 ganglioside. *J. Clin. Oncol.* **12,** 1036–1044.

Mitchell, E. P. (1998). Role of carcinoembryonic antigen in the management of advanced colorectal cancer. *Semin. Oncol.* **25,** 12–20.

Nestle, F. O., Alijagic, S., Gilliet, M., Sun, Y., Grabbe, S., Dummer, R., Burg, G., and Schadendorf, D. (1998). Vaccination of melanoma patients with peptide- or tumor lysate-pulsed dendritic cells. *Nature Med.* **4,** 328–332.

Old, L. J., and Chen, Y.-T. (1998). New paths in human cancer serology. *J. Exp. Med.* **187,** 1163–1167.

Press, O. W., Eary, J. F., Appelbaum, F. R., Martin, P. J., Badger, C. C., Nelp, W. B., Glenn, S., Butchko, G., Fisher, D., Porter, B., *et al.* (1993). Radiolabeled-antibody therapy of B-cell lymphoma with autologous bone marrow support. *N. Engl. J. Med.* **329,** 1219–1224.

Riethmuller, G., Schneider-Gadicke, E., Schlimok, G., Schmiegel, W., Raab, R., Hoffken, K., Gruber, R., Pichlmaier, H., Hirche, H., Pichlmayr, R., *et al.* (1994). Randomised trial of monoclonal antibody for adjuvant therapy of resected Dukes' C colorectal carcinoma: German Cancer Aid 17-1A Study Group. *Lancet* **343,** 1177–1183.

Rosenberg, S. A. (1995). Cell transfer therapy: Clinical applications. *In* "Biologic Therapy of Cancer" (V. T. DeVita, S. Hellman, S. A. Rosenberg, eds.), J. P. Lippincott, Philadelphia.

Stevenson, F. K. (1999). DNA vaccines against cancer: from genes to therapy. *Ann. Oncol.* **10,** 1413–1418.

Tumor Cell Motility and Invasion

J. Jouanneau
J. P. Thiery
Institut Curie, Paris, France

It has long been thought that the invasive behavior of tumor cells depends on their motility. Cell motility has been studied for many years in *in vitro* and *in vivo* model systems. Cytokine- and growth factor-induced cell motility is physiologically controlled by several processes, such as development and wound repair; however, these processes may be constitutively or inappropriately activated in the tumorigenic cascade of tumor progression. This article focuses on tumor cell-induced or -acquired motility and invasive properties that are a prerequisite for metastatic spreading.

I. CELL MOTILITY

A. Definition

Cell motility is the capacity of cells to translocate onto a solid substratum. This behavior is often a hall-mark of fibroblastic cells. In epithelial cells, cell motility occurs after the dissociation of a cell from its neighboring cell(s) and after the modification of its position relative to other cells or a solid substrate.

There is usually a cell phenotype associated with cell motility. Motile cells are polarized, and the actin cytoskeleton is a key modulator of cell polarity and cell motility. Although cellular polarity is a functional aspect of most cell types, the polarity of the motile cell is associated with the formation of pseudopods whose stabilization determines the directionality of the movement. Pseudopodal protrusion is associated with actin cytoskeletal dynamics because the continual extension of pseudopodia by the motile cell necessitates the polarized targeting of the proteins involved in the transduction of motility signals, the regulation of actin and microtubule cytoskeleton dynamics, the formation of cell substrate adhesion, and the localized degradation of the extracellular matrix (ECM) environment.

The study of the mechanisms underlying cellular motility is facilitated by culturing motile cells on a planar surface; however, cell movement *in vivo*

Encyclopedia of Cancer, Second Edition
Volume 4

requires the ability to degrade and to invade the extracellular matrix and is a prerequisite for tumor cell metastasis.

B. Experimental Analysis of Cell Motility

One of the simplest techniques for analyzing cell motility is the "wound healing method" in which a confluent cell monolayer is wounded and time-lapse photography is used to follow the closure of the wound by moving cells. The current technique allows the movement of individual cells or of cell clusters to be followed for long periods of time. Typically, cells are cultured in tissue culture dishes or glass window-sealed chambers and are maintained at 37°C in an air/CO_2-controlled environment on the stage of an inverted microscope. Programming the motorized microscope stage allows the repeated screening of several fields of the same culture, and a CDD camera allows each frame to be digitized. Appropriate software (such as Metamorph, Universal Imaging) can be used to analyze recorded image trajectories. The speed of movement of the dispersed motile cells can easily be established, as can other more refined parameters, including the duration of cell–cell contact, contact inhibition or induction of movements, filopodial or lamellipodial activities, and the strength of inducers. Digitized time-lapse videomicroscopy can also be used to follow the protein fluorescence in time and space, such as the localized polymerization of actin filaments within alive motile cells during the protrusion extension of the cell body (lamellipodia extension and membrane ruffling).

C. Cell–Cell Interactions: Adherent Junctions

Desmosomes and adherent junctions constitute the main adhesive junctions between epithelial cells; these junctions are disrupted during cell scattering and acquisition of motile phenotype. Desmosomes are specialized membrane junctions containing the transmembrane desmocollins and desmogleins, two members of the cadherin superfamily. These adhesive molecules are connected to plakoglobin and desmoplakins in the cytoplasm, which are connected to the cytokeratin network in turn. Adherent junctions are specialized regions of the plasma membrane in which the

transmembrane cell adhesion molecules, E-cadherin recognize and bind neighboring cells containing E-cadherin molecules in Ca^{2+}-dependent. E-cadherin is a 120-kDa transmembrane glycoprotein containing five immunoglobulin domains in the extracellular domain that are involved in the homophilic interaction. The short cytoplasmic domain is connected to β-cadherin, which binds to α-catenin in turn. The cadherin–catenin complexes can interact directly or indirectly with the actin microfilament network. This interaction is essential for the integrity of adherent junctions.

Any significant changes in the expression and/or the structure of the essential desmosome or adherent junction components can lead to junctional disassembly and, consequently, to invasive carcinoma cells.

Various types of human carcinomas have been examined for defects in one of the intercellular junction constitutents. A correlation has been shown between the dysfunction of E-cadherin-mediated cellular adhesion, due to downregulating E-cadherin expression or to mutations in the E-cadherin gene, and the invasive potential of many types of carcinomas. *In vitro*, the invasiveness of carcinoma cells with a fibroblastoid phenotype can be stopped by transfection with E-cadherin cDNA and can be reinduced by treating the transfected cells with anti-E-cadherin monoclonal antibodies. These findings indicate (1) that the loss of E-cadherin is a critical step in the dedifferentiation of epithelial cells and in the acquisition of invasive properties and (2) that E-cadherin acts as a tumor (invasive) suppressor. Nevertheless, in a few reported cases, alterations in cell–cell adhesion between carcinoma cells result from the loss of α- or β-catenin due to gene mutations. It has been suggested that unlike E-cadherin, N-cadherin may promote motility and invasion in some carcinoma cells and that this motility may be mediated by FGF (fibroblast growth factor) receptor signaling.

D. Cell–Matrix Integrins Are Cell Surface Matrix Receptors

Cadherins and integrins play a critical role in the maintenance of tissue integrity and normal organization. Integrins are cell surface matrix receptors. They are transmembrane heterodimers composed of α and β subunits, which possess binding sites for matrix proteins, such as collagens, fibronectin, and laminins, in their extracellular regions. The effect of matrix macromolecules on cell motility is well documented, and cell adhesion to the extracellular matrix is absolutely required for the cell movement.

Most of the adherent cells are dispersed under tension. This tension is mediated through integrins, which link the extracellular matrix to the adhesion complex and the actin cytoskeleton. Modulation of these cell–substratum interactions is a prerequisite for cell migration. Interaction of the cell with the extracellular matrix induces the formation of filipodia and lamellipodia and/or the assembly of focal contacts and associated stress fibers in many cell types.

Research has shown that these molecules participate in cell signaling. Integrins can convey signals from the extracellular matrix to intracellular regions; integrins and GTPases of the Rho family coordinate signaling processes and cytoskeletal reorganization, in general, and cancer cell growth and behavior, in particular. Cell behavior depends on specific induced transduction pathways, most of which lead to the activation of the MAP kinase pathway.

Different clinical and pathological studies have demonstrated qualitative and quantitative changes in cadherins and/or integrins in several malignancies, which correlate with decreased states of tumor differentiation and increased invasiveness.

E. Factors That Induce Cell Motility

There is increasing evidence that the cell adhesion machinery is regulated by several soluble factors that induce cell–cell dissociation, cell scattering, and cell motility, leading to the invasion of tumor cells and thus possibly promoting tumor metastasis.

Several factors are known to induce epithelial cell scattering. The most potent and general epithelial dissociating factor is hepatocyte growth factor/scatter factor (HGF/SF). HGF/SF signals through the c-met transmembrane tyrosine-kinase type receptor and has been implicated in several neoplasia. A variety of other growth factors, such as epidermal growth factor (EGF), transforming growth factor β (TGFβ), fibroblast growth factors (FGFs), cytokines, and motility factors produced by the tumor cells themselves, may accumulate within the tumor microenvironment and contribute to tumor growth, invasion, and metastasis through autocrine or paracrine mechanisms. In ep-

ithelial tumor cells, lamellipodia are extended within minutes of exposure to EGF or HGF.

Autocrine motility factor (AMF) has been identified as the phosphohexo isomerase (PHI) enzyme and is a tumor-secreted 55-kDa protein, which regulates cell motility *in vitro* and invasion and metastasis *in vivo*. AMF induces cellular responses by binding to its receptor, AMFR, a seven transmembrane 78-kDa glycoprotein, and subsequently activating a transduction cascade. AMF and its receptor have been postulated to play a role in tumor cell metastasis. Upregulation of AMFR expression is concomitant with the progression of bladder cancer and with the downregulation of E-cadherin, consistent with a shift from a sedentary to a motile cellular phenotype.

The stroma has been shown to contribute to tumor invasion. Migration stimulating factor (MSF), a 192-kDa protein, is produced by fibroblasts obtained from most breast tumors. MSF stimulates the synthesis of high molecular weight hyaluronic acid (HA), and it has been suggested that the observed effect of MSF on fibroblast migration is a consequence of its effect on HA synthesis by an unknown mechanism.

F. Cell Signaling Cascade Associated with Cell Motility and Invasion

The actin cytoskeleton is a dynamic filament network essential for cell movement. Cell activation by extracellular signals induces actin polymerization. The rapid movement of cells over a substrate requires coordinated actin-based protrusive activities with a supply of molecular components for the renewal of the pseudopodial domain. The assembly of molecular machinery at the site of pseudopodial protrusion must be an essential aspect of cell movement. It is now well known that these mechanisms are dependent on the activation of several small G proteins (see Fig. 1 for a general diagram).

Members of ras-related GTPases could serve as molecular switches regulating the polymerization of actin into distinct structures. Interplay among Rho, Rac, and Cdc42 activation generates specific GTPase cascades that regulate the actin cytoskeleton and cell behavior. Growth factor stimulation of Rho regulates the formation of actin stress fibers and of focal contacts. Rac stimulates the formation of membrane ruffles and lamellipodia, and Cdc42 stimulates the formation of filopodia. Furthermore, Rho, Rac, and

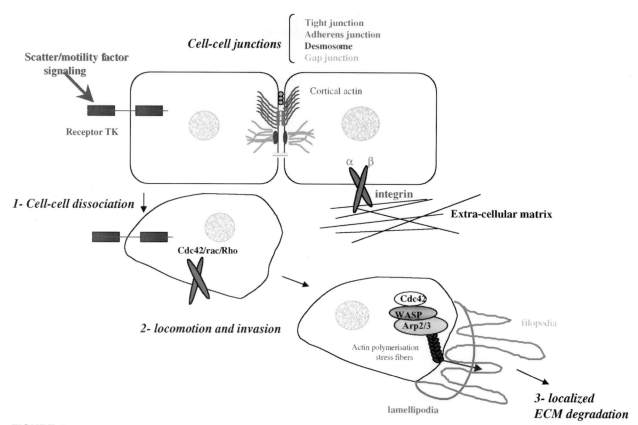

FIGURE 1 Adjacent epithelial cells are linked through different cell–cell junctions. These cells could be dissociated upon a scatter/motility factor signaling mainly through activation of specific transmembrane tyrosine kinase receptor (receptor TK). Cells also adhere to the extracellular matrix (ECM) via integrins which in turn could be activated. Actin polymerization into stress fibers is thus induced, allowing the assembly of a supramolecular machinery required for cell protrusions (lamellipodia and filipodia); these steps during locomotion and invasion are largely dependent on activation of several small G proteins (rho/rac/cdc42). Progression of the cell movement is concomitant with the degradation of the ECM by different specific proteases.

Cdc42 stimulate the formation of integrin-containing focal complexes and, therefore, their activation may directly affect integrin function.

The role of proteins acting as nucleation centers for cortical actin microfilaments is also well established; N-WASP is an adaptator protein that is bound to Cdc42, which is connected through its carboxy terminus to the Arp 2/3 complex that is responsible for the nucleation of actin polymerization. A similar complex machinery has been described for the integrin cytoplasmic domain, which is connected to zyxin; zyxin is related to the Act A protein, which is responsible for actin polymerization and thus allows intracellular motility of the pathogen *Listeria monocytogenes* following cell infection.

In addition to directly inducing cell scattering, growth factor signaling may also cooperate with adhesion molecules. The insulin-like growth factor receptor cooperates with the commonly expressed integrin, $\alpha v \beta 5$, to promote the dissemination of different types of malignant cells *in vivo*.

As indicated earlier, it appears that different cell signals are responsible for tumor cell motility and for the acquisition of invasive properties, which enable cells to integrate information originating from themselves and/or from the tumor microenvironment.

II. CELL INVASION

It was reported in the 1980s that enzymatic degradation of the basal lamina collagen is one of the critical determinants in tumor invasion and metastasis.

A. Definition

Invasion occurs when a tumor cell acquires properties that enable it to penetrate the surrounding tissue or basement membrane. It is becoming obvious that cell motility is the major rate-limiting step in invasion. Current research suggests that tumor cell motile responses to growth and scatter factors promote invasion through signals for motility.

Cancer cell detachment and migration require reduced adhesiveness of the cells either between themselves or from the basal lamina. Cancer cells must overcome anchorage dependence to move away from their original site and they must also be invasive and penetrate the basement membrane before becoming metastatic. This requires different conditions such as abrogation of cell–cell interactions and production of specific enzymes to degrade the basal lamina and matrix components. Some of the proteases produced by tumor cells and, more specifically, by highly metastatic cells are important for matrix degradation within their environment and also for the processing of several growth factors to active forms. In association with this concept, it has been proposed that distinct proteases may promote invasion through limited proteolytic activity and an increase in cell motility.

B. Testing the Invasive Properties of Cells

The active migration of tumor cells is usually tested *in vitro* by use of the Boyden chambers-type assay (Transwell, Costar, Inc.). Use of Transwell chambers allows the cell movement to be determined across a filter with defined pore size. Cells are deposited in the upper chamber on top of the filter and after a few hours the cells that have translocated to the lower chamber are counted. Alternatively, when induced motility is to be tested, the inducer or growth factor is placed in one or both chambers. In these experiments, cell translocation is accompanied with a change in cell shape because cells have to pass through narrow channels.

Clusters of coherent carcinoma cells, which are malignant cells of epithelial origin, may also invade the surrounding tissue. Experiments on gelatin-coated substrates have indicated that cohort migration is probably due to the modulation of cell–cell adhesion of the lower portion of the clusters through an E-cadherin– catenin-based mechanism.

C. Gene Expression Associated with Cell Invasive Properties

1. Proteases and Their Inhibitors

Matrix metalloproteases (MMPs) are proteases whose expression may be regulated in function of cell or tissue behavior. The expression of most MMPs is transcriptionally regulated by growth factors and cellular transformation. They contribute to tissue remodeling and have a key role in the migration of normal and malignant cells through the body. Their functions are associated with degradation of the extracellular matrix and of the basement membrane, which is a specialized matrix barrier essentially composed of type IV collagen, laminins, entactin glycosaminoglycans, and proteolycans. The breakdown of this lamina by MMPs is required for cell invasion and for metastatic process. MMP2 and MMP9, the so-called gelatinase-A and -B, are secreted type IV collagenases, mainly involved in the latter process. These MMPs may be produced by the tumor cells themselves, but there is growing evidence that the normal host stromal cells respond to tumor cells by inducing MMPs.

MMP activity is regulated at transcriptional and processing levels and can also be blocked by direct association of the protein and physiological MMP inhibitors, termed tissue inhibitor of metalloproteases (TIMP), generating an inactive MMP/TIMP complex. The degradative potential is the result of the balanced or imbalanced production of these molecules.

Evidence has shown that cells focus proteolytic activities at their cell surface and essentially at their leading edge to help remove extracellular matrix barriers for migration during their invasion. Membrane-bound MMPs, termed Mt-MMP, have been identified, and Mt1-MMP was shown to be predominantly localized in the invadopodia or lamellipodia of invading cells. Furthermore, Mt1-MMP could form cell surface complexes with TIMP that behave as MMP2 receptors.

2. Plasmin System uPA/uPAR/PAI

The plasmin cascade system, which allows plasminogen to be activated to plasmin, also appears to be a cell membrane-associated mechanism through a urokinase receptor, uPAR. The different molecules involved in this system are colocalized with integrins in focal contacts and at the leading edges of the migrating cells.

The physiological extracellular plasminogen-activator inhibitor PAI-1 forms a complex with activated uPA and is rapidly endocytozed from the cell surface. Different reports have revealed that uPAR is implicated in plasminogen activation and also contributes to cell adhesion and migratory processes in a nonproteolytic manner.

III. CONCLUDING REMARKS

Numerous laboratories are carrying out research to try to decipher the exact molecular control mechanisms of growth factor-induced motility. These investigations will probably help us determine the cascade of controlled or uncontrolled events that are the key to the clinical control of tumor invasion.

See Also the Following Articles

AUTOCRINE AND PARACRINE GROWTH MECHANISMS IN CANCER PROGRESSION AND METASTASIS • CELL–MATRIX INTERACTIONS • MOLECULAR MECHANISMS OF CANCER INVASION • VASCULAR TARGETING

Bibliography

Andreasen, P. A., Kjoller, L., Christensen, L., and Duffy, M. J. (1997). The urokinase-type plasminogen activator system in cancer metastasis: A review. *Int. J. Cancer* **72**, 1–22.

Beckerle, M. C. (1998). Spatial control of actin filament assembly: Lessons from *Listeria*. *Cell* **95**, 741–748.

Blobel, C. P. (1997). Metalloprotease-disintegrins: Links to cell adhesion and cleavage of TNF alpha and Notch. *Cell* **90**, 589–592.

Bonneton, C., Sibarita, J. B., and Thiery, J. P. (1999). Relationship between cell migration and cell cycle during the initiation of epithelial to fibroblastoid transition. *Cell Motil Cytoskel.* **43**, 288–295.

Brew, K., Dinakarpandian, and Nagase, H. (2000). Tissue inhibitors of metalloproteases: Evolution, structure and function. *Biochim. Biophys. Acta* **1477**, 267–283.

Brooks, P. C., Klemke, R. L., Schon, S., Lewis, J. M., Schartz, M. A., and Cheresh, D. A. (1997). Insulin-like growth factor receptor cooperates with integrin αvβ5 to promote tumor cell dissemination in vivo. *J. Clin. Invest.* **15**, 1390–1398.

Fini, M. E., Cook, J. R., Mohan, R., and Brinckerhoft, C. E. (1998). Regulation of MMP gene expression. In "Matrix Metalloproteinases" (W. C. Parks and R. P. Mecham, eds.), pp. 299–356. Academic Press, San Diego.

Frixen, U. H., Berhens, J., Sachs, M., Eberle, G., Voss, B., Warda, A., Lochner, D., and Birchmeier, W. (1991). E-cadherin mediated cell-cell adhesion prevents invasiveness of human carcinoma cells. *J. Cell Biol.* **113**, 173–185.

Hall, A. (1998). Rho GTPases and the actin cytoskeleton. *Science* **279**, 509–514.

Hazan, R. B., Phillips, G. R., Qiao, R. F,, Norton, L., and Aaronson, S. (2000). Exogenous expression of N-cadherin in breast cancer cells induces cell migration, invasion and metastasis. *J. Cell Biol.* **148**, 779–790.

Horwitz, A. R., and Parsons, J. T. (1999). Cell migration: Movin' on. *Science* **286**, 1102–1103.

Hynes, R. O. (1992). Integrins: Versatility, modulation, and signalling in cell adhesion. *Cell* **68**, 11–25.

Kawanishi, J., Kato, J., Sasaki, K., Fuji, S., Watanabe, N., and Nitsu, Y. (1995). Loss of E-cadherin-dependent-cell-cell adhesion due to mutation of the β-catenin gene in a human cancer cell line, HSC-39. *Mol. Cell Biol.* **15**, 1175–1181.

Kawanishi, K., Doki Shiozaki, H., Yano, M., Inoue, M., Fukuhi, N., Utsunomiya, T., Watanabe, H., and Monden, M. (2000). Correlation between loss of E-cadherin expression and overexpression of autocrine motility factor receptor in association with progression of gastric cancers. *Am. J. Pathol.* **113**, 266–274.

Keely, P., Parise, L., and Juliano, R. (1998). Integrins and GTPases in tumor cell growth, motility and invasion. *Trend Cell Biol.* **8**, 101–106.

Lauffenburger, D. A., and Horwitz, A. F. (1996). Cell migration: A physically integrated molecular process. *Cell* **84**, 359–369.

Liotta, L. A., Trygvason, K., Garbisa, S., *et al.* (1980). Metastatic potential correlates with enzymatic degradation of basement membrane collagen. *Nature* **284**, 67–68.

Murphy, G., and Gavrilovic, J. (1999). Proteolysis and cell migration: Creating a path? *Curr. Opin. Cell Biol.* **11**, 614–621.

Nabeshima, K., Inoue, T., Shimao, Y., Kataoka, H., and Koono, M. (1999). Cohort migration of carcinoma cells: Differentiated colorectal carcinoma cells move as coherent cell clusters or sheets. *Histol. Histopathol.* **14**, 1183–1197.

Nabi, I. R. (1999). The polarisation of the motile cell. *J. Cell Sci.* **112**, 1803–1811.

Nelson, A. R., Fingleton, B., Rothenberg, M. L., and Matrisian, L. (2000). Matrix metalloproteinases: Biological activity and clinical implications. *J. Clin. Oncol.* **18**, 1135–1149.

Nieman, M. T., Prudoff, R. S., Johnson, K. R., and Weelock, M. J. (1999). N-cadherin promotes motility in human breast cancer cells regardless of their E-cadherin expression. *J. Cell Biol.* **147**, 631–643.

Nobes, C. D., and Hall, A. (1995). Rho, rac and cdc42 GTPases regulate the assembly of multimolecular focal complexes associated with actin stress fibers, lamellipodia and filopodia. *Cell* **81**, 53–62.

Preissner, K., Kanse, S. M., and May, A. E. (2000). Urokinase receptor: A molecular organizer in cellular communication. *Curr. Opin. Cell Biol.* **12**, 621–628.

Rohatgi, R., Ma, L., Miki, H., Lopez, M., Kirchhausen, T., Takenawa, T., and Kirschner, M. (1999). The interaction between N-WASP and the Arp2/3 complex links Cdc42-dependent signals to actin assembly. *Cell* **97,** 221–231.

Schor, S. L. (1995). Fibroblast subpopulation as accelerators of tumor progression: The role of migration stimulating factor. *EXS* **74,** 273–296.

Shimizu, K., Tani, M., Watanabe, H., Nagamachi, Y., Niinaka, Y., Shiroishi, T., Ohwada, S., Raz, A., and Yokota, J. (1999). The autocrine motility factor receptor gene encodes a novel type of seven transmembrane protein. *FEBS Lett.* **456,** 295–300.

Shimoyama, M., Nagafuchi, A., Fujita, A., Gotoh, M., Takeichi, M., Tsukita, S., and Hirohashi, S. (1992). Cadherin dysfunction in a human cancer cell line: Possible involvement of loss of α-catenin expression in reduced cell-cell adhesiveness. *Cancer Res.* **52,** 5770–5774.

Silletti, C., and Raz, A. (1993). Autocrine motility factor is a growth factor. *Biochem. Biophys. Res. Commun.* **194,** 446–457.

Silletti, S., Yao, J. P., Pienta, K. J., and Raz, A. (1995). Loss of cell contact regulation and altered responses to autocrine motility factor correlate with increased malignancy in prostate cancer cells. *Int. J. Cancer* **63,** 100–105.

Takeichi, M. (1991). Cadherin cell adhesion receptors as a morphogenetic regulator. *Science* **251,** 1451–1455.

Takeichi, M. (1993). Cadherin in cancer: Implications for invasion and metastasis. *Curr. Opin. Cell Biol.* **5,** 806–811.

Van der Voort, R., Taher, T. E., Derksen, P. W., Spaargaren, M., van der Neut, R., and Pals, S. T. (2000). The hepatocyte growth factor/Met pathway in development, tumorigenesis and B-cell differentiation. *Adv. Cancer Res.* **79,** 39–90.

Wells, A. (2000). Tumor invasion: Role of growth factor-induced cell motility. *Adv. Cancer Res.* **78,** 31–101.

Tumor Necrosis Factors

Carl F. Ware

La Jolla Institute for Allergy and Immunology

GLOSSARY

apoptosis A regulated process of cell death characterized by membrane blebbing, nuclear condensation, fragmentation of DNA, and phagocytosis, also referred to as programmed cell death.

cachexia Wasting syndrome characterized by weight loss, anorexia, and anemia, often seen in patients with cancer or with chronic infectious disease.

death domain A linear sequence of 80 amino acids responsible for inducing apoptosis first defined in TNFR1 and Fas.

knockout mice Animals genetically deleted of a specific gene by homologous recombination.

shedding Loss of membrane proteins by proteolytic cleavage of the extracellular domain, often generating a soluble cytokine or receptor.

TNF receptor-associated factor (TRAF) A family of zinc RING/finger proteins containing a unique receptor-binding domain, the TRAF domain.

virokines and viroceptors Anti-immune response proteins that are viral versions of cytokines or their receptors.

Tumor necrosis factors are a family of membrane-anchored cytokines that mediate a broad range of processes in development and physiologic functions through a corresponding family of specific cell surface receptors. Many of the TNF-related cytokines are produced by cells of the immune system, which orchestrate innate and acquired host defenses to generate inflammatory processes against infectious and malignant diseases. Several members of this cytokine–receptor superfamily, including TNF and Fas ligand, induce cell death (apoptosis). Other members, such as CD40 or the p75 neurotrophin receptor, promote the survival of lymphocytes or neurons or mediate the effector functions of cellular immunity, whereas still others, such as lymphotoxin (LT)-α and β, are involved in the development of lymphoid organs. Two major families of signaling proteins, death domain proteins and TRAFs, which bind directly to the intracellular domain of the receptor, propagate signals that initiate cellular responses. Several distinct viruses have evolved specific genetic mechanisms to thwart or usurp the action of TNF receptors and their signaling proteins. Genetic mutations in certain members of the TNF superfamily are associated autoimmunity, immunodeficiency, and pathophysiologic states such as septic shock and wasting (cachexia) associated with chronic infectious diseases and cancer. The potent cell regulatory activities of the TNF superfamily mark these cytokines as targets for therapeutic intervention in cancer and autoimmune diseases.

I. INTRODUCTION

Cytokines control cell survival, death, and differentiation, which are integral processes necessary for tissue development and homeostasis. In the immune system, these include interferons, hemopoietins, cytokines, chemokines, transforming growth factors, and tumor necrosis factors. A prominent feature of the TNF cytokine family is the ability to induce apoptotic cell death. The regulation of cell growth and death is now a fundamental approach to the treatment of cancer and other proliferative diseases. TNF has a long history in the treatment of malignant disease that dates back to the beginning of the previous century as the likely element of Coley's toxins. Lymphotoxin (LT), another cytokine with cytotoxic activities similar to TNF, was shown to be structurally related to TNF, heralding the two prototypic members of this family, with most of the rest discovered since 1993 (Table I).

A parallel family of cognate TNF receptors (TNFR) emerged when two specific TNFR were cloned revealing extensive homology to CD27, CD40, and the low affinity nerve growth factor (NGF) receptor (NGFR; also known as the low affinity neurotrophin receptor). These receptors bind specifically to their respective ligands, which in turn generate signals inside the cell that change the function of the cell, in some cases leading to cell death or the induction of gene transcription. The mechanism propagating the

signals is via the binding of distinct cytosolic protein adaptors, which fall into two major classes, TRAFs and death domain proteins. A third group of receptors lack a cytoplasmic domain altogether and are secreted or anchored by a lipid linkage. These proteins capture the cytokine, circumventing binding to cell surface receptors, and act as decoys.

Several members of the TNF family are capable of protecting against cell death and enhancing cell growth. For example, signals from CD27 or TNFR2 enhance the proliferation of T lymphocytes that are activated through the T-cell antigen receptor. However, in contrast to a true growth factor, such as IL-2, neither TNF nor CD27L will sustain independent proliferation of T cells. Thus, some of the TNF-related ligands are classified as costimulatory or survival factors for cellular proliferation.

The determination of whether a cell will grow, die, or differentiate in response to these ligands depends on specific characteristics of the cell type. It is clear that infection with certain viruses can make normal cells sensitive to the apoptosis-inducing activity of TNF. Not all tumor cell lines are sensitive to cell death action of TNF. The mechanism(s) underlying resistance to cell death may be related to the induction of genes dependent on the transcription factor NF-κB. NF-κB is crucial for inducing resistance to TNF-induced apoptosis. TNF-induced genes, such as Mn superoxide dismutase or A20 zinc finger, and the inhibitors of apoptosis (IAP) are required for cellular resistance to the cytotoxic action of TNF, thus the cell must actively protect itself from the apoptotic effect of TNF. Because viruses can shut off host protein synthesis as a consequence of their parasitic action, the default pathway induced by TNF selectively initiates death of virus-infected cells, sparing normal cells. However, many viruses have evolved mechanisms to resist apoptosis.

II. STRUCTURAL FEATURES OF TUMOR NECROSIS FACTOR (TNF) LIGAND FAMILY

The TNF family of ligands are characteristically type II transmembrane proteins with the C terminus displayed on the outside of the cell, a retained transmembrane region, and short cytoplasmic tails (15–25

TABLE I
Members of the TNF-Related Cytokine-Receptor Superfamily

Receptor	Ligand	Signaling type	Function
TNFR60 (R1)	TNF/LTα3/LTα2β	Death domain	Apoptosis/inflammation
TNFR80 (R2)	TNF/LTα3/LTα2β	TRAF	Apoptosis/proliferation
LTβR	LTα1β2/LIGHT	TRAF	Lymphoid organogenesis
HVEM (HveA)	LIGHT/LTα3	TRAF	Herpesvirus entry/costimulation
Fas/CD95	Fas L	Death domain	Apoptosis
CD40	CD40 L	TRAF	B-cell survival
CD30	CD30 L	TRAF	Apoptosis/negative selection
CD27	CD27 L	TRAF	Costimulation
OX40	OX40 L	TRAF	Costimulation
41BB	41BB L	TRAF	Costimulation
p75NTR	Neurotrophins, NGF	TRAF	Neuron survival
TRAIL-R1 (DR4)	TRAIL	Death domain	Apoptosis
TRAIL-R2 (DR5)	TRAIL	Death domain	Apoptosis
TRAIL-R3	TRAIL	Partial death domain	Decoy receptor
TRAIL-R4 (DcR2)	TRAIL	GPI link	NF-κB
DR3	?	Death domain	Apoptosis
GITR	GITR L	TRAF	Cell survival
RANK (TRANCE-R)	RANK L (TRANCE)	TRAF	Osteoclast differentiation
Osteoprotegerin	RANKL TRAIL	Soluble receptor	Soluble regulator
DR3 (TRAMP)	VEGI (TL1)	Death domain	Costimulation
Fn14	TWEAK	TRAF	Angiogenesis
TACI	BAFF APRIL	TRAF/CAML	B-cell survival
BCMA	BAFF APRIL	TRAF	B-cell survival
DcR3	FasLigand LIGHT	Soluble	Decoy receptor
EDAR	EDA-A1	TRAF	Ectodermal dysplasias
XDAR	EDA-A2	TRAF	
DR6	?	Death domain	Apoptosis

[a]BAFF, B-cell-activating factor belonging to the TNF family; BCMA, B-cell maturation antigen; CD, cluster of differentiation; DR3, 4, and 5, death receptor -3, -4, and -5; EDA, ectodermal dysplasin; HVEM, herpes virus entry mediator; GITR, glucocorticoid-induced TNF receptor; LT, lymphotoxin; LIGHT, LT-like ligand competitive with gD-1 HSV for HVEM expressed on T cells; NTR, neurotrophin (nerve growth factor) receptor; TACI, transmembrane activator and CAML interactor; TNF, tumor necrosis factor; TRAIL, TNF-related apoptosis-inducing ligand; TRAMP, TNF receptor-associated membrane protein; TRANCE, TNF-related activation-induced cytokine; TWEAK, TNF-related ligand with weak apoptosis activity; TRAIL receptor without an intracellular domain; DcR, decoy receptor-1, -2, or -3; VEGI, vascular endothelial growth inhibitor.

residues in length). The TNF ligand family is defined by several discrete regions of conserved sequences in the primary structure located in the C-terminal domain involved in trimerization and binding receptor (Fig. 1). The overall homology of the sequences is modest (25–30%); however, there is a high level of conservation of the three-dimensional shape of these proteins. The primary structure of TNF-related ligands is a polypeptide chain that folds into an antiparallel β-sheet sandwich, with a characteristic "Greek key" topology. This subunit assembles into a compact trimer, with the end-to-face interaction about a threefold axis of symmetry. This generates a cone-shaped molecule with a large flat base and narrow top. Both the N and the C termini are located at the base, and thus the top of the TNF molecule is

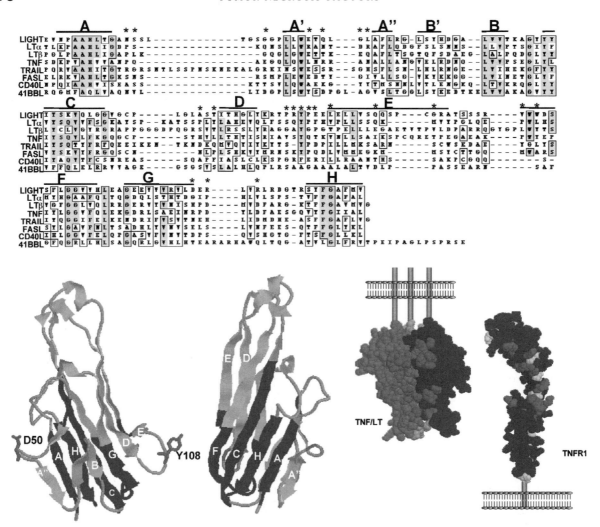

FIGURE 1 Structural features of TNF superfamily. (Top) Amino acid sequence alignment of several TNF-related ligands. Alignment generated ClustalW of the ligand-binding domains of the indicated ligands. Bars indicate β strands labeled A–H according to Eck *et al.* (1992). Eck, M. J., Ultsch, M., Rinderknecht, E., de Vos, A. M., and Sprang, S. R. (1992). The structure of human lymphotoxin at 1.9-A resolution. *J. Biol. Chem.* **267,** 2119. Residues in LTα that make contact with TNFR1 are shown with asterisks. (Lower left) Ribbon diagram of a single LTα subunit showing the β-strand structure, where conserved residues are shown in dark, and tyrosine 108 (Y108) and aspartic acid 50 (D50) are involved in receptor binding. The structure on the left shows the solvent exposed side, as in the trimer, and the structure on the right is rotated ~180° to reveal the interior face. (Lower right) Space-filling models of LTα trimer in the orientation, as it would exist as a membrane-anchored ligand, and a single TNFR1. TNFR1 is rotated ~180° to reveal contact residues. Contact residues on both LTα and TNFR1 are shown in dark gray. Banner, D. W., D'Arcy, A., Janes, W., Gentz, R., Schoenfeld, H. J., Broger, C., Loetscher, H., and Lesslauer, W. (1993). Crystal structure of the soluble human 55 kd TNF receptor-human TNF beta complex: Implications for TNF receptor activation. *Cell* **73,** 431.

thought to protrude outward from the cell surface. When these homology regions are identified in the three-dimensional structure of TNF, they line up adjacent to each other on the face of the internal β sheet, suggesting that all members of this family are trimers. This same structural feature is also found in the globular head of the first component of complement, C1q, suggesting that TNF-related ligands and C1q-related proteins are derived from a common an-

cestral gene. Soluble forms of several TNF-related cytokines are produced by cells using different mechanisms, including proteolysis, alternate splicing, or deletion. Proteolytic processing is a posttranslational feature common to certain members of this family. Human TNF is translated as a 26-kDa precursor and is processed by a cell surface proteinase (a member of the Adams family of disintegrin metalloproteinases) at the cell surface to yield the 17-kDa secreted form.

The surface form of LT is unique in this family. Surface LT is a heteromeric complex assembled from two subunits, LTα and LTβ, whereas all of the other ligands are homotrimers. The association between the two LT subunits occurs during biosynthesis, generating two types of heterotrimer; LTα1β2 and LTα2β1.

The genetic organization for members of this cytokine family indicate that gene duplication is an active mechanism generating diversity of this superfamily (Table II). The genes encoding TNF, LTα, and LTβ lie adjacent to each other as a cytokine locus of ~8 kb sandwiched between the HLA-B locus and complement proteins on human chromosome 6 (mouse chromosome 17). Each ligand is usually encoded by three or four exons. The last exon is the largest and encodes the majority of the extracellular, receptor-binding domain. Disease linkage of several ligand genes has been demonstrated (Table III). For instance, mutations in the CD40 ligand are the cause of X-linked immunodeficiency, known as hyper-IgM syndrome in humans. This immunodeficiency is associated with a failure of B cells to switch isotype classes to IgG, IgA, and IgE. FasL mutation in mice results

in generalized lymphoproliferative disorder *gld*. A similar phenotype is observed with mutations in Fas identified as lymphoproliferative defect *lpr*, an autoimmune-like condition in mice and humans (autoimmune syndrome with lymphproliferation, ALPS). However, the proliferation of T cells in *lpr* and *gld* mice, although extensive, is not malignant. None of the ligand genes show potential to function independently as oncogenes. The positioning of the LTβ/TNF gene locus in the MHC has fueled speculation of linkage to several of the MHC-associated diseases, such as rheumatoid arthritis.

Most of the TNF-related ligands are expressed by activated lymphoid and myeloid-derived cells, particularly T cells, but several are also produced by nonlymphoid tissue. TNF is a good example of a broadly expressed ligand. It is primarily produced by macrophages and T cells when activated by inflammatory or antigenic stimuli, but is also produced by fibroblasts, mast cells, and basophils. Ectopic expression in nonlymphoid tumors has also been observed. CD40L is expressed primarily by CD4[+] T helper cells, but platelets and basophils in response to activation

TABLE II
Chromosomal Location of TNF Ligands

Gene name	Human	Mouse	mRNA accession numbers		Ligand symbol
			Human	Mouse	
TNF	6p21.3	ch17 (19.06 cm)	NM_000594	M11731	TNFSF1A
LTα	6p21.3	ch17 (19.06 cm)	NM_000595	M16819	TNFSF1B
LTβ	6p21.3	ch17 (19.06 cm)	NM_002341	U16985	TNFSF3
OX40-L	1q25	ch1 (84.90 cM)	NM_003326	U12763	TNFSF4
CD40-L, CD154	Xq26	chX (18.0 cM)	NM_000074	X65453	TNFSF5
Fas-L	1q23	ch1 (85.0 cM)	NM_000639	S76752	TNFSF6
CD27-L, CD70	19p13	ch17 (20.0 cM)	NM_001252	Y13636	TNFSF7
CD30-L, CD153	9q33	ch4 (32.20 cM)	NM_001244	L09754	TNFSF8
4-1BB-L	19p13	ch17 (20.0 cM)	NM_003811	L15435	TNFSF9
TRAIL	3q26	Unknown	NM_003810	U37522	TNFSF10
RANK-L, OPG-L, TRANCE	13q14	ch14 (45.0 cM)	AF053712	AB008426	TNFSF11
TWEAK	17p13	Unknown	NM_003809	AF030100	TNFSF12
APRIL/TALL2	17P13.1	Unknown	NM_003808	AF294825	TNFSF13
BAFF, BLYS, TALL1	13q32-q34	Unknown	NM_006573	AF119383	TNFSF13B
LIGHT	19p13.3	ch17 (D-E1)	NM_003807	AF227533	TNFSF14
VEGI, TL1	9q33	Unknown	AF039390	Unknown	TNFSF15
GITRL, AITRL	1q23	Unknown	NM_005092	Unknown	TNFSF18
EDA1	Xq12-q13.1	chX (37.0 cM)	NM_001399	NM_010099	
EDA2	Xq12-q13.1	chX (37.0 cM)	AF061189	AJ243657	

TABLE III
Human Genetic Diseases Associated with TNF Superfamily

System	Disease	Mutation
TNFR1	Familial periodic fever	Mutation in first cysteine-rich domain
CD40 ligand	Hyper-IgM syndrome	Multiple mutations affecting receptor binding and processing
EDA	X-linked hypohidrotic ectodermal dysplasia	Multiple mutations affecting receptor binding, trimerization, and secretion
RANK	Familial expansile osteolysis	Mutation in the signal peptide
Fas	Autoimmunelymphoproliferative syndrome	Multiple mutation in Fas deletion

stimuli can also produce this ligand. LTαβ expression is restricted to activated T and B lymphocytes and natural killer (NK) cells. FasL and OX40L are expressed predominantly by T cells, yet FasL mRNA is detected in reproductive organs and epithelium of the eye. The nonlymphoid expression of FasL, with its dramatically potent apoptosis-inducing activity for T cells, such as in epithelial cells of the eye, provides an immunosuppressive function by destroying migrating inflammatory cells, thus creating an immunologically privileged site. Expression of TNF-related ligands is highly regulated at transcriptional, translational, and posttranslational control points. An example of one significant control point is the production of TNF mRNA by inflammatory cells. TNF mRNA transcription is induced in response to innate as well as antigen receptors. TNF mRNA is short lived, giving rise to transient expression of the protein. Degradation of TNF and LTα mRNA is controlled in part by an AU-rich element in the 3′-untranslated region. The soluble form of TNF is relatively unstable, but can be stabilized by binding a soluble, monovalent form of TNFR. TNF receptors are shed during cellular activation, primarily by proteases in the Adams family, which also process TNF. Soluble receptors accumulate and when levels increase to occupy two or three binding sites on the ligand, they inhibit (antagonize) binding to cell surface receptors and thus block the target cell from receiving the signal, acting like "decoys."

III. TNF RECEPTOR FAMILY

Members of the TNF receptor superfamily include proteins of mammalian and viral origin (Table I).

Noteworthy members include the low-affinity, 75-kDa neurotrophin (nerve growth factor) receptor (NTR) and the soluble TNFR-like proteins produced by poxvirus. Although NTR is a member of the receptor family, its ligands (nerve growth factor and the other neurotrophins) are structurally unrelated to the TNF ligand family. In addition to the virus and nervous system receptors, the major grouping contains receptors that function primarily in the immune system. Two distinct receptors of 55–60 kDa (CD120a; TNFR1 or TNFR60) and 75–80 kDa (CD120b; TNFR2, TNFR80) have been identified that bind both TNF and LTα. The two TNFR genes reside on distinct chromosomes, but there they are linked to several other members. The *TNFR2* gene locus is on human chromosome 1p36 (conserved synteny with mouse Chr 4) linked with several others. The *TNFR1* gene locus is on human Chr 12p13 (mouse Chr 6) linked to LTβR and CD27 genes (Table IV).

All of the cellular receptors are type I membrane proteins (N terminus on the cell exterior) with a single transmembrane-spanning region. The defining feature of this family is a highly conserved, cysteine-rich motif in the extracellular (ecto) ligand-binding domain. The cytoplasmic domains show little sequence homology, yet several of the receptors bind common signaling proteins and initiate similar types of activities. The extracellular portion of the receptor is the ligand-binding domain (Fig. 1). Based on the crystal structure of the TNFR1, the cysteine-rich motif is a tightly knit domain formed around three disulfide bonds creating an elongated molecule that binds the ligand. The signature sequence of the core motif is CxxCxxC; however, this varies among members. The crystal structure of TNFR1 and the LTαhomotrimer revealed that the elongated receptors lay along the

TABLE IV
Chromosomal Location of TNF Receptors

Gene name/aliases	Chromosomal location		mRNA accession numbers		Receptor symbol
	Human	Mouse	Human	Mouse	
TNFRp60, (R1)	12p13.2	ch6 (60.55cM)	NM_001065	M60468	TNFRSF1A
TNFRp80, (R2)	1p36.3-36.2	ch4 (75.5cM)	NM_001066	U29173	TNFRSF1B
LTβR	12p13	ch6 (60.4cM)	NM_002342	NM_010736	TNFRSF3
OX40	1p36	ch4 (79.4cM)	NM_003327	Z21674	TNFRSF4
CD40	20q12-q13.2	ch2 (97.0cM)	NM_001250	M83312	TNFRSF5
FAS, CD95	10q24.1	ch19 (23.0cM)	NM_000043	M83649	TNFRSF6
DcR3	20q13	Unknown	NM_003823	Unknown	TNFRSF6B
CD27	12p13	ch6 (60.35)	NM_001242	L24495	TNFRSF7
CD30	1p36	ch4 (75.5cM)	NM_001243	U25416	TNFRSF8
4-1BB	1p36	ch4 (75.5cM)	NM_001561	J04492	TNFRSF9
TRAILR-1, DR4	8p21	Unknown	NM_003844	Unknown	TNFRSF10A
TRAIL-R2, DR5	8p22-p21	Unknown	NM_003842	AB031081	TNFRSF10B
TRAILR3, DcR1	8p22-p21	Unknown	NM_003841	Unknown	TNFRSF10C
TRAILR4, DcR2	8p21	Unknown	NM_003840	Unknown	TNFRSF10D
RANK, TRANCE-R	18q22.1	Unknown	NM_003839	AF019046	TNFRSF11A
OPG, TR1	8q24	Unknown	NM_002546	AB013898	TNFRSF11B
TRAMP, DR3, LARD	1p36.3	Unknown	NM_003790	Unknown	TNFRSF12
TACI	17p11.2	ch11	NM_012452	AF257673	TNFRSF13B
HVEM, HveA, ATAR	1p36.3-p36.2	Unknown	NM_003820	Unknown	TNFRSF14
p75NTR, NGFR	17q12-q22	ch11 (55.6cM)	NM_002507	AF105292	TNFRSF16
BCMA	16p13.1	ch16 (B3)	NM_001192	AF061505	TNFRSF17
AITR, GITR	1p36.3	ch4 (E)	NM_004195	NM_009400	TNFRSF18
TROY, TAJ	Unknown	ch14	NM_018647	AB040432	TNFRSF19
EDAR	2q11-q13	ch10	NM_022336	AF160502	
XEDAR	X	Unknown	AF298812	Unknown	
Fn14	16p13.3	ch17	NM_016639	AF156164	
DR6	6P12.2-21.1	Unknown	NM_014452	AF322069	

cleft formed between adjacent ligand subunits with the receptor N terminus closest to the base of the ligand. In this, orientation requires that the receptor and ligand are on juxtaposed membranes. In TNF and LTα, the loops connecting the D-E and the A-A″ β strands, located on opposite sides of the solvent exposed surface, contain the major receptor-binding residues. Thus, in a homotrimer, each ligand has three equivalent receptor-binding sites. This has led to the idea that aggregation or clustering of the receptor by the ligand is a critical feature in initiating signal transduction.

Cellular expression and tissue distribution of the different receptors are varied. TNF receptors are expressed at extremely low levels on most cells: typically less than a few thousand per cell. Several receptors are tissue restricted, e.g., BCMA is expressed on B lymphocytes, whereas TNFR1 is expressed by most tissues and TNFR2 is on activated T and B lymphocytes. Naïve T cells from peripheral blood have no binding sites for TNF; however, when activated via the TCR or IL-2, the TNFR2 gene is transcribed, resulting in peak protein surface expression in 48–72 h. Activated T cells, when restimulated, rapidly (within minutes) downregulate TNFR2 by shedding, which releases a soluble extracellular receptor domain with ligand-binding activity.

IV. SIGNALING MOLECULES

At the surface of the target cell, the initiating event in signal transduction is the clustering of multiple receptors around the trivalent ligand. This is a complex process, probably involving receptors in a pre-oligomerized conformation. Ligand binding leads to a corresponding transmembrane clustering and reorientation of the cytoplasmic domains. The propagation of signals to enzymatically active proteins is mediated by two distinct sets of adaptor proteins: the death domain family and the TRAF family. These adaptors allow certain receptors to activate caspases that mediate apoptosis or transcription factors NF-κB and API, which regulate gene expression.

A. Death Domain

TNFR1 and Fas both contain homologous domains, designated death domain (DD), now recognized as a family of as many as 30 members in vertebrates. The DD homology region is an ~80 amino acid region that folds into six α helixes. The DD is a protein interaction motif that binds in a restricted fashion to other proteins that contain a DD (Fig. 2). The DD of Fas will associate with itself (homotypic interaction), but not with TNFR1, and can interact with other DD containing proteins, such as Fas-associated DD (FADD). Following ligand binding, FADD becomes associated with (recruited) Fas, forming a multicomponent signaling complex. FADD contains a second protein interaction motif, called a death effector domain, DED that allows it to couple directly to procaspase 8, a cysteine-based, aspartic acid-specific protease. Caspase 8 is known as an initiator caspase that becomes activated by proteolysis into an active enzyme that can directly cleave caspase 3 and other caspases, which then execute the terminal phase of apoptosis by the cleavage of critical cellular proteins. A point mutant in Fas DD is responsible for an autoimmune disease in mice and humans.

TNFR1-induced cell death requires an additional DD containing adaptor to signal apoptosis. A protein interacting specifically with TNFR1 is known as the TNFR-associated death domain (TRADD). TRADD serves as a specific adaptor for TNFR1 that can recruit FADD to induce apoptosis. TRADD can also interact

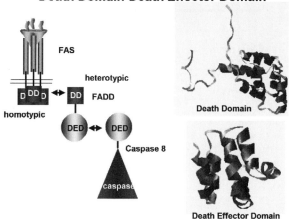

**Adaptor Schemes in TNFR Signaling:
Death Domain-Death Effector Domain**

FIGURE 2   Adaptor scheme in TNF receptor signaling: Death domain. (Left) Ligand-bound receptor in a clustered topography where the death domains are interacting with themselves (homotypic) and can interact with the death domain of FADD (heterotypic). FADD interacts with caspase 8 via a death effector domain. (Right) Ribbon diagrams of the six α helical death domain (Fas) and death effector domain (FADD).

with the other adaptor family, TRAFs. A third protein containing a DD, termed RIP, is a serine kinase. The current thought is that upon TNF binding to TNFR1, the clustered cytoplasmic domains recruit TRADD and RIP into a multicomponent signaling complex and RIP may function in the activation of procaspase 8.

B. TRAF

TNFR-associated factors (TRAF), the other major family of signaling adaptors, contain an N-terminal zinc RING and zinc finger motifs, followed by a coiled coil domain (isoleucine zipper) and a receptor association domain, or "TRAF" domain, the defining feature at the C terminus. The TRAF domain of a given TRAF can bind to several different receptors (Fig. 3). There are currently six members with distinct interaction patterns with members of the TNFR family that lack a DD, such as CD40, LTβR, TNFR2, and CD30. Additionally, TRAF6 has been implicated as the activator of NF-κB by IL-1 and thus represents an example of a TRAF molecule involved in a signaling pathway outside the TNFR family. TRAFs are trimers formed through their TRAF and coiled coil domains,

Adaptor Schemes in TNFR Signaling:
Receptor peptide-TRAF

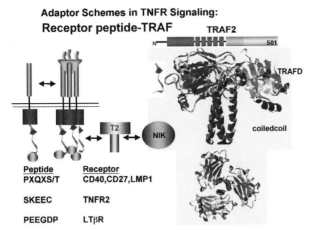

Peptide	Receptor
PXQXS/T	CD40,CD27,LMP1
SKEEC	TNFR2
PEEGDP	LTβR

FIGURE 3 Adaptor scheme in TNF receptor signaling: TRAF domain. (Left) Ligand-bound receptor in a clustered topography where TRAF2 interacts with a short peptide in the receptor and binds to the NF-κb inducing kinase, NIK. The TRAF-binding sequences of several members of the TNFR family are shown. Schematic diagram of TRAF2, with the RING finger located at the N terminus and multiple zinc fingers, and coiled coil region and the C-terminal TRAF domain. (Right) Ribbon diagram of the three-dimensional structure of TRAF2 in side view (and receptor peptide) and top view. Park, Y. C., Burkitt, V., Villa, A. R., Tong, L., and Wu, H. (1999). Structural basis for self-association and receptor recognition of human TRAF2. *Nature* **398**, 533–538.

which resemble a mushroom head and its stalk. TRAF-binding receptors contain a short proline anchored sequence that is responsible for binding directly to the mushroom head of various TRAFs. The TRAF domain is found in several other proteins, such as MUL, USP7, and SPOP, that interact with various TRAFs or have ubiquitin protease activity. These related proteins define a large family, called TRAF domain encompassing factors (TEFs), which have homologues throughout the eukaryotes, suggesting that this branch of the TRAF family arose from an ancient gene.

The function of the TRAF family is clearly involved in gene activation through NF-κB and AP1 and the regulation of apoptosis. LTβR and TNFR1, following ligand binding, both recruit TRAFs to their respective signaling complex, but differ in their mechanisms. TRAF2 binds directly to the receptor cytosolic domain of LTβR, whereas TRAF2 uses TRADD to couple to TNFR1. TRAF2 can interact with numerous other proteins, leading to the initiation of diverse signaling pathways. In mice, TRAF2 is essential for signaling JNK activation, but dispensable for NF-κB

activation when stimulated via TNF and TNFR1. In contrast, LTβR requires TRAF2 for NF-κB activation. Here, evidence indicates that TRAF2 binds the NF-κB inducing kinase (NIK), which is involved in the phosphorylation of p100 generating the p52 transcriptionally active form of NF-κB. The zinc RING motif in TRAFs, in general, appears to be involved as effector domains, as deletion causes loss of signaling function, and these mutants inhibit receptor signaling in a dominant fashion. The zinc RING of TRAF6 functions together with Ubc13 and Uev1A to catalyze the synthesis of unique polyubiquitin chains on ubiquitin that are essential for the activation of inhibitor of κB (IκB) kinase (IKK) and subsequent activation of NF-κB. Thus, TRAFs may participate in generating forms of ubiquitin that are essential in signal transduction independent of its role in proteosome-dependent degradation of proteins.

Genetic deletion of TRAF2, 3, or 6 results in abnormal development, as do some members of the DD family, indicating crucial roles in developmental process, where as TRAF 4, 5, and 1 are without developmental abnormalities (Table V). The phenotypes of TRAF-deficient mice are complex and, for several TRAFs, have not been clearly linked to signaling properties of specific TNFR.

V. BIOLOGICAL FUNCTIONS OF TNF SUPERFAMILY

The functions of the different members of this superfamily are diverse, but regulation of cell death and survival is a common theme that has emerged from various studies. Furthermore, these ligand–receptor systems play key roles in the development of organs and tissues and in controlling inflammation and immune responses. Perhaps the most insightful approaches are studies of naturally occurring mutations and those obtained through the development of gene deletion techniques creating gene "knockout" mice (Table VI). The TNF superfamily can be divided into discrete groups based on structural homology and shared ligand–receptor-binding patterns, and overlaid on this scheme are major functional properties, including inflammation, apoptosis, survival, and development.

TABLE V

Genetic Deficiency of TNFR Signaling Proteins in Mice

Gene	Phenotype
TRAF2	Normal at birth but become progressively runted and die. Atrophy of the thymus and spleen and depletion of B-cell precursors. TNF levels are elevated; severe reduction in TNF-mediated JNK/SAPK activation but a mild effect on NF-κB activation
TRAF3	Normal at birth but become progressively runted, with progressive hypoglycemia and depletion of peripheral white cells; die by 10 days. Fetal liver reconstitutes all hematopoietic lineages in lethally irradiated mice; however, impaired response to T-dependent antigen
TRAF5	No developmental effect. B-cell defects in proliferation and upregulation of CD23, CD54, CD80, CD86, and Fas in response to CD40 stimulation. *In vitro* Ig production reduced. CD27 costimulatory signal impaired.
TRAF6	Osteopetrotic with defects in bone remodeling and tooth eruption due to impaired osteoclast function. IL-1, CD40, LPS signaling defective. Immature B cells markedly reduced; no lymph nodes
relA	Embryonic lethality at 15–16 days with liver apoptosis. Cells defective in IκBα mRNA induction
relB	Multifocal, mixed inflammatory cell infiltration, myeloid hyperplasia, splenomegaly due to extramedullary hematopoiesis, and a reduced population of thymic dendritic cells
c-rel	Humoral immunity is impaired, and mature B and T cells were found to be unresponsive to most mitogenic stimuli
p50	No developmental abnormalities, but exhibit multifocal defects in immune responses involving B lymphocytes and nonspecific responses to infection
P52	Impaired in their ability to generate antibodies to T-dependent antigens, absence of B-cell follicles and FDC networks, inability to form germinal centers
Bcl-3	Impaired in germinal center reactions and T-dependent antibody responses to influenza virus. Altered microarchitecture of secondary lymphoid organs in mutant mice
FADD	Embryonic lethal day 11.5; cardiac failure and abdominal hemorrrhage
RIP	Neonatal lethal (days 1–3); apoptosis in both lymphoid and adipose tissue and dying at 1–3 days of age. No TNF activation of NF-κB
NIK	Alymphoplasia (aly) mutation (autosomal recessive), absence of secondary lymphoid tissues; disorganized splenic and thymic structures with immunodeficiency
IKKα	No impairment of TNF/IL-1 NF-κB activation, limb outgrowth impaired; epidermal hyperplasia
IKKβ	Embryonic lethal at 14.5 days; no TNF response; similar to p65- and p50-deficient mice

A. The Immediate TNF Family

The immediate family is defined by their shared ligand receptor-binding patterns and structural homology and represents a microcosm of all functional groupings. TNF, LTα, LTβ, and LIGHT define the core group of ligands within the larger TNF superfamily that binds four cognate cell surface receptors with distinct but significant overlapping specificity. TNF and LTα, as homotrimers, bind the same two receptors: TNFR1 (55–60 kDa) and TNFR2 (75–80 kDa). LTα assembles with LTβ to form the LTα1β2 heterotrimer, which binds exclusively to the LTβR. The LTβ-related ligand, LIGHT, engages the herpesvirus entry mediator (HVEM) and also binds the LTβR. HVEM binds LTα, but not to either the TNF or the LTαβ heterotrimer. The existence of a soluble binding protein for LIGHT, decoy receptor 3 (DcR3), which also binds the Fas ligand, underscores the multiple regulatory mechanisms designed to control the expression and function of these molecules.

Mice with TNFR1 gene deletion by homologous recombination are developmentally normal, but profoundly immune deficient in response to bacterial pathogens such as *Listeria monocytogenes*, a model for cellular immunity to an intracellular pathogen. TNF is a mediator of septic shock induced by bacterial lipopolysaccharide (LPS). TNFR1-deficient mice are resistant to low doses of LPS-induced shock after treatment of mice with D-galactosamine, but still succumb to high doses of LPS. Mice deficient in TNFR2 are less susceptible to *L. monocytogenes* than TNFR1-deficient mice, but they are unable to efficiently clear these pathogens. TNFR1-/- mice can clear cytomegalovirus (β herpesvirus) as efficiently as wild-type mice, but have a prolonged infiltration of organs with T cells. This indicates that TNFR

TABLE VI
Phenotypes of Mice Deficient in TNF Receptors

Receptor	Phenotype
TNFR1	Susceptibility to *L. monocytogenes*; resistant to toxic effects of LPS, no Peyer's patches, no germinal center formation
LTβR	No secondary lymphoid organs, deficiency in NK and NK T cells; no FDC formation, susceptible to herpesviruses
TNFR2	Milder phenotype of TNFR-1, normal lymphoid tissue; skin necrosis reaction to TNF
CD40	Failure to Ig class switch in response to T-cell-dependent antigens, no germinal centers following immunization
CD30	Elevated number of thymocytes, impaired negative selection
FAS	Lymphoproliferative syndrome, defective peripheral tolerance
CD27	Decreased T-cell memory, delayed response kinetics and reduction of CD8[+] virus-specific T-cell numbers; impaired primary CD4[+] and CD8[+] T-cell responses to influenza virus
OX40	T-cell survival defect, low frequencies of Ag-specific CD4 cells late in primary responses, lower frequencies of surviving memory cells
RANK	Osteopetrosis resulting from an apparent block in osteoclast differentiation; deficiency of B cells in spleen; no lymph nodes

plays a significant role in downmodulating immune responses.

The LTαβ cytokine system controls the development and organization of secondary lymphoid tissues. Mice with homozygous deletion of the LTα, LTβ, or LTβR genes have a complex phenotype, but most notably fail to develop lymph nodes and Peyer's patches, and also have a disorganized splenic architecture. Normally, T and B cells are located in distinct areas of the white pulp in the spleen, but this compartmentalization is disrupted in LTα -/- mice. Although T- and B-cell development is normal, NK cells and a specialized subset of T cells, called NK-T cells, fail to differentiate in LT-deficient mice. This result suggests that the LT system is required for the differentiation of crucial progenitors that give rise to these lineages.

LIGHT can interfere with herpes simplex virus entry and may play a role in lymphocyte activation and tumor immunity. Expression of LIGHT by transplanted tumors led to severe lymphocyte infiltration with enhanced T-cell cytotoxic and tumor necrosis. Consistent with this, inhibition of LIGHT with the soluble HVEM-Fc fusion protein reduced the severity of graft-versus-host disease. LIGHT transgenic animals exhibit abnormalities in lymphoid tissue architecture, as well as signs of severe inflammation of the intestine and tissue destruction of the reproductive organs. These results indicate that LIGHT may function as an important regulator of T-cell activation and implicate the LIGHT signaling pathways in tissue-specific inflammation.

B. Apoptosis and Death Domains

Fas, TRAIL receptors, DR3, and DR6 contain death domains that induce potent apoptosis in malignant and, in some cases, nontransformed cells. Fas and FasL have emerged as a critical system signaling T-cell apoptosis. Two naturally occurring mutants in Fas encoding *lymphoproliferative disorder (lpr)*, a gene disruption caused by a retrovirus insertion that expresses <1% of Fas and a point mutation lpr[cg], localized to the death domain encoding a valine to asparagine structural change. Both yield profound defects in immune regulation, leading to a progressive autoimmune syndrome. In *lpr*, animals have an excessive accumulation of T cells with an activated phenotype but are CD4/8 negative in their lymph nodes. A rapidly progressive and fatal disease occurs when *lpr* is on the MRL mouse background, whereas in some other strains of mice with a different genetic background, disease progression is slow or nonexistent. *gld* has a similar phenotype to *lpr*, but is a mutation in FasL. Studies of *lpr* and *gld* mice indicate a role of Fas/FasL in controlling T-cell differentiation in peripheral tissues, as thymic development is normal. Fas/Fas ligand is a critical armament of cytotoxic T cells (CTL), along with perforin and granzymes, that induces rapid destruction of cells harboring intracellular pathogens. Thus, the Fas ligand system serves as a potent mediator of tissue destruction by the action of CTL and NK cells by the elimination of pathogen-infected tissues, but also serves to dampen the immune system by the elimination of CTL and NK effector cells. Some tissues, such as the epithelium of the eye, express the Fas ligand, which can induce the death of infiltrating inflammatory cells, which express Fas, thus preserving integrity of the tissue.

The TRAIL cytokine system consists of four receptors, two with death domains and three decoy receptors. TRAIL was initially noted as an inducer of apoptosis that selectively killed tumor cells, suggesting its use as a potential cancer therapeutic. Deletion of TRAIL in mice does not lead to developmental abnormalities. Current evidence suggests that it may function as effector molecules for the destruction of tumor cells by NK cells selectively used in the liver.

DR3 and DR6 are orphan receptors that contains a death domain and induce apoptosis when overexpressed in tumor cells, yet little is know of its physiologic roles.

C. Cell Survival and Costimulation

Several members of the TNF family are involved in promoting the survival of lymphocytes that help protect their demise during and following cellular activation. These include CD27, 41BB, GITR, Ox40, and CD30 for T cells and CD40 and APRIL/BAFF systems for B cells. The term costimulation, often applied to these ligands, is operationally defined as a ligand that enhances the proliferation of cells at suboptimal (nonstimulating) doses of antigen, or antibodies directed to the T-cell antigen receptor. No disease linkage has been found for OX-40, CD27, CD30, and 4-1BB or their ligands. *In vitro* studies have suggested that these molecules may be involved as costimulators for full activation of T cells, acting as cell survival factors rather than as bona fide growth factors.

Ox40 is expressed on activated CD8$^+$ and CD4$^+$ T cells and interacts with Ox40L, which is expressed on dendritic, B, T, endothelial, and microglial cells. This interaction is not required for immune system development, as mice deficient in Ox40 or Ox40L show normal thymus, spleen, and lymph node organogenesis and have normal development of T and B cells. The most pronounced defect in mice deficient in the Ox40–Ox40L interaction is that their CD4 T-cell cytokine production and proliferative responses to lymphocytic choriomengiitis virus (LCMV), in-

fluenza virus, and soluble antigens were reduced. The Ox40–Ox40L system is important in autoimmune T-cell responses. When this interaction is blocked, autoimmunity was ameliorated in both experimental autoimmune encephalitis and inflammatory bowel disease models. The Ox40–Ox40L interaction serves primarily to modulate CD4 T-cell responses and may mediate signals from T cells into antigen-presenting cells. CD27 and its ligand, CD27L (CD70), function as a costimulatory system for T-cell activation, and also in B-cell activation, NK effector activity, and early thymic differentiation. 4-1BB is expressed by CD8$^+$ and CD4$^+$ T cells after they have been activated by antigen and by NK cells. The receptor interacts with the 41BB ligand, which is expressed on dendritic cells, skin Langerhan cells, activated B cells, and macrophages. While no human disease has yet been associated with a deficiency in 41BB or 41BBL, individuals with rheumatoid arthritis have a soluble form of 41BB in their serum. The 41BB–41BBL interaction serves as an costimulatory molecule for CD8$^+$ T cells (and, in some cases, CD4 T cells) by increasing T-cell proliferation and cytokine production.

First identified as a surface antigen on Reed–Sternberg cells in Hodgkin's disease, CD30 has since been studied in a variety of lymphomas and myelomas where it can induce proliferation or apoptosis in a lymphoma-specific manner. Mice deficient for CD30 show elevated numbers of thymocytes attributed to impaired thymic negative selection; however, positive selection remains intact. Consistent with the CD30 *null* phenotype, transgenic mice expressing CD30 in the thymus show increased negative selection. CD30L is expressed on activated T cells, as well as other leukocytes (e.g., mature human B cells), but its physiologic role is unclear. Together, these data suggest an important role for CD30/CD30L as negative regulators of T lymphocyte development.

Glucocorticoid induced related to TNF receptors (GITR) appears to mediate survival signals in T cells in response to glucocorticoid hormones, which, depending on the state of differentiation, can induce apoptosis of thymocytes.

CD40 was originally characterized as a cell surface molecule expressed on B lymphocytes that was crucial for T-cell-dependent B-cell immunity. The CD40 ligand (CD154) is expressed on T helper lymphocytes, which play a major role in helping B cells produce antibody. The significance of CD40–CD40 ligand signaling *in vivo* is exemplified by a heritable genetic syndrome in humans, called X-linked hyper-IgM syndrome, that is associated with CD40-L mutations. Afflicted patients show defects in immunoglobulin heavy chain class switching, which leads to deficiencies in serum levels of IgA and IgG, but causes elevated IgM levels, and thus fails to provide protection from reinfection at mucosal surfaces. An additional role for CD40 lies in the regulation of autoimmunity. Levels of CD40-L are elevated in the serum and on circulating T cells of patients with lupus. Blocking antibodies to CD40L have proven to be beneficial in multiple models of autoimmunity. However, activated platelets express the CD40 ligand on their surface, which unfortunately interfered in the treatment of patients with lupus using antibodies to CD40 ligand because of coagulopathy.

APRIL and BAFF are related ligands that interact with at least two distinct receptors, TACI and BCMA, involved in signaling cell survival. APRIL was identified as a growth stimulator for tumors of lymphoid, colon, and thyroid origin. BCMA and TACI recognize another TNF family member, BAFF, a B lymphocyte-activating factor. BAFF is implicated as an essential cytokine sustaining B-cell survival and, when overexpressed, may play a significant role in lupus-like autoimmune nephritis observed in NZB/WF1 mice. A soluble decoy form of BCMA that antagonizes the activity of APRIL inhibits the growth of tumors, which naturally overexpress APRIL. Similarly, the progression of lupus-like nephritis in NZB/WF1 mice was blocked with TACI-Fc protein implicating targeting BAFF or APRIL may yield new approaches for the treatment of cancer and autoimmune diseases.

D. Development and Morphogenesis

Several members of the TNF family are involved in the development of various organs, including LTαβ–LTβR (lymphoid organogenesis) and NGFR (neurons). EDA is the cytokine responsible for X-linked hypohidrotic ectodermal dysplasia, a defect in the development of hair, eccrine sweat glands, and teeth. EDA binds to EDAR, a TNFR family member; however, a two amino acid splice variant gives rise to a second ligand EDA-A2 that binds a distinct receptor, XEDAR.

RANK (receptor activator of NF-κB) and its ligand, RANKL (TRANCE), regulate osteoclastogenesis and bone resorption. Mutations in RANK cause familial expansile osteolysis, a rare, autosomal-dominant bone disorder characterized by focal areas of increased bone remodeling. Osteoprotegerin (OPG) is a soluble decoy found in plasma that regulates the bioavaliability of RANKL, expressed on osteoblasts, that signals via RANK on hematopoietic osteoclast precursor cells. The interaction of RANK and RANKL induces differentiation and maturation of osteoclast precursor cells to active osteoclasts capable of resorbing bone.

The vascular endothelial cell growth inhibitor (VEGI) is expressed predominantly in endothelial cells and may function as a costimulatory signal for T cells. TWEAK was initially defined as a weak inducer of apoptosis in some tumor lines and interacts with Fn14, a fibroblast growth factor 1-inducible gene, which contains a single cysteine-rich domain. TWEAK induces proliferation in a variety of normal human endothelial cells and in aortic smooth muscle cells. TWEAK induces a strong angiogenic response in a rat cornea model, suggesting a role in vasculature formation *in vivo*.

VI. VIRAL TARGETING OF TNF SUPERFAMILY

Several specific genetic mechanisms are used by distinct virus families to modify the activities of various members of the TNF superfamily. Adenovirus was the first virus recognized to have specific genes blocking the action of TNF in addition to its other anti-immune response genes. The E3 region of adenovirus contains three genes involved in regulating TNF superfamily responses. E1B (19 kDa) blocks the apoptotic action of TNF and Fas and is probably needed to counteract the proapoptotic action of E1A. E1A is the transforming protein for this DNA virus that stimulates cellular DNA synthesis promoting virus genome replication, and consequently increasing sensitivity to apoptosis (in the absence of TNF). E1A will also convert a cell normally resistant to the cell death action of TNF into a susceptible line. E3-10.4/14.5 and 6.7 genes form a membrane complex that mediates internalization of the death receptors, Fas and TRAILR1 and 2, blocking their cytotoxic effect. Poxvirus, including the former scourge smallpox, has three genes that encode soluble forms of the TNFR, a category of virus proteins known as viroceptors. The T2 protein of Shope fibroma virus, most homologous to TNFR2, binds and neutralizes both TNF and LTα, acting as a virus–receptor antagonist and was the initial model for the making of TNF inhibitors, such as Enbrel. The virus-infected cell is thought to secrete this protein so that it can help block the host defense alarms set off by TNF, but it also protects T cells from apoptosis as an internal protein. Human herpesviruses target several members of the TNF superfamily. Human cytomegalovirus encodes a membrane protein at orf UL144 with significant homology to HVEM and TRAILR, whereas the envelope glycoprotein of the avian leukosis virus binds to CAR1, an ortholog of TRAIL receptor. The Herpes Simplex virus infects T cells via the envelope glycoprotein D interaction with HVEM, a TNFR family member that binds LIGHT and LTα. The Epstein–Barr virus induces B lymphocyte activation and usurps the action of TRADD and TRAFs via the action of its dominant oncogene, LMP-1. The C-terminal tail of LMP-1 binds to TRAFs and TRADD, which in B cells signals cell survival through CD40. Other herpesviruses encode cytosolic proteins that block the coupling of FADD to caspase 8, a function analogous to FLIPs and thus block apoptosis signaling. Together, these examples show that viruses target nearly every step in the TNF signaling pathway, from ligand binding to activation of signaling cascades.

VII. TNF AND CANCER

TNF and malignant diseases are intimately linked historically, economically, and biologically. Stimulation of TNF production, or injection of recombinant TNF, causes a rapid necrotizing collapse of established tumors (4 cm diameter) within 24–48 h in mice. Indeed, this profound effect of TNF was part of the promise that fueled investment capital for the biotechnology industry during the early 1980s. The antitumor effect of TNF is not due to direct cytotoxic function, but rather from profound changes in tumor vasculature due, in part, to the effect of TNF on endothelium. In humans, systemic TNF administration is highly toxic at the doses required to achieve tumor regression.

Despite the beneficial role of TNF in immune defenses, TNF has a dark side in malignant disease. TNF is a recognized contributor to cachexia, a wasting syndrome characterized by weight loss, anorexia, anemia, and increased catabolism of proteins and lipids. Perhaps the most obvious symptoms of cachexia are anorexia and weight loss. TNF has been shown to be a mediator of these symptoms in animals studies, which indicate that chronic production of TNF is important for inducing the wasting state. Catabolism of proteins in cachexia is noteworthy because it can result in decreased mobility, decreased respiratory function, and eventually death. TNF has been shown to increase the rate of proteolysis in skeletal muscle and liver, which increases the concentration of acute-phase protein levels in the blood. Studies have shown that administration of TNF directly to the central nervous system (particularly the hypothalamus) is responsible for inducing fever and anorexia. TNF causes acute anorexia apparently by direct action on the feeding center of the hypothalamus, resulting in a decreased responsiveness of glucose-sensitive neurons. Anorexia induced by the direct action of TNF on the hypothalamus causes death much earlier than administration of TNF at a peripheral site.

The TNF superfamily plays several important roles in innate and acquired protective immune responses, homeostasis, and development, but also contributes significantly to pathophysiologic processes, such as cachexia. Because of the role TNF may play in cachexia, it is a potential site of therapeutic intervention. Approaches being taken to avoid the downside of TNF include humanized monoclonal antibodies that neutralize TNF and soluble receptors. Soluble TNFR are chimeric proteins consisting of the extracellular, ligand-binding domain of TNFR fused with the Fc region of IgG and is a potent antagonist. These reagents have a major impact on the inflammatory processes in arthritis (Enbrel and Infliximab) and are being explored in the treatment of several other diseases where TNF is implicated.

It is clear that basic research on TNF-related ligands in malignant disease is moving into a new phase.

The first translation of basic research on TNF was limited to its use as a chemotherapeutic agent to kill tumors. With our current understanding of the breadth of the actions of TNF as a potent physiologic modulator, the challenge is to translate this new knowledge into effective treatments for cancer. No longer do we think of TNF as a single cytokine, but one of several that regulate fundamental physiologic and developmental processes.

See Also the Following Articles

CASPASES IN PROGRAMMED CELL DEATH • HEPATITIS C VIRUS • CYTOKINES • INTERLEUKINS • MACROPHAGES • P-GLYCOPROTEIN AS A GENERAL ANTI-APOPTOTIC PROTEIN • TGFβ SIGNALING MECHANISMS

Bibliography

Banner, D. W., D'Arcy, A., Janes, W., Gentz, R., Schoenfeld, H. J., Broger, C., Loetscher, H., and Lesslauer, W. (1993). Crystal structure of the soluble human 55 kd TNF receptor-human TNF beta complex: Implications for TNF receptor activation. *Cell* **73**, 431–445.

Barry, M., and McFadden, G. (1998). Apoptosis regulators from DNA viruses. *Curr. Opin. Immunol.* **10**, 422–430.

Eck, M. J., Ultsch, M., Rinderknecht, E., de Vos, A. M., and Sprang, S. R. (1992). The structure of human lymphotoxin at 1.9-A resolution. *J. Biol. Chem.* **267**, 2119–2122.

Fu, Y.-X., and Chaplin. D. (1999). Development and maturation of secondary lymphoid tissues. *Annu. Rev. Immunol.* **17**, 399–433.

Lockesley, R. M., Killeen, N., and Lenardo, M. J. (2001). The TNF and TNF receptor superfamilies: Integrating mammalian biology. *Cell* **104,** 487–501.

Park, Y. C., Burkitt, V., Villa, A. R., Tong, L., and Wu, H. (1999). Structural basis for self-association and receptor recognition of human TRAF2. *Nature* **398**, 533–538.

Schneider, P., and Tschopp, J. (2000). Apoptosis induced by death receptors. *J. Pharm. Acta. Helv.* **74**, 281–286.

Smith, C. A., Farrah, T., and Goodwin, R. G. (1994). The TNF receptor superfamily of cellular and viral proteins: Activation, costimulation, and death. *Cell* **76**, 959–962.

Wajant, H., and Scheurich, P. (2001). Tumor necrosis factor receptor-associated factor (TRAF) 2 and its role in TNF signaling. *Int. J. Biochem. Cell. Biol.* **33**, 19–32.

Wallach, D., Varfolomeev, E. E., Malinin, N. L., Goltsev, Y. V., Kovalenko, A. V., and Boldin, M. P. (1999). Tumor necrosis factor receptor and Fas signaling mechanisms. *Annu. Rev. Immunol.* **17**, 331–367.

Ware, C. F., Santee, S., and Glass, A. (1998). Tumor necrosis factor-related ligands and receptors. *In* "The Cytokine Handbook" (A. Thompson, ed.), p. 549–576. Academic Press, San Diego.

Ware, C. F., VanArsdale, T. L., Crowe, P. D., and Browning, J. L. (1995). Cytokines and receptors of the lymphotoxin system. *Curr. Top. Microbiol. Immunol.* **198**, 175–218.

Tumor Suppressor Genes: Specific Classes

George Klein
Karolinska Institutet, Stockholm, Sweden

GLOSSARY

ARF Alternatively spliced product of the INK4a locus. When triggered by E1A, myc, E2F, or other illegitimately activated oncogenes, it binds MDM2. This leads to a rise of the p53 level, causing growth arrest and/or apoptosis.

carcinoma Malignant tumor of epithelial or other ectodermal origin.

immune rejection Cell-mediated immune response against tumor cells directed against tumor antigens. Virus-induced tumors provide the clearest examples.

leukemia Malignant proliferation of hemopoetic cells with an abnormally high cell count in the blood.

microarray Molecular technology that permits the simultaneous measurement of gene expression at a large number of loci.

sarcoma Malignant tumor of mesenchymal origin.

The term "tumor suppressor gene" is based on the idea that the expression of certain genes can antagonize the proliferative drive of illegitimately activated cells. "Illegitimate activation," e.g., by constitutively expressed or mutated oncogenes, generates an incessant drive toward a succession of S phases, and at least a relative resistance to normal regulatory controls. This creates potentially malignant cells that cannot express their tumorigenic potential, as a rule, unless antagonistic suppressor genes are inactivated at the structural or functional level. Suppressor genes thus contribute to tumor development and/or progression by their loss or permanent downregulation. This article presents the major classes of tumor suppressor genes that have been identified.

I. INTRODUCTION

The mutational basis of tumor development has been recognized already before the term "mutation" came into use. In 1909, Paul Ehrlich spoke about "aberrations" that may be expected to arise during fetal and postfetal development with an "extraordinary frequency." If most of them would not be checked by the defenses of the organism, many more tumors would develop. This statement is often quoted as the first formulation of the immune surveillance theory. In the light of our present knowledge, DNA repair appears as the first line of defense, however. Immune surveillance is mainly responsible for preventing the proliferation of virally transformed cells.

II. DNA REPAIR GENES

Impairment of DNA-correcting host mechanisms is often associated with a high tumor incidence. Xeroderma pigmentosum (XP) is the oldest known example. It is due to the deficiency of a single enzyme system that is normally responsible for the excision of thymidine dimers from UV-damaged DNA in epithelial cells. Exposure of XP patients to light leads to the appearance of hundreds of skin tumors.

Mutation or deletion of mismatch repair genes, such as MSH2 on human chromosome 2p or of the functionally similar MLH1 gene on chromosome 3p, leads to specific multicancer syndromes. Genomic instability at simple repeated sequences (SRS) may reflect up to thousandfold increases in mutation rates. It can be associated with both hereditary and sporadic cancers. Germline mutation of p53 is responsible for the Li–Fraumeni multicancer syndrome. Its experimental counterpart, the p53 knockout mouse, is also highly tumor prone. This can be seen in relation to the role of p53 as the "guardian of the genome" (see Section VII.B). DNA damage induces the stabilization of the normally short-lived p53. The protein binds to DNA and arrests the cell cycle in G_1. If the DNA is repaired during this arrest, the p53 level falls and the cell reenters the cycle. If the damage is too extensive, it dies by apoptosis. The p53 mutants found in many different tumors and in Li–Fraumeni patients do not bind to DNA and cannot induce growth ar-

rest. Spontaneous and induced mutations may remain uncorrected in the absence of normal p53. This permits the emergence of many new variants, including both preneoplastic and frankly neoplastic cells.

Other familial cancer syndromes caused by defects in DNA repair include ataxia-telangiectasia, Bloom's syndrome, and Fanconi's anemia. The breast cancer predisposing BRCA 1 and BRCA 2 mutations (see Section VII.D) are also believed to act at the level of DNA repair and the maintenance of genome integrity. Chromosomal and DNA changes are more frequent in tumors from BRCA1 and BRCA2 mutation carriers than in sporadic breast carcinomas. Germline mutation carriers show an increased tendency to develop ovarian, colonic, prostatic, and endometrial cancer as well.

These examples show that the impairment of normal DNA repair mechanisms can increase the risk of tumor development, sometimes dramatically. The important role of DNA repair enzymes in decreasing tumor development qualifies them as a separate class of tumor suppressor genes.

III. IMMUNE RESPONSE AND RELATED GENES

Ehrlich was thus right in principle but he or his later interpreters have overemphasized the role of immune defenses in preventing tumor development. They do have a role but it is largely restricted to the inhibition of virally transformed, potentially neoplastic cells. Congenital, infectious, and iatrogenic immunodeficiency may permit the growth of virus-induced or virus-associated tumors that would have been rejected in immunocompetent hosts. Horizontally transmitted DNA tumor viruses are particularly prominent in this context. The tumors that appear in immunodefectives are often referred to as "opportunistic," in analogy with opportunistic infections in immunodefectives. Three main categories have been noted in humans: EBV-carrying lymphomas, HPV-carrying papillomas and carcinomas, and Kaposi sarcoma, which is most probably due to HHV-8, also called KSHV.

Tumors of these categories express virally coded, transformation-associated, and potentially immunogenic proteins. Their recognition is dependent on the presence of appropriate MHC class I molecules in the host. Species that coexist with potentially tumorigenic, ubiquitous viruses are preselected for reactive MHC alleles. Pathogenicity is largely or entirely restricted to immunologically naive host species.

Genes responsible for the resistance of the natural host species against the proliferation of virally transformed cells may be regarded as an important special category of tumor suppressors.

There is no evidence that the incidence of nonviral tumors increases in immunodefective hosts. Both T- and non-T-cell effectors may protect the host against the outgrowth of disseminated tumor cells, however. It is also possible that contactual signals between normal and tumor cells and/or the interactions between tumor cells and inhibitory (or, the lack of stimulatory) cytokines play a role in protection of the host against the outgrowth of disseminated cells. Tumor cells may be also inhibited by contactual control from adjacent normal cells, probably through tight junctions or integrin-dependent signal transmission between cells.

IV. DIFFERENTIATION CONTROLLING GENES

Another important but largely unexplored area relates to the control of differentiation. Experiments with temperature-sensitive (ts) oncogene mutants have pointed the way. Cells of different lineages were transformed with ts mutants of v-*src* and v-*erbB*, respectively. At the permissive temperature, the transformed cells grew and failed to differentiate. Short-term incubation at the nonpermissive temperature triggered the irreversible differentiation of the originally undifferentiated myoblasts, chondroblasts, melanoblasts, and erythoblasts, respectively. These experiments showed that the growth of undifferentiated tumor cells was associated with, and perhaps due to, a differentiation block imposed by the oncogene. This block has prevented the transformed cells from maturing into terminally differentiated resting cells, as directed by their normal program. The mechanism of the block is not known, but it may be surmised that the activated oncogene drives the cell to divide by emitting constitutive "go signals" that prevent it from leaving the cycling compartment. Deregulated signals

of this type may originate from a defective receptor, a hyperactive kinase, a mutated signal transducer protein, or an illegitimately activated transcription factor. Experiments with the ts mutants have shown that even a temporary interruption of the deregulated signal may open the way toward the resumption of the original differentiation program. The process is irreversible, once it has started, and cannot be halted by the full reexpression of the oncogene at the permissive temperature. These experiments have also confirmed that activated oncogenes cannot drive cell division forward unless they are expressed in a specific window of differentiation. If the "oncogenic window" can be shifted, normal differentiation and associated growth arrest may follow.

Differentiation controlling genes can thus act as tumor suppressors. The balance between proliferation stimulating and differentiation inducing signals is decisive for the outcome in many other potentially or frankly neoplastic systems that are driven by unknown genes. Seemingly irreversible malignancies may be "tipped over" from a proliferating to a differentiating mode, after having received appropriate signals.

V. SUPPRESSION OF TUMORIGENICITY BY SOMATIC HYBRIDIZATION OF TUMOR WITH NORMAL CELLS

Cell fusion experiments have provided early information on tumor suppression. When normal and tumorigenic cells were fused in many different combinations, the resulting hybrids were nontumorigenic or only low tumorigenic, as a rule, provided that they have maintained a complete or nearly complete chromosome complement from both parents. Reappearance of tumorigenicity was associated with the loss of chromosomes from the normal parent. High malignant segregants were shown to lack specific chromosome pairs. In some combinations, suppression could be attributed to the imposition of a normal differentiation pathway by the normal parent cell on its malignant partner. Hybrids derived from the fusion of HeLa cells with normal keratinocytes are a case in point. The hybrid cells resembled the malignant parent *in vitro* and were still immortal, but nontumorigenic in immunodefective mice. In contrast to the progressively growing HeLa cells that showed no signs of maturation, the hybrids differentiated into squamous pearls *in vivo* and stopped growing.

Compelling as this and similar examples are, they cannot explain all cases of suppressed tumorigenicity. The hybrid cells may lack or not show any detectable morphological changes compared to the malignant parent and grow well *in vitro* but not *in vivo*. Genes responsible for this effect and their mechanism of action remain to be explored.

VI. REVERTANTS

Still another system of tumor suppression has been identified through the isolation and characterization of phenotypic revertants from cultures of transformed cells. They cannot be detected under ordinary culture conditions but are readily isolated if provided with a selective advantage, e.g., by turning cellular DNA synthesis in confluent cultures into a suicidal process. Photosensitizing cycling cells with bromodeoxyuridine or allowing them to incorporate highly radioactive thymidine are some of the methods that can provide revertants that have left the cycling compartment with a powerful selective advantage. Revertants may be also selected on the basis of their higher resistance to ouabain and other toxins. Both virally and chemically transformed cultures yielded revertants regularly by one of these approaches.

In a specific example, revertants isolated from fibroblast cultures transformed by the virally transduced Ki-*ras* gene still carried the transforming oncogene. Most of them were of the "postoncogene" type. They expressed the original transforming oncogene at a high level. It could be reisolated by helper rescue and had unchanged transforming activity. The revertants were resistant against retransformation attempts by activated ras and also by some other oncogenes. Different revertant phenotypes could be distinguished on the basis of their retransformability by a selected oncogene spectrum.

Several genes have been identified that can induce reversion when overexpressed in *ras*-transformed cells. K-rev-1 is a *ras*-related gene that shares an effector domain with transforming *ras*. It acts as a competitive antagonist. Another suppressor, *rsp-1*, may interact with ras-regulated proteins. Similar antagonists have been detected in relation to other oncogenes. Normal c-*erbA* can antagonize the transforming effect of the v-*erbA* oncogene. Transforming c-*src* mutants can be antagonized by nontransforming double mutants.

VII. MAJOR SUPPRESSOR GENES

Identification of the presently known major suppressor genes has started with two genes, RB and p53, that are still in the forefront of interest. Because they are covered in other articles, this article focuses only on some conceptual aspects. This is followed by a brief consideration of other suppressor genes.

A. RB

Discovery of the retinoblastoma gene stems from the serendipitous prediction of Alfred Knudson, based on the statistical analysis of age incidence curves of familial compared to sporadic retinoblastoma. Knudson's postulate that retinoblastoma arises when both alleles of the same gene are lost was fully confirmed by both genetic and molecular analysis. The analysis of the retinoblastoma system and the confirmation of Knudson's hypothesis were based on a comparison of normal and tumor cells from the same donor, with regard to the presence of heterozygous markers within the chromosomal region of interest. Consistent loss of a marker from the tumor (loss of heterozygosis, LOH) was taken to indicate the presence of a nearby suppressor gene.

Following cloning of the RB gene it was found that the protein (pRb) plays a crucial relay function in mediating cellular signal proliferation controlling signals to the nuclear transcription machinery. Cyclin-dependent G_1 kinases interact in mediating pRb phosphorylation, which leads to the release of the E2F transcription factor. E2F is actually a family of at least six related proteins that regulate the expression of several genes that play an important role for cell cycle progression. E2F overexpression induces quiescent cells to enter the S phase. This activity can be inhibited by either unphosphorylated pRb or its relatives, p107 and p130.

pRb phosphorylation and cell cycle progression require the activity of cyclin D-CDK4, which is, in turn, specifically inhibited by the p16 product of the INK4A cyclin-dependent kinase inhibitor (CKI) locus. p16 is also a tumor suppressor gene (see Section VII.C).

B. p53

p53 is the most frequently mutated gene in human tumors. Normal p53 has been called "the guardian of the genome." p53-induced growth arrest in cells with damaged DNA gives them time to repair their DNA or, if the damage has been too extensive, to exit by apoptosis, as already mentioned in Section II. In view of what has been said there, p53 may now be considered as one of several guardians of the genome, although a very important one. Most tumor-associated mutations occur in highly conserved regions. Mutated p53 is constitutively expressed at a high level, but it cannot bind to DNA and cannot arrest growth.

p53 mutations may contribute to tumor development in several ways. Certain dominant-negative mutants can drive cell proliferation, like oncogenes. Normal wild-type p53 qualifies as a tumor suppressor gene because its functional inactivation that sets growth-arresting downstream effectors (e.g., p21/WAF1) out of function can contribute to tumor development and/or progression. Wild-type p53 can also directly suppress malignant growth when expressed in tumor cells that contain mutant p53. As already mentioned in Section II, the inactivation of p53-dependent apoptosis causes genetic instability as also shown by the Li–Fraumeni syndrome that is due to germline p53 mutation. It is particularly noteworthy that apoptotic death induced by radiation or cytotoxic drugs requires p53. Loss of functional p53 may thus even contribute to therapy resistance.

p53 null mice develop multiple tumors at a young age. All die with tumors within 10 months. Thymic T-cell lymphomas are most frequent. B-cell lymphomas, soft tissue sarcomas, osteosarcomas, and testicular teratomas arise as well. In heterozygotes the tumors appear later, and both osteosarcomas and soft tissue sarcomas are more common than lymphomas. Some carcinomas appear as well. There is considerable similarity with the human Li–Fraumeni syndrome.

C. INK 4a and Related Loci

One product of this complex locus, p16, has been identified as a cell cycle inhibitor that is often homozygously deleted in melanoma, bladder, breast, kidney, and ovarian carcinoma and derived cell lines. The gene encoding p16 has been first designated MTS1 (multiple tumor suppressor 1). It is the first intrinsic component of the cell cycle machinery identified as a tumor suppressor. p16 binds to and inhibits CDK4, a kinase that complexes with the D group of cyclins. The complex is an effector of Rb phosphorylation and, consequently, cell cycle progression. p16 competes with the D cyclins.

Four other regulators, p15, p21, p24, and p27, can bind to and inhibit G_1/S cyclin–CDK complexes. They regulate the order of CDK activation during progression through G_1 (more about this in the next section). p15, also called MTS-2, has also been identified as a tumor suppressor gene. It is induced by TGF-β. Similar to p16, it binds to CDK4 and also to CDK6. It is more widely expressed in normal tissues than p16.

Changes of p16 and/or p15 were observed not only in cell lines but also in tumors, nonsmall cell lung carcinomas in particular. This predominant restriction to one histological subtype of lung carcinomas is intriguing. p15 and p16 are often homozygously deleted in glioblastoma multiforme, but not in medulloblastomas or ependymomas. Surprisingly, intragenic mutations are rare. This was taken to suggest that deletion is a more efficient mechanism for the simultaneous inactivation of both genes.

Homozygous deletions of both p15 and p16 have also been found in adult T-cell leukemia (ATL). Altogether, 27% of the examined ATL cases had lost the p15 and/or p16 gene. No point mutations were found in this system either. Germline p16 mutations have been detected in 9p21-linked familial melanoma.

p16 and, less frequently, p15 can be inactivated by DNA methylation as an alternative to deletion. Hypermethylation accounts particularly often for the loss of the cyclin D/Rb pathway in tumor cells with wild-type Rb.

An alternatively spliced product of the INK4a gene, p19ARF is an important upstream regulator of the p53-dependent growth arrest and apoptotic pathway. It also functions as a sensor for illegitimately activated oncogenes, such as c-myc, E2F, and E1A. They induce p19ARF-dependent degradation of MDM2. This leads to the stabilization of p53 with growth arrest and/or apoptosis as a consequence. There is thus a direct link between oncogene activation and tumor suppression, emphasizing the need for suppressor mutations in oncogenesis even further. It also illustrates how the same result may be attained through alternative pathways. ARF and p53 mutations can have the same effect, as also confirmed experimentally by the closely similar tumor spectra in p53 and in INK4a knockout mice.

D. Other CDK Inhibitors and the Choice between Growth Arrest and Apoptosis

Activation of other CDK inhibitors, such as p21 WAF1/CIP1, e.g., by p53, can inhibit the cell cycle and thereby block the final steps of growth stimulatory pathways. This leads to Rb dephosphorylation, E2F inactivation, and abrogation of c-myc-induced cell proliferation. The same oncogenes (including myc), growth factors, and other mitogenic stimuli can induce a proliferative (e.g., cyclin) signal and an antiproliferative (e.g., p21) signal. Because both processes may occur in the same cell, p21 induction must be eliminated to obtain a mitogenic response. Oncogenes may also upregulate p16, which also leads to growth arrest. p16 and ARF are usually induced in parallel. Loss of p53 or ARF may, however, uncouple the downstream proliferative signal from the apoptotic component.

The choice between p53-dependent growth arrest and an apoptotic program can be influenced by the extent of the DNA damage, levels of p53, cell type, cytokine, or growth factor concentrations. The cell cycle-arresting function of p53 is mediated largely by its effect on the transcription of an extensive array of growth regulatory genes.

Cells from p53 null mice are refractory to radiation-induced apoptosis. In crosses between oncogene (e.g., SV40-LT) transgenics and p53 null mice, tumor development is greatly accelerated. Basically similar results have been obtained with crosses between mammary tumor-prone Wnt-1 transgenic and p53-deficient mice and in crosses between c-ras transgenics and p53 null mice.

The balance between cell transformation and apoptosis is thus of decisive importance for the fate of the cell. Shifting the balance toward apoptosis may lead to tumor suppression. Within this dynamic system, activated oncogenes like myc may act as suppressor genes, not due to any change in expression or function, but because the cellular phenotype favors an apoptotic response.

E. APC, MCC, and DCC

Familial adenomatous polyposis (FAP) is a dominantly inherited colorectal cancer susceptibility disease caused by mutation of the APC gene, located on chromosome 5q21. Patients develop hundreds of colon polyps, some of which may progress to carcinoma. APC mutations occur also frequently in sporadic colon carcinomas.

The APC gene is large and complex. Its product is localized in the cytoskeleton and is suspected to have a signaling and/or adhesion function. Kinzler and Vogelstein have suggested that APC acts as a "gatekeeper" of colonic epithelial cell proliferation. Its loss may impair cell adhesion and other contactual interactions and promote proliferation. More than 100 different germline or somatic APC mutations have been described. Most of them result in the production of C-terminally truncated proteins.

Another 5q21-localized gene, designated MCC and located 180 kb from APC, is not mutated in the germline but can undergo somatic mutation in FAP and in colon cancer. It is also mutated in other cancers of the gastrointestinal tract, ovary, breast, lung, and prostate.

A third gene, DCC, localized on chromosome 18 is involved in the progression of colorectal adenomas to carcinoma and in the progression of nonsmall cell lung cancer. It encodes a cell adhesion molecule. Full-length DCC can suppress the tumorigenicity of carcinoma cells with a reduced DCC expression.

APC and DCC mutations (see later) may also contribute to the progression of nonsmall cell lung cancer and to the development of oral squamous cell carcinoma.

F. NF1 and NF-2

Several known or putative tumor suppressor genes are localized on the long arm of chromosome 17. NF-1, at 17q11.2, is a very large gene composed of 59 exons.

NF-2 is on chromosome 22. Germline mutations in one NF-1 allele, accompanied by the somatic loss or inactivation of the second allele, leads to neurofibromatosis. Malignant peripheral nerve sheath tumors show additional gene losses on 17p and 22q.

Loss of NF-2 can be related to neurofibromatosis type 2, with schwannomas of the eighth cranial nerve and other central nervous system tumors. The gene is homologous to a superfamily of membrane-organizing proteins.

G. BRCA1 and BRCA2

Mutations of either one of these two genes are associated with the majority of inherited breast cancer syndromes. BRCA1 is mutated in hereditary breast and ovarian cancer families and in sporadic ovarian tumors but not in sporadic breast carcinomas. About 40% of sporadic breast cancers and a similar proportion of ovarian cancers have allelic deletions at 17q where BRCA1 is also localized, but without somatic mutations in BRCA1. This indicates that an additional tumor suppressor gene may be localized nearby.

Superficially at least, this is reminiscent of the fact that APC and MCC, p16 and p15, and several putative suppressor genes on chromosome 3p are clustered as well. Moreover, the behavior of BRCA1 is reminiscent of the WTI tumor suppressor gene in Wilms' tumor, as the latter is mutated in most familial Wilms' tumors, but rarely in sporadic cases.

BRCA1 mutations are found in most families with multiple cases of both early onset breast and ovarian cancer and in about 45% of families with breast cancer only, but few if any families with both male and female breast cancer. Analyses of high-risk breast cancer families that were unlinked to BRCA1 have led to the localization of a second breast cancer susceptibility locus, BRCA2, to chromosome 13q12-13. BRCA2 confers a high risk for breast cancer but, in contrast to BRCA1, it does not increase the risk of ovarian cancer. In families where the risk of breast cancer is linked to BRCA2, the region of the latter is subject to LOH in the tumors, as a rule. The loss affects the wild-type allele that does not segregate with the disease in the family. These findings are consistent with the idea that both alleles of BRCA2 are inactivated in the tumors.

Taken together, mutations of the two genes, BRCA1 and BRCA2, are believed to contribute to approximately 80% of familial breast cancer cases, in equal proportions.

The mechanism of BRCA1 and BRCA2 action is far from clear, but there are strong indications that they participate together in pathways associated with the activation of double strand break repair and/or homologous recombination. Cells with mutated BRCA1 or BRCA2 are hypersensitive to ionizing radiation and are defective in DNA repair.

H. Other Tumor Suppressor Genes

WT1, an antagonist of a transcription factor, is involved in Wilms' tumor. VHL, an antagonist of elongin A and a potential mediator of RNA processing, is responsible for the von Hippel–Lindau syndrome. PTC, also called NBCS1, is involved in Gorlin syndrome; MEN 1 in multiple endocrine neoplasia type I; MEN 2, also called RET, a receptor tyrosine kinase, in multiple endocrine neoplasia type 2; and PTEN, also called MMAC1, in breast, brain, and prostate cancer. It encodes a dual specificity phosphatase. DPC4, a participant in TGF-β signaling, is biallelically inactivated in about 50% of all pancreatic cancers, but rarely in other human tumors.

The cell–cell adhesion protein E-cadherin is a candidate tumor suppressor gene in gastric, breast, endometrial, and ovarian cancer, whereas the cytoskeletal linker protein α-catenin is similarly implicated in prostate and lung cancer.

VIII. MULTISTEP SCENARIOS IN TUMOR DEVELOPMENT

Some of the major human carcinomas develop through a well-established series of changes. Colorectal tumors progress from hyperplasia, through different stages of adenomas, to malignant cancers. Two familial forms, hereditary nonpolyposis colon cancer (HNPCC) and familial adenomatous polyposis are initiated by germline mutations in mismatch repair genes in the former and the APC gene in the latter. Development of the hereditary forms is associated with the inactivation of the second allele and a series of sequential changes during somatic development. The latter are also found in the sporadic form. They include activation of Ki-ras or N-ras, inactivation of both copies of p53, and loss of a gene on chromosome 18 that is identical with or closely linked to DCC. Later stages of progression are associated with extensive aneuploidy, particularly in FAP and less in HNPCC-based tumors. The changes do not occur in the same order in different tumors, confirming the notion of alternative pathways.

About 15–20% of breast cancers have a family history. About 5% can be attributed to the dominant susceptibility genes BRCA1 and BRCA2. The development and biology of sporadic breast cancers are very diverse, indicating the existence of different progressional pathways. A gamut of growth factors and receptors (e.g., EGFR, HER-2/neu), signaling molecules (ras, src), and other intracellular growth regulators (e.g., myc, cyclin D) can be activated. Tumor suppressor genes (e.g., p53, RB1) and adhesion molecules (e.g., cadherin) may be set out of function. Many as yet unidentified genes may be involved in addition, as indicated by the numerous LOHs. Amplification of HER-2/neu is a bad prognostic sign. The protein product of the amplified gene can be used as a therapeutic target, however.

Prostatic carcinoma provides a similarly diverse panorama. In addition to the mutations of ras, p53, Rb, INK4b, and other known oncogenes and suppressor genes, cadherin downregulation and LOHs affecting chromosomes 5, 6, 8, 10, and 16 are often found as well. No single gene or chromosome region is affected in all prostatic carcinomas. Progression from hormone dependence to independence is often associated with the amplification of the androgen receptor gene on the X chromosome.

Lung carcinoma in heavy smokers is often a multifocal disease. Deletions affecting the short arm of chromosome 3 are found already at the hyperplastic or dysplastic precursor stage. Subsequent progression may feature 5q deletions, K-ras mutations, p16, FHIT, p53, and RB mutations. The deletions and rearrangements on chromosome 3 may become more extensive, probably affecting several genes within a cluster. During late stages of SCLC progression, amplification of myc family genes (c-, N-, or L-myc) is a bad prognostic sign.

Astrocytic tumors show an increasing number of changes with ascending grade. The least agressive forms show loss of wild-type p53 and a number of LOHs. Glioblastoma, the most malignant form, has a large number of genetic abnormalities. They include losses from chromosomes 6, 10, 13, and Y, gains on chromosomes 7 and 19, and structural abnormalities of chromosomes 1 and 9. Frequent double minutes indicate gene amplification. Homozygous deletions on 9p, affecting INK4a and INK4b (p15/16 and p19 ARF) loci, are found in 40–50% of cases. The inactivation of p15/16 deranges RB-dependent cell cycle control, whereas deletion of the alternatively spliced p19 product of the same gene cripples the p53-dependent apoptotic pathway.

Homozygous deletions of the p15-16-19 cluster are found in tumors that show no abnormalities of INK4, RB, MDM2, or p53 and vice versa. This illustrates the alternative modes of inactivating cell cycle regulating and apoptosis controlling genetic systems. This can be further exemplified by the fact that 90% of the glioblastomas have either no wild-type p16/p15 or no-wild type RB, or overexpress CDK4. In 75% of the glioblastomas, the apoptotic pathway is either inactivated by the lack of wild-type p53 or the inactivation of p19 ARF, or by overexpression of MDM2. Tumors with amplified MDM2 have two wild-type p53 alleles. These examples illustrate that different genetic aberrations may target different members of the same cellular control pathway and create similar phenotypes. Additional changes in glioblastomas include EGFR amplification and overexpression (35%) and allelic loss from chromosome 10 (90%), probably acting through the inactivation of PTEN/MMAC1 (>40%).

The hereditary form of renal carcinoma is often initiated by a mutation in the VHL gene at 3p26. The VHL gene is also frequently mutated in sporadic clear cell RCC. A cluster of as yet unidentified genes at 3p21.3 are frequently deleted during tumor progression in both the hereditary and the sporadic form. When an intact human chromosome 3 is introduced into mouse tumor cells and the monochromosomal hybrids are grown in immunodefective mice, a corresponding region, designated as CER1 (commonly eliminated region 1), is regularly eliminated, indicating the presence of one or several tumor-antagonizing genes. In contrast, a gene cluster at the telomeric end of the long arm (3q) is frequently retained. Hereditary papillary renal cell carcinoma (HPRC) shows no association with chromosome 3 losses or VHL mutations.

In skin cancer, allelic losses in basal cell carcinomas are almost entirely confined to the Gorlin locus at 9q. Squamous cell carcinomas show allelic losses in 25–30%, affecting chromosomes 3, 9, 13, and 17.

Pancreatic carcinoma shows a distinct mutation profile. K-ras is activated in 90% of the tumors by point mutations in codon 12. Among the suppressor genes, p16, p53, and DPC4 are frequently inactivated, RB1 less frequently. DPC4 is biallelically inactivated in almost 50% of all pancreatic cancers, but is only rarely affected in other tumors.

In endometrial cancer, microsatellite instability, K-ras, PTEN, and p53 mutations are most common. p53 overexpression is correlated with poor prognosis.

In carcinoma of the uterine cervix, the HPV-encoded transforming proteins E6 and E7 play an important early role. This is at least partly due to their inactivating effect on p53 and RB, respectively. This promotes genetic instability, counteracts apoptosis, and abolishes part of the cell cycle regulatory controls. In addition, amplification of myc and HER2neu, as well as loss of genes from chromosomes 1, 3, 5, and 11, may play an important role. 3p losses are particularly interesting because the same regions are deleted in renal, lung, and nasopharyngeal carcinomas.

In bladder cancer, chromosome losses are frequent. Monosomy of chromosome 9 is the most common abnormality. In addition, deletions are common on 9p, 17p, and 13q. p53 and RB mutations are correlated with poor prognosis. Multiple primary tumors may be generated by the spread and further progression of a single progenitor clone.

Hepatocellular carcinoma is often initiated by hepatitis B (HBV) or C type (HCV) infection. The virally encoded transactivator HBV-X is believed to induce the overexpression of several oncogenes. Sequential changes include p53 losses.

Hemopoetic tumors are often initiated by chromosomal translocation, leading to gene fusion (in CML and a wide variety of childhood leukemias) or juxtaposition of an oncogene to an Ig locus (B-cell lymphomas) or to a TCR locus (T-ALL). Sequential events affect mainly the apoptosis-regulating systems, with upregulation of bcl-2 or inactivation of p53, p19, ARF, or BAX. In T-ALL, p16 may remain unaffected, whereas ARF is disrupted or deleted. In the absence of ARF, p53 usually remains in wild-type configuration. A similar alternative mutational relationship has been found between p16 and RB as in other tumors.

See Also the Following Articles

APC • CELLULAR RESPONSES TO DNA DAMAGE • MISMATCH REPAIR: BIOCHEMISTRY AND GENETICS • NM23 METASTASIS SUPPRESSOR GENE • P16 AND ARF • PTEN • RETINOBLASTOMA TUMOR SUPPRESSOR GENE • TP53 TUMOR SUPPRESSOR GENE • VON HIPPEL–LINDAU DISEASE • WILMS TUMOR SUPPRESSOR WT1

Bibliography

Behrens, J. (1999). Cadherins and catenins: Role in signal transduction and tumor progression. *Cancer Metas. Rev.* **181,** 15–30.

Bishop, J. M. (1991). Molecular themes in oncogenesis. *Cell* **64,** 235–248.

Bodmer, W., Bishop, T., and Karran, P. (1994). Genetic steps in colorectal cancer. *Nature Genet.* **6,** 217–219.

Collins, V. P. (1998). Oncogenesis and progression in human gliomas. *In* "Brain Tumor Invasion" (T. Mikkelsen, ed.), pp. 71–86, Wiley-Liss, New York.

el-Deiry, W. S. (1998). Regulation of p53 downstream genes. *Semin. Cancer Biol.* **8,** 345–357.

Fearon, E. R., and Vogelstein, B. (1990). A genetic model for colorectal tumorigenesis. *Cell* **61,** 759–767.

Hanahan, D., and Weinberg, R A. (2000). The hallmarks of cancer. *Cell* **100,** 57–70.

Imreh, S. (1999). Genomic alterations in solid tumors. *Semin. Cancer Biol.* **9,** 241–325.

Imreh, S., Szekely, L., Wiman, K. G., and Klein, G. (1997). Oncogenes and tumour suppressor genes. *In* "Mechanisms of Oncogene Perturbation" (G. Peters, and K. Vousden, eds.), pp. 4–31. Oxford Univ. Press, Oxford.

Ingvarsson, S. (1999). Molecular genetics of breast cancer progression. *Semin. Cancer Biol.* **9,** 277–288.

Klein, G. (1997). Foulds' dangerous idea revisited: The multistep development of tumors 40 years later. *Adv. Cancer Res.* **72,** 2–23.

Klein, G., and Klein, E. (1985). Evolution of tumors and the impact of molecular oncology. *Nature* **315,** 190–195.

Mulligan, G., and Jacks, T. (1998). The retinoblastoma gene family: Cousins with overlapping interests. *Trends Genet.* **14,** 223–229.

Ried, T., Heselmeyer-Haddad, K., Blegen, H., Schrock, E., and Auer, G. (1999). Genomic changes defining the genesis, progression, and malignancy potential in solid human tumors: A phenotype/genotype correlation. *Genes Chromosomes Cancer* **25,** 195–204.

Selivanova, G., and Wiman, K. G. (1995). p53: A cell cycle regulator activated by DNA damage. *Adv. Cancer Res.* **66,** 143–180.

Whyte, P., Buchkovich, K. J., Horowitz, J. M., Friend, S. H., Raybuck, M., Weinberg, R. A., and Harlow, E. Association between an oncogene and an anti-oncogene: The adenovirus E1A proteins bind to the retinoblastoma gene product. *Nature* **334,** 124–129.

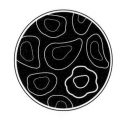

Vascular Targeting

Renata Pasqualini
Wadih Arap
The University of Texas M. D. Anderson Cancer Center

GLOSSARY

angiogenesis Formation of new blood vessels from established blood vessels.

biopanning Screening of a phage display peptide library on a target(s).

endothelial cells The main cell type forming the endothelium.

endothelium The layer of cells lining blood vessels.

phage random peptide library A large, random collection of peptides displayed as recombinant proteins on the surface of bacteriophage.

vascular map A ligand–receptor-based molecular map of blood vessels.

vascular targeting Targeting receptors in blood vessels with ligands derived from phage display screenings.

This article reviews several phage display targeting strategies (Fig. 1) that may enable the construction of a molecular map outlining vascular diversity in each organ, tissue, or pathological condition.

I. INTRODUCTION

Despite major progress brought about by the Human Genome Project, the molecular diversity of human blood vessels remains largely unexplored. Our research is aimed at targeting diagnostic and therapeutic agents to blood vessels by using probes that can bind to specific vascular addresses. Toward this goal, we have developed technologies to identify small peptides that

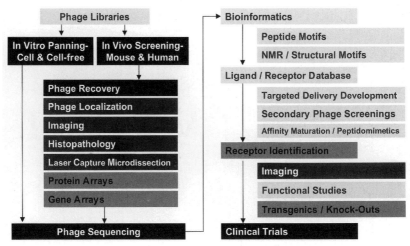

FIGURE 1 Vascular mapping outline. Strategies for targeting blood vessels are shown. They include phage display screenings on immobilized receptors (cell-free), on isolated cells, on animal models, and even in patients. Once the ligands are selected and validated, the corresponding receptor(s) can be found by biochemical or genetic methods. Ligands can serve as carriers for various diagnostic and therapeutic moieties. Imaging methods for blood vessels, analytical techniques, vascular receptor identification, and databases of ligand–receptor pairs must follow for vascular mapping to be ultimately validated in translational clinical trials that use this targeting concept. Shadings represent partners with expertise in different areas of such as cancer biology, molecular anatomy, chemistry, structural biology, and medical oncology.

target the endothelium. Different strategies are used to isolate peptides from large libraries displayed in the surface of bacteriophage.

Through this platform technology, we have uncovered various tissue-specific and angiogenesis-related vascular addresses. This complex system of ligand–receptor pairs will lead to a better understanding of tumor circulatory microenvironment, changes in blood vessels during tumor progression, and the localization of novel markers in cancer and other diseases with an angiogenesis component.

II. *IN VITRO* TARGETING

A. Cell-Free Screening on Isolated Receptors

Phage display involves genetically manipulating bacteriophage so that peptides or antibodies can be expressed on their surface (Fig. 2). Considerable progress has been made in the construction of phage display random peptide libraries and in screening methods. Ligands can be selected and isolated by "biopanning," a process in which phages that bind to a target molecule

are eluted and amplified in a host bacteria. Phage display random peptide libraries were designed to define binding sites of antibodies in isolated immunoglobulins. Later, many ligands for isolated receptors (including cell adhesion molecules, proteases, cell cycle regulators, viruses, oncoproteins, and tumor suppressor proteins, among others) were found by this technology.

This section presents a collection of the original phage display application as an example of a cell-free panning on isolated targets (e.g., immunoglobulins) with phage display peptide libraries (Fig. 3). Cancer patients can mount a humoral immune response (i.e., make antibodies) against vascular receptors that are also found in or presented by the nonmalignant cells of tumor blood vessels. Thus, panning on the pool of tumor-associated antibodies may lead to the discovery of new molecular addresses. In addition, targeting tumor antigens may lead to improved vaccines against tumors.

B. Screening the Molecular Diversity of Cell Surfaces

Probing the molecular diversity of cell surfaces is required for the development of targeted therapies. First,

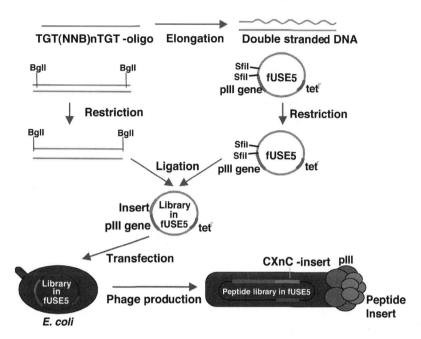

FIGURE 2 Phage library preparation. In order to construct a phage library, oligonucleotides encoding random peptides are individually fused to the phage genome, producing a large collection of phage particles (10^9 transducing units) displaying peptides as recombinant proteins in the phage surface. Shown is the construction of a library with peptides displayed on a coat protein (pIII) of an M13-derived bacteriophage vector. Each resulting phage clone will display three to five copies of a unique peptide. The preparation of phage libraries must be optimized to create the highest possible peptide diversity.

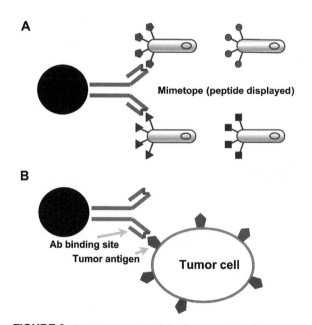

FIGURE 3 Panning on an immobilized receptor in a cell-free system. Phage display libraries were originally devised as a tool to define binding sites of antibodies. (A) It may be possible to fingerprint the repertoire of circulating tumor-associated antibodies by selection of a peptide library on immunoglobulins isolated from serum cancer patients. (B) Successive rounds of panning may select for peptides that mimic tumor surface antigens (and some of them may perhaps be vascular markers).

as opposed to purified receptors as discussed earlier, membrane-bound proteins are more likely to preserve their functional conformation, which can be lost upon purification and immobilization outside the context of intact cells. Second, many cell surface receptors require the cell membrane environment to function so that homo- or heterodimeric interactions may occur. Third, combinatorial approaches allow the selection of cell membrane ligands in an unbiased functional assay and without any preconceived notions about the nature of the cellular receptor repertoire; thus, unknown receptors can be targeted. Despite these advantages, it is often difficult to isolate specific ligands due to the high complexity of targets expressed simultaneously on a given cell population.

In recent years, a number of successful cell biopannings with phage display have been reported. Examples include cells expressing the urokinase receptor and the melanocortin receptor, fibroblasts and myoblasts, endothelial cells, neutrophils, T cells, head and neck carcinoma cells, and others. This relative success notwithstanding, the cell surface selection of phage libraries has been plagued by technical

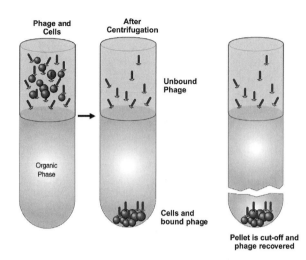

FIGURE 4 Biopanning and rapid analysis of selective interactive ligands (BRASIL). We have designed a novel strategy for panning on cells based on a binding assay in an aqueous phase followed by a separation of phage–cell complexes through an organic phase. This single-step centrifugation results in a hydrophobic passage in which only the phage bound to cells is recovered by infection, amplified, and used for another round of selection. A scheme of our method is shown. BRASIL can be performed with cultured cells or cells isolated from clinical samples.

difficulties. First, a high number of nonbinder and nonspecific binder clones are recovered when phage libraries are incubated with cell suspensions or monolayers. Moreover, removal of the background by repeated washes is both labor-intensive and inefficient. Finally, cells and potential ligands are frequently lost during the many washing steps required.

We have developed a new approach for the screening of cell surface-binding peptides from phage libraries. Biopanning and rapid analysis of selective interactive ligands (termed BRASIL) is based on differential centrifugation in which a cell suspension incubated with phage in an aqueous upper phase is centrifuged through a nonmiscible organic lower phase (Fig. 4). This single-step organic phase separation is faster, more sensitive, and more specific than current methods that rely on washing steps or limiting dilution. As a proof of principle, we screened human endothelial cells stimulated with vascular endothelial growth factor (VEGF) and constructed a peptide-based ligand–receptor map of that growth factor family. BRASIL may prove itself a superior method for probing target cell surfaces with a broad range of potential applications.

BRASIL is also of value for targeting and isolating ligand–receptor pairs in cell populations derived from clinical samples. The method may be used in tandem with fine-needle aspirates of solid tumors or fluorescence-activated cell sorting of leukemic cells obtained from patients. Moreover, because multiple samples and several rounds of preclearing and selection can be performed in a few hours with minimal loss, automation for high-throughput screening and clinical applications are likely to follow.

III. *IN VIVO* TARGETING

A. Vascular Targeting Technology

The molecular diversity of blood vessels has just begun to be uncovered. Many therapeutic targets may be expressed in very restricted—but highly specific and accessible—locations in the vascular endothelium. Thus potential targets for intervention may be easily overlooked in high-throughput DNA sequencing or in gene arrays because these approaches do not usually take into account cellular location, anatomical, and functional context.

We developed a selection method in which peptides that home to specific vascular beds are identified after administration of a random peptide library (Fig. 5). This section reviews our efforts toward the construction of a ligand–receptor map of the vasculature. This work may have broad implications for the development of targeted therapies. We have been using animal models of human cancer to discover addresses that are only present in tumor blood vessels but not in blood vessels of normal tissues. Based on previous work, we have found vascular receptors in tumor-bearing mice. Moreover, we have been able to show that they are also present in human tumors by staining human tissues with antibodies against the molecules. Thus, it is possible to use animal models to find molecular markers of human blood vessels. However, it is unknown whether targeted delivery will always be achieved in humans using mouse-derived probes. Data from the Human Genome Project indicate that the higher complexity of the human species relative to other species derives from protein expression patterns—at different tissue sites, levels, or times—rather than just a mere consequence of a greater number of genes. In fact, examples of species-specific differences in gene expression within the human vascular network have recently surfaced.

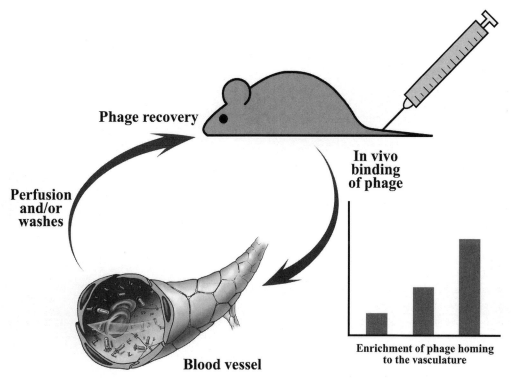

FIGURE 5 *In vivo* phage display. A random peptide library displayed on bacteriophage is also a source of ligands that can home to receptors on the vascular endothelium of blood vessels. Shown is an *in vivo* selection strategy for ligands that home to tissue-specific endothelium of certain organs or to angiogenesis-related vascular markers in activated blood vessels of tumors.

Thus, species-specific differences in protein expression caution that any vascular targeting data obtained in animal models must be carefully evaluated before extrapolation to human studies. Data from the preantibiotic era suggest that phage can be safely administered to patients. If so, screening phage display libraries in patients may enable the construction of a molecular map of vascular diversity in normal or diseased tissues.

B. Vascular Addresses in Blood Vessels

It is recognized that a tumor cannot get larger than 1 mm in diameter without new blood vessel formation. Tumor blood vessels are different from normal blood vessels, and we make use of those molecular differences in targeting anticancer therapies into cancers. Peptides selected from phage libraries have allowed the cloning of vascular receptors in normal and in angiogenic blood vessels. Vascular receptors are attractive targets for systemic delivery, in particular because such receptors are readily accessible through the circulation and often can mediate internalization of ligands by cells. A panel of endothelial cell surface receptors and homing peptides is presented in Table I, and many more ligand–receptor pairs are expected to emerge from screening phage libraries by the strategies described in this article.

IV. TARGETED THERAPIES

Many malignant, cardiovascular, and inflammatory diseases have a marked angiogenic component. In cancer, tumor vasculature is a suitable target for intervention because the vascular endothelium is composed of nonmalignant cells that are genetically stable but epigenetically diverse. Cancers appear to put an epigenetic molecular signature on their own blood vessels

TABLE I
Cell Surface Receptors and Homing Motifs Isolated by Phage Display Targeting[a]

Receptor	Function/class	Carrier?	Localization	Tissue	Homing motif
αv integrins	Cell adhesion	Yes	EC, tumor cells	Tumor	ACDCRGDCFCG
CD13	Aminopeptidase	Yes	EC, pericytes, tumor cells	Tumor	CNGRC
NG2/HMWMAA	Proteoglycan	N/D	Pericytes, tumor cells	Tumor	TAASGVRSMH LTLRWVGLMS
MDP	Dipeptidase	N/D	EC	Lung	CGFEC
MMP-2	Metalloproteinase	Yes	EC, tumor cells	Tumor	CRRHWGFEFC
MMP-9	Metalloproteinase	Yes	EC, tumor cells	Tumor	CTTHWGFTLC

[a]HMWMAA, high molecular weight melanoma-associated antigen; MMP, matrix metalloproteinase; MDP, membrane dipeptidase; EC, endothelial cells; N/D, not determined.

that targeted probes can use as a homing signal to deliver a drug into the vascular receptors

The biological basis for such vascular heterogeneity is still unknown. However, peptides selected by homing to blood vessels have been used to guide the delivery of cytotoxic drugs, proapoptotic peptides, metalloprotease inhibitors, cytokines, fluorophores, and genes. Generally, coupling to homing peptides appears to yield a targeted compound with a better therapeutic index than the untargeted parental compound. Taken together, these results show that it is possible to develop therapeutic strategies based on selective expression of vascular receptors.

V. CONCLUDING REMARKS

We are currently translating the phage display technology and molecular diversity of blood vessels into real clinical applications. We anticipate that by guiding anticancer compounds to tumor blood vessels, we will develop new, improved forms of targeted anticancer therapy. Aside from the therapeutic promise of peptide-guided therapy, this work outlines a road map of the molecular anatomy of blood vessels in cancer. In a larger sense, targeting the vasculature of normal and diseased organs may be the foundation of a new pharmacology for the treatment of malignant and inflammatory diseases by delivering drugs to blood vessels. Data reviewed here represent the latest advances toward a ligand-based map of the human vasculature.

Acknowledgments

We thank Marina Cardó-Vila, Ricardo J. Giordano, Johanna Lahdenranta, Paul J. Mintz, and Claudia I. Vidal for assistance with the illustrations. This work was funded in part by grants from NIH (CA90270 and CA8297601 to R.P., CA90270 and CA9081001 to W.A.) and awards from CaP CURE, the Gilson-Longenbaugh Foundation, the Susan G. Komen Breast Cancer Foundation, and the V Foundation (to R.P. and W.A.).

See Also the Following Articles

Anti-Vascular Endothelial Growth Factor-Based Angiostatics • Autocrine and Paracrine Growth Mechanisms in Cancer Progression and Metastasis • Molecular Mechanisms of Cancer Invasion • Tumor Cell Motility and Invasion

Bibliography

Arap, W., Pasqualini, R., and Ruoslahti, E. (1998). Cancer treatment by targeted drug delivery to tumor vasculature in a mouse model. *Science* **279,** 377–380.

Arap, W., Kolonin, M., Trepel, M., Baggerly, K., Lahdenranta, J., Giordano, R. J., Cardó-Vila, M., Yao, V., Mintz, P. J., Ardelt, P. U., Flamm, A., Valtanen, H., Weavind, L. M., Hicks, M., Troncoso, P., Pollock, R. E., Botz, G. H., Bucana, C., Koivunen, E., Cahill, D., Pentz, R. D., Do, K. H., Logothetis, C. J., and Pasqualini, R. (2002) Steps toward mapping human vasculature by in vivo phage display. *Nature Med.* **8,** 121–127.

Curnis, F., *et al.* (2000). Enhancement of tumor necrosis factor α antitumor immunotherapeutic properties by targeted delivery to aminopeptidase N (CD13). *Nature Biotechnol.* **18,** 1185–1190.

Ellerby, H. M., Arap, W., Ellerby, L. M., Kain, R., Andrusiak, R.,

Del Rio, G., Krajeswki, S., Lombardo, C. R., Rao, R., Ruoslahti, E., Bredesen, D., and Pasqualini, R. (1999). Anticancer activity of targeted proapoptotic peptides. *Nature Med.* **9,** 1032–1038.

Giordano, R, Cardo-Vila M, Lahdenranta J, Pasqualini R, Arap W (2001). Biopanning and Rapid Analysis of Selective and Interactive Ligands. *Nature Med.* **11,** 1249–1253.

Giordano, R. J., Cardó-Vila, M., Lahdenranta, M., Pasqualini, R., and Arap, W. (2001). Biopanning and rapid analysis of selective interactive ligands. *Nature Med.* **11,** 1249–1253.

Hong, F. D., and Clayman, G. L. (2000). Isolation of a peptide for targeted drug delivery into human head and neck solid tumors. *Cancer Res.* **60,** 6551–6556.

Koivunen, E., *et al.* (1999). Integrin-binding peptides from phage display peptide libraries. Integrin protocols. *Methods Mol. Biol.* **129,** 3–17.

Koivunen, E., Arap, W., Valtanen, H., Rainisalo, A., Medina, O. P., Heikkila, P., Kantor, C., Gahmberg, C. G., Salo, T., Konttinen, Y. T., Sorsa, T., Ruoslahti, E., and Pasqualini, R. (1999). Tumor-targeting with a selective gelatinase inhibitor. *Nature Biotechnol.* **8,** 768–774.

Koivunen, E., *et al.* (2001). Inhibition of β_2 integrin-mediated leukocyte cell adhesion by leucine-leucine-glycine motif-containing peptides. *J. Cell Biol.* **153,** 1–13.

Kolonin, M., Pasqualini, R., and Arap, W. (2001). Molecular addresses in blood vessels as targets for therapy. *Curr. Opin. Chem. Biol.* **5,** 308–313.

Pasqualini, R., McDonald D., and Arap, W. (2001). Targeting the vascular endothelium: Implications for antigen presentation and immune response. *Nature Immunol.* **2,** 567–568.

Smith, G. P., and Scott, J. K. (1990). Searching for peptide ligands with an epitope library. *Science* **249,** 386–390.

Vinca Alkaloids and Epipodophyllotoxins

Ritesh Rathore
Alan B. Weitberg
Roger Williams Medical Center/
Boston University School of Medicine

I. Vinca Alkaloids
II. Epipodophyllotoxins

GLOSSARY

cell cycle Multistep process in the life of each cell, including growth, resting, and division stages.
epipodophyllotoxins Chemical compounds used in cancer chemotherapy derived from the mandrake plant.
myelosuppression Reduction in white blood cell and platelet numbers.
topoisomerase II An enzyme in the nucleus responsible for DNA breakage and resealing.
tubulin Cellular component involved in mitosis.
vinca alkaloids Chemical compounds used in cancer chemotherapy derived from the pink periwinkle plant.

V inca alkaloids and epipodophyllotoxins are two distinct groups of plant-derived chemicals, which are commonly utilized in cancer chemotherapy. This article reviews the biological properties, clinical uses, and adverse effects associated with their use.

I. VINCA ALKALOIDS

A. Chemistry

Vinca alkaloids (vincristine, vinblastine, vinorelbine, and vindesine) are naturally occurring or semisynthetic compounds derived from the pink periwinkle plant (*Catharanthus roseus* g. Don). They have a large asymmetrical dimeric structure composed of a dihydroindole (vindoline) nucleus, which is the major alkaloid, linked to an indole (catharanthine) nucleus. Vincristine and vinblastine, the prototypic vinca alkaloids, have a single structural difference in the vindoline nucleus. Vindesine and vinorelbine are semisynthetic derivatives of vinblastine with differences in the indole nucleus.

B. Mechanism of Action

Vinca alkaloids are cell cycle-specific agents that block mitosis with metaphase arrest by binding to tubulin, which is a critical component of microtubules. Vinca alkaloids disrupt the mitotic apparatus after binding to tubulin, resulting in mitotic arrest in metaphase. This effect on the mitotic apparatus accounts for the cytotoxicity of these agents. However, other cellular functions depend on microtubular integrity as well (central nervous system function, neuromuscular transmission) and when affected account for the toxicity of these agents. Cross-resistance does not occur between vinca alkaloids, but has been observed with several antitumor antibiotics, suggesting a shared transport mechanism for cell entry.

C. Pharmacology

All vinca alkaloids bind extensively to plasma proteins and to all of the cellular elements of the blood, including platelets and lymphocytes. Differences in biologic and toxic effects have been related to their inherent pharmacologic differences. After intravenous injection of normal clinical doses, the peak concentration of vincristine and vinblastine is 0.4 μM. All vinca alkaloids have a multiphasic pattern of clearance and are principally metabolized in the liver. Biologically active derivatives of vinblastine and vinorelbine have been described. The major route of elimination of vincristine is biliary, with 70% of an administered dose appearing in the feces. In the case of other vinca alkaloids, fewer amounts are excreted in the feces and urine.

D. Clinical Indications

Vincristine is used in combination chemotherapy to treat a variety of solid and hematological malignancies, including acute lymphoblastic leukemia, Hodgkin's and non-Hodgkin's lymphoma, soft tissue sarcomas, Wilms' tumor, and neuroblastoma, with its greatest efficacy occurring in hematological malignancies. Vinblastine has a similar spectrum of clinical activity, although vincristine is more useful in lymphocytic leukemias, especially the acute variety in children, and vinblastine is more effective in the treatment of advanced testicular tumors. Vinorelbine is used as a single agent or in combination chemotherapy in the treatment of nonsmall cell lung cancer and breast cancer and has demonstrated activity in Hodgkin's and non-Hodgkin's lymphomas and ovarian carcinoma. Vindesine has demonstrated activity in nonsmall cell lung cancer and certain hematological and solid malignancies. However, there is no defined role for vindesine and it is available only for investigational use in the United States.

E. Adverse Reactions

Neurotoxicity, a major toxicity, is dose limiting for vincristine. Initially, peripheral neuropathies occur with a loss of deep tendon reflexes and distal paresthesias; continued administration can result in muscular weakness and sensory impairment. Autonomic neuropathies, including constipation, abdominal cramping, paralytic ileus, bladder atony, and orthostatic hypotension, can occur. Mental status changes, including confusion and coma, have been described. Neurotoxicity is both dose related and cumulative. Early toxicity is usually reversible, but motor deficits may persist. Patients receiving vincristine should be on a regimen of stool softeners and laxatives.

Myelosuppression, the other principal toxicity, is dose limiting for all except vincristine. Granulocyte nadir occurs at 7–10 days, with recovery completed by 14 days. Thrombocytopenia and anemia are of lesser incidence and severity. Reversible alopecia and mild nausea and vomiting occur less commonly. Greater toxicity is encountered in patients with hepatic dysfunction, and doses should be reduced in patients with biliary obstruction. A syndrome of hyponatremia secondary to the inappropriate secretion of antidiuretic hormone has been described with vincristine use. These agents are potent vesicants and care should be taken to avoid extravasation at injection sites.

II. EPIPODOPHYLLOTOXINS

A. Chemistry

Teniposide (VM-26) and etoposide (VP-16-213) are semisynthetic derivatives of podophyllotoxin, an extract of the mandrake plant (*Podophyllum peltatum*).

Chemical modification of podophyllotoxin by addition of the carbohydrate moieties β-D-thenylidene glucoside and β-D-ethylidene glucoside led to the development of teniposide and etoposide, respectively.

B. Mechanism of Action

Epipodophyllotoxins differ from the parent podophyllotoxins, which inhibit microtubule formation due to the glucoside moiety on the C ring of the molecule. They are cell cycle specific, arresting cells at the $S–G_2$ interface and causing single strand breaks in DNA. This is due to the inhibition of topoisomerase II, a nuclear enzyme responsible for the breakage and resealing of DNA. Epipodophyllotoxins also can inhibit nucleoside transport and impair incorporation of nucleosides into cellular nucleic acids.

C. Pharmacology

Oral administration is characterized by marked intrapatient and interpatient variability, with 40–50% of either drug being absorbed. Both teniposide and etoposide are highly protein bound. Following intravenous injection, etoposide has a biphasic clearance pattern with half-lives of 3 and 12 h. Forty-five percent of the dose is excreted in the urine (two-thirds unchanged and one-third as metabolites), and decreased clearance rates have been observed in patients with renal insufficiency requiring dose reduction. Hepatic dysfunction is not associated with significant changes in etoposide clearance and half-life. Fifteen percent is recovered in the feces, and less than 5% of the plasma concentration accumulates in the cerebrospinal fluid (CSF). Teniposide has a multiphasic pattern of clearance after intravenous injection. Approximately 45% of the drug is excreted in the urine, but unlike etoposide, most (80%) is recovered as metabolites. Less than 1% of the drug concentrates in the CSF. Teniposide undergoes some biliary elimination after conjugation with glucoronide or sulfate derivatives.

D. Toxicity

The toxicity profile is similar for both drugs, with myelosuppression being the dose-limiting toxicity. After intravenous administration, granulocyte nadirs are observed between 8 and 14 days and recovery is noted by 3 weeks. With continuous oral administration, granulocyte nadirs occur between days 21 and 28 with recovery by day 35. Thrombocytopenia is less frequent and usually is mild. Mild-to-moderate nausea and vomiting may occur in 30–40% of patients, with diarrhea, constipation, and stomatitis less commonly occurring. Mucositis is dose limiting at very high doses only (e.g., as used in bone marrow transplantation). Most patients develop complete but reversible alopecia. Hypersensitivity reactions (vasomotor, pulmonary, and gastrointestinal changes) occur uncommonly and may be prevented with antihistaminic premedications.

Therapy-related acute myeloid leukemias can appear relatively early after epipodophyllotoxin use (less than 5 years). They present without preceding myelodysplasia, are usually FAB subtypes M4–M5, and are characteristically associated with chromosomal 11q23 abnormalities. These leukemias are less responsive to standard antileukemic therapy and are associated with a poorer survival.

E. Clinical Indications

Etoposide, in combination with cisplatinum, is commonly used in the treatment of small cell and non-small cell lung cancer. It is used in combination chemotherapy for germ cell tumors, Hodgkin's and non-Hodgkin's lymphoma, acute and chronic leukemias, and other solid tumors. Teniposide has not been extensively used clinically but is effective in small cell lung cancer. Activity also is noted in acute lymphoblastic leukemia, neuroblastoma, and lymphomas.

See Also the Following Articles

ACUTE MYELOCYTIC LEUKEMIA • CELL CYCLE CONTROL • CISPLATIN AND RELATED DRUGS • RESISTANCE TO TOPOISOMERASE-TARGETING AGENTS • TAXOL AND OTHER MOLECULES THAT INTERACT WITH MICROTUBULES

Bibliography

Allen, L. M., and Creaven, P. J. (1975). Comparison of the human pharmacokinetics of VM-26 and VP-16, two antineoplastic epipodophyllotoxin glucopyranoside derivatives. *Eur. J. Cancer* **11**, 697–707.

Bender, R. A., Castle, M. C., Margileth, D. A., and Oliverio, V. T. (1977). The pharmacokinetics of (3H)-vincristine in man. *Clin. Pharm. Ther.* **22,** 430–435.

Drewinko, B., and Barlogie, B. (1976). Survival and cycle-progression delay of human lymphoma cells in vitro exposed to VP 16-213. *Cancer Treat. Rep.* **60,** 1295–1306.

D'Incalci, M., Rossi, C., Zucchetti, M., *et al.* (1986). Pharmacokinetics of etoposide in patients with abnormal renal and hepatic function. *Cancer Res.* **46,** 2566–2571.

Hande, K. R., Wolff, S. N., Greco, F. A., *et al.* (1990). Etoposide kinetics in patients with obstructive jaundice. *J. Clin. Oncol.* **8,** 1101–1107.

Jackson, D. V., Castle, M. C., and Bender, R. A. (1978). Biliary excretion of vincristine. *Clin. Pharm. Ther.* **24,** 101–107.

Krauhs, E., Little, M., Kempf, T., *et al.* (1981). Complete amino acid sequence of beta-tubulin from porcine brain. *Proc. Natl. Acad. Sci. USA* **78,** 4156–4160.

Miller, B. R. (1985). Neurotoxicity and vincristine. *JAMA* **253,** 2045.

Owellen, R. J., Hatke, C. A., and Hains, F. O. (1977). Pharmacokinetics and metabolism of vinblastine in humans. *Cancer Res.* **37,** 2597–2602.

Pui, C., Ribeiro, R. C., Hancock, M. L., *et al.* (1991). Acute myeloid leukemia in children treated with epipodophyllotoxins for acute lymphoblastic leukemia. *N. Engl. J. Med.* **325,** 1682–1687.

Ratain, M. J., Kaminer, L. S., Bitran, J. D., *et al.* (1987). Acute nonlymphoblastic leukemia following etoposide and cisplatin combination chemotherapy for advanced non-small cell carcinoma of the lung. *Blood* **70,** 1412–1417.

Robertson, G. L., Bhoopalam, N., and Zelkowitz, L. J. (1973). Vincristine neurotoxicity and abnormal secretion of antidiuretic hormone. *Arch. Intern. Med.* **132,** 717–720.

Ross, W., Rowe, T., Glisson, B., *et al.* (1984). Role of topoisomerase II in mediating epipodophyllotoxin-induced DNA cleavage. *Cancer Res.* **44,** 5857–5860.

Stewart, C. F., Pieper, J. A., Arbuck, S. G., *et al.* (1989). Altered binding of etoposide in patients with cancer. *Clin. Pharm. Ther.* **45,** 49–55.

Viral Agents

Wayne D. Lancaster
Wayne State University School of Medicine

José Campione-Piccardo
National Laboratory for Viral Oncology
Health and Welfare Canada

GLOSSARY

cis-acting A locus or protein that affects the activity only of DNA sequences on its own molecule of DNA.

episome Autonomously replicating circular, extrachromosomal DNA.

integration The insertion into a host genome of viral or another DNA covalently linked on either side to host sequences.

nucleocapsid The symmetric protein shell and the viral nucleic acid that it encloses.

oncogene A gene whose product has the ability to transform eukaryotic cells to tumor cells.

open reading frame A series of nucleotide triplets coding for amino acids without termination codons with the potential to be translated into protein.

protooncogene A normal gene that by mutation or overexpression can become an oncogene.

trans-acting Describing or relating to a locus or protein that affects the activity only of DNA sequences on another molecule of DNA.

tumor suppressor gene A gene whose product is needed for normal cell growth.

Human infections with selected RNA and DNA viruses are epidemiologically associated with certain forms of leukemias, lymphomas, and carcinomas. These virally associated cancers have long latency periods (decades), and the fact that cancers arise in only a small proportion of infected individuals suggests that these viruses contribute to the development of cancer in an indirect manner. Analysis of viral gene function at the molecular level supports this conclusion. The biological effects of virus infection appear to be a necessary step in a multistep carcinogenesis process and include perturbation of the immune response, alteration in cell growth control, and accumulation of cell mutations. Continued studies on the subtle interactions between host cell and viral functions will further our understanding of genetic and environmental factors that may contribute to malignancy.

I. INTRODUCTION

Teleologically, it is difficult to envision the evolutionary advantage for an organism to harbor cells that can escape normal growth restraints, invade their host as if they were independent organisms, and eventually cause the premature death of the host as well as their own death. Likewise, viral participation in oncogenesis shows no clear evolutionary advantage for the survival of the virus. It limits the survival of the host, and in most cases the malignant cell does not support the replication of viral progeny. It is likely that virus-associated malignancies arise from interactions between host cell functions and required viral processes that can, in some instances, unavoidably alter mechanisms of control of cellular replication. Whatever this mechanism of change represents, it must be unique because only a very few of the viruses infecting humans are linked to cancer induction. The diverse nature of these viruses would suggest that viral-associated oncogenesis is manifested through a number of mechanisms.

The discovery by Peyton Rous in 1911 that cell-free fitrates of certain avian cancers induced cancer in healthy birds was met with skepticism. However, many years later it was found that similar viruses could cause leukemias in chickens, rodents, monkeys, and many other species. These discoveries rationalized the foreignness of cancer and focused on the infectious nature of the disease in animals. The approach of extrapolating these results to human leukemias, and perhaps to other cancers, through a process of comparative pathology was attractive. Once a virus was identified as causing a human cancer it would be possible to prevent infection, and utimately the cancer, using vaccines. It is now felt that only a few human cancers are associated with virus infections. However, it is estimated that viruses are responsible for about 15% of all human cancers and represent the second most important risk factor for cancer next to tobacco use. For most, if not all, of these infections the virus participates only indirectly in the development of the cancer.

Experimental evidence has left no doubt about the oncogenic potential of human viruses in animals and in tissue culture cells. However, extrapolation of the data to human cancers is not always evident. For example, the small human papovaviruses JC and BK, adenovirus (types 12 and 18), and the poxvirus of molluscum contagiosum all exhibit cell transforming activity, but none have been regularly associated with human cancer. A more strict evaluation of an association of a virus with human cancer based on epidemiological evidence is that the virus represents a risk factor for tumor development. The nucleic acid of the virus should be present in tumor cells at high frequency, and, experimentally, the viral genome should be oncogenic. This evidence, along with the demonstration that the proliferative changes depend on functions exerted by the presistent viral nucleic acid, allows for the unambiguous identification of a tumor virus. A summary of human tumor viruses and the malignancies with which they are associated is present in Table 1.

II. HUMAN RETROVIRUSES AND HUMAN ONCOGENESIS

A. General Characteristics of Retroviruses

Retroviruses are characterized by an RNA genome composed of two identical single strands that replicate via a double-stranded DNA intermediate. Both RNA strands are homologous to viral mRNA transcripts (positive strands). These RNA strands are packaged into a nucleocapsid containing several structural nucleoproteins and a reverse transcriptase

TABLE I
Human Viruses and Associated Malignancies

Virus	Malignancy
Human T-cell lymphotropic virus (HTLV-I and HTLV-II)	Adult T-cell leukemia, T-cell lymphoma
Human herpes virus (HHV-8)	Kaposi sarcoma
Human immunodeficiency virus (HIV-1 and HIV-2)	Non-Hodgkin's lymphoma
Human papillomavirus (HPV)	Cervical cancer, skin cancer in epidermodysplasia verruciformis
Hepatitis B virus (HBV)	Hepatocellular carcinoma
Epstein-Barr virus (EBV)	Burkitt's lymphoma, nasopharyngeal carcinoma

(RNA-directed DNA polymerase). This enzyme is required for the retrotranscription of the double-stranded DNA intermediate. The nucleocapsid is surrounded by a cell-dervied membrane modified with viral glycoproteins. Retroviruses are classified into three subfamilies: Oncovirinae, Spumavirinae, and Lentivirinae. The family Oncovirinae is itself subclassified morphologically into A-, B-, and C-type viruses.

Each RNA strand packaged in the virion contains two transcriptional regulatory regions termed long terminal repeats (LTR) at both extremes flanking a 9–10 kilobase (kb) internal stretch with at least three gene encoding regions: Gag (group-specific antigen), Pol (reverse transcriptase), and Env (envelope proteins). Adjacent to the LTR is a primer binding site complementary to a specific tRNA that acts as primer for the initiation of reverse transcription (Fig. 1). Through the action of reverse transcriptase, strand switching, and the RNase H activity of the polymerase, two homologous strands of RNA are destructively transformed without net quantitative gain into two complementary strands of DNA.

Chromosomal integration of the double-stranded viral DNA is mediated by a nucleoprotein complex containing both viral and cellular enzymes involved in DNA replication and repair. The actual viral DNA molecules that are integrated correspond to linear double-stranded molecules with small 5′-end overhangs at both ends. Once integrated, the provirus is stable and is replicated and expressed as any other cellular locus. The LTR promoter directs polycistronic transcripts that, after differential posttranscriptional splicing, encode for the different precursor viral proteins. These precursors are, in turn, cleaved into the different functional or structural viral polypeptides. These polypeptides are designed with the letters p (protein) or gp (glycoprotein) followed by their estimated size in kilodaltons (e.g., p21, gp160).

Retroviruses have been related to the pathogenesis of a variety of malignancies in many animal species.

These include the viral etiology of leukemias and sarcomas in birds and rats, mammary tumors in mice, and leukemias and lymphomas in several mammalian species. The finding that feline and bovine leukemias were related to horizontally transmittable retrovirus infections paved the way for the search for human oncogenic retroviruses. The molecular mechanisms by which retroviruses induce these malignancies have been studied extensively. The high efficiency of transformation by some animal retroviruses has been attributed to specific genes that the virus appears to have retrotranscribed into intron-less DNA from mRNA before incorporating them into the viral genome. These transforming genes or oncogenes have been identified as normal cellular genes with normal function in intracellular signal transduction or control of the cell cycle, particularly during the early stages of ontogenesis. Their ability to transform normal cells is due to overexpression or expression of the oncogene at an inappropriate time of cell differentiation.

The majority of retroviruses, however, do not harbor oncogenes in their genome, and their mechanism of transformation is related to integration into the cellular genome and subsequent change in the control of expression of genes adjacent to the site of integration (in *cis*). Other retroviruses can induce transformation through the expression of viral genes able to act as transcription activators (in *trans*), influencing the transcription of cellular genes related to cellular growth. For some time the suspicion as well as the hope existed that retroviruses could be responsible for most if not all human malignancies. The first clear evidence associating a human retrovirus with cancer came with the ability to culture human lymphocytes susceptible to human lymphotropic retroviruses. This development occurred in 1975 with the discovery of interleukin-2 (IL-2) as a growth factor for T cells.

B. Human T-Lymphotropic Viruses

The human T-lymphotropic virus type 1 (HTLV-1) was the first human lymphotropic virus to be grown and isolated in the laboratory. It has since been shown to be strongly associated with adult T-cell leukemia (ATL) and some non-Hodgkin's lymphomas. ATL is an aggressive malignancy of varied cellular morphology

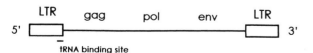

FIGURE 1 Genomic structure of a typical retrovirus.

often associated with skin (mycosis fungoides) and skeletal lytical lesions (hypercalcemia). Its highest incidence is observed in Japan and some Pacific and Caribbean archipelagos as well as in countries in western Africa. The incidence of T-cell malignancies in HTLV-infected persons is about 1–2 per 1000. ATL has also been linked with exposure to HTLV-I early in life and in particular to a syndrome characterized by generalized eczema and rhinitis probably related to immunosuppression caused by the HTLV-I primary infection of T cells early in childhood. In addition to ATL, HTLV-I has been related to B-cell chronic lymphocytic leukemia. This probably is the result of B-cell dysfunction caused by HTLV-I infection of T cells with B-cell regulatory function. HTLV-I has been occasionally related to other malignancies; however, these associations require further epidemiological support.

HTLV-II, the second member of the family of human lymphotropic viruses, was isolated from a case of T-hairy cell leukemia. The consistency of its association with this syndrome requires further documentation. This virus shows a higher prevalence among drug abusers as well as some Native Indian populations of South, Central, and North America and African bushmen. However, there is no epidemiological evidence of its pathogenicity in these populations. Both HTLV-I and HTLV-II are thought to be sexually transmitted as well as transmissible by parenteral injection. Thus, they show epidemiological associations with other malignancies related to sexual (anogenital carcinoma) and blood-borne (hepatocellular carcinoma) transmission.

HTLV-I and HTLV-II are tentatively classified as human C-type viruses in the family Oncovirinae. These viruses show the genomic architecture typical of most retroviruses. The Gag-precursor polypeptide is first myristylated and subsequently cleaved to yield polypeptides p14, p27, and p7 in HTLV-I and p15, p24, and p9 in HTLV-II. The Pol region encodes for the reverse transcriptase (p95). The Env-precursor polypeptide is glycosylated to yield the gp68 (HTLV-I) or gp62 (HTLV-II) precursors that are later cleaved into a transmembrane protein (p21) and a larger outer surface glycoprotein (gp46). The viral genome also encodes for a protease (p14) whose open reading frame overlaps portions of the Gag and Pol regions. These regions do not contain oncogenes but do contain several proteins that are encoded by open reading frames flanking or overlapping the Env region. These are p40 (*tax*), p27 (*rex*), and p21 (truncated *rex*) in HTLV-I and p37, p26, and p24 in HTLV-II. The *tax* product is considered to be a transcriptional activator, whereas the *rex* product is believed to be a posttranscriptional activator. Leukemogenesis by HTLV probably represents a multistep process in which the virus can participate in two ways: by disrupting immune surveillance mechanisms through direct phenotypic alteration of immunocompetent cells, and through the expression of the transcription trans-activation *tax* protein. This protein can trans-activate the expression of factors related to lymphocyte cell growth such as interleukin-2, its receptor, and cellular oncogenes such as c-*fos* and c-*sis*.

C. Human Immunodeficiency Viruses

Human immunodeficiency virus type 1 (HIV-1), first identified as a T-lymphotropic retrovirus by several investigators in 1983 and 1984, is currently accepted as the etiological agent of AIDS (acquired immunodeficiency syndrome). In 1986 a second immunodeficiency virus, HIV-2, was identified in West Africa that also causes AIDS. However, this virus does not serologically cross-react with HIV-1 in screening tests. HIV-1 is the topic of this discussion unless indicated otherwise. Through its disruption of the immune system, HIV may contribute to the pathogenesis of a variety of human malignancies (i.e., lymphoma, squamous cell skin carcinoma, melanoma, cervical carcinoma, hepatocellular carcinoma), many of which are primarily related to other human oncogenic viruses that may also share with HIV its epidemiology and modes of transmission. The *tat* protein of HIV may directly contribute to cellular transformation; however, the virus is more likely to play a role in oncogenesis through the disruption of immune surveillance mechanisms and, possibly, by induction of the aberrant expression of growth-promoting lymphokines.

Until the late 1970s Kaposi sarcoma was a rare skin malignancy restricted to older males of Mediterranean ancestry. In the late 1970s, the detection of an aggressive form of this sarcoma observed in never-married males was one of the first indications of the HIV epidemic. Since then, Kaposi sarcoma has been almost specific for HIV-infected gay males and very rare in parenterally infected individuals (i.e., hemophiliacs and intravenous drug users). However, cases of Kaposi sarcoma have been described in HIV-negative gay men. These features have pointed to the strong possibility of a concomitant infection with another sexually transmitted human oncogenic virus. Indeed, DNA sequences of a new herpesvirus have been detected in Kaposi sarcoma cells (see Section V.C). However, the *tat* protein, the transcriptional *trans*-activator of HIV, is suspected of playing a direct role in the proliferation of these cells. The sarcoma may result from immune depression as well as a true molecular oncogenic synergism between the two viruses.

HIV causes a lytic infection; however, the *tat* protein can be excreted and taken up by adjacent cells, where it could exert its transcriptional trans-activating function. HIV infection is also related to an increase in non-Hodgkin's lymphomas. The incidence of non-Hodgkin's lymphoma in AIDS patients is approximately 3.3 per 100. As therapy prolongs the life expectancy of immunosuppressed individuals, non-Hodgkin's lymphomas are expected to increase in HIV-infected individuals. Most of these tumors are undifferentiated B-cell Burkitt's-like lymphomas that in many cases show Epstein-Barr virus (EBV)-related c-*myc* rearrangements also involving immunoglobulin genes [i.e., t(8;14) translocations, see Section V,B].

HIV-1 and HIV-2 are related to the family Lentivirinae. The architecture of their genome also corresponds to that of most retroviruses. The Gag-precursor polypeptide (p53) is myristylated and then cleaved into p17 (capsid surface), p24 (major capsid component), and p15 which is subsequently cleaved into p7 and p9, and a RNA-binding protein probably related to packaging. The Pol-precursor polypeptide is cleaved into p10 (protease), p51/p66 (reverse transcriptase), and p32 (endonuclease). The gp160 Env-precursor is cleaved into the transmembrane glycoprotein (gp41) and the extracellular glycoprotein (gp120). Several open reading frames bind and overlap with the Env region and, through alternative splicing, give rise to several polypeptide products associated with viral protein expression, such as *tat* (transcription trans-activator), *rev* (posttranscriptional trans-activation), and *nef* (probably a GTP-binding negative regulator), or virion assembly, such as *vif, vpu* (HIV-1), or *vpr* and *vpx* (HIV-2).

III. HUMAN PAPILLOMAVIRUSES AND CERVICAL CANCER

With few exceptions, papillomaviruses are exclusively epitheliotropic and cause a self-limiting infection characterized by abnormal maturation and differentiation of epithelial cells. Virus infection is thought to begin in the basal layer of epithelial cells, presumably from virus released from infected, exfoliated cells that have lodged in microabrasions of the epithelium. The virus genome becomes stabilized as an episome after infection, either remaining latent (probably in basal cells without phenotypic changes in the maturing epithelial cells) or establishing an active infection of parabasal cells with subsequent morphological expression of early and late gene functions in differentiating squamous cells. Early gene functions are manifested histologically by an increase in the prickle cell layer (acanthosis), whereas late gene functions are characterized by the expression of intranuclear structural vital proteins in terminally differentiated keratinocytes. The late events that lead to viral capsid assembly are associated with degenerative changes in both the cytoplasm (vacuolization or koilocytosis) and nuclei (atypical sizes and shapes of pyknotic nuclei and binucleation). This process is sometimes referred to as koilocytotic atypia.

Viral capsid assembly (production of infectious virus) occurs predominantly in koilocytes located in the outer differentiating layers of the epithelium. In mucosal infections, localization of viral structural protein occurs only in selected koilocytes, and then in only up to half of the lesions tested. From these and other observations, particularly *in situ* hybridization studies for papillomavirus DNA and RNA transcripts, which are most often detected in differentiating keratinocytes, it is obvious that the life cycle of the virus is linked to the differentiation program of squamous epithelial cells. This probably accounts for the inability to devise a tissue culture system for their replication. However, there are some reports that papillomavirus-induced lesions grown in tissue culture occasionally produce virus particles.

Unique to these viruses is the extensive diversity of virus genotypes. More than 70 different human papillomavirus (HPV) types have been described that preferentially infect either cutaneous or mucosal epithelium. New virus type designations are assigned based on less than 90% nucleotide sequence similarity in certain genomic regions with previously identified HPV types. The papillomaviruses are small (55 nm diameter capsid), nonenveloped, and contain a circular, double-stranded DNA genome approximately 8000 base pairs (bp) in length. Transcription is from only one strand of the genome, which is divided into three distinct regions. Transcriptional regulatory elements reside in a large noncoding region (~1000 bp) followed by the early region containing genes expressed early in infection and the late region containing capsid genes. Early-region genes encode products involved in transcription regulation, DNA replication, and perturbation of the cell cycle.

The original description of the papilloma-to-carcinoma sequence in rabbits infected with the cottontail rabbit (Shope) papillomavirus appeared in the mid 1930s. In humans, HPV infection was previously regarded mainly as a cosmetic nuisance. However, evidence has accumulated that viral warts, in some instances, could become malignant. This observation was made in the rare inherited disorder epidermodysplasia verruciformis. This disease is characterized by disseminated polymorphic lesions that resemble flat warts or macules, some of which transform into skin cancer. The prominent role of human papillomavirus (HPV) (types 5, 18, 14, 17, and 20) in these lesions and associated cancers was verified using molecular cloning and hybridization studies.

Approximately one-third of the known HPV types preferentially infect metaplastic, keratinizing, and nonkeratining squamous epithelium of the genital tract. Epidemiological studies show that HPV infection is more widespread than previously thought and represents one of the most frequently acquired sexually transmitted diseases. Unfortunately, little is known about the factors that facilitate transmission or what determines the natural course of the infection. Many laboratory studies have found HPV DNA sequences from specific types in genital cancers, and epidemiological studies have shown the prominent role of the virus in cervical cancer. It is estimated that worldwide as many as 500,000 women die from cervical cancer every year. In the United States there are approximately 14,000 new cases and about 5000 deaths due to cervical cancer each year.

The genital tract HPV types produce benign genital warts, squamous intraepithelial neoplasia (premalignant lesions), or latent infections. The oncogenic potential of a subgroup of the viruses is reflected by the consistent association of certain types with low-grade and high-grade squamous intraepithelial lesions of the cervix and invasive cervical cancer. For example, HPV types 6 and 11 (as well as types 42, 43, and 44) are most often detected in benign condylomas and low-grade squamous intraepithelial lesions of the cervix. However, in high-grade squamous epithelial lesions of the cervix and in invasive cancers, HPV types 16 and 18 frequently are detected. HPV types 6 and 11 (and types 42, 43, and 44) are rarely, if ever, detected in invasive cancers of the cervix, and therefore they are thought to be so-called low-risk or no risk viruses. Nonetheless, some of the viruses within this group have been identified in verrucous carcinomas of the external genitalia. Based on their frequent association with malignant transformation, HPV types 16 and 18 along with types 45 and 56 could be considered high-risk viruses. However, in this group, differences have been seen with respect to the clinical description of the malignant lesion. The frequency of HPV-18, -45, and -56 in low-grade squamous intraepithelial lesion is disproportionately low when compared with the level in invasive cancers, suggesting that lesions associated with these viruses progress rapidly or that viral DNA levels are too low to detect in early lesions. Significantly, it was noticed that women with cervical cancers that are diagnosed after a recent normal Papanicolaou smear were three-fold more likely to have HPV-18 than HPV-16 detected. Moreover, HPV-18-associated cervical cancers tend to be associated with younger patient age, more frequent metastases, a higher recurrence rate, and a higher tumor grade. Another group of HPV termed intermediate-risk viruses (HPV types 31, 33, 35, 39, 51, 52, 58, 59, and 61) are closely related to HPV-16 but do not share the same distribution pattern in benign, premalignant, and malignant lesions of the cervix. These viruses are detected at a lower frequency in cervical cancers than in benign or premalignant lesions.

The specific role for HPV in cervical cancer has been derived from laboratory and epidemiological evidence. However, many observations have led to the opinion that these viruses are necessary but not sufficient to induce malignant transformation. About 90% of cervical cancers and their resultant metastases contain HPV sequences. These usually are represented by HPV-16 (~50% of cancers) and HPV-18 (~20% of cancers) and less frequently by HPV types 31, 33, and 35 (10–15% of cancers). Compared with squamous intraepithelial lesions, there is a change in the physical state of viral DNA in cancers. In biopsies of the former, autonomously replicating viral genomes at high copy number routinely are observed; however, a small fraction of high-grade premalignant lesions contain integrated viral genomes. Cervical cancers, however, frequently contain viral sequences integrated into the host genome, although episomal forms also are found in many instances. For this reason it is felt that integration may play a role in the pathobiology of HPV in cervical cancer.

Integration of viral DNA into the host genome appears to be random; however, the break in the viral genome occurs in the 3′ half of the early region, resulting in disruption of the regulation of early gene expression. This is thought to occur through transcription regulation exerted by the product of the E2 open reading frame. This open reading frame is either interrupted or placed in abnormal juxtaposition to the transcriptional regulatory region. The E2 product is a DNA-binding protein that recognizes DNA sequence motifs distributed throughout the noncoding region upstream of the "early" region genes, including one site immediately upstream of the early gene promoter. The binding of E2 to its recognition sequence at the early gene promoter downregulates transcription from the promoter, presumably through steric inhibition of formation of the transcription initiation complex.

Uniformly, the product of integration shows retention of the viral transcriptional regulatory region and two open reading frames (E6 and E7) immediately downstream. Analysis of cervical cancers and derived cell lines shows that these two open reading frames, encoding the putative viral oncoproteins, are expressed at high levels. The viral transcripts frequently extend into the flanking host sequences and use host polyadenylation signals for RNA processing. In cells harboring multiple integrated copies of virus DNA only a few appear to be transcriptionally active. This could be due to their peculiar integration pattern and may be under the control of a deregulated cellular promoter. In some cervical cancers HPV sequences have integrated near cellular protooncogenes. This raises the potential of cis-activation of host genes by the viral genome.

Both HPV-16 and HPV-18 DNA can morphologically transform various established rodent cell lines and extend the life span of primary fibroblast cultures. This effect depends on expression of the E6 and E7 open reading frames in most instances. These viruses (and HPV types 31, 33, and 35, but not 6 and 11) can immortalize primary human foreskin and exocervical keratinocytes. The cells are nontumorigenic in nude mice and show no differences in monolayer culture morphology compared with normal control keratinocytes. However, the immortalized cells show abnormal differentiation and stratification in organotypic cultures that morphologically mimic the histopathological appearance of squamous intraepithelial lesions. Immortalization of human keratinocytes requires expression of the E6 and E7 open reading frames. Biochemically, the E6 and E7 gene products may exert their effects on cell differentiation and proliferation by interacting with cellular proteins. The E7 gene product binds to the product of the retinoblastoma (*rb*) susceptibility gene. *In vitro*, the E6 protein binds to and destabilizes p53, a nuclear protein with transformation-suppressing activity. Because *rb* and p53 are associated with cell cycle control, inactivation of the proteins by viral gene products may lead to loss of cell growth control.

Blocking expression of the viral oncoproteins in cervical cancer cell lines inhibits cell growth. This suggests that these viral gene products are important in maintaining the malignant phenotype. However, cellular factors also play a role in control of proliferation of HPV-infected cells. Fusion of cervical cancer cells to normal cells revealed that cells retaining chromosomes from both donors were nontumorigenic. Malignant revertants correlated with the loss of normal chromosome 11, suggesting that expression of a gene on this chromosome controls cell proliferation regardless of the expression of viral E6 and E7 proteins. These proteins are expressed at equal levels in the parental tumorigenic cell line and the nontumorigenic fusion product.

The events required to convert an immortalized epithelial cell to a tumorigenic phenotype are not known. This progression has been refractile to physical and biochemical carcinogens. However, addition of an activated Harvey v-*ras* oncogene to HPV-immortalized keratinocytes renders them tumorigenic. Likewise, introducing the transforming region of the herpesvirus type 2 genome (*Bgl*II N fragment) also converts the cells to a tumorigenic phenotype. Neither gene had a demonstrable effect on normal keratinocytes. One keratinocyte line immortalized by HPV-18 DNA underwent tumorigenic conversion. For up to 12 passages, the cells were nontumorigenic in nude mice, but they became weakly tumorigenic after 32 passages and highly tumorigenic after 62 passages. Cytogenetic analysis revealed a correlation between tumorigenicity and chromosomal abnormalities. These results suggest that a stepwise progression of events is necessary for HPV-infected cells to convert from immortalized to fully transformed cells. The development of cancer likely arises from interactions of the viral oncoproteins with host tumor suppressor gene products. p53 is required for G_1 cell cycle arrest after DNA damage to allow for repair. E6 perturbs G_1 arrest after damage, presumably through its interaction with p53. This would allow accumulation of mutations that could eventually lead to the malignant phenotype.

Although papillomaviruses are not sufficient in themselves to induce malignant transformation, protection from infection by the virus or treatment of infected persons through vaccination with viral structural or nonstructural immunogens is feasible. Health care notwithstanding, development of such vaccines would be of significant financial benefit since it has been estimated that diagnosis and treatment of HPV-associated genital tract neoplasms cost many billions of dollars each year in the United States.

IV. HEPATITIS B VIRUS AND LIVER CANCER

Hepatitis B virus (HBV), a member of the Hepadnaviridae, is a hepatotropic DNA virus that causes acute and chronic liver cell damage and inflammation. The virus is a 42-nm particle consisting of a circular 3200-bp genome; the smallest of all known animal viruses. An endogenous DNA polymerase–reverse transcriptase activity is encased in a nucleocapsid that is surrounded by a glycoprotein envelope.

The DNA is gapped in one strand (the plus strand) and contains a terminal protein linked to the 5′ end of the complementary DNA minus strand. Replication of the viral genome occurs through an RNA pregenome produced by reverse transcription that involves the terminal protein during priming of DNA synthesis and is catalyzed by DNA polymerase–reverse transcriptase and RNase H activities.

The genome of the virus is so highly compact that much of the genome participates in multiple functions, such that the same nucleotides code for more than one protein and transcriptional regulatory elements are embedded within coding sequences. The virus genome (Fig. 2) contains four open reading frames on the minus strand. The C gene encodes the major nucleocapsid polypeptide. Three related viral surface–antigen polypeptides found in the virion envelope and in surface–antigen particles found in the serum of infected patients (HBV surface antigen or HBsAg) are encoded by the S gene. The P gene encodes the DNA polymerase–reverse transcriptase and RNase H activities and the terminal protein. The X gene encodes a polypeptide that activates transcription of the core promoter from the viral enhancer.

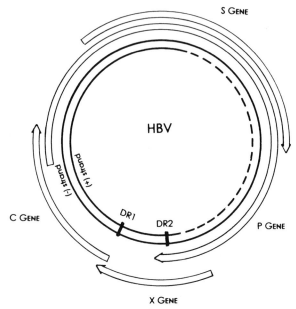

FIGURE 2 Structural organization of the HBV genome. The dashed line on the (+) strand represents the single-stranded region of the virus genome. Open arrows represent overlapping open reading frames.

After infection has occurred, there is approximately a 4-week incubation period before HBsAg is detected in the blood. For a while, the patient may remain healthy, but 60–180 days after infection clinical symptoms appear with elevated levels of serum aminotransferases. The clinical symptoms resolve in approximately 4 weeks with normalization of liver function and clearance of HBsAg from the blood. HBV infection at an early age is common, and the virus persists in populations where it is endemic such as eastern Asia and sub-Saharan Africa. Epidemiological studies have shown a geographic correspondence of rates of HBV infection and hepatocellular carcinoma (HCC). HBV is the major risk factor for development of HCC, and virus DNA sequences have been detected in about 85% of the cancers. Prospective studies indicate that 40% or more of middle-aged Chinese men with chronic HBV infection die of HCC. The chronic carrier state and risk for HCC is associated with persisting HBsAg in the blood. In a prospective study, the incidence of HCC was more than 200-fold higher in HBsAg carriers than among noncarriers in Taiwan. Although HBV sequences were found in HCC in some patients without other signs of HBV infection, most had HBV markers (anti-HBsAg antibodies or anti-hepatitis B core antigen antibodies, or both).

Infected hepatocytes contain episomal HBV DNA, integrated forms, or a combination of both. Episomal DNA is detected during the acute phase and some chronic stages of HBV infection. Integrated viral DNA generally is observed during chronic infection and especially in HCC. The presence of only episomal HBV sequences in HCC in the absence of integrated forms has not been reported. It is believed that integrated HBV sequences may be a pathogenic factor for tumor development. This is underscored by the fact that more than 90% of patients with HBsAg serum levels and HCC have clonally integrated HBV DNA in their cancers. These tumors must have arisen from clonal expansion of a cell containing a viral integrant. However, HCC usually have multiple clonal integrants, each at a different chromosomal site. There also exist contiguous linear HBV sequences without rearrangement in some HCC. This is in contrast to other HCC that appear to contain multiple integrated viral genomes with or without postintegration rearrangements.

It is unclear whether integrated HBV sequences play a direct role in HCC. An analysis of integration patterns of HBV sequences in tumors revealed that they were relatively simple in structure in that they did not show major rearrangements of virus DNA. Integration into the host genome appears to be random. One end of the integrated HBV DNA is near the 5′ end of DR1, one of two direct repeats present in the viral genome (Fig. 2). All HBV integrations are associated with deletion of approximately 10 bp of cellular DNA at the site of integration, although some show more extensive deletion of cell sequences. In most instances, rearrangements to either or both viral and flanking sequences can be observed. Other than the presence of free virus DNA, HBV integration patterns in livers of chronic carriers are similar to those seen in HCC; rearrangements to viral DNA and/or host flanking sequences usually are detected. These rearrangements thus appear to occur before malignant transformation. Furthermore, integrated rearranged HBV sequences in the absence of rearrangements of flanking cellular sequences suggest that deletions and rearrangements to the HBV genome may occur before integration.

Although integration of HBV DNA appears to be associated with HCC, the mechanism of integration and its effect on genetic expression are not well understood. However, HBV can act as an insertional mutagen and does cause frequent chromosome changes. In the woodchuck hepatitis virus model, integration of viral sequences in HCC in this species frequently is associated with activation of known oncogenes. The number of reports of integration of HBV near known oncogenes, however, are limited. Thus, cis-activation of protooncogenes in the development of HCC in humans may not play a major role in malignant transformation of infected hepatocytes. Although chromosomal abnormalities at the site of HBV integration are a common feature in HCC, the effect this has on genetic disruption is not known. However, HBV sequences have been found to be integrated in the coding sequences of the retinoic acid receptor B gene and the cyclin A gene. This integration could disrupt cell growth control. In addition HBV integration in HCC was identified on chromosome 17p, resulting in the loss of one allele of the tumor-suppressor gene p53. Although 30–60% of samples showed a loss of heterozygosity at the p53 locus, allelic loss also was observed at other chromosomal locations. Mutations of the p53 gene have been found in HCC. Most of these are single point mutations occurring in exons 5–8 and have been found in about 50% of HCC; this is similar to the frequency of p53 mutations detected in breast, lung, and colon cancers.

Hepatitis B virus, like many viruses, encodes functions that activate transcription from the viral promoter. The HBV X open reading frame encodes a transcriptional trans-activator that stimulates transcription from its own promoter and the promoters for the human interferon-β gene and the RNA polymerase II and III genes. This trans-activation appears to depend on protein–protein interactions between X and cellular transcription factors that interact with transcriptional regulatory elements, rather than direct binding of X to a particular DNA sequence. It is unlikely that this interaction alone explains the oncogenic potential of HBV. Integration of HBV frequently results in interruption of the X gene open reading frame. Fusion of HBV X to a downstream cellular gene that has DNA-binding activity could target the trans-activating activity of X to new transcriptional regulatory sequences, perhaps to a gene associated with cellular proliferation. The unscheduled expression of such a gene could result in uncontrolled cellular growth. The X protein has been found to have protein kinase activity. Phosphorylation of proteins by X through redirection of targeting also may have an impact on gene expression.

Hepatitis B virus sequences do not transform cultured primary hepatocytes. However, a line of immortalized nontumorigenic fully differentiated liver cells from a transgenic mouse carrying the simian virus 40 (SV40) T antigen under control of a heterologous promoter become tumorigenic in nude mice after transfection with HBV sequences. The tumors are differentiated or anaplastic and contain rearranged integrated viral sequences similar to those seen in human HCC. Most tumors and tumor-derived cell lines expressed the X gene product. However, it is unknown whether expression of the X gene confers tumorigenic potential in this system. Nevertheless, HBV gene expression (including that of the X gene) occurs for prolonged periods in infected hepatocytes *in vivo* without HCC formation. Thus X

gene expression for months or years appears insufficient to cause HCC. Moreover, the long latency for HCC suggests that an accumulation of mutational events is required for malignant phenotypic expression and that HBV may act indirectly.

Transgenic mice that overexpress the HBV envelope glycoprotein show liver cell injury, inflammation, and regenerative hyperplasia. In most animals, HCC follows with high levels of expression of the transgene. Hepatocyte regeneration would expand the proliferation of cells at high risk for mutations that deregulate cell growth. The finding that HBV transgene expression acts synergistically with hepatocarcinogens shows that, in these animals, liver regeneration is a factor in HCC malignant transformation. Chronic HBV infections in humans produces inflammation and cellular injury, resulting in mild cirrhosis. Cirrhosis from hepatitis C (an RNA virus that does not integrate) likewise places the patient at increased risk for HCC. The indolent nature of viral induced liver damage (resulting in hepatocyte regeneration and scarring after inflammation) provides evidence that the association of HBV with HCC may be more indirect rather than direct oncogenesis resulting from the interaction of viral sequences or gene products with the host genome. It has been established by epidemiological studies that chronic HBV infection is an important factor in the development of HCC. However, it is equally clear that the mechanism of HCC development as a result of HBV infection is not well defined. On the basis of the evidence thus far, HCC may be caused by a combination of direct viral effects and an accumulation of mutational events in liver cells undergoing reparative regeneration.

V. HERPESVIRUSES AND HUMAN CANCER

A. General Characteristics of Herpesviruses

Herpesviruses are composed of an icosahedral capsid surrounded by a cell-derived membrane modified with viral glycoproteins. The capsid contains a double-stranded unsegmented DNA genome of 90–200 kilobases (kb). The viral genome encodes several enzymes that participate in its own DNA replication and macromolecular metabolism. Several viral gene products act as trans-acting factors that affect gene expression. These factors activate or suppress the expression of other viral or cellular genes, and the different viral genes are expressed in a cascade manner, with some of them influencing in *trans* their own as well as the transcription and expression of other genes. The DNA is believed to replicate following a rolling-circle model without associating with cellular histones. Virus particles are assembled in the nucleus. A peculiarity of repetitive sequences flanking one or more unique large segments. In genomes containing more than one unique region flanked by these repeats, the unique segments are found in viral progeny in all possible reciprocal arrangements. This property is not a requisite for replication and is believed to be an epiphenomenon of intragenomic homologous recombination between the repetitive sequences.

On the basis of their biological properties the family Herpesviridae has been classified in three subfamilies, namely, the Alpha-, Beta-, and Gammaherpesvirinae. As a rule all herpesviruses are able to induce latency after infection of specific resting cells. Latency is associated with the expression of a small subset of the viral genes. Several animal herpesviruses have been known to be the etiological agent of lymphomas in fowl (Marek's disease) and renal adenocarcinoma in frogs (Lucké herpesvirus).

B. Epstein-Barr Virus

Epstein-Barr virus (EBV) is a member of the subfamily Gamma herpesvirinae. The viral genome is flanked by terminal repeats and five unique regions that are also bound by internal repeats. The viral genome is linear, but circular forms are often detected in latent infection. Permissive replicative infection takes place in epithelial cells of the oropharynx. It can also be induced in latently infected B cells *in vitro* by stimuli such as exposure to phorbol esters or induction of expression of the EBV ZEBRA polypeptide, a virus-encoded trans-acting factor that activates the EBV lytic cycle.

Epstein-Barr virus is the etiological agent of infectious mononucleosis, an acute disease related to the nonproductive latent infection of B lymphocytes. Although patients usually undergo a full clinical recovery, their B cells continue to harbor the virus in an episomal form. This latent infection is not without consequence to the biology of these cells, as they are readily stimulated to grow *in vitro*. In fact, artificial infection of peripheral lymphocytes with EBV is a common laboratory procedure for cellular lymphocyte immortalization. In most individuals EBV latency, infectious mononucleosis, and latent infection of B lymphocytes are not related to lymphoblastic proliferative disorders. However, EBV has been related to the pathogenesis of at least two human malignancies: Burkitt's lymphoma and nasopharyngeal carcinoma.

In B lymphocytes EBV causes latent infection characterized by a limited expression of its genes and tightly controlled DNA replication. Only 10 EBV genes are expressed during B-cell latent infection. Two of the genes (EBER-1 and EBER-2) are the most abundantly expressed and are the only ones transcribed by RNA polymerase III. Six others encode nuclear proteins (EBNA-1, -2, -3A, -3B, -3C, and -LP) and two correspond to membrane proteins (LMP-1 and -2). In general, similar genetic expression is observed in EBV genomes present in cultured cells from Burkitt's lymphomas or infectious mononucleosis. The EBERs and EBNAs, and particularly EBNA-LP, are considered to be trans-acting factors. The EBER RNAs are homologous to a cellular uracil-rich RNA involved in processing of pre-mRNAs. EBER RNAs are suspected to be involved in the regulation of alternate virus RNA splicing during latent infection. EBNA-1 interacts with EBV DNA at one of the two origins for DNA replication and is considered to be required for episome maintenance and replication. EBNA-2 is considered a trans-activator of viral gene expression. It activates the expression of cellular CD23 (a soluble autocrine lymphocytic growth factor). EBNA-LP is associated with EBV nuclear RNA and could play a role in posttranscriptional processing of RNA. B-Cell immortalization and growth are considered to be direct results of EBNA-2 activation of CD23 expression together with the association of LMP with membrane and cytoskeleton components. The presence of LMP in the cellular membrane also affects intracellular free calcium and the lymphoblast response to transforming growth factor-β (TGF-β). The viral genome persists in cell nuclei as a circular episomal element replicated by cell DNA polymerase. Replication occurs only once at the beginning of each S phase. In this circumstance the viral genome seems to associate itself with chromosomal proteins. The viral DNA can occasionally become integrated in the cellular genome.

Burkitt's lymphoma is endemic in children in areas of central Africa exposed to other tropical diseases, particularly malaria. These tumors contain specific reciprocal chromosomal translocations: 80% contain t(8;14)(q24;q32), and the remaining 20% show either t(2;8)(p11;q24) or t(8;22)(q24;q11). Interestingly, the genes for the immunoglobulin heavy chain map to 4q32, and those for the κ and λ light chains map to 2p11 and 22q11. More interesting is the fact that c-myc, the human homolog of the avian myeloblastosis virus oncogene v-myc, maps to 8q24. In all cases the translocation brings c-myc close to and under the transcriptional control of the promoter for an immunoglobulin gene constitutively activated in B cells. The chromosome break and juxtaposition are heterogeneous, but they are not random. Humoral immune diversity is the consequence of genetic shuffling carried out by the V–D–J joining system of recombination enzymes and by the process of isotype switching carried out by switching enzymes. Interestingly, both the V–D–J system and the switching enzymes are known to affect precisely the same sites involved in the reciprocal translocations seen in Burkitt's lymphoma. Chromosome 14 breaks occur in the VH, DH, and JH regions and in the switch regions Cμ, Cγ, and Cα. Breaks in chromosome 8 always occur near the c-myc 5′ end either before or within the first exon or intron. The second exon, which contains the functional ATG start codon, is always intact, and the c-myc polypeptide product is identical to the normal gene product (i.e., no chimeric protein is expressed). The lymphoma is believed to be the result of uncontrolled cellular proliferation secondary to the abnormal constitutive expression of c-myc within the B cell. EBV is believed to contribute to the cell phenotype by its immortalizing capabilities and promotion of chromosome rearrangements.

Nasopharyngeal carcinoma originates in the stratified nasopharyngeal epithelium of the pharynx and upper respiratory tract and, as such, represents a special type of squamous cell carcinoma. This malignancy is more frequent among individuals from Southern China, a fact that has raised suspicions about genetic and dietary factors such as the nitrosamines present in salted fish. The association of EBV with this malignancy is strong both epidemiologically and at the molecular level. The expression of EBV DNA in this cancer differs from that seen in Burkitt's lymphoma and infectious mononucleosis in two aspects. First, expression of the genes during latent infection is restricted to EBNA-1 and LMP, and several of the early viral genes that are normally expressed during permissive infection are also detected. Second, no cytogenetic alterations or abnormal protooncogene expression have been associated with these carcinomas.

In rare instances EBV infection and infectious monucleosis are associated with fatal diffuse lymphoproliferative disease and malignant lymphomas. One-half of these cases are seen in males with an X-linked immune defect (X-linked lymphoproliferative syndrome or XLPS).

C. Herpesviruses and Kaposi Sarcoma

Until the 1970s Kaposi sarcoma (KS) was a rare skin neoplasia observed only in older men of Mediterranean origin. The detection of a high incidence of this tumor in younger and never-married males was one of the first signs of the AIDS epidemic. An interesting epidemiological puzzle was the fact that KS is almost exclusively seen in HIV-positive gay men and is very rare in HIV-positive individuals infected transparenterally (non-gay intravenous drug users and hemophiliacs). This has pointed to the possibility of a concomitant non-blood-borne infectious agent transmissible by homosexual contact. Several viral agents had been suspected including two herpesviruses (cytomegalovirus and human herpesvirus 6), but no association could be substantiated. However, using polymerase chain reaction-based methods, a carefully conducted study provided evidence that KS cells of HIV-positive gay males contain DNA sequences that share homology with but are different from those of known herpes-viruses. The sequences were detected in over 90% of KS specimens and 15% of non-KS tissues from HIV-positive gay males. They were not detected in non-KS tissues from HIV-negative individuals. This virus has now been classified as human herpesvirus 8 (HHV-8). The conclusion is that these sequences correspond to a new herpesvirus that is fastidious but not particularly ubiquitous. The strongest genomic resemblance of this virus is to two other gammaherpesviruses of known oncogenicity: herpesvirus saimiri, a virus infecting squirrel monkeys, and EBV. More work is required to substantiate this claim, isolate the virus and postulate a plausible oncogenic mechanism. However, it can be speculated that the oncogenic potential of this virus may be synergistic with the induction by the HIV *tat* trans-activator protein of cytokines and other growth factors.

D. Herpes Simplex Virus and Cervical Cancer

In the 1970s, herpes simplex virus type 2 (HSV-2), a member of the subfamily Alphaherpesvirinae, was thought to be closely related to cervical cancer. This link was based mainly on seroepidemiological data showing that the prevalence of long-lasting anti-HSV-2 antibodies (indicative of incidence of past infection) was significantly higher in women with cervical cancer than in matched controls. However, the evidence for the presence of viral genomic sequences in transformed cells was never conclusive, and clear evidence for cell transformation has remained elusive. Some specific HSV-2 subgenomic DNA fragments artificially isolated and introduced into susceptible cells can induce morphological changes in cultured cells that alter their growth characteristics. However, the biological significance of these findings in human disease remains speculative since these viral fragments have never been consistently found in cervical cancer cells. In some specific resting cells HSV can modulate its own gene expression to control its growth and remain latent. However, for epithelial cells HSV is aggressively lytic. Natural transformation of these cells by HSV would require their exposure to virions defective for epithelial cell lysis. Although HSV replication under special *in vitro* conditions can generate such virions, their emergence and pathogenicity in a natural host remain speculative.

The association of HSV-2 with cervical cancer rests only on the strength of the seroepidemiological association and lacks a clear biological mechanism at the cellular and molecular level that could validate the association. It should be pointed out that HSV-2, unlike HPV, is not an independent risk factor for cervi-

cal cancer if one stratifies for risk factors of sexually transmitted diseases in general such as number of sexual partners. The compelling evidence on the role of some HPV types in the etiology of cervical cancer would suggest no peripheral role for HSV in this malignancy. Some groups persist in considering HSV as a cofactor with HPV in the causation of cervical cancer; however, the association of HSV-2 with these lesions is likely only circumstantial, reflecting similarities in the epidemiological patterns of these two sexually transmitted human viruses.

See Also the Following Articles

DNA Tumor Viruses: Adenovirus • Epstein-Barr Virus and Associated Malignancies • Hepatitis B Viruses • Hepatitis C Virus • HIV • Human T-Cell Leukemia/Lymphotropic Virus • Papillomaviruses • Retroviruses

Bibliography

Blattner, W. W. (1991). Human retroviruses and malignancy. *In* "Origins of Human Cancer: A Comprehensive Review" (J. Brugge, T. Curran, E. Harlow, and F. McCormick, eds.), p. 199. Cold Spring Harbor Laboratory, Cold Spring Harbor, New York.

Chang, Y., Cesarman, E., Pessin, M. S., Lee, F., Culpepper, J., Knowles, D. M., and More, P. (1994). Identification of herpesvirus-like DNA sequences in AIDS-associated Kaposi's sarcomas. *Science* **266,** 1865.

Daefler, S., and Wong-Staal, F. (1991). Molecular biology of human retroviruses and their relation to cancer. *In* "Molecular Foundations of Oncology" (S. Broder, ed.), p. 229. Williams & Wilkins, Baltimore, Maryland.

Gauwerky, C. E., and Croce, C. M. (1993). Chromosomal translocations in leukaemia. *Semin. Cancer Biol.* **4,** 333.

Knowles, D. M. (1993). Biologic aspects of AIDS-associated non-Hodgkin's lymphoma. *Curr. Opin. Oncol.* **5,** 845.

Lancaster, W. D., and Reid, R. (1994). Human papillomavirus. *In* "Obstetric and Gynecologic Infectious Disease" (J. G. Pastorek, ed.), p. 555. Raven, New York.

Lutwick, L. I. (1991). Hepatitis B virus. *In* "Textbook of Human Virology" (R. B. Belsche, ed.), 2nd Ed., p. 719. Mosby Year Book, St. Louis, Missouri.

Miller, G. (1990). Epstein-Barr virus: Biology, pathogenesis and medical aspects. *In* "Fields' Virology" (B. N. Fields and D. M. Knipe, eds.), p. 1921. Raven, New York.

Robinson, W. S. (1994). Molecular events in the pathogenesis of hepadnavirus-associated hepatocellular carcinoma. *Annu. Rev. Med.* **45,** 297.

zur Hausen, H. (1994). Molecular pathogenesis of cancer of the cervix and its causation by specific human papillomavirus types. *Curr. Top. Microbiol. Immunol.* **186,** 131.

von Hippel–Lindau Disease

William G. Kaelin

Dana-Farber Cancer Institute and Harvard Medical School

GLOSSARY

hemangioblastoma A slowly growing benign tumor made up of proliferating capillary vessel-forming endothelial cells.

hypoxia-inducible factor A sequence-specific DNA-binding transcription factor that binds to DNA as a heterodimer with the aryl hydrocarbon nuclear translocator protein.

pheochromocytoma A tumor derived from adrenal medullary tissue, often capable of secreting catecholamines.

proteasome A large cytosolic multiprotein complex that degrades proteins.

retinal angioma A blood vessel tumor of the retina with histopathologic features of a hemangioblastoma.

ubiquitin A specific 76 residue polypeptide.

ubiquitination Covalent attachment of ubiquitin to a target protein via the formation of an isopeptide bond. Subsequent attachment of additional ubiquitin molecules as a result of ubiquitin–ubiquitin covalent bonds leads to a polyubiquitin chain that is recognized by the proteasome.

G ermline mutations of the *VHL* tumor suppressor gene cause the von Hippel–Lindau (VHL) hereditary cancer syndrome, and somatic VHL mutations are important in sporadic kidney cancer and sporadic central nervous system hemangioblastoma. This article briefly reviews the clinical features of the VHL syndrome and describes our current understanding of the biochemical and cellular activities of the VHL gene product, pVHL.

I. VON HIPPEL–LINDAU (VHL) SYNDROME

A. Clinical Features

The von Hippel–Lindau hereditary cancer syndrome was first described in the medical literature approximately 100 years ago. In some VHL families it has been possible to trace the origins of VHL disease to as early as the 18th century. The hallmark features of this disease are retinal angiomas and central nervous system hemangioblastomas (particularly of the cerebellum and spinal cord). Histopathologically, retinal angiomas and central nervous system hemangioblastomas are indistinguishable from one another and consist of proliferating blood vessels admixed with a poorly understood stromal cell. Some VHL patients also develop additional tumors, including clear cell carcinomas of the kidney, pheochromocytomas, islet cell tumors of the pancreas, and endolymphatic sac tumors (Table I). VHL patients also frequently develop benign cysts of various viscera, including the kidneys, liver, and pancreas. The majority of VHL patients will present in early adulthood and die in the third to fifth decade. Hemangioblastoma and renal cell carcinoma are the two leading causes of death.

B. Genetics

Clinically, VHL disease displays an autosomal-dominant pattern of inheritance and affects approximately 1/35,000 individuals. Linkage analysis of VHL kindreds shows that the VHL susceptibility gene resides at chromosome 3p25, a region of the genome that is frequently altered in sporadic kidney cancers. Using this information, a consortium headed by Marston Linehan, Michael Lerman, and Bert Zbar at the National Cancer Insitute and Eamon Maher at the University of Cambridge cloned the *VHL* gene in 1993. The authenticity of this gene was established by showing that germline mutations of the *VHL* gene segregated with the development of VHL disease in VHL families. Essentially all individuals with a clinical diagnosis of VHL disease carry a germline mutation of the *VHL* gene if one employs a battery of screening methodologies, including direct DNA sequence analysis and quantitative Southern blot analysis. The latter is important for detecting those individuals in which the entire maternal or paternal VHL allele is deleted from the germ line.

TABLE I
VHL-Associated Neoplasms

Retinal angioma
Central nervous system hemangioblastoma
Clear cell renal carcinoma
Pheochromocytoma
Endolymphatic sac tumor
Epididymal cystadenoma

At the molecular level, VHL disease conforms to the "Knudson two-hit model" insofar as the development of pathology is linked to the somatic inactivation or loss of the remaining wild-type *VHL* allele in a susceptible cell. Biallelic inactivation of *VHL* can be demonstrated in the epithelial cells that line the renal cysts observed in VHL disease. It is presumed that additional genetic alterations are required to convert these cyst epithelial cells into frank carcinomas. Likewise, loss of the remaining wild-type *VHL* allele has been demonstrated in the stromal cell compartment of VHL-associated angiomata and hemangioblastomas.

In keeping with the Knudson two-hit model, *VHL* mutations are common in sporadic (nonhereditary) clear cell renal carcinomas and sporadic hemangioblastomas. In addition, some renal carcinomas and hemangioblastomas that retain a wild-type *VHL* allele fail to produce *VHL* mRNA due to hypermethylation of the *VHL* locus. One would also expect to find *VHL* mutations in sporadic pheochromocytomas, but this is rarely the case. Why the Knudson two-hit model is seemingly violated in this setting is not clear.

Genotype–phenotype correlations are emerging in VHL disease. VHL families can be subdivided into those with low risk (type 1) and high risk (type 2) of developing pheochromocytoma. Type 2 families almost always harbor a *VHL* missense mutation, whereas type 1 families may have *VHL* mutations that lead to gross alterations in pVHL or a complete absence of pVHL. Type 2 VHL disease can be further subdivided based on the risk of renal cell carcinoma (where type 2A denotes low risk and type 2B denotes high risk). A variant of VHL disease has been described (type 2C) in which individuals develop pheochromocytomas but are at a low risk for hemangioblastomas and renal cell carcinomas. The association of missense mutations with the development of pheochromocytoma may reflect a "gain of function" by certain pVHL mutants. Alternatively, complete loss of pVHL function may not be tolerated by the precursor cells that give rise to these tumors

II. VHL GENE STRUCTURE AND EXPRESSION

The human *VHL* gene consists of three exons and an unusually long 3′-untranslated region that contains multiple Alu repeat sequences. The promoter lacks a TATA box and contains binding sites for multiple transcription factors, including SP1, nuclear respiratory factor 1, and PAX. *VHL* homologues have also been identified in mouse, rat, and drosophila.

The human *VHL* gene gives rise to two mRNA transcripts due to alternative splicing. The long form, which is ~3.5 kb in length, is encoded by exons 1, 2, and 3. The short form lacks exon 2. Because some renal carcinomas produce only the short VHL mRNA, it is assumed that this VHL mRNA isoform lacks tumor suppressor function (at least with respect to the kidney). The *VHL* gene is ubiquitously expressed during development and in the adult. In particular, *VHL* expression is not restricted solely to those tissues affected in VHL disease.

VHL +/− mice develop normally and do not appear to be tumor prone. *VHL* −/− mice die at embryonic days 10.5–12.5 due, at least partly, to abnormal placental development. *VHL* −/− embryos also exhibit defects in extracellular matrix formation. Disruption of *VHL* function in drosophila by RNA interference leads to abnormal tracheal development. The drosophila tracheal system and mammalian vasculature are thought to be evolutionarily related.

III. VHL PROTEIN

A. Primary Sequence

The *VHL* mRNA gives rise to two protein isoforms due to the use of alternative in-frame translation initiation sites. The long form of the protein consists of 213 amino acid residues and migrates with an apparent molecular mass of ~28–30 kDa. The short form of the protein, resulting from internal translational initiation from codon 54, migrates with an apparent molecular mass of ~18 kDa. Why cells produce two VHL proteins is not clear, as they appear to be similar in the biochemical and biological assays performed to date. Of note, disease-associated VHL missense mutations always map C-terminal to codon 54, suggesting that both isoforms must be inactivated for tumors to develop. The similarity among VHL proteins from different species is greatest in the region 54–213, which again underscores the functional significance of the short form of the VHL protein. For the remainder of this article, the term "pVHL" is used generically when referring to both long and short VHL gene products.

The pVHL protein sequence is not highly similar to other known proteins and, in particular, does not contain any immediately recognizable structural motifs. The N terminus of the long form contains an acidic pentameric repeat of unknown significance. The long form of pVHL also contains multiple potential casein kinase II phosphorylation sites, and phosphorylation of the long form of pVHL can be detected in cells. The significance of pVHL phosphorylation is unknown.

B. Subcellular Localization

pVHL resides primarily in the cytoplasm, but significant amounts of pVHL can also be detected in nuclei and in association with membrane fractions. pVHL can shuttle between the nucleus and the cytoplasm. pVHL export requires sequences encoded by exon 2, is Ran mediated, and requires ATP hydrolysis. Blockade of RNA polymerase II function leads to nuclear accumulation of pVHL. pVHL variants that cannot shuttle by virtue of fusion to heterologous nuclear import or export sequences can no longer inhibit the accumulation of hypoxia-inducible mRNAs (see later).

C. Cellular Functions

Reintroduction of either the short or the long form of pVHL suppresses the tumor growth of pVHL-defective renal carcinoma cells in nude mouse xenograft studies consistent with its purported role as a tumor suppressor protein. In monolayer cultures, loss of pVHL leads to an impaired cell cycle exit in response to growth factor deprivation, and in spheroid growth assays, pVHL leads to decreased cellular proliferation and enhanced cellular differentiation. Cells lacking pVHL accumulate inappropriately high levels of the α subunits of the HIF (hypoxia-inducible factor) in the presence of oxygen and consequently overproduce a variety of hypoxia-inducible mRNAs, including those encoding VEGF, the GLUT1 glucose transporter, and the PDGF β chain. The biochemical basis for HIF deregulation in pVHL-defective cells is described later. A number of other pVHL target genes have been identified (see Table II). For some of these targets, it is not known whether the observed effects of pVHL are due, directly or indirectly, to changes in HIF. For example, pVHL downregulates the production of matrix metalloproteinase mRNAs and upregulates the production of tissue inhibitors of metalloproteinase mRNAs. This activity has been linked to the suppression of cellular invasiveness in response to hepatocyte growth factor/scatter factor by pVHL. pVHL also regulates the production of TGFα and TGFβ, both of which can affect renal epithelial cell growth.

D. Biochemical Activities

1. Binding to Elongins and Cul2

pVHL forms stable multimeric complexes that contain elongin C, elongin B, and Cul2 (Fig. 1). Elongin C binds directly to pVHL. Cul2 binds to elongin C, and the complex is stabilized by elongin B. Elongin C resembles the yeast protein Skp1 and Cul2 resembles the yeast protein Cdc53. In yeast, Skp1 and Cdc53 likewise bind to one another in conjunction with an "F-box protein" (so named because of a collinear motif first identified in cyclin F) to target specific proteins for ubiquitin-dependent proteolysis. The F-box

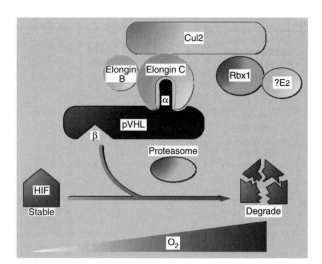

FIGURE 1   Model for pVHL action. pVHL contains two subdomains called α and β. The α domain binds to elongin C, which, in turn, binds to elongin B and Cul2. Cul2 binds to a protein called Rbx1 (or Roc1), which likely recruits an as yet unidentified ubiquitin-conjugating enzyme (E2). The β domain is a substrate-binding domain. In the presence of oxygen, the pVHL complex binds to HIF, leading to HIF ubiquitination. Ubiquitinated HIF is then destroyed by the proteasome. From Kaelin, W. G. (1999). *Nature* **399**, 203–204, with permission.

TABLE II
VHL Target Genes

VEGF, vascular endothelial growth factor
GLUT-1, glucose transporter 1
AK-3, adenylate kinase 3
TGF-β1, transforming growth factor β1
TGF-α, transforming growth factor α
ALD-A, aldolase
PGK-1, phosphoglycerate kinase
PFK-C, phosphofructose kinase C
LDH-A, lactate dehydrogenase A
PDGF-B, platelet-derived growth factor B chain
CA12, carbonic anhydrase 12
CA9, carbonic anhydrase 9
TIMP-1, tissue inhibitor of metalloproteinase
TIMP-2, tissue inhibitor of metalloproteinase
MMP-2, matrix metalloproteinases 2
MMP-9, matrix metalloproteinases 9

component of SCF (Skp1-Cdc53-F-box) complexes binds directly to the protein that will be ubiquitinated, whereas the Skp1/Cdc53 proteins recruit the ubiquitination machinery.

The crystal structure of pVHL bound to elongins B and C has been solved. It reveals that pVHL contains two structural subdomains that are frequently mutated in VHL disease. The α domain consists of three helices that bind to a helix in elongin C to form an intermolecular four-helical bundle. One of the pVHL helices, corresponding to residues 157–172, loosely resembles an F-box motif and *in vitro* is necessary and sufficient for elongin binding. The β domain, described in greater detail later, was inferred to be a substrate docking site because many VHL-associated mutations lead to alterations of surface residues within this region of the protein. Finally, the structure of elongin C resembles that of Skp1.

2. Ubiquitination of HIF

Currently, the best understood targets of the pVHL/elongin/Cul2 complex are the related proteins HIF1α and HIF2α. These two transcription factors are normally degraded under well-oxygenated conditions. In the absence of oxygen, these proteins become stable and activate transcription by binding to specific DNA sequences as heterodimers with ARNT. Cells lacking pVHL are unable to degrade HIF. In the presence of oxygen, HIF binds directly to the pVHL β domain and is ubiquitinated. Ubiquitinated HIF can then be degraded by the proteasome. All VHL mutants associated with classical VHL disease tested to date demonstrate an impaired ability to ubiquitinate HIF. *In vitro*, ubiquitination of HIF by pVHL is blocked in the presence of iron chelators, which have been used in the past as hypoxia mimetics, as well as by synthetic peptides that block the association of pVHL with the elongins and Cul2.

3. Binding to Fibronectin

pVHL binds to fibronectin. This interaction appears to take place in association with the endoplasmic reticulum. The structural requirements for this interaction are unknown. All disease-associated pVHL mutants tested to date have lost the ability to interact with fibronectin. pVHL-defective tumor cells, as well as VHL −/− mouse embryo fibroblasts, display profound defects in the formation of an extracellular fibronectin matrix. Whether and how the biochemical interaction of fibronectin with pVHL affects its subsequent ability to form extracellular fibrillar arrays is unknown. There is currently no evidence that pVHL is, itself, a secreted protein. A possible role of pVHL in the clearance or surveillance of proteins in the endoplasmic reticulum is supported by the finding that pVHL-defective cells are very sensitive to treatments that cause an accumulation of malfolded or malprocessed proteins in the endoplasmic reticulum.

4. Folding by CCT

pVHL interacts with the cytosolic chaperonin complex CCT through sequences encoded by exon 2. The interaction with CCT is likely important for the proper folding of the pVHL/elongin complex. pVHL folds poorly in the absence of elongins. In cells, however, elongins appear to be in vast excess of pVHL and thus it is likely that all of the pVHL is in complex with elongins B and C. pVHL mutants that cannot bind to the elongins are retained on CCT.

5. Binding to PKC

pVHL can bind to atypical PKC isoforms via pVHL residues 73–122. It should be noted that the interaction of pVHL with PKC has thus far only been detected using overproduced binding partners, and some disease-associated pVHL mutants retain the ability to bind to PKC. It has been suggested that pVHL may inhibit PKC function, perhaps through a sequestration mechanism. Inhibition of PKC function downregulates VEGF production in cells, perhaps through changes in Sp1 phosphorylation (see also later).

6. Binding to Sp1

A pVHL subdomain comprising residues 96–122 can bind to Sp1. As was true for PKC, the interaction of pVHL and Sp1 has thus far only been observed in overproduction studies, and some disease-associated pVHL mutants retain the ability to bind to Sp1. It has been suggested that inhibition of Sp1 may contribute to the ability of pVHL to downregulate the VEGF promoter.

IV. SUMMARY AND CONCLUSIONS

von Hippel–Lindau disease is a hereditary cancer syndrome in which blood vessel tumors (hemangioblastomas) of the central nervous system and retina are cardinal features. Some VHL patients also develop other tumors, including clear cell carcinomas of the kidney and pheochromocytomas. The disease is caused by germline mutations in the *VHL* tumor suppressor gene. The product of the *VHL* gene, pVHL, forms multiprotein complexes that target members of the HIF transcription factor family for ubiquitin-dependent proteolysis. Deregulation of HIF target genes, such as the gene encoding VEGF, is likely responsible for the vascular nature of VHL-associated neoplasms. pVHL has also been implicated in the control of extracellular matrix deposition and turnover, as well as in the control of cell cycle exit and differentiation.

See Also the Following Articles

NEUROBLASTOMA • RETINOBLASTOMA TUMOR SUPPRESSOR GENE • TUMOR SUPPRESSOR GENES: SPECIFIC CLASSES

Bibliography

Adryan, B., Decker, H.-J. H., Papas, T. S., and Hsu, T. (2000). Tracheal development and the von Hippel-Lindau tumor suppressor homolog in Drosophila. *Oncogene* **19,** 2803–2811

Cockman, M., Masson, N., Mole, D., Jaakkola, P., Chang, G., Clifford, S., Maher, E., Pugh, C., Ratcliffe, P., and Maxwell, P. (2000). Hypoxia inducible factor-alpha binding and ubiquitylation by the von Hippel-Lindau tumor suppressor protein. *J. Biol. Chem* **275,** 25733–25741.

Cohen, H., Zhou, M., Welsh, A., Zarghamee, S., Scholz, H., Mukhopadhyay, D., Kishida, T., Zbar, B., Knebelmann, B., and Sukhatme, V. (1999). An important von Hippel-Lindau tumor suppressor domain mediates Sp1-binding and self-association. *Biochem. Biophys. Res. Commun.* **266,** 43–50.

Feldman, D., Thulasiraman, V., Ferreyra, R., and Frydman, J. (1999). Formation of the VHL-elongin BC tumor suppressor complex is mediated by the chaperonin TRiC. *Mol. Cell* **4,** 1051–1061.

Gorospe, M., Egan, J., Zbar, B., Lerman, M., Geil, L., Kuzmin, I., and Holbrook, N. (1999). Protective function of von Hippel-Lindau protein against impaired protein processing in renal carcinoma cells. *Mol. Cell Biol.* **19,** 289–300.

Groulx, I., Bonicalzi, M., and Lee, S. (2000). Ran-mediated nuclear export of the von Hippel-Lindau tumor suppressor protein occurs independently of its assembly with cullin-2. *J. Biol. Chem.* **275,** 8991–9000.

Kaelin, W. G. (1999). Cancer. Many vessels, faulty gene. *Nature* **399,** 203–204.

Lee, S., Neumann, M., Stearman, R., Stauber, R., Pause, A., Pavlakis, G., and Klausner, R. (1999). Transcription-dependent nuclear-cytoplasmic trafficking is required for the function of the von Hippel–Lindau tumor suppressor protein. *Mol. Cell Biol.* **19,** 1486–1497.

Maher, E., and Kaelin, W. G. (1997). von Hippel-Lindau disease. *Medicine* **76,** 381–391.

Maxwell, P., Weisner, M., Chang, G.-W., Clifford, S., Vaux, E., Pugh, C., Maher, E., and Ratcliffe, P. (1999). The von Hippel-Lindau gene product is necessary for oxgyen-dependent proteolysis of hypoxia-inducible factor a subunits. *Nature* **399,** 271–275.

Ohh, M., and Kaelin, W. G. (1999). The von Hippel-Lindau tumour suppressor protein: new perspectives. *Mol. Med. Today* **5,** 257–263.

Ohh, M., Park, C. W., Ivan, M., Hoffman, M. A., Kim, T.-Y., Pavletich, N, Huang, L. E., Chau, V., and Kaelin, W. G. (2000). Ubiquitination of HIF requires direct binding to the von Hippel-Lindau protein beta domain. *Nature Cell Biol.* **2,** 423–427.

Okuda, H., Hirai, S., Takaki, Y., Kamada, M., Baba, M., Sakai, N., Kishida, T., Kaneko, S., Yao, M., Ohno, S., and Shuin, T. (1999). Direct interaction of the beta-domain of VHL tumor suppressor protein with the regulatory domain of atypical PKC isotypes. *Biochem. Biophys. Res. Commun.* **263,** 491–497.

Stebbins, C. E., Kaelin, W. G., and Pavletich, N. P. (1999). Structure of the VHL-Elongin C-elongin B complex: implications for VHL tumor suppressor function. *Science* **284,** 455–461.

Stolle, C., Glenn, G., Zbar, B., Humphrey, J., Choyke, P., Walther, M., Pack, S., Hurley, K., Andrey, C., Klausner, R., and Linehan, W. (1998). Improved detection of germline mutations in the von Hippel-Lindau disease tumor suppressor gene. *Hum. Mutat.* **12,** 417–423.

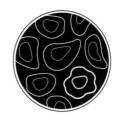

Wilms Tumor: Epidemiology

Norman E. Breslow
University of Washington, Seattle

GLOSSARY

incidence rate Measure of disease occurrence equal to the number of new cases diagnosed per person per unit of time.

relative risk Measure of association between disease occurrence and exposure to a "risk factor"; equal to the ratio of incidence rates for exposed vs nonexposed.

nephrogenic rests Remnants of embryonal kidney tissue that persist into childhood and that are likely precursors of malignancy.

somatic mosaicism A mixture of cells in the body such that different cells contain different genetic information, usually in reference to a specific gene or chromosomal region.

telomerase An enzyme that adds nucleotide repeats to telomeres, compensating for the loss of DNA that occurs with cellular replication.

Wilms tumor, also known as nephroblastoma, is an embryonal tumor of the kidney that on a worldwide basis affects approximately 1 child in every 10,000 before the age of 15 years. Since the advent of combination chemotherapy in the mid-1960s, the great majority of Wilms tumor patients have been cured of their disease. Epidemiologic studies comparing occupations of the fathers of patients and controls have yielded inconsistent results. The fact that incidence rates vary more with ethnicity than with geography suggests that genetic risk factors are likely to play a more important role in etiology than environmental risk factors. Differences in age at onset and in rates of bilateral disease in subgroups of patients having specific congenital anomalies or precursor lesions indicate heterogeneity in pathogenesis. The epidemiologic features further suggest that somatic mosaicism or genomic imprinting, rather than a germline mutation, may be responsible for some of the bilateral and multifocal cases. The genetics of Wilms tumor is relatively complex, with four or more genes implicated so far. Molecular biology has helped explain some of the epidemiology and pathology, but understanding of all the molecular events involved in Wilms tumorigenesis is far from complete.

I. INTRODUCTION

Epidemiology is the study of disease occurrence in human populations. By comparing the disease incidence in subgroups defined by their degree of exposure to an environmental agent or the presence or absence of a particular genetic trait, information on causative risk factors is gained that facilitates the planning of preventive strategies. Epidemiology also provides clues to etiology and pathogenesis. Systematic study of the age incidence patterns of human malignancy, for example, has contributed substantially to modern theories of carcinogenesis that are used both to guide laboratory studies and to make predictions that influence public health policy.

The epidemiology of Wilms tumor and most other childhood cancers is less well developed than that of adult epithelial tumors due to the relatively low incidence of childhood cancer and the consequent difficulty of gathering samples of sufficient size for rigorous statistical analysis. Much of the information presented here comes from two major sources. The International Agency for Research on Cancer (IARC) coordinates the collection of incidence data from population-based cancer registries around the world. Publication of these data in the series "Cancer Incidence in Five Continents" provides epidemiologists with essential descriptive information on the geographic distribution of malignant disease. The U.S. National Wilms Tumor Study Group (NWTSG) registers approximately 400 patients annually from over 200 treatment centers, an estimated 80% of the total national incidence. Although the NWTSG was established in 1969 with the primary goal of improving therapy, the 8000 cases registered to date are of increasing value for epidemiology and as a case-finding resource for molecular biologists.

II. INCIDENCE AND AGE AT ONSET

Wilms tumor is primarily a disease of children. Only 5–6% of Wilms tumors in the United States occur at ages over 14 years, although rare cases may occur in adults aged 50 years or more. On a worldwide basis, the annual incidence rate in children under 15 is about 7 cases per million population. Thus 1 child in 10,000 will eventually develop a Wilms tumor. Wilms tumor accounts for 6–7% of all childhood malignancies in the United States.

Because of its relatively constant incidence rate, Wilms tumor was once considered an "index" tumor of childhood against which the occurrence of other pediatric tumors could be compared. Although there is no evidence of a secular trend in incidence since the mid-1970s, the disease does occur more frequently in some population groups than others. Rates in several African populations are about threefold greater than those in Asian populations, with European populations occupying an intermediate position (Fig. 1). Nevertheless, the geographic variation is substantially less than that of adult epithelial tumors, for instance of lung or liver, where the ratios of incidence rates between high and low risk areas may exceed 20. Wilms tumor lacks another common characteristic of adult malignancies, which is the tendency for incidence to change in migrant populations. Incidence rates for 1975–1995 for the approximate 10% of the US population covered by the government's Surveillance Epidemiology and End Results (SEER) program were 7.9 cases per million population per year for whites, 9.8 for blacks, and about 3.7 for Asians and Pacific Islanders. These rates are similar to those for the same ethnic groups in other countries.

While most registries worldwide report a sex ratio close to 1, rates for girls in the United States are 22% higher than for boys. NWTSG female registrants are slightly older than males, those with unilateral disease having a median age at onset of 42 months vs 35 months for males (Fig. 2). Age at diagnosis varies according to ethnicity, with NWTS blacks being diagnosed at slightly older ages (median 41 months) and Asians at somewhat younger ones (30 months) compared to whites (37 months). Internationally, both incidence rates and age distributions vary more with ethnicity than with geography. This, together with the lack of observable time trends in incidence, suggests that environmental factors are unlikely to play a major role in the causation of Wilms tumor.

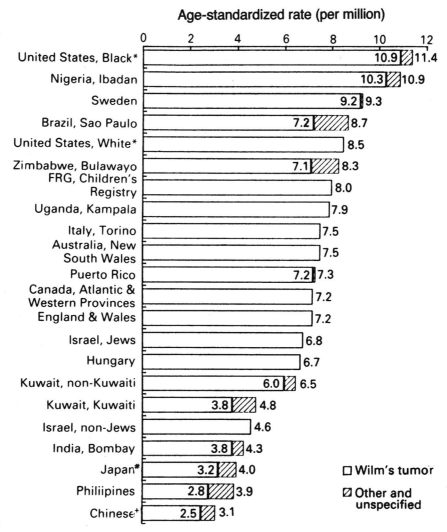

FIGURE 1 Age standardized rates per million persons per year of Wilms tumor and other unspecified kidney tumors (except carcinomas) in childhood. Reproduced from Stiller C. A. and Partkin, D. M. (1990). International variations in the incident of childhood renal tumors. *Br. J. Cancer* **62**, 1026.

III. PATHOLOGY, CLINICAL EPIDEMIOLOGY, AND PROGNOSIS

A. Prognosis with Modern Treatment

Wilms tumor is exquisitely sensitive to treatment with combination chemotherapy. The improvement in patient survival since the 1960s is one of the major success stories of modern cancer treatment. When the German surgeon and pathologist Max Wilms published his classic treatise on embryonal kidney tumors in 1899, gathering together under a single rubric a collection of histologically distinct neoplasms that

had been regarded previously as separate entities, the only available treatment was nephrectomy. Most children who survived the operation quickly succumbed to recurrent or metastatic disease. Improvements in surgical technique and the introduction of adjuvant radiation therapy increased survival rates somewhat, but it was not until the introduction of single agent chemotherapy with dactinomycin or vincristine sulfate in the mid-1960s that a majority of patients were cured of their disease. During the tenure of the NWTSG, the overall survival rates at 5 years from diagnosis increased from 60 to 90%, with 95% survival

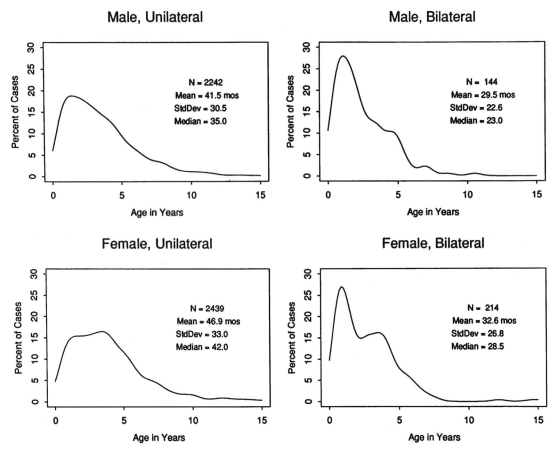

FIGURE 2 Age-at-onset distributions by gender and bilaterality. Reproduced from Breslow, N. E., *et al.* (1993). Epidemiology of Wilms tumor. *Med. Pediatr. Oncol.* **21,** 172.

in certain subgroups. Survival to 5 years is considered tantamount to cure for Wilms tumor, as very few tumor-related deaths occur after that time. Today most Wilms tumor patients are treated with a combination of dactinomycin and vincristine, without radiation therapy, so that the risk of long-term radiation effects such as second tumors has been reduced. Radiation and additional drugs, such as doxorubicin and cyclophosphamide, are used selectively in patient subgroups having a less favorable prognosis. Histology and stage (extent) of disease identify the subgroups of high-risk patients that require more aggressive therapy.

B. Pathology

Wilms tumors are believed to arise from mesenchymal renal stem cells or metanephric blastema that nor-

mally disappear early in embryogenesis but persist into infancy in certain individuals. Typical tumors comprise a mixture of blastemal, epithelial, and stromal tissue. While the epithelial component is a partially differentiated product of the malignant blastema, the stromal component may be either a differentiation product or a remnant of the original nephrogenic mesenchyme. In some tumors, one or the other of these three components predominates. Two distinct, monophasic sarcomas of the kidney have been identified, each comprising only 3% or less of patients, that tend to occur in the very young and that have a poor prognosis. One of these, the rhabdoid tumor of kidney, frequently recurs in the irradiated bed or metastasizes to the lung or liver, and is associated with the development of primary brain tumors. The other, clear cell sarcoma, is characterized by its tendency to metastasize to bone. The prognosis for patients with clear cell sarcoma has improved in recent years, most likely due to the increased use of doxorubicin as part of the treatment. Although these monophasic sarcomas are often grouped with Wilms tumors for reporting of incidence data, they are now regarded by clinicians and pathologists as distinct entities. A third histologic subgroup with an unfavorable prognosis comprises Wilms tumors with anaplasia present either diffusely throughout the tumor or localized to certain foci. NWTSG patients with true Wilms tumor and no anaplasia, who account for 88% of the total, are said to have favorable histology. Their survival is substantially better than for the unfavorable histology patients (Fig. 3).

C. Other Prognostic Factors

Prognosis is also highly dependent on the stage of disease at diagnosis. Patients with bilateral disease are classified as stage V. The presence of metastatic disease at diagnosis, typically in the lung (>90%) but occasionally also or instead in the liver, qualifies a patient with unilateral disease as stage IV. The next most important prognostic indicators are the presence of tumor in regional lymph nodes, in the peritoneum or in the margin of surgical resection (stage III). Patients who have none of these features but whose disease is discovered to have penetrated outside the kidney, e.g., into the renal vein or the perirenal fat, are stage II, provided that all of it has been surgically removed. Those whose disease is completely confined to the resected kidney qualify as stage I. Five-year survival percentages for favorable histology patients by stage are I, 96%; II, 94%; III, 87%; IV, 76%; and V, 85%. The greatest improvement in survival over the past several decades has occurred among stage III and IV patients. Current attempts to further refine therapy are oriented toward the identification of biological markers of poor prognosis. There is some suggestion that patients whose tumors show loss of heterogygosity (LOH) at chromosome 16q, or show high levels of expression of the

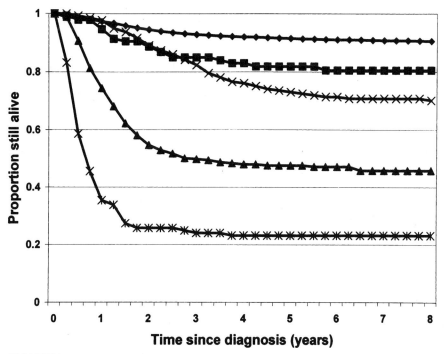

FIGURE 3 Survival of NWTSG patients (1969–1999) by histologic type, with numbers of patients in parentheses: ◆, favorable histology (6928); X, clear cell sarcoma (271); ■, focal anaplasia (140); ▲, diffuse anaplasia (422); *, rhabdoid tumor of kidney (131). Courtesy of NWTSG.

enzyme telomerase, may be at higher risk of relapse. Further study is needed, however.

D. Late Effects of Treatment

The occurrence of a second malignant neoplasm (SMN) in patients who have been cured of Wilms tumor is the most feared consequence of their possible genetic susceptibility or of the anticancer therapy they received. The cumulative risk of an SMN in NWTS survivors during the first 10 years following nephrectomy is 1%, some eightfold higher than for children in the general population. Four NWTSG patients, among 1364 who were followed at least 10 years, developed hepatocellular carcinoma some 12–16 years after receiving abdominal irradiation. Four female patients who received chest irradiation for metastatic Wilms tumor diagnosed shortly before puberty later developed breast cancer. The presence of a genetic corisk factor for these events cannot be excluded. Four case reports of pleural malignant mesothelioma, diagnosed 14–41 years after the Wilms tumor, are of interest because the Wilms tumor gene, *WT1* is expressed in developing mesothelium.

Cumulative rates of serious cardiac toxicity, including congestive heart failure and cardiomyopathy, are similar to those for SMNs. The cardiac events occur almost exclusively in patients who were treated with doxorubicin, especially if they also received radiation therapy, and are more prevalent among females. Renal failure is rare among patients with unilateral disease who are cured by modern front-line treatment protocols and who have none of the congenital anomaly syndromes associated with Wilms tumor (see later). In contrast, it affects the majority of patients with the Denys–Drash syndrome and, after puberty, the majority of those having the Wilms tumor-aniridia syndrome. Female patients who received whole abdominal radiation as part of their treatment for Wilms tumor are usually sterile. Those who received radiation treatment to the tumor bed and remain fertile have higher rates of adverse reproductive outcomes compared with normal controls. Lower rates of chronic toxicity are expected in the future, however, as fewer patients now receive radiation as part of the initial treatment plan.

IV. ENVIRONMENTAL RISK FACTORS

Despite the lack of support for the concept from descriptive epidemiology, cancer epidemiologists have attempted to correlate the occurrence of Wilms tumor with parental environmental exposures that could affect the germ cells or the developing foetus. Some small studies reported that fathers of Wilms tumor patients were more likely to be employed as machinists, vehicle mechanics, or welders than were fathers of control children. Other studies failed to confirm this suggestion. In view of the inherent limitations of observational studies, it is perhaps not surprising that the environmental epidemiology to date has produced an array of inconsistent findings. No studies involved more than 150 cases of Wilms tumor and virtually all attempted to link those cases with a large number of different occupational and exposure categories. Studies that involve a multiplicity of statistical comparisons will predictably turn up some "statistically significant" associations by chance alone. When a priori hypotheses based on previous findings were stated at the outset of a study, they were generally not confirmed. Consequently, a summary interpretation of epidemiologic data on environmental risk factors is not possible at this time.

V. GENETIC EPIDEMIOLOGY

A. Congenital Syndromes and Anomalies

The genetic epidemiology of Wilms tumor, in contrast, has produced many strong and consistent associations and appears to be a fertile ground for further research. The disease occurs in conjunction with several congenital syndromes and anomalies, including congenital aniridia, the Beckwith–Wiedemann syndrome (BWS; gigantism, macroglossia, omphalocele, renal medullary dysplasia), and the Denys–Drash syndrome (male pseudohermaphroditism, degenerative renal disease, and Wilms tumor) (see Table I). Congenital aniridia and hemihypertrophy are extremely rare in the general population, affecting about 1 and 3 children per 100,000, respectively. Male genitourinary anomalies are more common (5–12 boys per 1000),

Frequency (%) of Congenital Syndromes and Anomalies Observed
in Wilms Tumor Patients

Congenital syndrome or anomaly	UK (1971–1977) $n = 549$	France (1955–1989) $n = 501$	NWTS (1980–1999) $n = 6890$
Aniridia	2.2	0.8	0.8
Beckwith–Wiedemann	0.7	0.6	1.1
Denys–Drash	—	—	0.4
Sporadic hemihypertrophy	2.9	5.2	2.5
Genitourinary	1.8	2.2	—
Hypospadias	—	—	2.0[a]
Cryptorchidism	—	—	4.7[a]

[a]Rate for males only ($n = 3200$).

but occur at an even greater frequency in children with Wilms tumor. Patients with congenital aniridia often have other associated defects that form part of the WAGR (Wilms' tumor, aniridia, genitourinary, mental retardation) syndrome. Most WAGR patients have a constitutional deletion at chromosome 11p13 that is detectable by cytogenetics and that provided the first clue as to the location of the first Wilms tumor gene, *WT1*. Only about one-third of the cases of congenital aniridia, which is fully penetrant and a marker for the syndrome, develop Wilms tumor.

B. Precursor Lesions

Remnants of embryonal tissue known as nephrogenic rests, considered to be precursors of tumor, are found in the surgically removed kidneys of some 30–40% of NWTSG patients. Intralobar nephrogenic rests (ILNR), which occur in the interior of the renal lobe and are often adjacent to the tumor, are usually solitary. Perilobar nephrogenic rests (PLNR) may occur in multiplicity at the periphery of the renal lobe. PLNR are a relatively frequent (1%) incidental necropsy finding in infants under 3 months, whereas ILNR are exceptionally rare in the general population. Tumors arising in association with PLNR are composed primarily of blastemal or epithelial tissue, with differentiated elements that mimic the late stages of nephrogenesis. ILNR-associated tumors, which are stromal predominant, recapitulate the entire spectrum of renal histogenesis and frequently contain heterologous tissue such as skeletal muscle, squamous epithelium, or neuronal tissue in addition to the usual blastemal, epithelial, and stromal elements.

About 6% of NWTS patients have bilateral disease at diagnosis and another 1% develop new disease in the contralateral kidney after treatment for unilateral Wilms tumor. A further 10% have multiple tumors occurring in a single kidney. The four factors—multiple tumors, precursor lesion, congenital anomaly, and age at onset—are strongly associated. Aniridia and genital anomalies occur in association with ILNR. Bilaterality, multicentricity, and BWS are associated with both precursors, and sporadic hemihypertophy is linked to PLNR. The youngest patients at diagnosis are those with bilateral disease, aniridia, INLR, or a genital anomaly. Those with sporadic hemihypertophy are older. The age distribution for PLNR cases is particularly distinctive, with a peak at 4 years of age rather than at 2 or 3 years. Babies with PLNR, although rare, are much more likely to develop disease in the contralateral kidney than other patients.

Epidemiology and pathology data strongly suggest heterogeneity in the pathogenesis of Wilms tumor. ILNR-associated cases appear to arise from an initiating event early in embryogenesis that almost invariably leads to a Wilms tumor, usually at an early age and often in conjunction with aniridia and/or a genital anomaly. The events leading to PLNR appear to occur later in nephrogenesis and do not invariably lead to Wilms tumor, but if they do it is likely to be diagnosed at a later age, sometimes in conjunction with hemihypertrophy. Molecular genetic data support this proposed distinction. Reduced levels of *WT1* expression are found almost exclusively in Wilms tumors that contain regions of the heterologous tissue characteristic of ILNR-associated tumors. Mutations in *WT1* are found primarily in patients with the Denys–Drash syndrome or with genital anomalies. It is anticipated that when the putative second Wilms tumor gene *WT2* located at chromosome 11p15.5 is cloned, it may likewise help explain the occurrence of the PLNR cases and their association with hemihypertrophy.

C. Familial Wilms Tumor

Familial Wilms tumor is rare, on the order of 1–2% of cases. Only 93 of 6209 (1.5%) of NWTSG patients diagnosed during 1969–1994 were known to have a relative with Wilms tumor, but there may be some underascertainment (Table II). Most such families had only one member with a confirmed diagnosis in addition to the proband, but there were six families with confirmed disease in five or six relatives. The affected relative is usually a sibling or cousin, both parents being normal. Indeed, in several pedigrees there are multiple cases among cousins with none in the preceding generations. Figure 4 shows one such family. The concept of a "premutation" has been invoked

to explain this phenomenon, but no specific genetic basis has been identified.

Some relevant characteristics of NWTSG cases with familial disease are listed in Table II. While they tend to have younger ages at diagnosis and are more likely to have bilateral disease than their nonfamilial counterparts, there is no clear association with any of the typical congenital anomalies. The rarity of familial cases, however, precludes definitive statements. Linkage analysis of Wilms tumor in several large, multiple case pedigrees has identified one familial Wilms tumor locus (*FWT1*) on chromosome 17q that affects two families and another (*FWT2*) on chromosome 19q that affects at least five families. Penetrance of the familial Wilms tumor genes is variable, having recently been estimated at 20% for *FWT1*.

NWTSG data provided indirect evidence that a *de novo* germline mutation is responsible for some nonfamilial Wilms tumor cases. There was an excess of fathers over 55 years of age at patient's birth (9 observed vs 4.5 expected) and, in comparison to the general population, a slight excess in the average age of both father and mother at the time of the patient's birth. The excess is particularly striking for patients whose tumor occurred in conjunction with the male GU anomalies or with ILNR but not, surprisingly, for those with bilateral disease. If 10% of Wilms' tumor cases resulted from a germline mutation that had 20% penetrance and that was dominantly inherited, the recurrence risk in offspring would be $0.10 \times 0.20 \times 0.5 = 1\%$. This estimate is consistent with the four cases of Wilms tumor that have been reported among 343 live born offspring of survivors of unilateral disease, two of which occurred in a single family. Among 71 NWTSG patients with a twin sibling, of which 35 were dizygotic, 31 monozygotic, and 5 unknown zygosity, only one twin pair was concordant for Wilms tumor and that pair was dizygotic. Thus, while some Wilms tumors clearly arise from germline mutations, their frequency may not be great. In contrast, as many as 35–40% of retinoblastomas are germline mutants.

D. Wilms Tumor and the Two-Stage Model

The two-stage mutational model for retinoblastoma and other childhood tumors, developed by geneticist Alfred Knudson to explain the available statistical data

TABLE II

Characteristics of Wilms Tumor Patients with Familial Versus Nonfamilial Disease: NWTSG Data for 1969–1994

	Familial	Nonfamilial
No. of patients	93	6116
Median age at diagnosis (months)	25	38
	Frequency of congenital anomalies (%)	
Aniridia	3.2	0.7
Hemihypertrophy	5.4	3.3
Beckwith–Wiedemann syndrome	3.2	0.9
Cryptorchidism and/or hypospadias[a]	10.6	6.2
	Distribution of bilaterality/ multifocality (%)	
Bilateral at onset	15.1	6.3
Late bilateral	1.1	0.8
Unilateral, multifocal	8.6	9.6
Unilateral, unifocal	73.1	83.2

[a]Percentage of males.

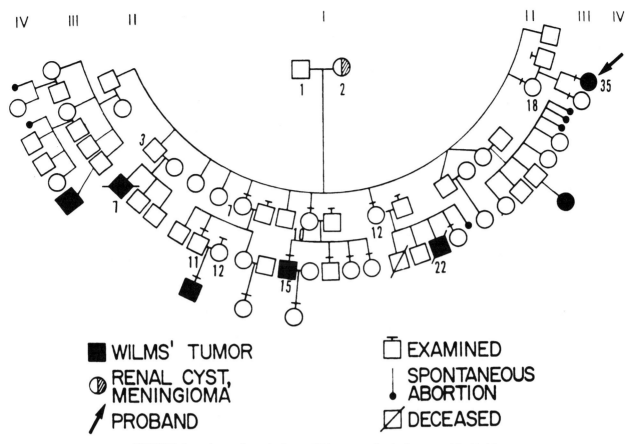

FIGURE 4 Pedigree of a multiple case Wilms tumor family. Courtesy of Dr. Fred Li.

relating familiality, bilaterality, and age-at-onset distributions, has strongly influenced the thinking of both epidemiologists and molecular biologists. According to the model, two rate-limiting mutational events occur as part of a causal chain leading to tumor development. In hereditary cases, identified phenotypically by familiality, a multiplicity of tumors, or the presence of specific congenital anomalies, the first mutation occurs in or is inherited via the germ cell while the second occurs in a somatic cell. The fact that all cells are at risk for the second event provides a mechanism for the occurrence of multiple (bilateral or unilateral, multifocal) tumors. The need for only a single mutation in a somatic cell explains their early ages at onset. Both mutations occur in somatic cells in sporadic cases.

This simple model explains much if not all the occurrence of retinoblastoma, where the two mutational events were identified as an initial mutation or deletion in the *RB* gene followed by loss of the wild-type allele. A similar mechanism is responsible for selected cases of bilateral Wilms tumors: inheritance of a *WT1* mutation followed by reduction to homozygosity or hemizygosity at this locus in the tumor cells. Epidemiologic data, however, suggest that other cases of bilateral and multifocal disease are most likely due to another mechanism. The unilateral, multifocal cases are more numerous than the bilaterals, whereas the reverse would be expected if both kidneys were equally at risk of receiving a "second hit" in patients carrying the germline mutation. The ages at onset for unilateral, multifocal cases are intermediate (median 33 months) between those of the bilateral (27 months) and unilateral, unifocal cases (39 months). The fact that the frequency of bilaterality in familial cases is only modestly increased in comparison to nonfamilial cases (Table II) conflicts with the notion that all bilateral or multifocal tumors are necessarily hereditary. If one uses familial cases to estimate the prevalence of bilateral disease among carriers of the germline mutation to be 16%, and further assumes that all bilateral cases are carriers, the proportion of Wilms tumor patients who are carriers is estimated as $0.07 \div 0.16 = 44\%$. If the bilateral and unilateral, multifocal cases are grouped together as hereditary cases in making the calculation, the estimated fraction of Wilms tumors that are hereditary increases to $0.16 \div 0.25 = 64\%$. These estimates are much higher than the 10% figure assumed earlier and are difficult to reconcile with the low recurrence risk observed in offspring of survivors and the low prevalence of familial disease.

A possibly alternative explanation for the occurrence of multiple tumors in the same patient is an event early in embryogenesis giving rise to somatic mosaicism. Genetic mosaicism involving 11p markers has been observed in the normal tissue of some Wilms tumor patients. In other cases, the mosaicism may involve loss of maternal imprinting of genes at the 11p15 locus. The degree of mosaicism and the specific timing of the event that led to it could account for both unilateral, multifocal and bilateral cases, as well as provide a genetic basis for the differences in incidence and ages at onset between girls and boys.

E. Heterogeneity in the Pathogenesis of Wilms Tumor

The study of Wilms tumor patients led to identification of the insulin-like growth factor gene *IGF2*, located at chromosome 11p15, as the first gene known to be imprinted in humans. Whereas normal tissues express only the paternal copy, loss of the imprint resulting in the expression of both paternal and maternal *IGF2* alleles occurs in perhaps 70% of Wilms tumors that do not show LOH at chromosome 11p13. Intriguingly, birth weights for NWTSG patients as a whole, and particularly for those whose Wilms tumors develop in conjunction with BWS, with hemihypertrophy, or with PLNR, are elevated in comparison with those for the general U.S. population. Thus, molecular and epidemiologic data both suggest that prenatal growth factors may have a role in Wilms tumorigenesis.

It is now well known from epidemiology, pathology, and genetics that Wilms tumor is heterogeneous as a pathogenetic entity. Mutation or deletion of the *WT1* gene at 11p13 leads to the WAGR syndrome, to the Denys–Drash syndrome, and to some ILNR-associated Wilms tumors. Mutation and/or loss of imprinting of genes located at 11p15, the putative *WT2* locus, may lead to Wilms tumors associated with overgrowth disorders and PLNR. The genetic events leading to tumors in several large, multiple case families take place elsewhere than at the two loci already identified for *FWT1* and *FWT2*. It is anticipated that additional molecular genetic pathways to Wilms tumorigenesis will be discovered.

See Also the Following Articles

MULTISTAGE CARCINOGENESIS • NEUROBLASTOMA • PEDIATRIC CANCERS, MOLECULAR FEATURES • RHABDOMYOSARCOMA, EARLY ONSET • TELOMERES AND TELOMERASE • WILMS TUMOR SUPPRESSOR WT1

Bibliography

Beckwith, J. B., Kiviat, N. B., and Bonadio, J. F. (1990). Nephrogenic rests, nephroblastomatosis, and the pathogenesis of Wilms Tumor. *Pediatr. Pathol.* **10**, 1.

Breslow, N. E., Olshan, A., Beckwith, J. B., and Green, D. M. (1993). Epidemiology of Wilms tumor. *Med. Pediatr. Oncol.* **21**, 172.

Green, D. M., Breslow, N. E., Beckwith, J. B., Finklestein, J. Z., Grundy, P. E., Thomas, P. R. M., Kim, T., Shochat, S. J., Haase, G. M., Ritchey, M. L., Kelalis, P. P., and D'Angio, G. J. (1998). Comparison between single-dose and divided-dose administration of dactinomycin and doxorubicin for patients with Wilms tumor: A report from the National Wilms' Tumor Study Group. *J. Clin. Oncol.* **16**, 237.

Knudson, A. G. (1993). Introduction to the genetics of primary renal tumors in children. *Med. Pediatr. Oncol.* **21**, 193.

Pritchard-Jones, K., and Hastie, N. D. (1990). Wilms' tumor as a paradigm for the relationship of cancer to development. *Cancer Surv.* **9**, 555.

Wilms Tumor Suppressor WT1

Ricky W. Johnstone
The Peter MacCallum Cancer Institute, East Melbourne, Australia

Yang Shi
Harvard Medical School

GLOSSARY

apoptosis A mechanism of cell death characterized morphologically by DNA fragmentation and the formation of membrane blebs.

cell cycle A series of events that an eukaryotic cell follows in order to divide. It consists of four phases: G_1/G_o, S, G_2 and M.

oncogene A gene encoding a dominantly acting protein that promotes cell growth and transformation.

posttranslational modification Covalent attachment of carbohydrates, fatty acids, lipids, or phosphate onto specific amino acids of a protein after translation.

promoter A DNA sequence adjacent to the coding sequence of a gene that directs and controls transcription.

RNA splicing Deletion of intron sequences from transcribed RNA to produce mature messenger RNA.

transcription Synthesis of RNA from a DNA template.

transcription factors Proteins that bind to specific DNA sequences to mediate RNA synthesis.

translation The synthesis of polypeptide from a specific messenger RNA.

tumor suppressor gene A gene whose protein product is a negative regulator of growth and counteracts the transformation action of oncogenes.

Wilms tumor Pediatric kidney cancer characterized by inefficient differentiation of the embryonic mesenchyme.

WT1 is a transcription factor that functions as a tumor suppressor. The *WT1* gene is infrequently mutated in Wilms tumor, a pediatric kidney cancer. Much has been written about the mutations of *WT1* found in Wilms tumors and the role of WT1 in development of the urinogenital system. This article focuses on our current understanding of the molecular basis of the tumor suppressor function of WT1, as well as posttranscriptional events that regulate the activity of WT1.

I. INTRODUCTION

Wilms tumor, or nephroblastoma, is a pediatric kidney cancer affecting approximately 1 in 10,000 children, making it one of the most frequent solid tumors in children. Wilms tumors arise following the inability of the embryonic metanephric mechanchym to differentiate, resulting in a disorganized array of epithelial, mesenchymal, and stromal cells. Wilms tumors are also associated with other congenital defects, including Beckwith–Wiedemann syndrome, Denys–Drash syndrome, WAGR syndrome and Perlman syndrome.

The gene encoding WT1, the Wilms' tumor suppressor protein, was originally isolated by a positional cloning approach over a decade ago. The *WT1* gene is located on chromosome 11p13 and is thought to be one of at least three genes that are Wilms tumor predisposition genes. *WT1* is approximately 50 kb, consisting of 10 exons, and can give rise to four WT1 mRNA isoforms through alternative splicing. These four mRNA isoforms encode four highly related protein isoforms, WT1 A–D (Fig. 1). The first splice variant includes exon 5 encoding 17 amino acids upstream of the first zinc finger, whereas the use of an alternative splice donor site within exon 9 results in the insertion of three amino acids (Lys-Thr-Ser, KTS) between the third and fourth zinc fingers (Fig. 1). All four protein isoforms appear to be present in cells that express WT1. However, their molecular and biological functions may differ markedly (discussed later).

In addition to RNA splicing, alternative WT1 isoforms may be produced following RNA editing at position 839 of the WT1 RNA, which replaces leucine 280 with a proline residue. To further add to the complexity of WT1 expression, it has also been reported that an in-frame internal initiation codon, or a novel non-AUG initiation codon 204 bases upstream and in-frame with the initiator AUG, may be used to produce shorter or longer WT1 isoforms, respectively. It is therefore possible that the *WT1* gene gives rise to 24 different naturally occurring protein isoforms, each of which may have slightly or vastly different functions (Table I). In addition to the production of multiple different protein isoforms, WT1 is also subjected to posttranslational modifications, such as phosphorylation, which contributes to an even larger repertoire of WT1 proteins.

The predicted molecular mass of WT1 is approximately 49 kDa. The structural hallmarks of the WT1 protein include four Cys_2-His_2 type zinc fingers located at the C terminus responsible for binding spe-

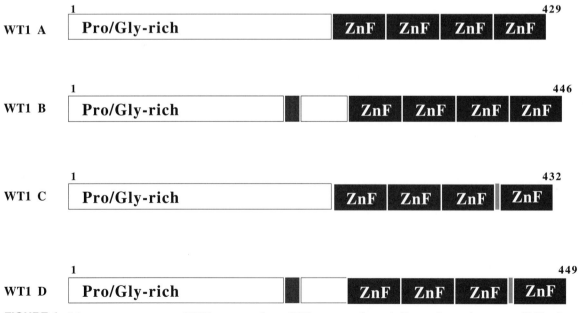

FIGURE 1 Schematic representation of WT1 protein isoforms. WT1 protein isoforms A–D arise due to alternative mRNA splicing. The four zinc fingers with DNA-binding activity are shown to the right. The lysine, threonine, and serine insertion between zinc fingers three and four is shown in light gray. The 17 amino acid insertion encoded by exon 5 is shown in dark gray.

TABLE I

WT1 Protein Species[a]

Isoform	Size (amino acids)	Properties/function
WT1 A	429	DNA binding (strong), transcription activation/repression, tumor suppression, regulation of apoptosis, RNA binding (weak), RNA splicing factor binding (weak)
WT1 B	446	DNA binding (strong), transcription activation/repression, tumor suppression, regulation of apoptosis, RNA binding (weak), RNA splicing factor binding (weak)
WT1 C	432	DNA binding (weak), transcription activation/repression, tumor suppression, regulation of apoptosis, RNA binding (strong), RNA splicing factor binding (strong)
WT1 D	449	DNA binding (weak), transcription activation/repression, tumor suppression, regulation of apoptosis, RNA binding (strong), RNA splicing factor binding (strong)
WT1 A (L264P)	429	DNA binding, transcription repression (weak)
WT1 B (L281P)	446	NT
WT1 C (L264P)	432	NT
WT1 D (L281P)	449	NT
LWT1 A	497	Transcription repression
LWT1 B	514	NT
LWT1 C	500	NT
LWT1 D	514	NT
SWT1 A	302	Transcription activation (strong), no transcription repression, induction of apoptosis
SWT1 B	319	NT
SWT1 C	305	NT
SWT1 D	322	NT
LWT1 A (L332S)	497	NT
LWT1 B (L349S)	514	NT
LWT1 C (L332S)	500	NT
LWT1 D (L349S)	514	NT
SWT1 A (L167S)	322	NT
SWT1 B (L184S)	319	NT
SWT1 C (L167S)	305	NT
SWT1 D (L184S)	322	NT

[a]Multiple WT1 protein species arise due to mRNA splicing (WT1 A-D), alternative translational start codons giving rise to longer (L) or shorter (S) mRNA transcripts, or RNA editing replacing a leucine residue with a proline residue at position 280.

cific DNA sequences, and a glutamine and proline-rich amino-terminal region at the N terminus that is believed to be important for the transcriptional activity of WT1. In cell culture, WT1 has been shown to suppress cell growth, an activity expected of a tumor suppressor protein.

Although WT1 has been extensively studied over many years, identification of its physiological functions and the molecular mechanisms underpinning these functions are still the topics of many debates. The current model suggests that WT1 functions predominantly as a transcription factor that regulates genes important for cell proliferation and differentiation. This article discusses advancement in understanding how WT1 exerts its tumor suppressor function through its ability to regulate transcription and how its transcriptional activities may be regulated in normal and tumor cells.

II. WT1 AS A TRANSCRIPTION FACTOR

Purified recombinant WT1 protein was used to identify a specific DNA-binding site from a pool of degenerate oligonucleotides. The binding sites obtained were similar to the sequence recognized by the early growth response-1 (EGR-1) gene product. Interestingly, addition of the KTS residues within the zinc finger DNA-binding domain altered the affinity of WT1 to its consensus DNA element. This suggested for the first time that the different WT1 protein isoforms might have distinct molecular targets and thus different and biological activities. Like many transcription factors, WT1 has a modular structure with a C-terminal DNA-binding domain, a transcriptional activation domain in the middle of the molecule (amino acids 181–250), an amino-terminal repression domain (amino acids 85–124), and two separate dimerization domains (amino acids 8–37 and 158–183). When bound to target genes, WT1 has been shown to either repress or activate transcription dependent on the promoter context.

It has long been thought that the ability of WT1 to repress transcription is correlated with its ability to function as a tumor suppressor. However, experiments from several laboratories suggest that the activation function of WT1 may be crucial for its tumor suppressor function. This suggestion is based on studies of several different aspects of WT1: the transcriptional activities of both wild-type and naturally occurring WT1 proteins, as well as the physiological target genes of WT1 as discussed later.

A. WT1 Is a Transcriptional Activator as Well as a Repressor

Initial experiments demonstrated that binding of WT1 to promoters containing EGR consensus sequences resulted in transcriptional repression. The cellular genes that were identified as WT1 targets include growth factor, and growth factor receptor genes (Table II) were consistent with the idea that transcriptional repression function is important for the tumor suppressor activity of WT1. However, the majority of naturally occurring WT1 mutants isolated from Wilms tumor samples carry mutations in the zinc finger DNA-binding domain, resulting in a loss of the ability of WT1 to bind to its DNA targets. Therefore, it is difficult to assess whether a specific loss of the transcriptional repression activity is critical for the loss of the tumor suppression function of WT1. Functional mutations in WT1 outside the zinc finger domain resulting in a serine-to-glycine substitution at codon 273, a glycine-to-aspartic acid mutation at codon 201, and deletion of exon 2 due to aberrant

TABLE II
Putative WT1 Target Genes[a]

Gene	Function	Effect on transcription by WT1
EGR1	Transcription factor	Activation
WT1	Transcription factor	Activation
c-myc	Transcription factor	Activation
Bcl-2	Apoptosis inhibition	Activation
Syndecan-1	Differentiation	Activation
RbAP46	Binds pRb	Activation
Amphiregulin	EGFR ligand	Activation
HSP70	Protein chaperone	Activation
P21[CIP1/WAF1]	Cyclin-dependent kinase inhibitor	Activation
Dax-1	Nuclear hormone receptor/ transcription repression	Activation
E-cadherin	Cell signaling	Activation
Pax2	Transcription factor	Repression
c-Myb	Transcription factor	Repression
ODC	Enzyme involved in synthesis of polyamines	Repression
Gαi-2	Protooncogene	Repression
Insulin receptor	Growth factor receptor	Repression
Midkine	Growth factor	Repression
IGF-2	Growth factor	Repression
IGF1R	Growth factor receptor	Repression
Inhibin	Ovarian differentiation	Repression
PDGF-A	Growth factor	Repression
CSF-1	Growth factor	Repression
TGF-β1	Growth factor	Repression
EGFR	Growth factor receptor	Repression
NovH	IGF-binding protein/ protooncogene	
MDR1	Drug resistance	Repression

[a]The name of each gene is shown in column 1 and the defined function of the protein products of each gene in column 2. The effect of WT1 binding to the promoters of each gene is shown in column 3.

mRNA splicing have been identified. Importantly, these mutations resulted in the loss of WT1-mediated transcriptional repression and subsequent transcriptional activation of the EGR1 site and correlated with an inability of these mutant proteins to suppress tumor cell growth. These data strengthened the hypothesis that transcription repression by WT1 correlated with tumor suppressor function.

A series of studies have challenged the notion that the tumor suppression function of WT1 is correlated with its transcriptional repression activity. The first clue that WT1 may have additional activity important for its biological activity came from the study demonstrating that WT1 can efficiently activate transcription. A number of naturally occurring WT1 mutants (amino acid 112, F to W; amino acid 129, P to

L; amino acid 154, F to S) have been shown to be defective for their transcriptional activation function but their repression activity is left intact. Significantly, all these mutants are partially defective in growth suppression assays. These findings suggest strongly that the transcriptional activation function of WT1 may be critical for the growth suppression function of WT1.

Gene expression profiling experiments have provided another important line of evidence that supports the idea that the transcriptional activation function of WT1 is important for its biological activity. These experiments identified a number of genes, including *amphiregulin*, *HSP70*, and *p21WAF1/CIP1*, as WT1 target genes that are transcriptionally activated by WT1. That fact that the negative cell growth regulator p21[CIP1/WAF1] is activated by WT1 is consistent with the growth suppression function of WT1. Interestingly, none of the growth factor or growth factor receptor genes previously shown to be negatively regulated by WT1 have been isolated as genes downregulated by WT1 in these experiments. Collectively, these studies find no clear correlation between transcriptional repression and growth suppression of WT1. However, it is still possible that in a physiological setting the ability of WT1 to activate and repress transcription are both essential for its overall tumor suppression function.

III. REGULATION OF WT1-MEDIATED TRANSCRIPTIONAL ACTIVITIES

As stated earlier, WT1 can function as a transcription activator or repressor. WT1 function can be regulated at a number of different levels, including RNA splicing and editing, posttranslational modification, and interaction with other cellular proteins.

A. RNA Splicing, Use of Alternative Translation Start Codons, and RNA Editing

While there are DNA sequences that can bind to all four splice variants of WT1, it has become increasingly clear that RNA splicing, in particular the insertion of the KTS tripeptide within the zinc finger domain of WT1, can dramatically affect DNA binding

(Table 1). The two splice isoforms containing the KTS insertion have a generally lower affinity for DNA than the other two isoforms, and in fact, confocal studies performed in the laboratory of Nick Hastie have demonstrated that the presence of the KTS sequence can alter the subnuclear expression of WT1. The −KTS isoforms were found to be diffusely expressed in the nucleus and colocalized with other transcription factors such as SP1 and PAX6. In contrast, the +KTS isoforms were expressed in a speckled pattern within the nucleus and colocalized with splicing factors, including U2B, U2AF, U1-70, and p80 coilin. These observations led to the hypothesis that WT1 may also function as a RNA-binding protein. This theory is supported by experiments showing that both WT1 +KTS and −KTS isoforms were capable of binding to an RNA probe derived from exon 2 of the *Igf-2* gene and that the zinc finger region of WT1 was required for the protein/RNA interaction. Interestingly, and in keeping with nuclear localization observations, −KTS isoforms have a higher affinity for RNA than −KTS isoforms. These observations have subsequently been strengthened by the identification of an RNA recognition motif (RRM) homologous to that found in the U1-A small nuclear ribonuclearprotein using three-dimensional modeling.

At present, the physiological relevance of these findings is still uncertain and no functional effect of WT1 binding to RNA has been demonstrated. However, the treatment of cells with RNase causes the release of WT1 from the nucleus, whereas DNase treatment appears to have no effect. While the circumstantial evidence supporting a functional role for WT1 in RNA splicing, stability, folding, or elongation is mounting, there is currently a lack of experimental data to conclusively endorse the functional significance of these hypotheses.

The *WT1* mRNA also undergoes RNA editing to produce protein isoforms with a single amino acid change. Editing of a thymidine residue at position 1222 in the human WT1 mRNA to a cytosine results in an amino acid change from a leucine to a proline. WT1 A (L264P) isoforms appears to be able to bind to a consensus WT1 DNA element, but its ability to repress transcription is decreased by 25–30%. Analysis of Wilms tumor samples revealed that RNA editing does not appear to be a frequent mechanism of WT1 alteration during tumorigenesis.

It has been reported that shorter and longer WT1 protein isoforms can be produced due to the use of an internal AUG translation start codon or upstream non-AUG start codon, respectively (Table I). The use of an internal AUG for translation results in truncated WT1 protein isoforms of 302–322 amino acids that lack a full repression and dimerization domain at the N terminus but does not particularly alter the *in vivo* half-life of the proteins. Interestingly, the smaller WT1 isoform (SWT1 A) is not capable of repressing transcription, but has enhanced transactivation activity compared to wild-type WT1 A. The functional activities of the larger WT1 protein isoforms have not been extensively studied. A chimeric protein consisting of a large WT1 isoform (LWT1 A) with its zinc finger region replaced by the yeast GAL4 DNA-binding domain could repress transcription from a CAT reporter gene containing GAL4 DNA-binding sites within the promoter region. It is presently unclear whether large or small WT1 isoforms can affect the expression of known WT1 target genes or whether aberrant expression of these molecules is involved in Wilms tumorigensis.

B. Posttranslational Modification

Although earlier studies failed to demonstrate significant *in vivo* phosphorylation of WT1, it has been demonstrated that the protein can be phosphorylated and that this modification might alter the function of WT1. Two separate groups reported that WT1 is phosphorylated by PKA on serine residues within the zinc finger DNA-binding domain. Significantly, phosphorylation of these sites drastically decreased the affinity of WT1 for DNA but did not alter the RNA-binding activity. Moreover, phosphorylation of WT1 also results in the retention of WT1 in the cytosol. In addition to cAMP-dependent protein kinase-mediated phosphorylation of WT1, the c-Abl oncoprotein has also been demonstrated to phosphorylate the EWS/WT1 fusion protein. The EWS/WT1 fusion oncoprotein found in desmoplastic small round cell tumors is produced following the t(11;22)(p13;q12) translocation and contains 21 EWS amino acids from the N-terminal domain fused to WT1 zinc fingers 2–4. Phosphorylation of EWS/WT1 by c-Abl inhibits DNA binding by this chimeric protein, although the

exact sites of phosphorylation have not been mapped. These studies demonstrate that in addition to mutations of *WT1*, the function of WT1 may also be regulated by posttranslational modification. It remains to be seen whether altered expression or activation of protein kinases results in aberrant phosphorylation of WT1 and altered expression of downstream cellular genes.

IV. WT1-BINDING PROTEINS

As with many transcription factors, WT1 can physically interact with a number of other cellular proteins (Table III). These interactions may have a twofold effect: (i) the partner proteins might regulate the expression or function of WT1 and (ii) WT1 might affect the expression or function of the partner proteins. The best studied example of a WT1-binding protein that both regulates the function of WT1 and is reciprocally affected by WT1 is the p53 tumor suppressor protein. Binding of p53 to WT1 converts WT1 from a transcriptional activator to a repressor. In contrast, WT1 enhances p53-mediated transcriptional activation and reduces its repression function. The interaction of WT1 with p53 stabilizes p53 and extends its *in vivo* half-life.

The significance of the WT1/p53 interaction in tumorigenesis is still unclear, as Wilms tumors are not associated with mutations in p53, although p53 mutations are correlated with anaplastic Wilms tumors. It has been shown that WT1 can interact with the newly identified p53 family members p63/KET and p73. Unlike p53, p73 is not stablized by WT1. Binding of WT1 to p73 inhibits p73-mediated transcriptional activation. Reciprocally, p73 inhibits DNA binding and transactivation by WT1.

Another protein shown to interact with WT1 *in vivo* and *in vitro* is the prostate apoptosis response gene product, par-4. Par-4 was first isolated from rat prostate as a gene that is upregulated during apoptosis. Par-4 binds to the zinc finger domain of WT1, inhibits transactivation, and augments the transrepression activities of WT1. Interestingly, par-4 does not interact with the EWS/WT1 fusion protein, which is a dominant oncoprotein. It is therefore possible that the ability of par-4 to negatively regulate WT1 acti-

TABLE III
WT1-Interacting Proteins[a]

Interacting protein	Site of interaction	Function consequence
p53	C terminus	WT1 stabilizes p53, enhances transcriptional activation, reduces repression, and inhibits p53-mediated apoptosis. p53 converts WT1 from transcriptional activator to repressor
p73	C terminus	p73 inhibits DNA binding and transcriptional activation by WT1
par-4	C terminus	WT1 inhibits par-4-mediated apoptosis. Par-4 augments WT1 transrepression, inhibits transactivation, and rescues cells from WT-mediated growth suppression
Ciao-1	C terminus	Ciao-1 inhibits WT1-mediated transactivation
Splicing factors (U2AF65, U170K, U2B, p80 coilin)	C terminus (U2AF65)	Unknown
UBC 90	N terminus	Unknown
HSP-70	N terminus	HSP-70 facilitates WT1-mediated growth suppression
SF-1	N terminus	WT1 and SF-1 form a functional complex to bind the *MIS* promoter and activate *MIS* transcription

[a]Cellular proteins shown to interact with WT1 are shown in column 1, and the region of WT1 necessary for the interaction is shown in column 2. The functional consequence(s) of the protein–protein interactions is shown in column 3.

vation activity may be important for the homeostasis of the WT1 biological activity.

In contrast to p53 and par-4, which both interact with the C-terminal zinc finger region of WT1, the heat shock protein HSP70 and testis-specific orphan nuclear receptor steroidogenic factor 1 (SF-1) both bind the N terminus of WT1. Intriguingly, SF-1 only interacts with those WT1 isoforms lacking the KTS insertion, and interaction of WT1 to SF-1 results in the transcriptional activation of male-specific genes, including Mullerian inhibitory substance (MIS). In this model, WT1 competes with the Dax-1 protein for binding to SF-1 to enable *MIS* activation. Interestingly, *DAX-1* is a transcriptional target of WT1, indicating the presence of a negative feedback loop to control *MIS* expression. This is an elegant example of how the relative levels of different proteins may regulate gene expression and may give a clue as to how the functional interaction between WT1 and other cellular proteins may be regulated.

V. ROLE OF WT1 IN REGULATING CELL GROWTH AND APOPTOSIS

Consistent with its role as a tumor suppressor protein, WT1 has been demonstrated to regulate cell growth, differentiation, and survival. At present, a number of different studies demonstrate a role for WT1 in inducing or inhibiting cell growth and/or survival depending on the cell type used, the isoforms of WT1, the expression vector used, and the assays performed.

A. Regulation of Cell Growth by WT1

Initial studies demonstrated that expression of either of the four most common WT1 isoforms (WT1 A-D) correlated with a decrease in RM1 (Wilms tumor) cell line growth. Significantly, the expression of WT1 mutant proteins found in Wilms tumor samples did not induce inhibition of cell growth. The growth suppression effect of WT1 was demonstrated to be dependent on the cell type used, with simultaneous experiments performed in SM2 rhabdoid tumor cells demonstrating no effect of WT1 on cell growth. Numerous other groups have since shown that the expression of different WT1 protein isoforms correlates with the induction of cellular differentiation and/or a reduction in cell proliferation. The question of how this occurs has mainly been tackled by studying the target genes transcriptionally regulated by WT1 (Table II). As discussed earlier, the p21[CIP1/WAF1] cyclin-dependent kinase inhibitor has been shown to be transcriptionally upregulated by WT1 in a p53-independent manner. Importantly, p21[CIP1/WAF1] expression correlates with the expression of WT1 in the sites of cellular differentiation in the kidney, indicating that this may be a physiological pathway leading to WT1-mediated differentiation.

However, WT1 has also been show to repress many growth factors and their cognate receptors, which are correlated with the inhibition of cell proliferation. Once again, there are inconsistencies between different groups as to whether WT1 is a positive or negative regulator of cell proliferation and which genes are the important downstream targets to mediate a cellular response. Analyses of gene-targeted mice with the *WT1* gene functionally mutated demonstrate that WT1 is necessary for kidney development and is particularly important in epithelial differentiation. Just what the true physiological target genes of WT1 are, and how they mediate a cellular response to WT1 expression, remain the topic of much debate.

B. Regulation of Apoptosis by WT1

In addition to its role in mediating cell growth and differentiation, WT1 has also been shown to regulate apoptosis. There are conflicting reports as to whether WT1 induces or inhibits apoptosis. Two laboratories independently demonstrated that WT1 induces apoptosis. Significantly, both groups showed that WT1-mediated cell death could be rescued by expression of the epidermal growth factor receptor (EGFR). The *EGFR* is a target gene of WT1 and has been demonstrated to be transcriptionally repressed *in vitro* by WT1. Importantly, EGFR expression in renal precursor cells declines with the onset of WT1 expression, suggesting that this pathway may contribute to the kidney development by WT1.

In addition to its role in inducing cell death, WT1 may also inhibit apoptosis mediated by WT1-binding proteins such as p53 or par-4. Interestingly, WT1 can inhibit p53-mediated apoptosis but does not affect p53-induced growth arrest. p53 promotes apoptosis in part by activating proapoptotic genes such as *bax*, whose protein product induces apoptosis by deregulating mitochondrial function. It seems somewhat counterintuitive that WT1 would inhibit p53-mediated apoptosis but at the same time enhance the transcriptional activation activity of p53. Interestingly, WT1 can upregulate transcription of the *bcl-2* protoonco-

gene, which is a functional antagonist of bax. Thus, it is possible that positive regulation of the transactivation function of p53 by WT1 through physical interaction can result in either cell cycle arrest or apoptosis. However, due to the ability of WT1 to directly upregulate antiapoptotic genes such as *bcl-2* and cell cycle control genes such as $p21^{WAF1/CIP1}$, the end result is growth suppression rather than apoptosis.

VI. CONCLUDING REMARKS

WT1 functions as a transcriptional regulator and a tumor suppressor. Current experimental results support the notion that the tumor suppressor function is correlated with the transcriptional activation function of WT1. It appears likely that WT1 promotes growth suppression by activating the transcription of genes encoding proteins that inhibit cell proliferation. However, a role for the transcriptional repression activity of WT1 in tumorigenesis and development cannot be ruled out. WT1 can also induce apoptosis or inhibit p53-mediated apoptosis. It is possible that the ability of WT1 to induce apoptosis may be related to its tumor suppression function. However, suffice it to say that much is to be learned about the physiological relevance of the pro- and antiapoptotic activities of WT1.

WT1 is expressed as multiple isoforms, some of which have been suggested to be involved in RNA processing. It remains to be determined whether the nontranscriptional activities of WT1 are essential for its tumor suppressor function. Finally, the transcriptional and growth regulatory activities of WT1 may be regulated at a number of different levels that include RNA splicing and editing, translation, posttranslational modifications, and physical interactions with other cellular proteins. Perhaps the culminated variables of the regulated expression of different protein isoforms, coupled with phosphorylation and the interactions with other proteins, is the manner in which WT1 function is controlled in physiological settings.

See Also the Following Articles

WILMS TUMOR: EPIDEMIOLOGY

Bibliography

Call, K., Glaser, T., Ito, C., Pelletier, J. Haber, D., Rose, E., et. al. (1990). Isolation and characterisation of a zinc finger polypeptide gene at the human chromosome 11 Wilms tumor locus. *Cell* **60**, 509–520.

Coppes, M. J., Campbell, C. E., and Williams, B. R. G. (1993). The role of WT1 in Wilms tumorigenesis. *FASEB J.* **7**, 886–895.

Davies, R. C., Calvio, C., Bratt, E., Larsson, S. H., Lamond, A. I., and Hastie, N. D. (1996). WT1 interacts with the splicing factor U2AF65 in an isoform-dependent manner and can be incorporated into spliceosomes. *Genes Dev.* **12**, 3217–3225.

Englert, C., Hou, X., Maheswaran, S., Bennett, P., Ngwu, C., Re, G. G., Garvin, A. J., Rosner, M. R., and Haber, D. A. (1995). WT1 suppresses synthesis of the epidermal growth factor receptor and induces apoptosis. *EMBO J.* **14**, 4662–4675.

English, M. A., and Licht, J. D. (1999). Tumor-associated WT1 missense mutants indicate that transcriptional activation by WT1 is critical for growth control. *J. Biol. Chem.* **274**, 13258–13263.

Haber, D. A., Park, S., Maheswaran, S., Englert, C., Re, G. G., et. al. (1993). WT1-mediated growth suppression of Wilms tumor cells expressing a WT1 splicing variant. *Science* **262**, 2057–2059.

Hewitt, S. M., Hamada, S., McDonnell, T. J., Rauscher, F. J., III, and Saunders, G. F. (1995). Regulation of the proto-oncogenes bcl-2 and c-myc by the Wilms' tumor suppressor gene WT1. *Cancer Res.* **55**, 5386–5389.

Johnstone, R. W., See, R. H., Sells, S. F., Wang, J., Muthukkumar, S., Englert, C., et. al. (1996). A novel repressor par-4 modulates transcription and growth suppression functions of the Wilms tumor suppressor WT1. *Mol. Cell. Biol.* **16**, 6945–6956.

Kennedy, D., Ramsdale, T., Mattick, J., and Little, M. (1996). An RNA recognition motif in Wilms' tumour protein (WT1) revealed by structural modelling. *Nature Genet.* **12**, 329–331.

Larsson, S. H., Charlieu, J. P., Miyagawa, K., Engelkamp, D., Rassoulzadegan, M., et al. (1995). Subnuclear localization of WT1 in splicing or transcription factor domains is regulated by alternative splicing. *Cell* **81**, 391–401.

Lee, S. B., Huang, K., Palmer, R., Truong, V. B., Herzlinger, D., Kolquist, K. A., Wong, J., Paulding, C., Yoon, S. K., Gerald, W., Oliner, J. D., and Haber, D. A. (1999). The Wilms tumor suppressor WT1 encodes a transcriptional activator of amphiregulin. *Cell* **98**, 663–673.

Little, M. H., Prosser, J., Condie, A., Smith, P. J., Van Heyningen, V., and Hastie, N. D. (1992). Zinc finger point mutations within the WT1 gene in Wilms tumor patients. *Proc. Natl. Acad. Sci. USA* **89**, 4791–4795.

Madden, S. L., Cook, D. M., Morris, J. F., Gashler, A., Sukhatme, V. P., and Rauscher, F. J., III. (1991). Transcriptional repression mediated by the WT1 Wilms tumor gene product. *Science* **253**, 1550–1553.

Maheswaran, S., Englert, C., Bennett, P., Heinrich, G., and Haber, D. A. (1995). The WT1 gene product stabilizes p53 and inhibits p53-mediated apoptosis. *Genes Dev.* **9**, 2143–2156.

Maheswaran, S., Englert, C., Zheng, G., Lee, S. B., Wong, J., et al. (1998). Inhibition of cellular proliferation by the Wilms tumor suppressor WT1 requires association with the inducible chaperone Hsp70. *Genes Dev.* **12**, 1108–1120.

Maheswaran, S., Park, S., Bernard, A., Morris, J. F., Rauscher, F. J., III, Hill, D. E., and Haber, D. A. (1993). Physical and functional interaction between WT1 and p53 proteins. *Proc. Natl. Acad. Sci. USA* **90**, 5100–5104.

Menke, A. L., Shvarts, A., Riteco, N., van Ham, R. C., van der Eb, A. J., and Jochemsen, A. G. (1997). Wilms' tumor 1-KTS isoforms induce p53-independent apoptosis that can be partially rescued by expression of the epidermal growth factor receptor or the insulin receptor. *Cancer Res.* **57**, 1353–1363.

Nachtigal, M. W., Hirokawa, Y., Enyeart-VanHouten, D. L., Flanagan, J. N., Hammer, G. D., and Ingraham, H. A. (1998). Wilms' tumor 1 and Dax-1 modulate the orphan nuclear receptor SF-1 in sex-specific gene expression. *Cell* **93**, 445–454.

Park, S., Schalling, M., Bernard, A., Maheswaran S., Shipley, G. C., Roberts, D., et. al. (1993). The Wilms tumor gene WT1 is expressed in murine mesoderm-derived tissues and mutated in human mesothelioma. *Nature Genet.* **4**, 415–493.

Park, S., Tomlinson, G., Nisen, P., and Haber, D. A. (1993). Altered trans-activational properties of a mutated WT1 gene product in a WAGR-associated Wilms' tumor. *Cancer Res.* **53**, 4757–4760.

Rauscher, F. J. (1993). The WT1 Wilms tumor gene product: A developmentally regulated transcription factor in the kidney that functions as a tumor suppressor. *FASEB J.* **7**, 896–903.

Reddy, J. C., Hosono, S., and Licht, J. D. (1995). The transcriptional effect of WT1 is modulated by choice of expression vector. *J. Biol. Chem.* **270**, 29976–29982.

Sakamoto, Y., Yoshida, M., Semba, K., and Hunter, T. (1997). Inhibition of the DNA-binding and transcriptional repression activity of the Wilms' tumor gene product, WT1, by cAMP-dependent protein kinase-mediated phosphorylation of Ser-365 and Ser-393 in the zinc finger domain. *Oncogene* **15**, 2001–2012.

Sharma, P. M., Bowman, M., Madden, S. L., Rauscher, F. J., III, and Sukumar, S. (1994). RNA editing in the Wilms' tumor susceptibility gene, WT1. *Genes Dev.* **8**, 720–731.

Wang, Z. Y., Qiu, Q. Q., and Deuel, T. F. (1993). The Wilms' tumor gene product WT1 activates or suppresses transcription through separate functional domains. *J. Biol. Chem.* **268**, 9172–9175.

Ye, Y., Raychaudhuri, B., Gurney, A., Campbell, C. E., and Williams, B. R. (1996). Regulation of WT1 by phosphorylation: Inhibition of DNA binding, alteration of transcriptional activity and cellular translocation. *EMBO J.* **15**, 5606–5615.

Wnt Signaling

Jan Kitajewski

Columbia University, New York, New York

GLOSSARY

adenomatous polyposis coli (APC) A tumor suppressor gene encoding a protein that functions to control the growth of epithelial cells in the colon; loss of APC is associated with colon cancer development.

β-catenin A protein that functions both to maintain cell–cell adhesion and to act as a signal transducing molecule.

growth factor A polypeptide that binds specifically to a cell surface receptor and thus regulates cell proliferation and differentiation.

oncogene A gene whose protein product can promote tumor development.

serine/threonine kinase An enzyme that catalyzes the transfer of γ-phosphate from ATP to serine or threonine residues on proteins.

signal transduction The transmission of a signal, originating from the outside of a cell, to the intracellular compartment and, ultimately, the nucleus.

tumor suppresor gene A gene that function to suppress cell growth; loss of a tumor suppressor gene by mutation leads to tumor development.

T he *Wnt* gene family encodes growth factors that were originally identified by their ability to induce mammary gland tumors in mouse model systems. Wnts are involved in cell growth and cell fate determination during embryogenesis, organogenesis, and oncogenesis. Aberrant Wnt signaling is common to several human tumors, most notably colon cancer and melanoma, where mutations are found in the *APC* and *β-catenin* genes that lead to Wnt signal activation. Wnt proteins utilize a signal transduction pathway that involves Frizzled, the receptor, Dishevelled, a protein of unknown activity, glycogen synthase kinase-3, a serine/threonine kinase, and adenomatous polyposis coli, a tumor suppressor. The focus of the signaling pathway is the regulation of the steady-state levels and activity of the β-catenin protein.

Copyright 2002, Elsevier Science (USA).
All rights reserved.

I. INTRODUCTION

The *Wnt* gene family encodes growth factors that were originally identified by their ability to induce mammary gland tumors in mouse model systems. The *Wnt-1* gene (originally *int-1*) was identified as a frequent target for insertional activation by mouse mammary tumor virus (MMTV), a virus known to cause mammary gland tumors in mice. Inappropriate expression of either *Wnt-1* or *Wnt-3* leads to epithelial proliferation in the mammary gland and eventually tumors. These findings originally placed *Wnt* genes in the family of oncogenes involved in tumor development.

Most *Wnt* genes have been isolated by cloning genes homologous to *Wnt-1* and they encode cysteine-rich, secretory glycoproteins from 350 to 380 amino acids. Studies of the biochemical properties of Wnt proteins have largely been carried out with cultured cells programmed to express exogenous Wnt proteins. These studies suggest that Wnt proteins act as diffusible secreted factors that are tightly associated to extracellular proteins, making the levels of extracellular, soluble Wnt proteins low. Analysis of wingless (wg) protein function, the *Drosophila* homologue of Wnt-1, suggests that it acts in a paracrine fashion. These observations have led to the model that Wnt proteins are local-acting factors, i.e., they function to signal cells adjacent to or near the site of Wnt production. Biologically active, soluble wg or Wnt-1 proteins have been generated as conditioned media preparations; however, despite such progress, purification of active Wnt or wg proteins has yet to be accomplished.

The normal functions of *Wnt* genes have been analyzed in organisms amenable to genetic analysis of early development. The *Wnt-1* orthologue in *Drosophila* is the segment polarity gene *wingless*. Genetic and biochemical analyses suggest that the wg protein functions as a local-acting, secreted factor that triggers a cascade of molecular events that assist in directing body plan organization of the *Drosophila* embryo and organization of structures such as the limbs and wings. In the frog, *Xenopus laevis*, several different *Wnt* genes have been shown to contribute to the experimental induction of dorsal mesoderm tissue and subsequent establishment of the body axis. This induction can lead to complete duplication of the body axis.

II. Wnt SIGNALING PATHWAY

The nature of the signaling events triggered by Wnt proteins has become apparent. Genetic and biochemical analyses of the wg signal transduction pathway in *Drosophila* embryos and cultured insect cells suggest a cascade of events distinct from any previously described signal transduction pathway. The elements of the pathway defined genetically in *Drosophila* have been conserved in vertebrates, such as mouse or man. An elementary model for the Wnt signaling pathway is schematized in Fig. 1.

Wnts interact with the Frizzled cell surface receptor. Frizzled proteins contain a conserved amino-terminal cysteine-rich domain and seven putative transmembrane segments. Genetic analysis in *Drosophila* shows that Frizzleds are required for Wnt signaling, and biochemical studies have established that Frizzled proteins can bind Wnts. Within the target cell, the cytosolic Dishevelled protein is the first known intracellular component in Wnt-mediated signaling. However, the specific function of Dishevelled has not

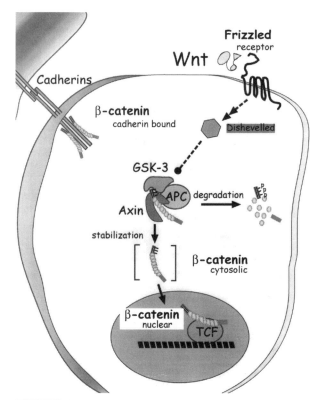

FIGURE 1 Wnt signaling pathway. See text for details and description of components of the pathway.

yet been established. Downstream of Dishevelled is the serine/threonine protein kinase, glycogen synthase kinase 3 (GSK-3), whose activity must be suppressed to transmit Wnt signals. In cells where Wnt/Frizzled signals are not on, GSK-3 continually phosphorylates β-catenin. This phosphorylation marks β-catenin as a target for proteolytic degradation. Suppression of GSK-3 kinase activity leads to dephosphorylation and increased stability of cytosolic β-catenin protein.

Several proteins have been proposed to form a large complex within the cytosol whose goal is to recognize the phosphorylated form of β-catenin and target the protein for destruction. A notable component of this complex is the tumor suppressor adenomatous polyposis coli or APC. APC likely mediates the targeting of β-catenin to the ubiquitin-mediated proteolysis pathway. Another protein in this complex is Axin. Axin is a protein structurally similar to RGS proteins (regulators of G-protein signaling) and to Dishevelled. Disruption of this gene in the mouse germ line causes embryonic axis duplication, a response similar to the effect of excess Wnt in *Xenopus* embryos, which leads to axis duplication. This remarkable finding in mouse studies suggests that Axin functions as a negative regulator of Wnt signaling, a proposal born out after analysis of Axin function in several organisms from flies to frogs. When the targeting activity of this GSK-3/APC/Axin complex is suppressed, the levels of cytosolic β-catenin increase dramatically. This increase in the steady-state levels of β-catenin promotes the transit of β-catenin to the nucleus and the formation of a complex with the TCF/LEF-1 family of transcription factor. β-Catenin/TCF complexes form in the nucleus and directly regulate the expression of target genes of the Wnt signaling pathway.

III. β-CATENIN, THE CENTRAL PLAYER IN SIGNAL TRANSDUCTION

Most of the identified proteins within the Wnt signaling pathway are involved in regulating the activity and levels of β-catenin. Thus, β-catenin functions as the central mediator of Wnt signaling and is the key protein responsible for conversion from the "signal off" state to "signal on." Catenins exist in three isoforms, α, β, and γ, which form a complex with cadherins. This complex resides at the cytoplasmic

tail of the membrane-spanning cadherins (Fig. 1). Cadherin–catenin complexes are essential for cell–cell adhesion. Within cells, the majority of β-catenin is found in association with cadherins at the membrane. The signaling form of β-catenin is not associated with cadherins and resides in the cytosol or nucleus.

To focus on β-catenin as a signal transduction protein, one can analyze the fate of β-catenin. Cytosolic β-catenin responds to Wnt signals, whereas cadherin-bound β-catenin does not. Operationally, this is accomplished by evaluating the membrane-bound and cytosolic forms of β-catenin. Cells to be analyzed are Dounce homogenized, and high-speed centrifugation is used to separate a supernatant fraction (cytosolic) and a pellet (membranous). The resultant fractions are then analyzed by immunoblotting using anti-β-catenin antibodies. To date, this is one of the most sensitive assays for Wnt signaling.

To study the mechanism of action of β-catenin and Wnt signaling in colon cancer cells, we established that β-catenin is constitutively stabilized in cells with APC or β-catenin mutations (see Section IV for a description of mutations). DLD-1 is a colon cancer cell line that expresses a truncated APC and displays increased TCF transcriptional activity. HCT116 is a colon cancer cell line that expresses mutated β-catenin that lacks Ser-45 and also displays increased TCF transcriptional activity. When analyzed for cytosolic β-catenin levels in HCT116 and DLD-1, we found that in both colon cancer cells lines β-catenin was constitutively stabilized in the cytosol and Wnt-1 expression did not increase cytosolic β-catenin (Fig. 2). As a positive control, the β-catenin response in the colon cancer lines was

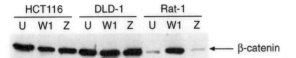

FIGURE 2 Levels of cytosolic β-catenin in colon cancer cell lines. DLD-1 is a human colon cancer cell line that expresses a truncated APC. HCT116 is a human colon cancer cell line that expresses mutated β-catenin. HCT116, DLD-1, or Rat-1 cells were either mock infected (U) or infected with either adenovirus vectors expressing Wnt-1 (W1) or LacZ (Z). Cells were Dounce homogenized, and centrifugation was used to prepare a high-speed supernatant, designated cytosolic fraction. Antibodies against β-catenin were used to generate immune complexes from the cytosolic fraction, and the complexes were analyzed by immunoblotting for β-catenin.

compared to the response found in rat-1 fibroblasts. Normal rat-1 fibroblasts have low cytosolic levels of β-catenin and thus are in the "signal off" state, whereas Wnt-1-stimulated rat-1 cells have elevated levels of cytosolic β-catenin, or "signal on."

IV. HUMAN CANCERS AND APC/β-CATENIN

Several genes involved in Wnt signaling act as oncogenes or tumor suppressor genes. The *APC* gene functions as a tumor suppressor, i.e., it encodes a protein that normally functions as a growth suppressor in colon epithelium. APC was originally implicated in the Wnt signaling pathway based on its ability to associate with β-catenin and GSK-3. Earlier work established that loss of *APC* is correlated with cancer progression in the colon. This loss can be acquired in an individual through inheritance of a mutated *APC* gene. Such individuals have familial adenomatous polyposis (FAP) syndrome manifested by numerous colonic polyps that develop into carcinoma. Loss of *APC* can also be acquired through somatic mutation of the gene, also leading to colon cancer development. Mutations of *APC* almost always lead to the expression of a truncated APC protein missing much of the domain of APC that has been defined as necessary for binding to β-catenin.

The link between loss of *APC* and activation of Wnt signaling by excess β-catenin is compelling. Colon carcinoma cells devoid of APC contain elevated β-catenin levels (Fig. 2) and a β-catenin–TCF complex that is constitutively active. Thus, constitutive transcription of TCF target genes can be caused by loss of APC function, suggesting that activation of the Wnt signaling pathway is a key event in the transformation of colonic epithelium.

Genetic defects that result in the deregulation of β-catenin play a role in melanoma progression. Abnormally high levels of β-catenin due to missplicing or missense mutations of the *β-catenin* gene were detected in several human melanoma cell lines. Other melanoma lines are missing APC or contain structurally altered APC proteins. These alterations are associated with constitutive activation of β-catenin–TCF transcription complexes.

Mutation of the *β-catenin* gene has been reported for a variety of other human tumors. Most of the identified mutations affect one of the putative GSK-3 phosphorylation sites of β-catenin (S33, S37, T41, and S45 amino acid residues in human β-catenin). Mutations in the *β-catenin* gene have been found in colorectal adenoma, colorectal carcinoma, melanoma, endometrial carcinoma, gastric carcinoma, hepatocellular carcinoma, malignant fibrous histiocytoma, medulloblastoma, ovarian carcinoma, pilomatricoma, prostate cancer, synovial sarcoma, and uterine cancer. *β-catenin* is thus a target for oncogenic mutations in a wide variety of human tissues.

APC mutations are most highly correlated with colon cancer and such mutations are less frequently found in other tumor types. Interestingly, although Wnt signaling promotes mammary tumors in mouse models, mutations in *APC* or *β-catenin* genes in human breast cancer are rare. Mutation of APC is also found in another human tumor type, aggressive fibromatosis.

V. ONCOPROTEIN PATHWAYS THAT INTERSECT Wnt SIGNALING

With the rapid progress in the molecular analysis of the Wnt signaling cascade, new players in the pathway have been identified. The variety of signaling components is described in several comprehensive reviews of the pathway and some are noted in Fig. 3. Many of these new components participate in distinct signaling cascades known to function in cancer development. The Wnt/Frizzled cascade that regulates β-catenin also regulates other cellular targets. It is clear from *Drosophila* analysis that the *Drosophila* homologue of RhoA p21 GTPase has been genetically tied to Frizzled function. Vertebrate RhoA affects the JNK kinase signaling cascade, a pathway that regulates cellular proliferation. It is not clear how Wnt/Frizzled interaction ultimately regulates the RhoA/JNK cascade, but it is clear that the regulation is mediated through Disheveled. The GSK-3 binding protein (GBP), a new component of the pathway, regulates GSK-3 activity and is related to the human *FRAT* gene (frequently rearranged in advanced T-cell lymphomas). Analysis in *Xenopus* embryos of the Wnt cascade suggests a key role for Ca^{2+} signaling for some

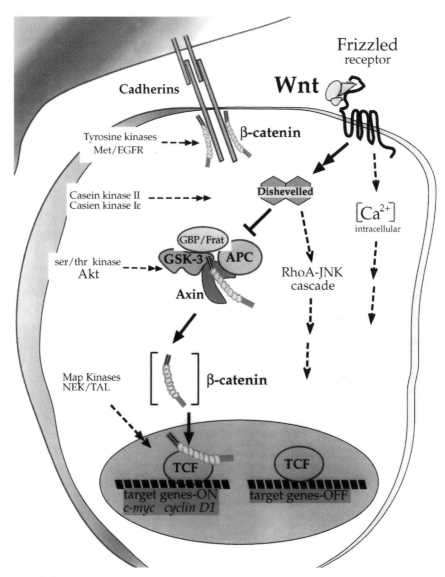

FIGURE 3 Intersection of mitogenic signaling pathways with Wnt signaling cascade. Wnt signal OFF represents the pathway in the absence of Wnt. Wnt signal ON represents Wnt-activated events, leading to β-catenin stabilization and activation of TCF target genes, *c-myc* and *cyclin D1*. Dotted arrows represent either intersecting pathways (Met, EGF receptor, casein kinase II, casein kinase Iε, Akt, NEK, TAL) or parallel pathways (RhoA-JNK and intracellular Ca²⁺).

Wnt/Frizzled signaling functions. The Ser/Thr kinase Akt is involved in regulating cellular proliferation and can be regulated by the PTEN tumor suppressor. Akt also phosphorylates and suppresses GSK-3 activity, but the link between PTEN/Akt and the Wnt signaling cascade has not been firmly established.

Other kinase cascades involved in cellular proliferation can target components of the Wnt cascade. The tyrosine kinases Met and epidermal growth factor receptor (EGFR) phosphorylate β-catenin on tyrosine residues. The consequences of this phosphorylation are unclear. The serine/threonine kinases, casein kinase II and Iε, phosphorylate Dishevelled. It is well established that casein kinase Iε directly affects Wnt signaling when analyzed in *Caenorhabditis elegans* and *Xenopus*. Components of the mitogen-activated protein kinase (MAPK) cascade of *C. elegans*, NEK and TAL, have been implicated in phosphorylation and regulation of the TCF transcription factor. All these studies suggest that Wnt signaling is responsive to signals from other growth regulatory signaling cascades. The nature of the integration of such diverse signaling cascades in a cell is not understood, but may be key to understanding the ultimate growth state of any given cell.

Wnt signaling can also transcriptionally activate cellular oncogenes. The *C-MYC* and *cyclin D1* genes are transcriptional targets of β-catenin/TCF. *C-MYC* expression is linked to a variety of human cancers and is essential for cell survival signals. Cyclin D1 promotes cell cycle progression, and aberrant expression of cyclin D1 is also linked to human tumors. Current models propose that Wnt/Frizzled signals may ultimately target several other growth-promoting gene products.

VI. MOUSE MODELS OF Wnt FUNCTION IN ONCOGENESIS

Mouse models have illuminated the normal function of Wnt genes in many tissues. Although Wnts are clearly essential for induction and cell specification in both invertebrates and vertebrates, many of the mouse models point to a role for Wnts in promoting cellular proliferation. There are four illustrative target tissues where Wnt proliferative functions have been defined through experimental analysis using mouse: the colon, mammary gland, uterus, and the developing central nervous system.

Mouse models for loss of *Apc* have arisen in nature, the Apc min mouse, or have been engineered using gene-targeting strategies. In these models, loss of APC leads to excess proliferation of intestinal epithelial cells and the development of numerous intestinal tumors. In intestinal epithelium, a member of the TCF transcription family, TCF-4, likely mediates the Wnt response. Loss of Tcf-4 in mice leads to a reduced proliferation of intestinal stem cells. It is likely that loss of APC leads to constitutive TCF-4/β-catenin activity promoting uncontrolled intestinal cell proliferation and intestinal tumors. Thus, in both mouse and man the Wnt sig-

naling pathway via APC/β-catenin/TCF is key to normal and abnormal proliferation of colonic epithelium.

In the mouse, the role of Wnts in mammary gland development and mammary oncogenesis is coming to light. Aberrant expression of either *Wnt-1* or *Wnt-4* does not solely convert the mammary ductal epithelium into carcinoma but induces hyperplasia and excess branching of the epithelial ducts. Other mutational events contribute further to tumor development. Studies *in vitro* with cultured mammary epithelial cells suggest that Wnts can act as both proliferative and morphogenic factors to promote epithelial tube formation, thus directing both growth and patterning. Endogenous *Wnt-2*, *Wnt-4*, *Wnt-5a*, *Wnt-5b*, *Wnt-6*, and *Wnt-7a* genes are expressed in the mammary gland during growth and differentiation (in virgin and pregnant mice), but are not expressed in lactating glands, when the gland is no longer growing. Furthermore, the expression of several *Wnt* genes appears to be hormonally regulated. These two findings taken together suggest that the regulated expression of *Wnt* gene products plays a role in the normal expansion or differentiation of the mammary epithelium before lactation. Because mutation of APC and β-*catenin* genes in human breast cancer is very rare, mouse models do not prove predictive for human breast cancer mutations involving Wnt signaling genes. However, as new components of the signaling pathway are defined and divergent pathways emerge, a role for Wnt signaling in human breast cancer may yet emerge.

Reproductive tract development and function are regulated by circulating steroid hormones such as estrogenic compounds that direct aspects of uterine gland formation and epithelial differentiation. The use of the synthetic estrogenic compound diethylstilbestrol (DES) in the 1950s on pregnant women to prevent possible miscarriage had the unexpected effect of inducing a range of gynecological problems, including malformed reproductive tracts and a higher incidence of reproductive tract cancer in daughters of these women. Studies in the mouse have identified Wnts as signaling proteins with a role during uterine development and adult function. For one member of the *Wnt* gene family, *Wnt-7a*, deregulation in mice in response to prenatal exposure to DES leads to uterine abnormalities reminiscent of the human condition. These malformations are also exhibited in a mouse lacking the *Wnt*-7a gene. These advances point to an important role for the *Wnt* gene family in various reproductive tract pathologies, including cancer.

In the central nervous system (CNS), Wnts promote the development of several structures or regions of the brain, including the cerebellum and hippocampus. In each of these regions, loss of the appropriate *Wnt* gene (*Wnt*-1 for cerebellum and *Wnt*-3a for hippocampus) leads to reduced cellular proliferation. Wnt signaling is also essential for the proliferation of neural crest and CNS progenitor cells.

Acknowledgments

The author acknowledges support from NIH RO1 CA75353 and the Marilyn Bokemeier Sperry Fund. I thank Colleen Craig and Inca Chui for critical reading of the manuscript. This review is dedicated to the memory of Stanley Buturla.

See Also the Following Articles

APC (ADENOMATOUS POLYPOSIS COLI) TUMOR SUPPRESSOR • INTEGRIN RECEPTOR SIGNALING PATHWAYS • KINASE-REGULATED SIGNAL TRANSDUCTION PATHWAYS • MAP KINASE MODULES IN SIGNALING • SIGNAL TRANSDUCTION MECHANISMS INITIATED BY RECEPTOR TYROSINE KINASES • TGF-BETA SIGNALING MECHANISMS

Bibliography

Arias, A. M., Brown, A. M., and Brennan, K. (1999). Wnt signaling: Pathway or network? *Curr. Opin. Genet. Dev.* **9,** 447–454.

Cadigan, K. M., and Nusse, R. (1997). Wnt signaling: A common theme in animal development. *Genes Dev.* **11,** 3286–3305.

Kinzler, K. W., and Vogelstein, B. (1998). Landscaping the cancer terrain. *Science* **280,** 1036–1037.

Kitajewski, J., and Sassoon, D. (2000). The emergence of molecular gynecology: Patterning genes in the reproductive tract. *Bioessays* **22,** 902–910.

Miller, J. R., Hocking, A. M., Brown, J. D., and Moon, R. T. (1999). Mechanism and function of signaling transduction by the Wnt/beta-catenin and Wnt/Ca^{2+} pathways. *Oncogene* **18,** 7860–7872.

Nusse, R., and Varmus, H. E. (1992). *Wnt* genes. *Cell* **69,** 1073–1087.

Schlosshauer, P., Eisinger, K., Guglielminetti, E., Hendrick-Ellison, L., Parson, R., Brown, S., and Kitajewski, J. (2000). A human breast cancer cell line with an APC mutation and elevated β-catenin. *Carcinogenesis* **21,** 1453–1456.

Uyttendaele, H., Soriano, J., Montesano, R., and Kitajewski, J. (1998). Notch4 and Wnt-1 proteins function to regulate branching morphogenesis of mammary epithelial cells in opposing fashion. *Dev. Biol.* **196,** 204–217.

Young, C. S., Kitamura, M., Hardy, S., and Kitajewski, J. (1998). Wnt-1 induces growth, cytosolic β-catenin, and Tcf/Lef transcriptional activation in rat-1 fibroblasts. *Mol. Cell. Biol.* **18,** 2474–2485.

Index